"Pioneers in pediatric hypnosis - Drs. Kohen & Olness's 'Hypnosis with Children' is an essential reference, a source of ongoing inspiration for every pediatric professional, and a wonderful read!"

**Dr. Leora Kuttner** *(Clin.Psych.); Clinical Professor, Faculty of Medicine, Pediatric Department, BC Children's Hospital and University of British Columbia*

"It is truly unimaginable that the field of pediatric hypnosis would not be anchored by this seminal text by Drs. Daniel Kohen and Karen Olness. Our colleagues have again provided a newer and greater edition for clinicians at every skill level. Drs. Kohen and Olness continue to excel at updating their book, helping those who help children learn how to help themselves."

**Bob Deutsch**, *PhD*

"Daniel Kohen and Karen Olness are the 'founding parents' of pediatric hypnosis worldwide. In this classic handbook, they use their outstanding expertise to provide the reader with an excellent overview of the principles of hypnotherapy in children and its scientific evidence, combined with numerous practical case studies."

**Arine M. Vlieger**, *MD, PhD; Pediatrician, Department of Pediatrics, St. Antonius Hospital Nieuwegein, The Netherlands; and Co-founder and Chair, Dutch Foundation for Pediatric Hypnosis*

# HYPNOSIS WITH CHILDREN

Updated and revised in response to developments in the field, this fifth edition of *Hypnosis with Children* describes the research and clinical historical underpinnings of hypnosis with children and adolescents, and presents an up-to-date compendium of the pertinent world literature regarding this arena.

The authors focus on the wide variety and scope of applications for therapeutic hypnosis; including an integrated description of both clinical and evidence-based research as it relates to understanding approaches to various clinical situations, case studies of practical aspects, and how-to elements of teaching therapeutic hypnosis skills to clients. This new edition includes new chapters on helping children in disasters and pandemics with hypnosis, and helping parents.

This book is essential for therapists and students who wish to gain a complete overview of hypnosis with children and adolescents.

**Daniel P. Kohen, MD**, is a retired professor of Pediatrics and Family Medicine and Community Health at the University of Minnesota, a former director of Developmental-Behavioral Pediatrics at the University of Minnesota, and a former president of the American Board of Medical Hypnosis. He is a Fellow of the American Academy of Pediatrics, the American Society of Clinical Hypnosis, and the Society for Clinical and Experimental Hypnosis. He is Co-Founder of and Director of Education for the National Pediatric Hypnosis Training Institute (NPHTI).

**Karen Olness, MD**, is a professor of Pediatrics, Family Medicine, and Global Health at Case Western Reserve University, as well as a Fellow of the American Academy of Pediatrics, the American Society of Clinical Hypnosis, and the Society for Clinical and Experimental Hypnosis. She is also a former president of the American Board of Medical Hypnosis, the American Society of Clinical Hypnosis, the Society for Clinical and Experimental Hypnosis, and the International Society of Hypnosis.

# HYPNOSIS WITH CHILDREN

Fifth Edition

*Daniel P. Kohen and Karen Olness*

Routledge
Taylor & Francis Group
NEW YORK AND LONDON

Cover image: Getty Images

Fifth edition published 2023
by Routledge
605 Third Avenue, New York, NY 10158

and by Routledge
4 Park Square, Milton Park, Abingdon, Oxon, OX14 4RN

*Routledge is an imprint of the Taylor & Francis Group, an informa business*



First edition published by Grune & Stratton 1981
Fifth edition published by Routledge 2022

ISBN: 978-1-032-15068-0 (hbk)
ISBN: 978-1-032-15338-4 (pbk)
ISBN: 978-1-003-24368-7 (ebk)

DOI: 10.4324/9781003243687

Typeset in Bembo
by MPS Limited, Dehradun

Access the Support Material: www.routledge.com/9781032153384

# CONTENTS

# NOTE TO THE FIFTH EDITION

After over 40 years of applying therapeutic clinical hypnosis strategies toward helping children and adolescents help themselves, I remain immensely grateful and privileged to co-author this fifth edition of what we evolved to now call *Hypnosis with Children* with my dear friend and colleague, Karen Olness. I have never tired of my ongoing review of the vast array of research and clinical papers that have contributed so substantially to our understanding of hypnosis with children. I am thrilled to know that today, around the world, therapeutic hypnosis with children is evidence-based medicine, that it has grown so substantially in scope and practice and that hypnosis is indeed mainstream and in many places no longer considered alternative and complementary medicine; and yet there is still much to be learned.

I am grateful to Karen Olness for her ongoing creativity, humble and steady leadership, and continued visionary and optimistic approach and belief in what she told me when we first met over 44 years ago: "We create our own reality." I offer thanks especially to my earliest teachers and friends and colleagues – may they rest in peace – Kay Thompson, Bob Pearson, Franz Baumann, Bertha Rodger, Harold Golan, and many incredible others. Their words and models as clinicians and mentors live on in the successes and growth of so many young people I have had the opportunity to meet, teach, and help. Special thanks continue to go to all of the children, adolescents, young adults, and their families through whose learning of hypnosis I have continued to be inspired and through some of whose stories this volume teaches what really is possible.

I dedicate this book to my family as it continues to grow: to the memory of my parents, Benjamin L. and Roselea Kohen (Z"L), and my sister-in-law, Janet Kohen (Z"L), whose love always supported me; my brother Andy who has always been there for and with me, his children and grandchildren and my sister Naomi, and her children and grandchildren. To our children, Aaron and Sarah, and Joshua and Jessica for their independence, creativity, love, and confidence in one another and me; to our grandson, Chai, a truly bright light and incredible person for whom even the sky is not a limit; and to our newest grandchildren, Josh and Jessica's two daughters, Sophia Rae (almost 2-year-old) and Eden Belle (5 weeks old as I write this) whom I believe will each take the world by storm; and to my partner and wife of 53 years, Harriet, for her love, unwavering kindness to all, wise counsel, guidance, and sustained belief in my endeavors.

**Daniel P. Kohen, MD, FAAP, ABMH**

As we have done for previous editions of this book, as soon as the last is completed we begin compiling new articles on hypnosis research with children and adolescents and also listening to our colleagues who share their wonderful experiences teaching hypnosis to children. This sharing happens in casual conversations and also through the NPHTI listserv that remains very active. I am so grateful to the many colleagues who share and validate how children enhance their personal sense of competency and coping when they use self-hypnosis. I am also grateful to the adults who were once my child patients learning hypnosis and who let me know that this tool is still helping them.

I give thanks to those on whose shoulders I stand, such as Walter Majewski MD who told me that he wished to give me a gift, the gift of self-hypnosis. He was so right, although I was dubious at first. I have been privileged to pass the gift on. I am grateful for all the teaching I received from Franz Baumann MD, Erik Wright MD, PhD, Esther Bartlett MD, Bertha Rodger MD, Bill Kroger MD, Harold Golan DDS, Kay Thompson DDS, Bob Pearson MD, Selig Finkelstein DDS, Erika Fromm PhD, Josephine Hilgard MD, PhD, Philip Ament DDS, PhD, and many amazing others. They were often regarded as iconoclasts for teaching hypnosis; they were all courageous, positive people. Blessed be their memories. And, once again, it has been a great pleasure to work on this project with my long-time colleague and dear friend, Dan Kohen. He puts his heart and soul into everything he does. This has benefited thousands of children who have experienced his remarkable skill as a teacher of hypnosis.

I am thrilled to see younger colleagues teaching hypnosis with children throughout the United States and in many other countries, and I am grateful for their efforts.

I dedicate this book to Hakon Torjesen, my husband of 60 years, who has long been the wind beneath my sails with his continuing love, his laughter, his encouragement and advocacy.

**Karen Olness MD, ABMH**

# PREFACE

The first edition of the book was published in 1981. The authors were G. Gail Gardner, a clinical child psychologist, and Karen Olness, a pediatrician. They separately became interested in the possibilities of helping children with hypnosis. When they first met in the 1970s, most child health professionals believed that children either could not learn hypnosis or that this was not an appropriate treatment for them.

Drs. Gardner and Olness scoured the literature and found a few American health professionals who did teach hypnosis to children. These included Milton Erickson, a psychiatrist who was a creative therapist and taught hypnosis to both adults and children, and Franz Baumann, a pediatrician who worked in San Francisco. Gardner and Olness began teaching hypnosis workshops together in the seventies as interest and knowledge expanded, in the United States and elsewhere. Eventually they decided that the available information warranted a comprehensive text on the subject and they wrote the first edition of this book.

The second edition was published in 1988. Co-author of the third edition in 1996, and first author of the fourth edition in 2011 was Daniel P. Kohen, a pediatrician who has helped children with hypnosis since 1977.

Hypnosis has been taught to children for more than 200 years. In 1959, Dr. Andre Weitzenhoffer published a *Bibliography of Hypnotism in Pediatrics,* which contained 86 references, many in French and German, that spanned the years 1886–1959. In 1980 Gardner published a bibliography of 114 references dating from 1955 to 1980, almost entirely limited to publications in American journals.

Training in hypnosis with children has expanded greatly in the past 30 years. In 1987, the Society for Developmental and Behavioral Pediatrics began offering an annual 3-day workshop on clinical hypnosis with children. In 2010, the National Pediatric Hypnosis Training Institute (NPHTI) was founded by Daniel P. Kohen and Pamela Kaiser, child psychologist and pediatric nurse practitioner. NPHTI organized annual workshops in Minnesota until the COVID-19 pandemic. Since then NPHTI has offered many virtual seminars and one virtual 2-day workshop for child health professionals who had completed an Introductory (Fundamentals) workshop in child hypnosis. Child health professionals from other countries have attended the NPHTI workshops and there are several workshops available in Europe on hypnosis with children. NPHTI has also organized workshops on training faculty to teach the next generation.

The purpose of this fifth edition is to update all chapters with respect to recent research publications, to increase recommendations for utilization, to expand guidelines on how to teach child hypnosis, to share information about global education and research in child hypnosis, and to add sections on how children in disasters may be helped with hypnosis and how to help parents.

There remains a great need for more research in how most effectively to teach children hypnosis and for long-term follow-up research. Our clinical experience, after 40–50 years of teaching hypnosis to children, is that many retain their self-regulation skills into adulthood. How does this benefit their overall lives? Hopefully, another generation or two of researchers will let us know.

# PART I

# Introduction

# 1

# SCENES OF CHILDHOOD

## Introduction

To help the reader more fully understand our approach to hypnosis, we present some themes of child development that form the rationale for our methods with children.

## The Urge for Experience

Beginning at birth, babies seek stimulation. In the first days of life, they prefer to focus their gaze on something and prefer a more complex visual stimulus (e.g., a striped pattern) to a simple one (e.g., a solid red square). Most of all, they enjoy gazing at a human face. Very soon, children define all objects as *things to find out about*, and they make maximal use of sensory and motor development to experience themselves and their world. They do this first with mouths and eyes, then with hands, and finally with their whole bodies. If the results of such experiences are generally pleasurable, they continue to explore in more complex ways, using to their own advantage such developing ego functions as motility and coordination, language, perceptual skills, memory, ability to distinguish between reality and fantasy, and social skills. Temperamental and environmental factors combine to shape and often to put limits on the child's urge for experience, but only rarely can these cancel the urge altogether. For example, in the case of the frightened child who retreats to a corner on the first day of school, a patient teacher usually finds that the child prefers to stand facing the room rather than facing the wall. For such children, visual exploration often leads to positive school adjustment as efficiently as motor exploration for other children. As Fromm (1972) pointed out, it is very important not to confuse behavioral passivity with ego passivity. On the other hand, Kagan's work (Kagan, 1994) has documented that there is substantial capacity for change in temperament and behavior between 2 and 7 years. Evidence of an inhibited personality in infancy does not necessarily predict the adolescent or adult personality.

## The Urge for Mastery

Right on the heels of the urge for experience comes the urge for mastery, both of the self and of the environment. Objects and people become *things with which to do something.*

DOI: 10.4324/9781003243687-2

Ego activity and behavioral activity join forces, sometimes to the dismay of parents who find the contents of the dresser drawers on the floor. It is sheer pleasure to share with young children in the mastery process. As children grow older, they continue to experience the same drive for mastery, unless this aspect of ego functioning is seriously derailed by environmental or physical or mental handicaps.

## The Urge for Social Interaction

Children are social creatures. Even at birth, their favorite visual stimulus is a human face. Children develop language not only for its own reward of mastery but also because it vastly increases possibilities for social interaction. The endless "why" questions of the toddler are often less a request for information than for social play, just as endless requests for peek-a-boo or chase-around-the-tree serve to exercise social as much as sensory and motor needs. Social interaction is more than social control, more than merely a way to have needs satisfied; for the child, it is a pleasure in itself. Children progress from interaction with parents to interaction with peers, and in this way they develop social skills that may provide pleasure for the rest of their lives. Again, socialization skills can be derailed by physical or mental disabilities or by abusive adults, but most children manage to remember that at least some relationships are safe and may be a means to pleasure. Although some children may be slow to warm up in new relationships, very few choose to remain totally isolated.

## The Urge for the Inner World of Imagination

Just as children enjoy increasing the range of their experiences in and with their everyday external world, so they also delight in the realms of their inner experience – that is, what they call *pretending*, *daydreaming*, or *imagination* and what we call *fantasy*. These internal activities serve useful functions. Children may explore unconsciously several possible actions in their fantasies before selecting the apparent best behavioral choice, thus saving time and energy. They spontaneously may use such fantasy to modify unpleasant situations, to gratify unmet needs, or to prepare for creative activities and new achievements (J.R. Hilgard, 1970; Olness, 1985b). Imaginative involvement, of course, may be pleasurable in its own right. For example, a group of 15 4-year-olds were asked to report dreams. After the first child described what was probably a nocturnal "monster" dream, the rest excitedly jumped in with variations. It was obvious that, for the most part, these other reports were not dreams but instead were entries into a quite conscious competition to see who could create the wildest monster story. All had happy, masterful endings, again following the lead of the first child who managed to throw her dream monster out the window. Such fantasies are typical of countless stories and fairy tales that have existed for many centuries throughout different cultures. The development of imagery in the thinking processes of children is an important part of child development, related to play patterns and creativity as well as, ultimately, to adult activity. Image-generated effects on physiology, nutrition, behavior, performance, and disease, formerly not understood to be subject to voluntary modulation, have been investigated by many researchers (Felt et al., 1998; Hall, Minnes, Tosi, & Olness, 1992; Olness, 1985b; Wang & Morgan, 1992). In our laboratory, we (Lee & Olness, 1995) have documented changes in cardiac rate dependent on shifts in the imagining of children.

Inasmuch as we recognize a basic need for nocturnal dreams, we could postulate a similar need and value for waking fantasy and imagining. There is valid current concern that the images provided by television, internet gaming, smartphone "apps" have negative effects on childhood development and that especially violent images may impact negatively on a young child's value system. Part of the damage of these media may be that they steal from spontaneous, creative imagining time for children and adolescents. In fact, we wonder whether Western culture's devaluation of fantasy during adolescence may not contribute to some of the conflict and strife typical of that developmental period.

## The Urge for Wellness

Under most circumstances, children choose to be healthy rather than sick, comfortable rather than distressed. Children like to be well. When physically stressed, the body automatically adapts in an effort to restore integration; thus, platelets and white cells rush to the site of a wound to stop bleeding and prevent infection. Likewise, when psychologically distressed, the individual uses various defense mechanisms and coping devices to handle the situation as adaptively as possible. Maladaptive behavior serves a purpose, conscious or unconscious or both. But, almost always, there is some part of the person that would gladly trade maladaptive behavior for behavior that serves the same purpose in a more constructive and truly self-satisfying way. In the case of maladaptive behavior in children, there is the added advantage of a higher degree of ego resiliency and flexibility than is often seen with adults. Children have still another advantage in their search for wellness – namely, their generally greater comfort in seeking help, learning new skills, and allowing a certain degree of adaptive regression that is inherent in a successful helping relationship.

## Implications for Hypnotherapy

In our therapeutic work, we recognize that we are not treating problems; we are treating and helping children who happen to have problems. No matter how severe the problems of our child patients, we address ourselves to their striving for experience, for mastery, for social interaction, for the inner world of imagination, and for wellness. Thus, we gain an ally in that part of the child that wants to experience life to the fullest, and this alliance forms the foundation of treatment.

When we select hypnosis as the treatment of choice for a particular child's problem, we emphasize specific therapeutic techniques and strategies that enhance and strengthen healthy strivings. Invitation (often also called Induction) approaches are selected partly on the basis of experiential satisfaction as well as the developmental stage and learning style of each child. Treatment is conducted in the context of a safe, comfortable relationship in which the child is invited to capitalize on imagery skills to enhance and promote feelings of control and mastery and, in so doing, to recover a state of wellness to the greatest extent possible. Treatment should not require passive submission but, rather, active and joyful participation. In the final analysis, we see ourselves as guides, coaches, and teachers. It is the children who bring healing to themselves.

## References

Felt, B.T., Berman, B., Broffman, G., Coury, D., Dattner, A., French, G., Hall, H., Kohen, D.P., Schmidt, W., Young, M.H., & Olness, K. (1998). Wart regression in children: comparison of relaxation-imagery to topical treatment and equal time interventions. *American Journal of Clinical Hypnosis, 41*(2), 130–138.

Fromm, E. (1972). Ego activity and ego passivity in hypnosis. *International Journal of Clinical and Experimental Hypnosis, 20*, 238–251.

Hall, H.R., Minnes, L., Tosi, M., & Olness, K. (1992). Voluntary modulation of neutrophil adhesiveness using a cyberphysiologic strategy. *International Journal of Neuroscience, 63*, 287–297.
Hilgard, J.R. (1970). *Personality and Hypnosis: A Study of Imaginative Involvement.* Chicago, IL: University of Chicago Press.
Kagan, J. (1994). *Galen's Prophecy*. New York: Basic Books.
Lee, L. & Olness, K. (1995). Impact of imagery changes on autonomic reactivity in children [abstract]. *Archives of Pediatrics and Adolescent Medicine, 149*, 47.
Olness, K. (1985b). Little people, images, and child health. *American Journal of Clinical Hypnosis, 27*, 169–174.
Wang, Y. & Morgan, W.P. (1992). The effect of imagery perspectives on the psychophysiological responses to imagined exercise. *Behavior and Brain Research, 52*, 167–174.

# 2

# EARLY USES OF HYPNOSIS WITH CHILDREN

## Introduction

The use of hypnotic-like techniques with children goes back to ancient times. Both the Old and New Testaments contain accounts of ill children responding to healing methods based on suggestion and faith (I Kings XVII:17–24; Mark IX:17–27). Children in primitive cultures have employed trance phenomena in initiation rites and other ceremonies (Mead, 1949).

## Franz Anton Mesmer (1734–1815)

The modern history of hypnosis begins with Mesmer, an Austrian physician whose interest in the healing power of magnetic influence was a logical extension of attention to magnetic forces among astronomers and physicists of that time. In 1766, Mesmer wrote a dissertation entitled *The Influences of the Planets on the Human Body* (cited in Tinterow, 1970).

During the next decade, Mesmer developed his theory of animal magnetism. Briefly, the theory held that all objects in the universe are connected by and filled with a physical fluid having magnetic properties. When the fluid is out of balance in the human body, disease occurs. Certain techniques can be employed to restore the fluid to proper equilibrium and thus heal the patient. Mesmer's techniques included staring into his patients' eyes and making various "hand movements" over their bodies, using his own "magnetic influence" to promote a cure. While living in Vienna, Mesmer (Tinterow, 1970) reported his use of animal magnetism to cure several patients, including children and adolescents. Though details of his methods with specific patients are sketchy, verbal instructions and suggestions seem to have been minimized in favor of the "hand movements" that supposedly restored the patient's own magnetic fluid to proper balance.

One of Mesmer's patients was Miss Ossine, an 18-year-old girl whose problems included tuberculosis, melancholia, fits, rage, vomiting, spitting up blood, and fainting. She recovered after treatment with animal magnetism. Another patient, also 18 years old at the time of treatment, was Miss Paradis, who had been blind since age 4 and who suffered melancholia "accompanied by stoppages in the spleen and liver" that often brought on fits of delirium and rage. Most significant is Mesmer's awareness of the extent to which parental interference can sabotage treatment. Following restoration of the girl's sight by animal magnetism, a public dispute developed over

DOI: 10.4324/9781003243687-3

whether she could really see or was just faking. Moreover, the father became fearful that his daughter's disability pension might be stopped. He terminated her treatment, whereupon she soon relapsed into frequent seizures and later into blindness. The father then changed his mind and asked that Mesmer resume treatment. Intensive treatment for 15 days again controlled the seizures and restored the girl's vision, after which she returned home. Subsequently, the family claimed that she had again relapsed. Mesmer thought the girl was being forced to imitate her maladies, but he could not obtain further follow-up. At the same time, Mesmer described his treatment of Miss Wipior, age 9, who had a tumor on one cornea, rendering her blind in that eye. He stated that animal magnetism resulted in partial removal of the tumor so that the child could read sideways. He anticipated a full cure, but circumstances interrupted the treatment.

Following his work with these and other patients, Mesmer became discouraged by his colleagues' repeated charges that animal magnetism was no more than quackery. In 1778, Mesmer moved to Paris, where he initially enjoyed good favor and, in 1779, published his famous *Dissertations on the Discovery of Animal Magnetism*. His fame spread rapidly, and he began treating patients in large groups, using more and more dramatic methods. His colleagues again charged quackery, and local scientific societies refused to acknowledge his discoveries. Once more discouraged, Mesmer left Paris, but "mesmerism" continued to flourish in the hands of his disciples, especially Charles d'Eslon.

## The Franklin Commission

In 1784, King Louis XVI appointed a commission to investigate mesmerism and, particularly, the claims of the disciple d'Eslon (Tinterow, 1970). The president of the commission was Benjamin Franklin, then the American Ambassador to France. Other distinguished members included the chemist Lavoisier and the physician Guillotin. The commissioners agreed that some patients were cured by mesmerism, but they questioned the underlying theory of the existence of magnetic fluid.

In experiments designed to test the theory, the commissioners took pains to include several children, particularly from the lower classes, so as to minimize the effects of prior knowledge and expectation. One of these was Claude Renand, a 6-year-old boy with tuberculosis. Unlike other patients, who had usually experienced pain, perspiration, and convulsions during mesmeric treatment, little Claude reported no sensation at all. Another child subject was Genevieve Leroux, age 9, suffering convulsions and chorea; she, too, felt no sensation. Procedures used with these and other subjects included passes made with iron rods and hand or finger pressure on various body parts, sometimes for several hours. An assistant played rapid piano music for the purpose of enhancing the likelihood of a "convulsive crisis."

Because Mesmer had claimed that he could transfer magnetic influence to inanimate objects and that patients could then be healed merely by touching these objects, the commission tested this aspect of the theory, again with a naive child as subject. On the extensive grounds of Franklin's estate outside Paris, d'Eslon magnetized a certain apricot tree. A 12-year-old boy, known to be susceptible to the more common methods of animal magnetism, remained indoors, unaware of which tree was magnetized. The commissioners reported their observations in detail.

> The boy was then brought into the orchard, his eyes covered with a bandage, and successively taken to trees upon which the procedure had not been performed, and he embraced them for the space of two minutes, the method of communication which had been prescribed by M. d'Eslon.

> At the first tree, the boy, being questioned at the end of a minute, declared that he had perspired in large drops, he coughed, spit, and complained of a slight pain in his head; the distance of the tree which had been magnetized was about twenty-seven feet.
>
> At the second tree he felt the sensations of stupefaction and pain in his head; the distance was thirty-six feet.
>
> At the third tree, the stupefaction and headache increased considerably, and he said that he believed he was approaching the tree which had been magnetized. The distance was then about thirty-eight feet.
>
> In line with the fourth tree, one which had not been rendered the object of the procedure, and at a distance of about twenty-four feet from the tree which had, the boy fell into a crisis, he fainted, his limbs stiffened, and he was carried on to a plot of grass, where M. d'Eslon hurried to his side and revived him.
>
> The result of this experiment is entirely contrary to the theory of animal magnetism. M. d'Eslon accounted for it by observing that all the trees, by their very nature, participated in the magnetism, and that their magnetism was reinforced by his presence. But in that case, a person, sensitive to the power of magnetism, could not hazard a walk in the garden without the risk of convulsions, an assertion which is contradicted by the experience of every day. The presence of M. d'Eslon had no greater influence here than in the coach, in which the boy came along with him. He was placed opposite the coach and he felt nothing. If he had experienced no sensation even under the tree which was magnetized, it might have been said that at least on that day he had not been sufficiently susceptible. However, the boy fell into a crisis under a tree which was not magnetized.
>
> The crisis was therefore the effect of no physical or exterior cause, but is to be attributed solely to the influence of imagination. The experiment is therefore entirely conclusive. The boy knew that he was about to be led to a tree upon which the magnetical operation had been performed, his imagination was struck, it was increased by the successive steps of the experiment, and at the fourth tree it was raised to the height necessary to produce the crisis. (quoted in Tinterow, 1970, pp. 108–109)

The commissioners thus rejected the theory of animal magnetism and concluded that the results of these and other experiments "are uniform in their nature, and contribute alike to the same decision. They authorize us to conclude that the imagination is the true cause of the effects attributed to the magnetism" (p. 114).

## John Elliotson (1791–1868)

Charges and countercharges raged between Mesmer's disciples and others who agreed with the Franklin Commission report. The controversy between proponents of animal magnetism and those of imagination spread to England, where the defense of animal magnetism was led by John Elliotson, a distinguished physician whose achievements included introducing the stethoscope to his country. Hoping to convince his colleagues, Elliotson decided in 1842 to edit a journal, *The Zoist*, concerned with information about cerebral physiology and mesmerism. The 13 volumes of this journal, published from 1842 to 1856, contain several references to the use of mesmerism in the management of childhood problems. Apparently, Elliotson lacked the scientific sophistication of the 1784 Commission, for much of his argument in support of the theory rested on evidence that patients could be cured after mesmerism, a point never contested by the Commission. Like Mesmer and d'Eslon, Elliotson was denounced by the medical profession, and the practice of mesmerism was prohibited in many English hospitals. The doctor and his pupils, unwilling to submit papers to traditional medical journals where they would not have been accepted, reported many successful cases in *The Zoist*. Failures were not reported.

Elliotson (1843a) reported an 18-year-old boy with rheumatism and delirium with convulsions, probably associated with fever. The boy made little progress during the first month of medical treatment, which included bleeding, opium, purgatives, head shaving and application of lotions to the scalp, quinine, musk, creosote, iron, prussic acid, and arsenic. His behavior was so violent that he was tied with ropes across his bed and further restrained by three strong men. At this point, Elliotson visited the patient. In the first session, 45 minutes of mesmeric passes had no effect. Elliotson turned the case over to one of his former pupils. The following evening's session lasted over 2 hours; the doctor noted that the convulsive attack, which usually occurred in the evening, ended a bit sooner than usual. Medication was continued in reduced doses. Mesmeric treatment continued each evening, with gradual improvement noted. After 1 week, the doctor reported that the boy was becoming attached to him. To our knowledge, this is the earliest reference to the transference aspects of the therapeutic hypnosis relationship. The transference was reported almost in passing, and its role in the curative process was not fully recognized. Eleven days after mesmeric treatment began, the patient's violent attacks ceased, and treatment stopped. The patient continued to sleep poorly for several weeks, a problem which Elliotson attributed to premature termination of treatment.

In the same paper, Elliotson reported successful mesmeric treatment in eight cases of chorea, of which six were children ranging in age from 9 to 17 years. Duration of treatment ranged from 1 day to 2 months. With the exception of iron, other medications were discontinued, most of them doing more harm than good.

In 1843, Elliotson published a book entitled *Numerous Cases of Surgical Operations without Pain in the Mesmeric State* (1843b), describing both his own work and that of his colleagues. Here he mentioned several cases of painless dental extractions in children. He reported that after 5 minutes of mesmeric passes a colleague had opened a large abscess behind the ear of a 12-year-old boy. The patient was comfortable throughout the procedure. He also reported a colleague's operation on a 17-year-old girl to release knee contractures while she was in a mesmeric trance. She experienced no pain and was unaware that the procedures had been accomplished until she saw spots of blood on the sheets of her hospital bed.

Elliotson concluded from his clinical experience that his favorable results were attributable to mesmeric passes, and he continued to deny most vehemently that imagination played any role in the cures. He apparently never understood that his methods could not provide any evidence in favor of one theory or the other.

## James Braid (1795–1860)

Braid was an English surgeon, a contemporary of Elliotson, who began investigating mesmerism as a complete skeptic. Unlike Elliotson, when he saw that such phenomena as induced catalepsy and analgesia were real, he elected to avoid diatribes and to be open minded with regard to the underlying theoretical explanation, although he leaned toward imagination as a good possibility. In 1843, Braid wrote of his techniques:

> I feel we have acquired in this process a valuable addition to our curative means; but I repudiate the idea of holding it up as a universal remedy, nor do I even pretend to

> understand, as yet, the whole range of diseases in which it may be useful. … Whether the extraordinary physical effects are produced through the imagination chiefly, or by other means, it appears to me quite certain, that the imagination has never been so much under our control, or capable of being made to act in the same beneficial and uniform manner, by any other mode of management hitherto known.
>
> *(Braid, 1843/1960)*

Braid, however, rejected the idea that imagination alone could produce trance.

Both for theoretical and for practical reasons, Braid discarded the whole idea of animal magnetism, and he avoided the word "mesmerism." Thinking of trance phenomena as some sort of nervous sleep, he coined the term "hypnosis" from the Greek word *hypnos*, meaning sleep. He abandoned the use of passes and, instead, required his subjects to fix their gaze on an object and concentrate attention on a single idea (monoideism). Braid's elucidation of the psychological aspects of hypnosis was a major contribution, and his theories were subsequently adopted by Broca, Charcot, Liebault, and Bernheim.

Braid was impressed by the ease and rapidity with which a trance could be induced, and he took careful notice of instances in which some individuals went into a trance state without any formal induction. In an 1855 work, he reported an anecdote in which an elderly man discovered a boy who had climbed up into one of his apple trees and was in the midst of stealing an apple:

> At this moment the gentleman addressed the boy in a stern manner, declaring that he would fix him there in the position he was then in. Having said so, the gentleman left the orchard and went off to church, not doubting that the boy would soon come down and effect his escape when he knew the master of the orchard was gone. However, it turned out otherwise; for, upon going into the orchard on his return from church, he was not a little surprised to find that the boy had been spell-bound by his declaration to that effect – for there he still remained, in the exact attitude in which he left him, with his arm outstretched, and his hand ready to lay hold of the apple. By some farther remarks from this gentleman the spell was broken, and the boy allowed to escape without further punishment.
>
> *(Braid, 1855)*

In this and other anecdotes, Braid recognized the power of mind over body, and he pointed out that children were frequently "sensitive" in this regard. He failed to recognize these instances as spontaneous hypnosis, describing them instead as waking phenomena. Holding to the idea that hypnotic phenomena were produced by formal visual and mental fixation, he said, "In cases of children, and those (adults) of weak intellect, or of restless and excitable minds whom I could not manage so as to make them comply with these simple rules, I have always been foiled, although most anxious to succeed" (Braid, 1843/1960). He made this comment in spite of the fact that, in the same paper, he reported inducing light hypnosis with arm catalepsy in 32 children at once by making them stand and sit over a period of 10–12 minutes. It seems that, like Mesmer and Elliotson before him, Braid made the mistake of defining hypnotic phenomena by the techniques he used to produce them.

Braid seemed tantalizingly close to the step of recognizing the independence of trance phenomena from particular induction methods. He fully recognized that the operator involved in trance production did not communicate any magnetic, electrical, or other force from his own body but, rather, acted as an engineer, using various modes to direct vital forces within the patient's body. He recognized the importance of the patient's faith and confidence in the process. He even recognized the possibility of self-hypnosis, using it to manage his own pains, but it would be several more years before his speculations about the role of imagination in hypnosis would be deliberately applied to child patients.

## Charles Dickens (1812–1870) and Chauncey Hare Townshend (1798–1868)

The first of the three volumes of *Great Expectations* by Dickens was "affectionately inscribed" to Chauncey Hare Townshend, who was a wealthy minister, poet, and art collector. Charles Dickens first met him in 1840 as a result of their common enthusiasm for "hypnotism." Townshend published a book, *Facts in Mesmerism*, in 1840. Two books about Dickens describe his interest in and use of hypnosis (Pearson, 1949; Pope-Hennessey, 1946). His primary teacher was John Elliotson. Later, in *Dickens and Mesmerism* (Kaplan, 1975), the author noted that Dickens' interest in hypnosis impacted several of his novels. As described in a more recent book by Wendy Moore, John Elliotson became the family doctor for Dickens and they were very close friends (Moore, 2017). These biographies describe several of Dickens' clinical experiences with hypnosis, including his treatment of a friend who had suffered pain following a concussion and a woman with facial tics and anxiety.

## Jean-Martin Charcot (1835–1893)

Charcot, a distinguished French neurologist, began his investigation of hypnosis at the School of the Salpetriere in 1878. His descriptions of hypnosis in neurological terms gave it a new measure of scientific respectability. By 1882, the subject appeared regularly in the best medical journals as well as in the lay press. Scientific journals devoted entirely to hypnosis sprang up in both France and Germany (Tinterow, 1970). In spite of – or perhaps because of – Charcot's having his own clinic with ample numbers of assistants to work with patients, he really did little to advance understanding of hypnosis, especially in the case of children. He conceived of hypnosis as a pathological state, a form of hysterical neurosis, able to be produced more easily in women than in men. He considered all children unsusceptible. According to a biography about Guillain (cited in Tinterow, 1970), Charcot failed to check the work of his assistants and never personally hypnotized a single patient. Having developed a theory, he unwittingly restricted his experimental work in such a way that the data could only support his ideas. Late in his life, in the face of increasing criticism, he saw the need to revise his theory, but by this time he was quite ill, and he died without beginning the actual work of revision.

## Auguste Ambrose Liebault (1823–1904) and Hippolyte Bernheim (1840–1919)

At about the same time that Charcot founded the School of the Salpetriere, Liebault founded another French school devoted to the investigation of hypnosis, the School of Nancy. He was soon joined by Bernheim, and together they developed theories and gathered data that opposed those of Charcot and have since proved to be more accurate. Specifically, they conceived of hypnosis as an entirely normal phenomenon based chiefly on suggestion and imagination, thus clarifying and extending the earlier speculation of Braid. In 1888, Bernheim wrote, "I define hypnotism as the induction of a peculiar physical condition which increases the susceptibility to suggestion. Often, it is true, the sleep that may be induced facilitates suggestion, but it is not the necessary preliminary. It is suggestion that rules hypnotism" (in Tinterow, 1970, p. 454). He concluded that hypnosis occurs as a result of various induction methods "acting upon imagination."

As might be expected on the basis of their theories, Liebault and Bernheim found that most children were quickly and easily hypnotized, as long as they were able to pay attention and understand instructions. Their method consisted of eye fixation with repeated suggestions for eye closure and sleep. They did not insist on sleep if the subject showed no such inclinations, but they

**TABLE 2.1** Norms of Hypnotizability

| *Age (Years)* | *Somnambulism (%)* | *Less Deep Hypnotism (%)* | *Refractory (%)* |
|---|---|---|---|
| 0 6 | 26.5 | 73.7 | — |
| 7–13 | 55.3 | 44.4 | — |
| 14–20 | 25.2 | 64.2 | 10.3 |
| 21–27 | 13.2 | 77.4 | 9.1 |
| 28–34 | 22.6 | 71.2 | 5.9 |
| 35–41 | 10.5 | 81.1 | 8.2 |
| 42–48 | 21.6 | 65.9 | 12.2 |
| 49–55 | 7.3 | 87.9 | 4.4 |
| 56–62 | 7.3 | 78.0 | 14.4 |
| 63+ | 11.8 | 74.3 | 13.5 |

*Source*: Adapted from Bramwell, J.M., *Hypnotism: Its History, Practice and Theory*, Julian Press, New York, 1956 (original work published in 1903).

manually pushed down the eyelids if the subject's eyes remained open for more than a few minutes. Any resistance was met by more forceful commands.

More than their predecessors, Liebault and Bernheim recognized individual differences in response to hypnotic suggestions. Hypnosis was not an all-or-none phenomenon but could be manifested at varying degrees of depth. The deepest level, somnambulism, and each of the lighter levels had characteristic features, although there were individual differences in response within each level as well as between levels. Once they made these advances toward greater scientific sophistication, the next step was to carry out normative studies on a large scale. According to Bramwell (1903/1956), Liebault compiled data from 755 subjects and found no differences in hypnotizability between males and females. The data were then restated in order to focus on age differences across the whole range from young children to the elderly. As shown in Table 2.1, the highest percentage of somnambules occurred in children 7–14 years of age. No subject in this age group or in the group of children younger than 7 years was entirely refractory.

## J. Milne Bramwell (1852–1925)

Bramwell was an English psychotherapist who began to use hypnosis in 1889. In 1903, he published *Hypnotism: Its History, Practice, and Theory*, a comprehensive review that was widely quoted as the major text in the field for many years. From vignettes of his own cases and those of his colleagues, we get a good idea of the range of childhood disorders treated with therapeutic hypnosis at the turn of the century. These disorders included behavior problems (e.g., stealing, lying, masturbation, insolence), chorea, eczema, enuresis, headaches, hyperhidrosis (excessive sweating), nail biting, night terrors, seizures, and stammering (Bramwell, 1903/1956). The success rate was reportedly very high, but we are not sure whether all failures were reported. The children described ranged in age from 3 to 19 years.

## The Beginning of Child Hypnosis in America

So far as we know, the first publication concerning child hypnosis in a major American journal was a paper in *Science* entitled "Suggestion in Infancy" (Baldwin, 1891). The author discussed the idea that the rise of interest in hypnosis had opened the way for increased understanding of infant behavior beyond mere physiological or reflex reactions. Such behavior could now be understood in terms of environmental influences, especially what he called *ideomotor suggestions*; for example, he described his use of reward and punishment to extinguish scratching behavior in a 3-month-old infant. He also discussed the child's development of imitative behavior, beginning at about 8 months. Baldwin did not use hypnosis *per se* but, rather, understood the possibility of understanding hypnotic phenomena as a point of departure for the study of consciousness, an idea that came back into sharp focus with the work of Hilgard (E.R. Hilgard, 1977).

Lightner Witmer, who coined the term *clinical psychology* and opened the first American psychological clinic in 1896 at the University of Pennsylvania, published a sharply critical paper about hypnosis in the 1897 volume of *Pediatrics* (Witmer, 1897). When he expressed his alarm that pedagogical uses of hypnosis were often considered a panacea, he was referring not only to the use of hypnosis in formal education but also to any hypnotic treatment in which suggestions were given chiefly for the purpose of educating the patient – for example, to expend constructive effort in work or to desist from objectionable habits. Like Charcot, Witmer thought that "the susceptibility to hypnotic influence is itself a stigma of neuroticism, perhaps of hysteria" (p. 26). He believed that hypnosis weakened the will and fostered impulsivity, adding that "mental tonic is what such persons need, not such mental perversion as hypnotism is" (p. 27).

R. Osgood Mason (1897) replied to Witmer's editorial with matching vehemence in support of pedagogical hypnosis, especially in the case of children. He described the beneficial effects of hypnosis for a wide variety of pediatric problems. He denied that he considered it a panacea, or that it weakened the patient's will or capacity for independent judgment. Countering Witmer's notion of hypnosis as a phenomenon seen chiefly in hysterics, Mason cited Bernheim's hypnotic research with large numbers of normal subjects.

Citing his own case records, Mason reported successful therapeutic hypnosis with a 15-year-old girl suffering from lack of concentration and poor memory for schoolwork, a 7-year-old boy who was too frightened to cooperate with necessary medical treatment, a 5-year-old girl suffering frequent night terrors, and a 16-year-old boy referred because of masturbation and cigarette smoking. In each case "the treatment was essentially educational – the dismissal of the abnormal hurtful or evil ideas and tendencies and the restoration or introduction of new, normal, and helpful ones in their place" (p. 104). Treatment time varied from one session to a long series of visits.

By 1900, in both America and Europe, interest in child hypnosis was waning and would not revive again for nearly half a century. Then it got off to a slow start, not becoming a major research area until the late 1950s and early 1960s. During the two World Wars, interest in adult hypnosis increased briefly, as a result of pressure to get disabled soldiers back on the battlefield quickly. From the experiences of injured soldiers much was learned about how self-hypnotic anesthesia works. Injured soldiers would dissociate spontaneously and reduce discomfort. This was an important observation in the evolution of understanding about child hypnotic pain control. But, during these periods, little else was learned that was relevant to the treatment of children. When interest in child hypnosis increased again in the 1950s, researchers and clinicians began essentially where they had left off half a century before.

During the 1960s, a few publications were related to children and hypnosis, including some related to child hypnotizability. Increased numbers of pediatricians, child psychiatrists, and child psychologists were teaching children self-hypnosis in the 1970s and beginning research on hypnosis and children. The first workshop devoted solely to child hypnosis took place in 1976. Subsequently, the American Society of Clinical Hypnosis and the Society for Clinical and Experimental Hypnosis sponsored workshops related to hypnosis with children. A small group of faculty had developed by the 1980s, and in 1987 they held a three-day workshop on hypnosis with children with sponsorship from the Society for Developmental and Behavioral Pediatrics. These workshops continued for 24 years. In 2010, the workshop was developed by the faculty group of what was to become the National Pediatric Hypnosis Training Institute (NPHTI) and co-sponsored by the University of Minnesota and the Minnesota Society of Clinical Hypnosis. NPHTI has since become an independent volunteer organization that has organized training in child hypnosis each year. During the COVID-19 pandemic, NPHTI has organized successful virtual workshops and webinar series.

Since the 1980s hundreds of research studies and clinical reports have involved children and hypnosis. When preparing the third edition of this book in 1996, it was still possible for us to reference all pediatric research studies involving hypnosis, but this was no longer possible for the fourth or fifth editions.

## Conclusions

Early reports of hypnosis with children were primarily anecdotal, often in the context of emotional appeals to support or refute current theories and speculations about various aspects of human behavior. Nevertheless, by the end of the 19th century, those who had studied the field carefully already knew that children were suitable hypnotic subjects, that the peak of hypnotizability occurred in middle childhood, and that hypnotic techniques were applicable to a wide variety of childhood medical and psychological problems. By the end of the 20th century, pediatric hypnosis had begun to become evidenced based, with a multitude of compelling clinical reports being reinforced by a growing number of solid research studies describing the significant effectiveness of hypnosis in and for many pediatric conditions, illnesses, and problems – including its superiority to conventional or traditional and pharmacologic therapies in selected conditions and circumstances. The first decades of the 21st century have proved to be increasingly productive in describing exciting controlled research studies documenting the efficacy of hypnosis in a variety of child health and illness conditions and the increasing research laboratory discoveries of physiologic correlates of the hypnotic experience in children.

## References


Baldwin, J.M. (1891). Suggestion in infancy. *Science, 17*(421), 113–117.

Braid, J. (1855). *The Physiology of Fascination and the Critics Criticized.* Manchester, U.K.: Grant & Co.

Braid, J. (1960). *Neurypnology; or the Rationale of Nervous Sleep.* New York: Julian Press (original work published 1843; revised as *Braid on Hypnotism*, 1889).

Bramwell, J.M. (1956). *Hypnotism: Its History, Practice, and Theory* (reissued with new introduction). New York: Julian Press (original work published 1903).

Elliotson, J. (1843a). Cases of cures by mesmerism. *The Zoist, 1*, 161–208.

Elliotson, J. (1843b). *Numerous Cases of Surgical Operations without Pain in the Mesmeric State.* Philadelphia, PA: Lea & Blanchard.

Hilgard, E.R. (1977). *Divided Consciousness: Multiple Controls in Human Thought and Action.* New York: John Wiley & Sons.

Kaplan, F. (1975). *Dickens and Mesmerism: The Hidden Springs of Fiction.* Princeton, NJ: Princeton University Press.

Mason, R.O. (1897). Educational uses of hypnotism: a reply to Prof. Lightner Witmer's editorial in *Pediatrics* for January 1, 1897. *Pediatrics, III*(3), 97–105.

Mead, M. (1949). *Male and Female: A Study of the Sexes in a Changing World.* New York: William Morrow.

Moore, W.E. (2017). *The Mesmerist, the Society Doctor Who Held Victorian London Spellbound.* London: Weidenfeld & Nicolson.

Pearson, H. (1949). *Dickens: His Character, Comedy and Career.* New York: Harpers.

Pope-Hennessy, U. (1946). *Charles Dickens.* London: Lewes.

Tinterow, M.M. (1970). *Foundations of Hypnosis: From Mesmer to Freud.* Springfield, IL: Charles C. Thomas.

Townshend, C.H. (2004). *Facts in Mesmerism, with Reasons for a Dispassionate Inquiry into It.* Whitefish, MT: Keissigner Publishing (original work published 1840).

Witmer, L. (1897). The use of hypnotism in education. *Pediatrics, III*(1), 23–27.

# 3

# NORMS OF HYPNOTIC RESPONSIVITY IN CHILDREN

## Introduction

The question of degrees of hypnotizability in children is not new. In the 1880s, Liebault (Tinterow, 1970), struggled with it in his studies of hypnotizability that included subjects from early childhood to over 60 years of age. In a recent book (Moore, 2017) Wendy Moore chronicles the friendship between Charles Dickens and the British Surgeon, John Elliotson and the conflict between Thomas Wakley who required scientific proof and John Elliotson, including reports of Elliotson's successful work with children.

In the 1930s, Hull (1933) and his students, especially Messerschmidt (1933a, b), studied children's responses to waking suggestibility items. Although they did not equate suggestibility with hypnotizability, the two traits were positively correlated. The results of the early studies were quite similar to more recent studies. That is, early research concluded that hypnotizability and suggestibility are quite limited in young children, increase markedly in the middle childhood years from about 7 to 14, and then decrease somewhat in adolescence, becoming quite stable throughout early and mid-adulthood and tailing off again in the older population.

With all normative studies reaching essentially the same conclusion, one is tempted to review them rather briefly and then move on to other issues. The major problem is that these research findings are at variance with a growing body of clinical data indicating that children of preschool age, and perhaps even younger, do in fact respond positively to what is described as the therapeutic use of hypnosis. The issues involved in this controversy are complex; thus, we choose to confront them head-on in order to leave the reader with some measure of the complexity of what appears on the surface to be an easy answer. We begin with a critical review of recent normative studies and then deal with the special problem of hypnotizability in young children.

## Normative Studies

Stukat (1958) and Barber and Calverley (1963) administered tests of suggestibility to children at various ages. Because they did not claim to be using hypnotic techniques, we will not review their studies in detail. It should be noted that their findings for suggestibility are similar to studies measuring hypnotizability, as can be seen in Figure 3.1, which compares their results with normative data for hypnotic susceptibility in children. One can conclude either that the traits

DOI: 10.4324/9781003243687-4

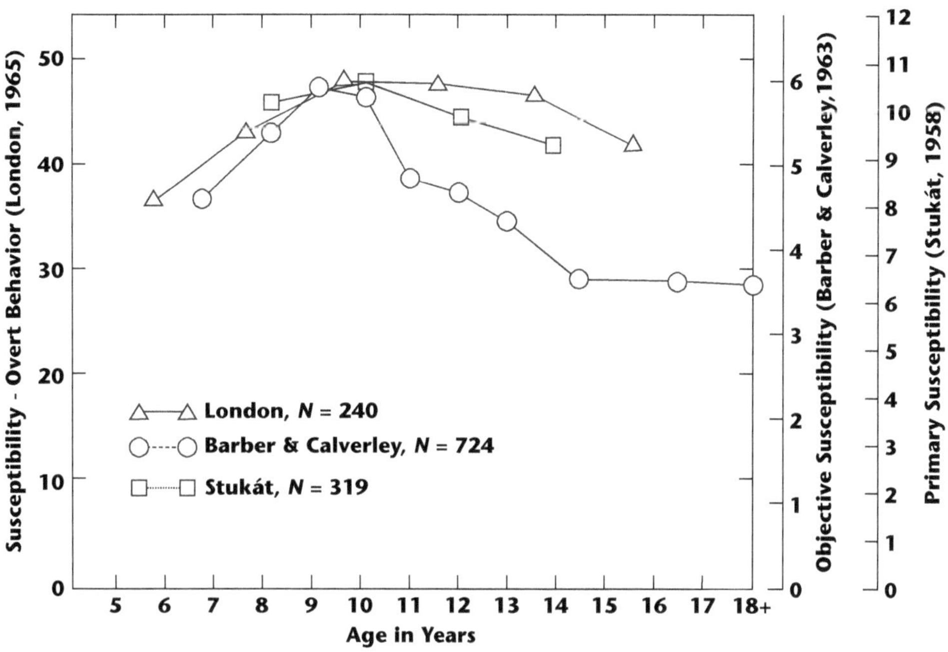


FIGURE 3.1 Changes in suggestibility with age. Barber and Calverley's and Stukat's suggestibility scales (not involving hypnosis) correlate highly with hypnotic performances. London did use hypnotic techniques

*Source*: Adapted from Hilgard, E.R., in *Minnesota Symposia on Child Psychology*, Vol. 5, Hill, J.P., Ed., Lund Press, Minneapolis, MN, 1971. With permission.

measured by the three scales are highly correlated or that suggestibility, as measured by these tests, and hypnotic susceptibility are essentially the same trait.

Commenting on Tromater's (1961) review of early studies of childhood hypnotizability, London (1962) observed that early efforts to assess hypnotizability in children were in general agreement that children, as a group, are more susceptible than adults and that there is a curvilinear relationship between age and susceptibility, with a peak in the 8–12-year age range. London noted methodological problems in these early studies, especially the lack of an operational definition of susceptibility and imprecise measuring devices, and he set out to remedy these problems.

London (1963) developed a test known as the Children's Hypnotic Susceptibility Scale (CHSS) that was based on the items in the Stanford Hypnotic Susceptibility Scale (SHSS), Form A (SHSS, Form A) (Weitzenhoffer & Hilgard, 1959). The CHSS contains 22 items in two parts; Part I is parallel in content to SHSS, Form A, and Part II contains some more difficult items such as visual hallucinations and thirst and taste hallucinations. Administration of the scale requires 45–60 minutes for each child.

Because some children in the pilot studies (London, 1962) appeared to be faking or "playing along" with the instructions, the subjects received two scores for each item, one based on their overt behavioral response (OB) and the other based on the examiner's impression of the extent of the subjects' subjective involvement (SI) – that is, whether they appeared to be (1) faking or role-playing, (2) partially involved, or (3) deeply involved in the item. The product of these two scores yielded a total score (TOT). Usually, the score ultimately derived for a subject is the total for Part I and Part II combined. Sometimes the emphasis can be on a part score; for example, if one wants to make comparisons with the SHSS, Form A, a 12-item test scored on the basis of the subject's overt behavior, then one would score the CHSS only for Part I, which contains the 12 parallel items, and only for overt behavior. Interscorer reliability, based on a pilot sample of 36 children retested after 1 week, was 92, indicating consistent performance in children similar to that found for adults.

Using data from 57 children, London (1962) found that children were more often successful on almost all CHSS items, as compared with adults on the SHSS, lending further credence to the notion that children are more susceptible. London was unable to establish a significant curvilinear relationship between age and susceptibility, although there was a trend in that direction. He predicted that the trend would become statistically meaningful when the sample size was increased, but he thought the curve would remain a shallow one, indicating that the relationship between susceptibility and age cannot be accounted for simply on the basis of age. He noted that "there is probably more variability among children at any given age than between children of any two successive ages" (p. 87).

To study the possibility that role-playing might account for high scores among some children, London (1962) selected a new sample of 40 children, ages 5–11 years, the group in which role-playing tended to occur. After performing six "playlets," each subject was engaged in a simulation task, following the motivation instructions for adults designed by Orne (1959). In his classic studies of hypnotic simulation, Orne compared non-hypnotizable subjects who were told to simulate hypnosis with highly hypnotizable subjects and found that even well-trained examiners could not tell which subjects belonged to which group. London's instructions to each child in his simulation study (1962) were as follows:

> We are going to be alone in this room for a few more minutes and then I am going to get Mrs. X. When she comes in, she will think that I have hypnotized you, and that you are in a deep hypnotic trance. Do you know what that means? Well, what I want you to do is make her think that you are really hypnotized, and to do everything she tells you as if you were hypnotized. The things will be very easy for you, and the only thing you need to know is that, when she comes in, your eyes should be closed, and always keep them closed unless she tells you to open them.
>
> Now, she may be a little bit suspicious that you aren't hypnotized because she knows that there will be one or two kids in here who are just faking, and she will wonder a little if it is you. If she thinks that you are faking, she will stop what she is doing right away – but as long as she keeps on going, you will know that you are fooling her into thinking you are hypnotized. (p. 87)

For children in this limited age range, there is a linear relationship between age and simulation ability. The simulation scores on the CHSS, Part II, were lower than those for hypnotic subjects below age 8 years but merged thereafter. In other words, simulation was obvious below age 8 years, but it was indistinguishable from hypnotic performance at higher ages. Noting that the youngest subjects were poor simulators and that older adolescents tend to be too honest to simulate on hypnotic susceptibility tests, London was left with the conclusion that "children in the middle group achieve peak scores because they can communicate simulated performances with the same effectiveness that they do real performances and we cannot tell them apart" (p. 90). This does not mean that all children in this group simulate, and those who do may do so only on selected items. Yet, when these children do simulate, it is not likely to be noticed, even by trained examiners. London concluded that the evidence for curvilinearity is weak and is even further weakened by the insensitivity of the CHSS to the simulation of individual items. London noted that the subjects in these studies were chiefly from upper-middle-class backgrounds but did not speculate about the impact of social class distribution on his results.

London (1965) standardized his scale on a group of 240 children, ages 5–16 years, with ten boys and ten girls at each year level. These subjects came from a group of 303 children whose parents had responded to a form letter, and again the sample was markedly skewed toward upper-middle-class professional and managerial backgrounds. For this new sample, inter-scorer reliability for the full-scale CHSS ranged from .88 to .97 for the three obtained scores (overt behavior, subjective involvement, and total). Test–retest reliability ($N = 50$) after 1 week ranged from .75 to .84. As in the pilot studies, a modest curvilinear relationship between age and susceptibility was observed, with the peak in the 9–12-year range. And, again, the standard deviations were large at all ages. London (1965) noted that "the extent of susceptibility or the lack of it among different children within a single age group is more impressive than are changes across ages" (p. 195).

The mean score of the standardization sample of 240 children (8.16) was significantly larger than the mean score of college students (5.25) in the normative data for the SHSS, Form A. When scores were grouped into high, medium, and low categories for children, the largest group fell in the range of high susceptibility; for adults, the largest group fell in the range of low susceptibility. These data again support the notion that children are more responsive to hypnosis than adults (London & Cooper, 1969).

Cooper and London (1971) reported longitudinal data for a subset of the standardization sample. The intercorrelations across time periods, ranging from 1 week to 2 years, were significantly positive but by no means perfect. Moreover, the correlations for younger children were lower than those for older children. These results are similar to those obtained in the measurement of intelligence; namely, it is more difficult to predict from obtained scores to future scores for younger children than for older children. Results of this longitudinal study were similar to those of the cross-sectional studies, leading the authors to conclude that changes in susceptibility do occur with age and that these changes are extremely stable.

Morgan and Hilgard (1973) reported a massive study of age differences in hypnotic susceptibility for 1,232 subjects, ranging in age from 5 to 78 years. Again the subjects clustered in the middle socioeconomic class. The results for children, based on a slightly modified SHSS, Form A, were similar to those cited earlier, with a peak in the preadolescent years and a gradual decline thereafter. Morgan and Hilgard did not comment on the issue of simulation. No significant sex differences in hypnotic susceptibility were observed in any of these studies or in the report of Cooper and London (1966), which specifically addressed this issue.

The normative study of Morgan and Hilgard (1979) came to the same conclusions regarding age and hypnotizability as did the earlier studies. Its significance lies in the fact that the score is based on a short scale, the Stanford Hypnotic Clinical Scale for Children (SHCS-C), that can be administered in 20 minutes. This scale can be found in its entirety in the Appendix in the fourth edition of this text. The brevity of the scale makes it feasible to use in a primarily therapeutic setting, although 20 minutes is a long time in most managed care settings.

Over the years, many clinicians have argued that the use of a scale to measure hypnotizability was, at best, irrelevant and at worst, improper. They argued that clinical hypnosis and laboratory hypnosis are two different entities with little or no connection, and they argued that, even if a scale could measure the kind of hypnotizability that is observed in a clinical setting, patients subjected to such a scale would experience frustration and failure that would both interfere with rapport and compromise therapeutic progress. Contrary to the assumptions of the first argument, E.R. Hilgard and Hilgard (1975) found that adult subjects who score higher on a hypnotizability scale tend to respond more effectively to suggestions for pain control, both in experimental and in clinical settings. Contrary to the assumptions of the second argument, Morgan and Hilgard (1979) did not find any marked concerns about failure in the context of their permissive induction and suggestions. If a child began to apologize for a failed item, the examiner immediately countered with, "We are just as interested in what people don't experience as we are in what people do experience." Children in the clinical setting were told, "Not everybody does the same things. We have to find those things that are best for you, some you will find much more interesting than others. There will be some that we can build on" (Morgan & Hilgard, 1979, p. 154).

The Morgan and Hilgard (1979) study makes another major contribution to the field of hypnosis. Unfortunately, the authors make no mention of it, and we would like to take this opportunity to give them the credit they deserve. For the first time in the series of studies reported here, the term *susceptibility* has been omitted and the term *responsivity* used in its place. This shift reflects a growing awareness that the capacity to experience hypnosis is chiefly a skill or talent of the subject and not a phenomenon created by the clinician or researcher facilitating the hypnosis. The so-called hypnotist is a teacher or coach rather than a controlling force; thus, the term *hypnotic virtuoso* describes the behavior of the subject, not the hypnotist. This change in terminology reflected the change over the last few decades from an authoritarian to a permissive approach in hypnosis and what we are now calling therapeutic hypnosis. We are in full agreement that the locus of control should be and is in the subject; therefore, in this book, we use the term *responsiveness* or its equivalent except when referring to historical matters. Additionally, we avoid use of the word *hypnotist*, as it tends to connote to readers what we believe to be a mistaken and outdated image of an all-powerful, all-controlling person whom we have now come to understand quite differently.

The SHCS-C includes one form for children 6–16 years old and another form for children 4–8 years old. The form for older children is based on an eye closure–relaxation induction followed by seven test items. The form for younger children is based on an active imagination induction, as young or immature children often respond negatively to suggestions for eye closure. This form contains six test items. In both forms, the items are intrinsically interesting to children, allow some success at all ages, and have direct relevance for choice of therapeutic techniques. The test correlated .67 with the longer SHSS, Form A, modified slightly for use with children.

In these early stages of its development, the SHCS-C consisted of only one form, utilizing an eye closure–relaxation induction. The second form (active imagination) was created when the authors discovered that the younger children failed most or all items in the relaxation condition but passed some of the same items in the imagination condition. At that time, exhibiting a degree of flexibility not seen in earlier studies, the authors modified the induction for younger children so they could pass more items. The awareness of this need for flexibility now takes us into a new area, guaranteed to confuse more than to clarify what has already become a muddied field in the area of norms of hypnotizability in children.

Peter and colleagues in Germany (2015) administered the German version of the Harvard Group Scale of Hypnotic Susceptibility, Form A, to 99 German adolescents, aged 15–19 years. Twenty-nine percent of these students reported prior experiences with relaxation techniques. Scores ranged from 0 to 12, and the mean score was 6.11. There were no gender differences in the results. Authors concluded that the data did not differ significantly from testing of adults in other countries.

## Hypnosis as a Function of Induction and Measurement Techniques

Historically, the measurement of hypnotic susceptibility (responsivity) has consisted of a hypnotic induction emphasizing relaxation and eye closure followed by a number of test items reflecting various phenomena that most people agree typify hypnotic behavior. Subjects who score very low on these scales are said to not be hypnotizable. Moreover, some researchers (e.g., Barber, 1979) have taken the position that, if there is no formal hypnotic induction, the subject cannot be said to be in hypnosis at all. We disagree with Barber's position. As yet, there is no absolute knowledge of the boundaries that define hypnosis. Instead, we take the position that certain kinds of behavior

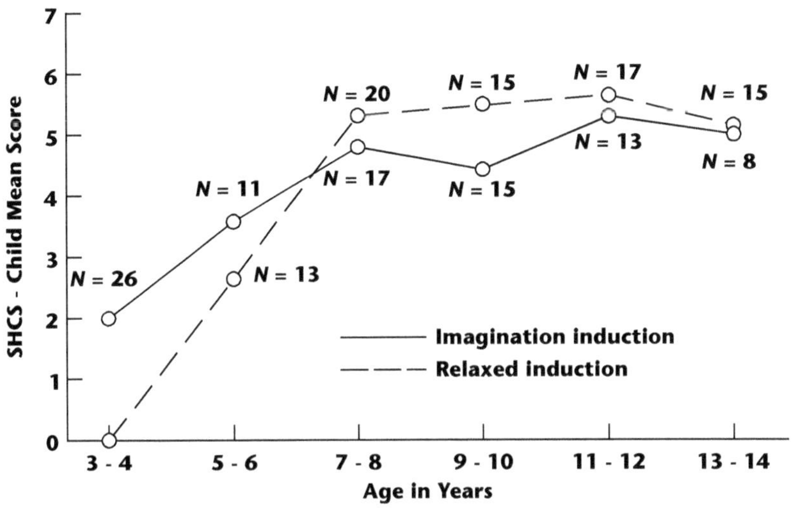


**FIGURE 3.2** Mean scores by age on seven items of the SHCS-C. Imagination induction is compared with relaxation induction

*Source*: Adapted from Morgan, A.H. and Hilgard, E.R., *American Journal of Clinical Hypnosis*, 21, 148–169, 1979. With permission.

can be described as hypnotic behavior, whether they are induced or occur spontaneously. These behaviors include, but are not limited to, the behaviors elicited by standard scales of hypnotizability. It is important to note that people vary in terms of their ability to experience different hypnotic phenomena; for example, two individuals with identical scores on a hypnotizability scale may have passed different kinds of items in order to obtain those scores. We also believe that people vary in terms of the antecedent conditions that are necessary in order to experience hypnosis. In this regard, we find it refreshing that Morgan and Hilgard (1979) directed their research to show that some children respond positively to test items following one kind of induction but not another. Figure 3.2 shows the mean scores for their subjects following eye closure–relaxation and imagination inductions.

When children obtain different scores following different induction procedures, one might ask which scores are the "true" scores. We answer simply whichever scores are higher, as the purpose of a scale of hypnotic responsiveness is to allow the subjects to demonstrate their skills. The findings of Morgan and Hilgard (1979), however, suggest that, in measuring hypnotizability, we have put some children in a position, through inappropriate induction techniques, where they do not do what they really can do. We then may come to the false conclusion that they are not responsive to hypnosis.

The situation is analogous to forcing a child into a sitting position and then measuring height by the distance of the child's head from the floor. Or, we could picture tying a child's hands behind his or her back and then concluding that he or she is not mature enough to tie his or her own shoes. We can only wonder what the normative data of London and Cooper and others would look like, particularly for younger children, if they modified the hypnotic induction in such a way as to maximize the child's ability to respond to the test items.

If the nature of hypnotic induction can affect the scores on a responsivity scale, then the nature of the test items themselves will clearly also affect the scores. Logically, some items will be passed at virtually all ages, some at one age but not another, and some items might not be passed by children of any age. The test scores will depend on which kinds of items and how many of each kind and which difficulty levels are included. As with intelligence, ultimately the meaning of hypnotizability is reduced to what precisely is tested by the test.

Hilgard and colleagues (E.R. Hilgard, Weitzenhoffer, Landes, & Moore, 1961) recognized the need for an operational definition when they wrote that "what we shall mean by hypnotic susceptibility for the purpose of our investigations is a relatively persistent tendency to yield the phenomena historically recognized as belonging to the hypnotic trance, when the opportunity to yield these phenomena is given under standard conditions" (p. 1). Adult scales of hypnotizability sample a variety of hypnotic phenomena, with items placed roughly in order of difficulty and high scores considered more "susceptible" than low ones.

In the case of children, degrees of item difficulty are not the same as those for adults or even for children of different ages; therefore we must at least pause before we conclude that, on a particular scale of children's hypnotic responsiveness, a specific score necessarily means the same thing that it does on an adult scale. We must question whether the "broad sample of hypnotic phenomena" approach is as appropriate for children as it is for adults; that is, some so-called traditional hypnotic phenomena may be traditional for adults but not for children or for certain groups of children because of developmental issues. To use another analogy, we do not administer the same types of intelligence test items to young children that we use for adults on the Stanford–Binet, recognizing that certain language and abstract reasoning skills are simply not developed in the young child; that is, we define intelligence somewhat differently for young children than for adults.

Moreover, if we want the concept of hypnosis to mean roughly the same thing for children as for adults, then we should be reasonably confident that a given item is tapping the same quality in children as for adults, in addition to tapping the same quality in children of different ages. Such item equivalence is probably not the case in some instances, as evidenced by data relating age to item difficulty on scales of hypnotic responsiveness in children. London and Cooper (1969) reported item difficulty for their standardization sample of 240 children for the CHSS, and they compared percent passing each item with the equivalent data for adults on the SHSS, Form A. In Table 3.1, we have adapted these data and rank ordered each item in terms of relative difficulty for children and for adults.

**TABLE 3.1** Item Difficulty for Children on the CHSS and for Adults on the SHSS, Form A

| | *Rank Order of Difficulty*[a] | |
|---|---|---|
| *Item* | *Children* | *Adults* |
| Auditory hallucination | 1.0 | 6.0 |
| Postural sway | 2.0 | 3.0 |
| Hands together | 3.0 | 2.0 |
| Hands lowering | 4.0 | 1.0 |
| Finger lock | 5.0 | 8.0 |
| Posthypnotic suggestion | 6.5 | 5.0 |
| Amnesia | 6.5 | 8.0 |
| Arm rigidity | 8.0 | 8.0 |
| Verbal inhibition | 9.0 | 11.0 |
| Eye catalepsy | 10.0 | 10.0 |
| Arm immobilization | 11.0 | 12.0 |
| Eye closure | 12.0 | 4.0 |

*Source*: Adapted from London, P. and Cooper, L.M., *Developmental Psychology*, 1, 113–124, 1969.

*Note*

a 1 = easiest item, 12 = hardest item.

When these data are studied, the most striking finding is that eye closure is the most difficult item of all for children, whereas it is relatively easy for adults. We suspect that, in the case of children, suggestions for eye closure trigger negative attitudes and concerns about sleep and that these issues preclude the sort of detached interest in motor phenomena that most likely predominates for adults. If the item is tapping something in children that has little or nothing to do with hypnosis, then it really does not belong in the test.

Moore and Cooper (1966) commented on the difficulty with eye closure for children as compared to adults. They noted that the CHSS employs a Chevreul pendulum for this item with the instruction to hold the chain, look at the ball, and try to prevent it from moving. The parallel adult item (SHSS, Form B) requires the subject merely to look passively at a fixed target. They concluded that "for children, it may be that the interesting activity of trying to hold the attractive plastic ball stationary is less conducive to eye closure than focusing the gaze on a target some distance away" (p. 320). If this is true, then again, the two items are not measuring the same thing. To give another example, children find the auditory hallucination item very easy (89% pass), whereas for adults it is moderately difficult (35% pass). In this case, we have a notion that the item probably is measuring the same ability in children as in adults, with children simply being more skilled at this particular task. Moore and Lauer (1963) studied item difficulty for a sample of 48 children, ages 6–12 years, and compared their data to adult scores, with essentially the same results as the sample of London and Cooper (1969).

Questions about the meaning of test items become even more interesting when we look at the data in Table 3.2, showing the relative difficulty of each item for children at different ages.

**TABLE 3.2** Relative Item Difficulty on the CHSS across Age Levels (N = 240)

| | *Age (years)*[a] | | | | | |
|---|---|---|---|---|---|---|
| *Item* | *5–6* | *7–8* | *9–10* | *11–12* | *13–14* | *15–16* |
| Amnesia | 1.0 | 11.5 | 13.0 | 10.0 | 16.0 | 12.0 |
| Auditory hallucination | 2.0 | 2.0 | 2.0 | 1.5 | 1.0 | 4.5 |
| Hands together | 3.5 | 6.0 | 5.0 | 12.5 | 4.5 | 3.0 |
| Cold hallucination | 3.5 | 4.0 | 5.0 | 7.0 | 8.0 | 6.0 |
| Postural sway | 5.0 | 9.0 | 8.5 | 3.5 | 2.5 | 1.5 |
| Television | 6.5 | 6.0 | 3.5 | 5.5 | 8.0 | 10.0 |
| Visual hallucination | 6.5 | 1.0 | 1.0 | 1.5 | 4.5 | 8.5 |
| Finger lock | 8.0 | 8.0 | 8.5 | 12.5 | 6.0 | 12.0 |
| Hand lowering | 9.0 | 3.0 | 11.5 | 10.0 | 8.0 | 4.5 |
| Taste hallucination | 10.0 | 6.0 | 5.0 | 3.5 | 10.0 | 15.5 |
| Arm rigidity | 11.0 | 11.5 | 10.0 | 16.0 | 19.0 | 19.5 |
| Verbal inhibition | 13.0 | 15.5 | 16.0 | 18.0 | 13.5 | 19.5 |
| Smell hallucination | 13.0 | 10.0 | 17.0 | 8.0 | 16.0 | 8.5 |
| Dream | 13.0 | 13.0 | 3.5 | 5.5 | 2.5 | 1.5 |
| Posthypnotic suggestion II | 15.0 | 15.5 | 14.5 | 21.0 | 18.0 | 17.0 |
| Arm immobilization | 16.0 | 18.0 | 19.5 | 17.0 | 13.5 | 19.5 |
| Eye closure | 17.5 | 21.0 | 22.0 | 22.0 | 21.0 | 15.5 |
| Posthypnotic suggestion I | 17.5 | 15.5 | 11.5 | 10.0 | 11.0 | 12.0 |
| Eye catalepsy | 19.5 | 15.5 | 14.5 | 20.0 | 16.0 | 22.0 |
| Anesthesia | 19.5 | 19.5 | 19.5 | 19.0 | 20.0 | 19.5 |
| Regression | 21.5 | 19.5 | 21.0 | 14.5 | 12.0 | 7.0 |
| Posthypnotic suggestion III | 21.5 | 22.0 | 18.0 | 14.5 | 22.0 | 14.0 |

*Source*: Adapted from London, P. and Cooper, L.M., *Developmental Psychology*, 1, 113–124, 1969.

*Note*

a 1 = easiest item, 22 = hardest item.

Although we have not attempted any statistical analysis of these data, we are struck by several instances of marked shifts in difficulty level from one age group to another; for example, it is astonishing that the amnesia item is the easiest of all for the 5–6-year-olds, whereas it is moderately difficult for children at all other ages and for adults. We strongly suspect that, although the item taps problems of memory retrieval for subjects beyond age 6, it taps problems of memory storage in the very young child. Because memory storage is not really what the item is designed to measure, it should probably not be in the test for this young age group.

Thus, we agree with E.R. Hilgard and colleagues (1961). If a scale purports to sample hypnotic phenomena, then it should do that and not something else. We would therefore anticipate some sort of revision of the CHSS in the same way and for the same reasons that intelligence tests or aptitude tests are subjected to item analysis and revised according to the data obtained.

After having dealt with some of the more formal problems involved in test construction, we now turn to the relevance of a hypnotic responsiveness scale of a therapeutic situation. Morgan (1974) and Morgan and Hilgard (1979) both addressed this issue. Morgan noted that the factor analytic studies on the SHSS, Form A, yielded three main factors: (1) factor I included challenge items (e.g., arm immobilization, finger lock); (2) factor II included direct suggestion items (e.g., hand lowering, eye closure); and (3) factor III included cognitive items (e.g., fly hallucination, posthypnotic amnesia). Morgan noted that challenge items are relatively difficult for children and place the locus of control outside the child. Moreover, such items may encourage young children to balk because they have not yet resolved developmental issues in which oppositional behavior is a major response style. Morgan concluded that use of such items is probably undesirable in a treatment situation. On the other hand, direct suggestion items are easy for children, are readily converted to autosuggestions, and may therefore be especially appropriate in the context of treatment. Likewise, cognitive items are easy and may provide information that is useful in treatment. Morgan and Hilgard (1979) applied these conclusions advantageously in the development of their short clinical scale for children. In other words, general hypnotic responsivity is not the same as the particular kind or kinds of responsivity that may be appropriate and relevant in a clinical situation. One should be able to predict something about treatment response from the latter but not necessarily from the former.

## Hypnosis and the Young Child

Available scales have indicated that 5- and 6-year-old children are not very responsive as compared with older children, and it is generally assumed that children too young for the scales would score even lower than the 5-year-olds from whom data are available. Several clinical reports, however, have described the effectiveness of hypnotherapy with preschool children for such diverse problems as easing induction of anesthesia (Antitch, 1967; Cullen, 1958), alleviating distress and reducing pain (Gardner, 1978b; Kuttner, 1991; LaBaw, 1973; Olness, 1981b), controlling enuresis and encopresis (Olness, 1975, 1976), adjusting to contact lenses (Olness & Gardner, 1978), and asthma (Kohen & Wynne, 1988).

The recent short clinical scale (Morgan & Hilgard, 1979) reaches down to age 4 years, and we have virtually no research information about children ages 3 years and younger. Because we must assume that subjects who are not "hypnotizable" (as defined by the available scales) could not profitably utilize hypnosis in the course of treatment, we must either conclude that the claims for hypnotherapeutic efficacy are based on some aspect of the therapeutic relationship or process other than hypnosis, or we must revise our assumptions about the nature of hypnotizability.

Gardner (1977a) reviewed the question of hypnosis with infants and pre-school children in some detail, noting that the primary problem lies in how one defines hypnosis:

> The tendency has been to look at a score on a scale, or to consider a response to some sort of formal hypnotic induction, or at least to assess the subject's verbal report of his own experiences. These criteria are not applicable to very young children; we have no scales below age 4, generally recognized formal induction methods do not exist below about age 4, and the youngsters do not have adequate verbal fluency to describe their experiences in acceptable detail.
>
> In the absence of the usual criteria for defining hypnosis, one must rely on observations of certain behaviors of the young child which are similar to behaviors associated with hypnosis in adults. These include (1) quiet, wakeful behavior, which may or may not lead to sleep, following soothing repetitive stimulation, which is a primary characteristic of most formal induction procedures; (2) involvement in vivid imagery during induction in children beyond infancy; (3) heightened attention to a narrow focus with concomitant alterations in awareness; (4) capacity to follow post-hypnotic suggestions as evidenced by behavior which deviates from what is known to be the child's usual behavior in a particular situation. (pp. 158–159)

Gardner (1977a) reviewed clinical evidence supporting the notion that small children develop reliable ways of soothing themselves such as rocking or talking rhythmically. She noted that parents also find reliable ways of calming their young children. Specific examples include stroking some part of the body, playing music, turning on a vacuum cleaner, and putting an electric shaver near the child. She found that the sound of a small hair dryer has the same quieting effect on a fretful infant. She described young patients who responded positively to rhythmic stimulation. She noted studies of hypnosis (Morgan, 1973; Ruch, 1975) in which the authors suggest that hypnotic talent may be present from a very young age or even from birth, and she also reported pertinent studies in child development that show children as young as 2 years having the capacity for fantasy and rapport and the desire for mastery intrinsic to the hypnotic situation.

Bowers and LeBaron (1986) discussed the importance of developmental factors in assessing hypnotic responsivity. They noted that most 7-year-old children have the cognitive ability to experience most aspects of hypnosis reported by adults. They also observed that many children find hypnotic suggestions to be as natural as play. LeBaron (1983) found a significant relationship between the occurrence of fantasy-oriented activities in children's family environments and their hypnotic susceptibility. One can also speculate on the possibility that neurobiological differences produce some parents who are fantasy oriented and are able to provide their children with both the genetic and environmental resources for enjoyment of fantasy. Furthermore, preschoolers are often in states equivalent to if not hypnosis when they are in fact active, noisy, and moving about, especially when they are play acting or role-playing.Hilgard

Gardner (1977a) suggested developing a scale that might tap hypnotic potentialities in very young children, adding that hypnotherapy might be more appropriate for this age group than hitherto recognized. A test of hypnotic responsiveness may be conceptualized as a work sample; for any subject, one must be sure that the work sample is relevant to available behavior and abilities. Rather than insisting that hypnotic responsiveness is present only if a large number of hypnotic phenomena can be elicited, it might be more useful in the case of very young children to start from a position closer to Bartlett's (1968) definition of hypnosis as "a control of the normal control of input (information) for the purpose of controlling output (behavior)" (p. 69). Some hypnosis researchers seem to be moving in this general direction; for example, Hilgard and Morgan (1978) noted the following:

> First, for the young child, approximately the age group of four to six, with as always a few exceptions, it is inappropriate to rely upon formal hypnotic procedures. These procedures

> involve two major elements: (a) the implied difference between voluntary and involuntary action, and (b) the expectation of distraction through self-controlled fantasy. Instead, this group is more responsive to a kind of proto-hypnosis, in which the distraction has at first been set up in the external situation. That is, the very young child is better able to be distracted by listening to a story or by participating in a verbal game with a friendly adult than by removing himself from the scene through his own fantasy or through reliving an earlier game or experience on his own. Gradually the content of the external stimulation can be altered in such a way that the child achieves the control. From the beginning, the primary goal is to give the control to the child. This technique of distraction works with children who are unable to use formal hypnosis; such a group also includes some of the older children. (p. 286)

In a later chapter (Morgan & Hilgard, 1979), the same authors concluded that "the child under 6 is hypnotizable, but not according to the sample practices commonly used with older children" (p. 154). They noted the rather poor response of the youngest children to hypnotic suggestions for pain and anxiety control during such major medical procedures as spinal taps and bone marrow aspirates. We would add that, even if these results follow from the use of fully appropriate induction techniques and suggestions, the fact that the young subjects did not respond much to hypnosis for this purpose does not mean they might not respond positively in some less threatening situation. General hypnotic responsiveness and responsiveness in a particular laboratory or clinical setting may be two very different things.

In the case of young children, the field is wide open for advances in the study of hypnotic responsivity and its clinical applications. Recently, nursing researchers sought to develop a children's imagery questionnaire with the hope of utilizing it to discern in advance of painful medical procedures, for example, those children who score "high" and who might be more likely to benefit from "guided imagery," particularly to obviate anxiety and discomfort in association with otherwise painful medical procedures. The resulting Kids Imaging Ability Questionnaire (KIAQ) (Kwekkeboom, Maddox, & West, 2000) was developed as a modification of an adult-focused scale, the Imaging Ability Questionnaire (IAQ) (Kwekkeboom, 2000). This 17-item scale has thus far been tested with a small sample ($N = 55$) and, although it was not found to be culturally relevant, it was deemed to be reliable and to have content validity sufficient to warrant additional development and testing (Kwekkeboom, 2000).

This scale is referred to as a guided imagery scale that is a "cognitive–behavioral intervention defined as concentrated focusing on images formed in the mind, through which the patient is helped to relax, focus, and develop mental images that result in an alteration of perceived pain or distress," but we believe that, for all intents and purposes, this is the same as hypnosis. Indeed, the KIAQ as it is defined includes 17 items appropriate for children between 6 and 14 years, and it has two subscales, measuring absorption and image generation skills. The absorption subscale was designed to assess responsivity to engaging stimuli, enhanced cognition, synesthesia, oblivious/dissociative involvement, and vivid reminiscence. The imagery subscale (seven items) was designed to assess skill at generating mental images, and children are asked to imagine a particular image and rate its vividness as "can't see it at all" (0), "can kind of see it" (1), and "I can really see it well" (2). Higher scores are said to indicate greater imaging ability (Kwekkeboom et al., 2000). Further testing of this scale will help discern both its utility as a research tool and its value in clinical care.

## Conclusions

We have strayed far from the simple curvilinear relationship, with its peak in the middle childhood years, that is often assumed to describe accurately the norms of hypnotizability in children. Major problems include the difficulty in identifying instances in which subjects in middle childhood simulate hypnosis, use of samples limited to the middle socioeconomic class, very large standard deviations, weaknesses in test construction, frequent use of induction techniques that may interfere with hypnotic responsiveness, use of items to measure hypnotizability that may actually be measuring something quite different, and lack of data and methods for assessing hypnotizability in very young children.

The truth is that we really cannot say very much with confidence concerning hypnotic responsiveness in children. Although there is obviously a tremendous need for more research, we believe we can conclude two things. First, most studies err on the side of underestimating children's hypnotic talent. Second – and this conclusion derives from the first – the lack of solid evidence concerning children's hypnotic responsiveness does not imply that we should abandon our clinical efforts to help children through hypnotherapy. On the contrary, in a context of proper modesty, we should continue to expand both research and clinical efforts and thereby enlarge the data bank. Many children do respond to therapeutic hypnosis, and many reports conclude that the crucial element in treatment is hypnosis and not something else. In a field where the state of the art is not as primitive as it is in child hypnosis, such an argument would, at best, be considered very weak. In this field, however, it seems to be the only reasonable place to stand for the time being.

## References


Antitch, J.L.S. (1967). The use of hypnosis in pediatric anesthesia. *Journal of the American Society of Psychosomatic Dentistry and Medicine, 14*, 70–75.

Barber, T.X. (1979). Suggested ("hypnotic") behavior: the trance paradigm versus an alternative paradigm. In E. Fromm & R.E. Shor, Eds., *Hypnosis: Developments in Research and New Perspectives*, 2nd ed. (pp. 217–271). Hawthorne, NY: Aldine.

Barber, T.X. & Hahn, K.W., Jr. (1962). Physiological and subjective responses to pain producing stimulation under hypnotically-suggested and waking imagined "analgesia." *Journal of Abnormal and Social Psychology, 65*, 411–418.

Bartlett, E.E. (1968). A proposed definition of hypnosis with a theory of its mechanism of action. *American Journal of Clinical Hypnosis, 11*, 69–73.

Bowers, K.S. & LeBaron, S. (1986). Hypnosis and hypnotizability: implications for clinical intervention. *Hospital and Community Psychiatry, 37*, 457–467.

Cooper, L.M. & London, P. (1971). The development of hypnotic susceptibility: a longitudinal (convergence) study. *Child Development, 42*, 487–503.

Cullen, S.C. (1958). Current comment and case reports: hypno-induction techniques in pediatric anesthesia. *Anesthesiology, 19*, 279–281.

Gardner, G.G. (1977a). Hypnosis with infants and preschool children. *American Journal of Clinical Hypnosis, 19*, 158–162.

Gardner, G.G. (1978b). The use of hypnotherapy in a pediatric setting. In E. Gellert, Ed., *Psychosocial Aspects of Pediatric Care*. New York: Grune & Stratton.

Hilgard, E.R. & Hilgard, J.R. (1975). *Hypnosis in the Relief of Pain*. Los Altos, CA: William Kaufman.

Hilgard, J.R. & Morgan, A.H. (1978). Treatment of anxiety and pain in childhood cancer through hypnosis. In F.H. Frankel & H.S. Zamansky, Eds., *Hypnosis at Its Bicentennial: Selected Papers*. New York: Plenum Press.

Hilgard, E.R., Weitzenhoffer, A.M., Landes, J., & Moore, R.K. (1961). The distribution of susceptibility to hypnosis in a student population: a study using the Stanford Hypnotic Susceptibility Scale. *Psychological Monographs, 75(8, Whole No. 512)*.

Hull, C.L. (1933). *Hypnosis and Suggestibility: An Experimental Approach*. New York: D. Appleton-Century Co.

Kohen, D.P. & Wynne, E. (1997). Applying hypnosis in a preschool family asthma education program: uses of storytelling, imagery, and relaxation. *American Journal of Clinical Hypnosis, 39*, 2–14.

Kohen, D.P. & Wynne, E. (1988). A preschool family asthma education program: Uses of storytelling, imagery, and relaxation. presented at the 11th International Congress of Hypnosis and Psychosomatic Medicine, The Hague, The Netherlands.

Kuttner, L. (1991). Helpful strategies in working with preschool children in pediatric practice. *Pediatric Annals, 20*(3), 120–127.

Kwekkeboom, K.L. (2000). Measuring imaging ability: psychometric testing of the imaging ability questionnaire. *Research in Nursing and Health, 23*, 301–309.
Kwekkeboom. K.L., Maddox, M.A., & West, T. (2000). Measuring imaging ability in children. *Journal of Pediatric Health Care, 14*, 297–303.
LaBaw, W.L. (1973). Adjunctive trance therapy with severely burned children. *International Journal of Child Psychotherapy, 2*, 80–92.
LeBaron, S. (1983).Fantasies of children and adolescents: implications for behavioral intervention in chronic illness. In D. R. Copeland, B. Pfefferbaum, & A. Storall, Eds., *The Mind of the Child Who Is Said to Be Sick*. Springfield, IL: Charles C. Thomas.
London, P. (1962). Hypnosis in children: an experimental approach. *International Journal of Clinical and Experimental Hypnosis, 10*, 79–91.
London, P. (1963). *Children's Hypnotic Susceptibility Scale*. Palo Alto, CA: Consulting Psychologists Press.
London, P. (1965). Developmental experiments in hypnosis. *Journal of Projective Techniques and Personality Assessment, 29*, 189–199.
London, P. (1966). Child hypnosis and personality. *American Journal of Clinical Hypnosis, 8*, 161–168.
London, P. & Cooper, L.M. (1969). Norms of hypnotic susceptibility in children. *Developmental Psychology, 1*, 113–124.
Messerschmidt, R. (1933a). Responses of boys between the ages of five and sixteen years to Hull's postural suggestion test. *Journal of Genetic Psychology, 43*, 405–421.
Messerschmidt, B. (1993b). The suggestibility of boys and girls between the ages of six and sixteen years. *Journal of Genetic Psychology*, 43, 422-437.
Moore, R.K. & Cooper, L.M. (1966). Item difficulty in childhood hypnotic susceptibility scales as a function of item wording, repetition, and age. *International Journal of Clinical and Experimental Hypnosis, 14*, 316–323.
Moore, R.K. & Lauer, L.W. (1963). Hypnotic susceptibility in middle childhood. *International Journal of Clinical and Experimental Hypnosis, 11*, 167–174.
Moore, W. (2017). *The Mesmerist: The Society Doctor Who Held Victorian London Spellbound*. London: Orion Books.
Morgan, A.H. (1973). The heritability of hypnotic susceptibility in twins. *Journal of Abnormal Psychology, 82*, 55–61.
Morgan, A.H. (1974). Hypnotizability in Children as a Function of the Nature of the Suggestion Item, paper presented at the 82nd Annual Meeting of the American Psychological Association, New Orleans, LA.
Morgan, A.H. & Hilgard, E.R. (1973). Age differences in susceptibility to hypnosis. *International Journal of Clinical and Experimental Hypnosis, 21*, 78–85.
Morgan, A.H. & Hilgard, E.R. (1979). The Stanford Hypnotic Clinical Scale for children. *American Journal of Clinical Hypnosis, 21*, 148–169.
Olness, K. (1975). The use of self-hypnosis in the treatment of childhood nocturnal enuresis: A report on forty patients. *Clinical Pediatrics, 14*, 273–279.
Olness, K. (1976). Autohypnosis in functional megacolon in children. *American Journal of Clinical Hypnosis, 19*, 28–32.
Olness, K. (1981b). Imagery (self-hypnosis) as adjunct care in childhood cancer: clinical experience with 25 patients. *American Journal of Pediatric Hematology/Oncology, 3*, 313–321.
Olness, K. & Gardner, G.G. (1978). Some guidelines for uses of hypnotherapy in pediatrics. *Pediatrics, 62*, 228–233.
Orne, M.T. (1959). The nature of hypnosis: artifact and essence. *Journal of Abnormal and Social Psychology, 58*, 277–299.
Peter, B., Geiger, E., Prade, T., Vogel, S., & Piebergen, C. (2015). Norms of German adolescents for the Harvard group scale of hypnotic susceptibility, form A. *The International Journal of Clinical and Experimental Hypnosis, 63*, 92–109.
Ruch, J.C. (1975). Self-hypnosis: the result of heterohypnosis or vice-versa? *International Journal of Clinical and Experimental Hypnosis, 23*, 282–304.
Stukat, K.G. (1958). *Suggestibility: A Factorial and Experimental Analysis*. Stockholm: Almquist & Wiksell.
Tromater, F.T. (1961). Some Developmental Correlates of Hypnotic Susceptibility, unpublished Master's thesis, University of Illinois, Urbana.
Weitzenhoffer, A.M. & Hilgard, E.R. (1959). *Stanford Hypnotic Susceptibility Scale, Forms A and B*. Palo Alto, CA: Consulting Psychologists Press.

# 4

# CORRELATES OF CHILDHOOD HYPNOTIC RESPONSIVENESS

## Introduction

Researchers and clinicians have wrestled with the problem of determining why children, as a group, are more responsive to hypnosis than adults. Some suggested answers are based on research, others are derived from theories of child development, and still others are derived from informal observations of children. In this chapter, we discuss a wide variety of possible correlates and evaluate the available data. A few correlates have already been discussed, and we mention them briefly for the sake of completion.

## Variables

### *Age*

The relationship between age and hypnotic responsivity is very complex. The repeated finding of a modest curvilinear relationship, with its peak in middle childhood, may or may not be entirely accurate. Some of the correlates postulated below are derived from the assumption that the results of the normative studies are truly a reflection of reality.

### *Sex*

We have noted that there are no significant differences in hypnotic responsiveness between boys and girls at any age; therefore, it is reasonable to combine data for both sexes in discussing research and clinical findings.

## Nature of the Induction and of the Suggestion Item

Children of different ages respond best to different kinds of inductions, and specific items may measure different dimensions at one age than at another. The reader will have to bear this in mind when evaluating clinical findings presented in later chapters.

DOI: 10.4324/9781003243687-5

## Genetics

Morgan, Hilgard, and Davert (1970) studied the hypnotic responsiveness of 76 pairs of twins, together with their parents and siblings close in age, using the Stanford Hypnotic Susceptibility Scale, Form A (SHSS, Form A) (Weitzenhoffer & Hilgard, 1959). Morgan (1973) later increased the twin sample to 140 pairs, including the original 76. Because larger samples yield more reliable data, we report data only from the more recent study. The twins' age range was 5–22 years. Zygosity of the twin pairs was based primarily on the mothers' reports, this method having been found to correlate very highly with serological methods. Both members of a twin pair were taught hypnosis simultaneously, in separate rooms, in order to avoid experimenter bias or communication between the twins. Parents also completed a questionnaire, rating each child for similarity to father and to mother on 11 personality and temperamental variables.

The correlations for monozygotic twins were statistically significant for both males ($r = .54$) and females ($r = .49$). Correlations for dizygotic twins and for sibling nontwin pairs were not different from zero ($r = .08$–$.25$). Moreover, the correlation for monozygotic pairs ($r = .52$) was significantly higher than the correlation for like-sexed dizygotic pairs ($r = .18$). These data, together with a computed heritability index of .64 and a low but significant correlation between midparent and mean child susceptibility, were consistent with the interpretation of a genetic contribution.

Personality resemblance, as rated by the parents, was positively related to hypnotizability scores for either sexed child and the like-sexed parent. No such interaction existed for either sexed child and the opposite-sexed parent. Morgan (1973) interpreted these results as suggesting an environmental contribution to hypnotizability, based mainly on identification with the liked-sexed parent and modeling of that parent's behavior. She concluded that "hypnotizability thus appears to be the product of both a genetic predisposition and subsequent environmental influences, as well as their interaction" (p. 61).

The capacity for eidetic imagery (photographic memory) is known to exist in approximately 6% of children in the Western world but is also known to be nearly universal in certain tribal groups in Africa. This may be a genetic trait that would relate to the capacity for hypnotic responsiveness; however, this phenomenon has not been studied. It has been our clinical experience that children who have eidetic imagery learn and apply self-hypnosis very easily.

## Cognitive Development

London (1965) correlated hypnotizability scores on the Children's Hypnotic Susceptibility Scale (CHSS) (London, 1963) with intelligence test scores for a group of 42 children, ages 8–12 years, taken from his standardization sample, and for a group of 54 children, ages 6–12 years, participating in the Pels Institute Longitudinal Study. For the first group, IQ scores were extrapolated from scores on the Vocabulary subtest of the Wechsler Intelligence Scale for Children (WISC) (Wechsler, 1949). For the Pels group, complete WISC scores were available. The relationship between hypnotizability and intelligence was positive but modest. Comparing the difference in the correlation coefficients for the two samples, London concluded that standardization sample $r = .43$.

Jacobs and Jacobs (1966) studied the hypnotizability of 64 school children, ages 4–17 years, who were referred because of poor school achievement associated with a variety of factors, including manifest brain injury, mental retardation, delinquency, behavior disorders, and psychoses. No standardized scale of hypnotizability was utilized. The subjects were considered to be in hypnosis "when eye closure with rhythmic eyeball movements, increased and forceful swallowing, masked facies, regular slow respiration and muscular relaxation were obtained, followed by a catalepsy of the eyelids or extremities" (p. 270). Sixty of the children were given one or more of several individual intelligence tests, either privately or by a school psychologist. The IQ distribution was skewed toward the lower end, with five subjects scoring from 50 to 70 and five subjects below 50. Only three subjects scored above 130. Visual inspection of the data indicated that those with the highest IQs achieved a trance state more often than those rated below average or retarded. No tests of statistical significance were performed. The large incidence of severe neurological and emotional disorders and the likelihood that the children came from a wide range of social class backgrounds make it impossible to compare these data meaningfully with the data of London (1965).

At this time, therapists are not trained to adapt therapeutic hypnosis or other forms of communication to the specific learning capabilities of each child. It is possible that some children would respond better to visual or nonverbal teaching strategies than to talk strategies. It is hoped that research will provide screening assessments to guide therapists in their choice of teaching strategies.

## Child Behavior

Although clinicians utilizing therapeutic hypnosis generally agree that usual teaching strategies are ineffective with children who have an attention-deficit or attention-deficit/hyperactivity disorder, such children may focus very well on hypnotic invitations that include physical movement or provide appealing biofeedback. A study by Kohen and colleagues (Kohen & Ondich, 1992) found no correlation between the SHCS-C and the Achenbach Child Behavior Checklist and its subscales with 100 children. For the present, we cannot predict hypnotic responsiveness based on specific behaviors of children.

## Electroencephalographic Patterns

Children's electroencephalographic (EEG) patterns have been studied in hopes of finding some relationship to hypnotizability. Cooper and London (1976) and London (1976) studied a sample of 35 normal children, ages 7–16 years. Hypnotic susceptibility was significantly correlated with alpha duration ($r = .29$) when the children's eyes were open. Although the alpha duration increased as expected when the children were told to close their eyes, the relationship between alpha and hypnotizability vanished ($r = -.09$). The authors (Cooper & London, 1976) noted that alpha represents a relatively alert state of consciousness in children, and they surmised that:

> ... since it is well known also that young children do not like to keep their eyes shut for long, the relatively higher incidence of alpha duration in the Eyes Closed condition of this study may represent exactly the opposite of what it would represent in an adult study; namely, that the children are more alerted when their eyes are closed than when they are open. (p. 146)

They concluded that it might have been more appropriate to study theta waves. The data were further confused by the finding that the magnitude of the correlations varied markedly from one experimenter to another.

Jacobs and Jacobs (1966) found, in their study of a group of children with poor school achievement, that children with markedly abnormal EEGs showed poor responsiveness to hypnotic induction. As noted in the section on intelligence, many of their subjects manifested mental retardation and frank brain damage, thus making the data even more difficult to interpret.

D. Walters, E. Green, and A. Green (pers. comm.) at the Menninger Clinic developed an EEG biofeedback unit that produces alpha, beta, and theta feedback concurrently and also provides a quantitative measure of various brain wave percentages. In piloting these units, we have noted that the brain wave measures vary rapidly and directly according to the type of thinking that a child is asked to do. Children are also able to develop skill in changing brain wave pattern voluntarily. These units have been used therapeutically in working with children who have attention-deficit disorders and seizures.

## Response to Thermal Biofeedback Training

Several studies of adults have found no relationship between scores on various hypnotizability scales and response to biofeedback training for control of peripheral skin temperature (Engstrom, 1976; Frischholz & Tryon, 1980; Roberts, Schuler, Bacon, Zimmerman, & Patterson, 1975). Engstrom (1976), however, found that when subjects attempted to change skin temperature using hypnosis alone, with no biofeedback, low hypnotizable subjects failed while highly hypnotizable subjects succeeded.

Children respond to thermal biofeedback training (Hunter, Russel, Russell, & Zimmerman, 1976; Lynch, Hama, Kohn, & Miller, 1976). We know of no studies of children in which success in such training has been correlated with hypnotic responsiveness. Dikel and Olness (1980) studied control of peripheral skin temperature in children ages 5–15 years. Most children succeeded at this task. There were no differences in temperature control between children who used hypnotic imagery alone and those who combined hypnosis with biofeedback training. Moreover, neither of these two groups differed from a third group, with no previous hypnosis training, that achieved temperature control using biofeedback alone. Because some children in the third group reported using spontaneous thermal imagery (e.g., putting their hands into snow) similar to the imagery offered to the first two groups by the experimenters, it seemed possible that the third group had actually used hypnotic techniques in spite of the effort to control for this variable. A few children who achieved little temperature change using hypnosis alone were much more successful when biofeedback was added. Although the authors did not measure hypnotic responsiveness, it is possible that these subjects were at the lower end of that continuum. Subjects who responded minimally to biofeedback alone were not offered the opportunity to see whether they might do better with hypnosis training.

We attempted to correlate skill in peripheral temperature control in two clinical studies (Olness & Singher, 1989; Olness, MacDonald, & Uden, 1987). These involved training in self-regulation of pain in children with cancer and with juvenile migraine. No correlations were observed between ability to control peripheral temperature and ability to demonstrate pain control in a clinically useful manner. This was because the majority of children demonstrated rapid, significant changes in peripheral temperature, as has been described in other studies. The variation in this ability was not sensitive enough to provide a predictor with respect to application of skills in self-hypnosis.

King and Montgomery (1980) discussed complex methodological problems in evaluating the results of thermal biofeedback training. Given the additional complexities of measuring hypnotic responsiveness in children, we anticipate that it will be some time before there is clarification of the relationship between the two skills. Our hunch is that the two skills are unrelated in children as well as in adults. We wonder whether children whose locus of control is external may respond better to biofeedback training, whereas those who tend more toward internal locus of control may be able to change skin temperature more easily with hypnosis. As cyberphysiological (self-regulatory) skills, however, biofeedback training may be applied clinically in a variety of complementary ways (Culbert, Reaney, & Kohen, 1994).

## Control of Tissue Oxygen

A pilot study by Olness and Conroy (1985) did show that some children were able to control tissue oxygen using self-hypnosis techniques, but it did not conclude that self-hypnosis was a causative factor or essential to success in such control.

## Achievement Motivation

In 1966, London despaired of ever finding personality variables that would correlate with hypnotizability in children. Later reports (Cooper & London, 1976) were somewhat more optimistic with respect to achievement motivation. In a study of 35 children, in which EEG data were also reported, the subjects were asked to solve puzzles 1 week after the CHSS was administered. They were asked to try to get the solution independently, although they could request parental help if they wished. Children with the highest hypnotic susceptibility scores tended to wait the longest before requesting help, indicating higher achievement motivation. London suggested that these findings reflected variations in child-rearing practices, especially with respect to independence training.

The research on hypnotizability and achievement motivation is consistent with clinical impressions that children's natural desire for mastery of skills and for understanding of, and participation in, their environment is directly related to their responsiveness to hypnosis (Erickson, 1958b; Gardner, 1974a). Clinicians capitalize on these qualities when they introduce hypnosis to a child as "something new you can learn how to do – not everybody knows how to do it, just as not everybody knows how to ride a bike."

## Role-playing

London (1962) observed that some subjects seemed to be faking on the CHSS, especially those in the 8–12-year age group. This observation was supported by the ability of children in this age group to simulate hypnosis when instructed to do so. In further examination of these findings, especially in the context of Sarbin's (1950) role theory of hypnotic susceptibility, Bowers and London (1965) compared the abilities of 40 children, ages 5–11 years, on two role-playing tasks. One was a measure of dramatic acting skill; the other was a hypnotic simulation test. When age and intelligence were held statistically constant, there was no correlation between the two measures.

Madsen and London (1966) then explored the relationship of these two skills to hypnotic susceptibility scores on the CHSS. The subjects were 42 middle-class children ages 7–11 years. The dramatic acting test measured the extent to which the children could portray the cultural stereotype of such familiar roles as mother, bully, teacher, and sheriff. The hypnotic simulation test was the one described in the earlier London (1962) studies. All subjects were given the CHSS, followed 1 week later by the two role-playing tests. Hypnotizability scores were significantly correlated with scores on the simulation test, but there was no relationship between CHSS scores and dramatic acting ability. Thus, role-playing is a complex behavior, made up of several skills that may or may not be related to each other and to other variables. Madsen and London (1966) noted that children who scored low on the CHSS scored about five points higher on the simulation test given a week later. For high scores on the CHSS, the later simulation score was essentially unchanged. The authors postulated a possible rehearsal effect for the low susceptibility children and designed another study to test that hypothesis.

In the second study (London & Madsen, 1968), 34 children, ages 7–11 years, were given the same tests as in the first study, but this time the order was reversed, with the CHSS following the role-playing tests. Unlike the earlier (1966) study of these authors, there was no significant correlation between hypnotic simulation and hypnotic susceptibility. In other words, if the subjects were familiarized with the various phenomena on the CHSS, they could role-play the part of a hypnotized person with some proficiency, but they could not simulate a set of behaviors about which they knew very little. With respect to overt behavior scores, prior simulation experience had virtually no effect on the later CHSS scores; however, to the surprise of the experimenters, prior simulation experience led to a significant decrease on CHSS subjective involvement scores measuring the degree to which the experimenters thought the subjects were really involved in the items.

The experimenters concluded that attempting deliberately to act like a hypnotized person inhibits the ability to become deeply involved in a similar task. To put it in another framework (Fromm, 1977), approaching a task in the context of ego activity may interfere with later ability to perform the task in a more ego-receptive mode.

## Imaginative Involvement

Several studies of child development have clearly established that children in the 2–5-year age range not only are capable of imagery and fantasy but also spend a great deal of their time engaged in various types of imaginative behavior (Gould, 1972; Murphy, 1962; Singer, 1973, 1974). Kosslyn, Margolis, Barrett, Goldknopf, and Daly (1990) conducted a study in which they compared mental processing of visual images by 5-year-olds, 8-year-olds, 14-year-olds, and adults on four imagery tasks. These included image generation, image maintenance, image scanning, and image rotation (for example, deciding which pieces could be loaded into a car trunk). All tasks were computer-administered, and subjects generally responded by pressing the appropriate key on the keyboard. Adults and 14-year-olds were tested in a single session, but younger children were tested in two separate sessions. Subjects were asked to memorize uppercase block letters as they appeared drawn in 4 × 5 grids, and later they were asked to look at two X marks in an empty grid. They were to decide whether a specified uppercase letter would cover both marks if it were present in the grid as previously seen. Ten letters were used; five were relatively simple (L, C, U, F, H). Five (P, J, O, S, G) were relatively complex. Twenty trials were used. Response times were slower with younger children. Male children took relatively more time to generate images of complex letters than did female children. In an image maintenance task, younger children were as adept at holding images as the older children. For a scanning task, the 5- and 8-year-olds were slower than the 14-year-olds and adults, but 8-year-olds were very adept at accurately generating images of simple letters.

This is one of the first studies of mental processing of images in children and is important; however, whether or not it is relevant to spontaneous use of imagination in children is not known. The researchers defined a visual image. Letters may not be familiar to all 5-year-olds; this may have given an advantage to older children. Letter reversals are also frequent in many 5-year-olds, and this may have impacted on the results; however, the finding that the female children were superior in generating and maintaining images as defined in this study is worth noting. No studies have been done relating sex to image preferences in children or to hypnosis teaching strategies for children.

The idea that imagination is an important factor in hypnotic responsiveness is at least as old as the commission that investigated Mesmer's theories in 1784. The positive relationship between various kinds of imaginative involvement and hypnotizability in adults is now well established, particularly as a result of careful investigations by J.R. Hilgard (1970). In her elaborate study of young adults, she found that highly hypnotizable subjects engaged in a variety of imaginative involvements as adults, and these subjects – in contrast to those who were low on susceptibility tests – more frequently had engaged in imaginative experiences in childhood, according to their own reports. In the highly hypnotizable subjects, imagination was typically related to stimuli outside the person rather than autistic or inner-stimulated imagination. Parents either reinforced fantasy or at least did not interfere with it. LeBaron's study (1983) showed a significant relationship between fantasy-oriented activities in the family environment and children's hypnotic responsiveness.

Many child clinicians are convinced that the readiness with which children respond to hypnosis is related to their imaginative skills and involvements (Ambrose, 1961; Boswell, 1962; Erickson, 1958b; Gardner, 1974a; Jacobs, 1962; Kohen & Olness, 1993; Kuttner, 1988, 1991; Olness & Gardner, 1978). Gardner (1974a) described several aspects of cognitive and emotional development in children that are probably related to both imaginative involvement and hypnotizability. These include (1) capacity for intense concentration, immersion, focused attention on a limited stimulus field, and full absorption in the immediate present; (2) a tendency toward concrete, literal thinking; (3) limited reality testing, love of magic, and readiness to shift back and forth between reality and fantasy; (4) intensity of feeling states, often in an all-or-nothing way; and (5) openness to new ideas and delight with new experiences in a context of felt safety and trust.

Some writers have offered explanations of changes in hypnotic responsiveness with age largely in terms of development and decline of imaginative skills. E.R. Hilgard (1971) made the following interpretation:

> Hypnosis reaches its height in the preadolescent period because by that time language and experience have stimulated imagination and given it content, so that those characteristics described as child-likeness have had a full opportunity to bloom. … [In late adolescence] reality-orientations conflict with the free enjoyment of a life of fantasy and adventure, and for many people this means a reduction in their hypnotizability. (p. 38)

J.R. Hilgard (1970) commented similarly on declining hypnotizability with age:

> One may hazard the guess that the conditions of increasing rational sophistication and the needs for competency and achievement bring with them a decline in wonderment; these changes with age somehow counteract the imaginative involvements so important in hypnosis and substitute for them interactions on a reality level that make hypnosis increasingly difficult … . (p. 189)

Whether this is true, or whether the change in imaginative involvement with age makes hypnosis different with increasing age, rather than more difficult, is unclear.

In London's study (1966) of a large number of personality variables in relation to childhood hypnotizability, he included information about the children's tendency to be imaginative and to engage in an active fantasy life, obtaining his data through interviews with parents of 111 children. Specific questions concerned imaginary playmates, extent of dreaming, whether the child talked to him- or herself much, and whether the child played imaginative games either alone or with other children. None of these items – alone or in combination – correlated with CHSS scores, although they correlated positively with each other; however, a certain moderating effect of imagination on age and susceptibility was observed. There was a significant correlation between age and susceptibility for children low in imagination but no age – susceptibility relationship for children whose imagination scores were high. Considering the very large number of variables studied, London was hesitant to make very much of these findings.

LeBaron, Zeltzer, and Fanurik (1988) conducted two pilot studies to assess the relationship between hypnotizability in children and the extent of involvement in fantasy-related activities during early childhood. They developed a structured interview questionnaire regarding fantasy activities that occurred between ages 4 and 7 years. These included questions such as: "What were your favorite games and activities?"; "What games or activities did you like best when you were all alone?"; and "Did your parents ever read to you or tell you stories?" They administered the SHCS-C and the fantasy questionnaire to 30 children with medical problems, ages 6–18 years, and to 37 healthy children, ages 6–12, years from a school population. They found that the distribution of fantasy scores was approximately normal, but, as has been true in many other studies, the hypnotizability scores were strongly skewed toward the high end of the scale. They found that there was a correlation of .42 ($p < .03$) between fantasy and SHCS-C scores in the children with medical problems and .39 ($p < .02$) for the healthy children. They recognized a confounding variable that the older subjects might have had difficulty in recalling imaginative involvement from childhood or be more reluctant to reveal childhood interests to the interviewer. The authors noted a problem in the SHCS-C in that criteria allow for passing the "fantasy" items such as a dream with a minimum of detail, so that the total score does not distinguish between children who are able to experience richly detailed fantasies and those who report only a few images.

Plotnick, Payne, and O'Grady (1991) reported a study using the fantasy questionnaire used in the LeBaron study, the Children's Social Desirability Questionnaire (CSDQ), the Zeltzer and LeBaron (1984) revision of the Stanford Hypnotic Clinical Scale for Children (SHCS-C-R), and the Children's Fantasy Inventory: Absorption and Vividness Scales (CFI:A&V). This study had recruiting difficulties; the investigators ultimately studied 42 children from 26 families and sent the script of the SHCS-C to the parents before they brought their children in for the study. This could have resulted in contamination of results. The authors found that absorption in imaginary involvements in children (CFI:A) related significantly to the hypnotizability scores for Observed Behavior ($r = .42$, $p < .01$). Scores on the vividness of imagery scale (CFI:V) and involvement in fantasy play also correlated positively with hypnotizability scales for Observed Behavior, Realness, and SHCS-C-R ($p < .01$). Social desirability scores did not relate to hypnotizability scores for Observed Behavior, Realness, or SHCS-C-R. Authors noted that several children appeared to be somewhat wary of the procedures, and they suspected that some of the children did not consider it socially desirable to respond. They suggested that the Attitude Toward Hypnosis Scale of Spanos, Lush, Smith, and deGroh (1986) should be adapted to children and used in future similar studies.

A weakness of the reported studies is that the terms *fantasy* and *imagery* are interpreted to refer to visual mental constructions. It would be important to determine whether or not subjects prefer auditory imagery to visual or kinesthetic to visual images. Some children enjoy olfactory imagery. We use a simple imagery questionnaire that is useful clinically in developing hypnotic inductions for children (see Appendix B in the fourth edition of this text). We welcome the use of this questionnaire or a modification in future clinical studies.

## Attitudes toward Adults

Gardner (1974a) has hypothesized that children may be especially responsive to hypnotic suggestions because they are generally predisposed to trust adults, responsive to social influence and authority, and comfortable about engaging in help-seeking behavior. Most children feel safe when they experience regressive aspects of hypnosis in the presence of a presumably competent adult. In most cases, they do not experience the degree of anxiety about control that often interferes with hypnotic responsiveness in adults. There has been no research to test these hypotheses.

## Parent–Child Interaction

Several psychoanalytic writers (Ambrose, 1963, 1968; Boswell, 1962; Call, 1976; Krojanker, 1969) have focused on transferential and regression aspects of the hypnotic relationship. In this context, it becomes possible to specify the kinds of parent–child relationships most conducive to hypnotic responsiveness in the child. For example, Call (1976) theorized that, while in hypnosis, the child subjectively experiences a relationship with the powerful, internalized parent image; therefore, the child who has had a past experience with a well-defined, powerful, omnipotent parent would be more responsive to hypnosis than a child who had less well-defined parental influences.

Results of two retrospective studies of young adults (Hilgard, 1970; Hilgard & Hilgard, 1962) found that subjects who identified with the work habits and attitudes of neither parent were low in hypnotizability. The same was true for identification with parental temperament. In both studies, highly hypnotizable subjects identified most strongly with the opposite-sex parent. The families of highly hypnotizable subjects were characterized by a combination of warmth and strict discipline, a setting in which the likelihood of clear identifications and strong ego development was optimized. Hilgard (1970) hypothesized that the hypnotizable subject may later incorporate the clinician guiding the therapeutic hypnosis in the same way that the parents were incorporated, with a certain readiness to conform to authority even if it seems rather illogical.

In a longitudinal study, children who had initially been studied in kindergarten were tested for hypnotizability and related behaviors when they reached their senior year in high school (Nowlis, 1969). The results indicated that "a rather stern, restrictive, and punitive home environment at the time the children were in kindergarten was related to higher susceptibility to hypnotic-like experience when the children reached the twelfth grade in high school" (p. 114). In these comparisons, "hypnotic-like experience" was measured by Shor's Personal Experiences Questionnaire, Form L (Shor, 1960; Shor, Orne, & O'Connell, 1962), an inventory of trance-like experiences in everyday life that predicts hypnotizability but is not itself a test of hypnotizability. On an actual hypnotizability scale, the Harvard Group Scale of Hypnotic Susceptibility, Form A (Shor & Orne, 1962), only the antecedent child-rearing variable was significantly related to hypnotizability – namely, pressure for conformity with table standards. In view of the many variables studied, the author concluded this one finding should probably be attributed to chance.

In the only study in which parent–child relationships and childhood hypnotizability have been studied concurrently, Cooper and London (1976) found that parents of highly hypnotizable subjects tended to rate themselves as more strict, anxious, and impatient than parents of low hypnotizability subjects. When these parents offered help to their children on a puzzle task, the suggestions given by parents of highly susceptible children were more abstract and constructive than the suggestions given by parents of low susceptibility children. Cooper and London suggested caution in interpreting these results because of the large number of variables studied.

Despite methodological differences and difficulties in the studies of Hilgard (1970), Nowlis (1969), and Cooper and London (1976), the results of all three point in the same direction leading to a position of greater credence than would have been possible from any of the studies taken alone.

## Factors that May Compromise Hypnotic Responsiveness

In an extensive review of correlates of hypnotic responsiveness in childhood, it is necessary to go beyond the developmental issues that have concerned us so far. We will discuss several variables not directly related to hypnotic talent but that may enhance or impede hypnotic responsiveness.

## Misconceptions about Hypnosis

We have found that many children (as well perhaps as their parents) approach clinical therapeutic hypnosis with a great deal of misinformation. Often they may believe that they will somehow be put to sleep or, as commonly depicted in cartoons, be "put into a trance" and then be under the absolute control of the "hypnotist" and not remember anything that transpires during the hypnotic session. While sometimes children get these notions from parents and other adults, more often they come from television, movies, or, these days, YouTube. One children's program, for example, portrayed a mad scientist who used a shiny ring to bring various people under his spell. When his victims wore the ring, they walked around in an obvious trance-like state and followed his instructions, including engaging in embarrassing and antisocial behavior while muttering "Yes, master." They had no memory of their behavior when the trance was lifted by removal of the scientist's ring. The popular film *Aladdin* portrayed hypnosis in such a fashion – that is, as a controlling power used by the sinister bad guy to further his cause of evil. Films (e.g., *The Manchurian Candidate, Get Out!*) and television shows (e.g., *The X-Files*) perpetuate the old mythology of hypnosis as brainwashing, wherein people are instructed in hypnosis to perpetrate a serious crime (e.g., murder) or assume an alternative identity for which they would then have amnesia. Although many – including the film industry – might argue that this makes good entertainment, we would not only take serious issue with that but also decry this misrepresentation of this powerful clinical skill.

Sometimes the effect of programs like *Aladdin* is more positive than negative with respect to children's willingness to experience hypnosis. They are more intrigued by the magic portrayed than they are concerned about being controlled or made to engage in unacceptable behavior. However, for therapeutic as well as for educational reasons, we strongly advise that any first hypnotic invitation or experience be preceded by a didactic session in which children's (and parents) prior ideas (and fears or worries) about hypnosis are solicited and understood, misconceptions are clarified, and myths put to rest. We are aware of one 12-year-old boy who initially refused hypnosis on religious grounds because he thought it involved some sort of demonology or witchcraft. Only after being assured that neither he nor the therapist was possessed by demons did he consent to therapeutic invitation to hypnosis.

Some children refuse therapeutic hypnosis despite all efforts at clarification. In a few cases, the children have even demonstrated that they are hypnotizable but still refuse to apply their skills to a particular problem. Reasons for these examples of apparent resistance are not always clear, but they may include (1) being unwilling to give up a symptom because of secondary gains; (2) equating hypnosis with loss of autonomy and choice; (3) equating freedom from pain and anxiety with death, in severe illness; (4) being unwilling to give up a symptom that serves a major defensive function against debilitating depression or psychosis; (5) experiencing anxiety with certain induction techniques that compromise coping mechanisms – for example, resisting dissociative imagery because of a need for cognitive mastery during medical procedures; and (6) having had a previous negative experience with another clinician teaching hypnosis.

When the therapist understands the resistance, sometimes further clarification or modification of technique will be helpful; at times, the therapist will decide that therapeutic hypnosis is contraindicated. Occasionally, the therapist will be unable to understand the apparent reluctance, and the child will remain (seemingly) refractory to hypnosis. And, sometimes what seems like resistance may simply represent a mismatch between therapist and child patient. In such cases, rather than abandon the (potential) use and value of hypnosis, the therapist may opt to refer the child to a colleague who also uses therapeutic hypnosis strategies and with whom the child may well connect more easily or positively. This, of course, remains a matter of personal judgment by each clinician.

## Attitudes of Significant Adults

Some clinicians treating children despair of attempting therapeutic hypnosis with children because of presumed negative attitudes on the part of the patients' parents, teachers, clergy, and other adults from whom children get their concept of reality and of appropriate behavior.

## Attitudes in Institutional Settings

Misconceptions, negative attitudes, and a lack of information about hypnosis among child health professionals not only limit the number of children who might be referred for clinical therapeutic hypnosis but also can sabotage ongoing therapeutic hypnosis done by a qualified professional with a motivated and capable child. It is disheartening to give postsurgical child patient hypnotic suggestions for increased and comfortable food intake only to discover that someone else has put the emesis basin closer to the child than the dinner tray! Another common problem in hospitals is that colleagues may consider using therapeutic hypnosis but only as a last resort when a child has developed severe conditioned fear and anxiety about procedures in general. Although such children can benefit greatly from therapeutic hypnosis and overcome their conditioned negative responses, this usually takes multiple therapy sessions. When the hypnotherapist is called 30 minutes prior to the procedure and cannot deliver a calm child to the treatment room, the naive colleague will say, "It doesn't work." Although this has the logic of complaining that a child's throat still hurts after one dose of penicillin, the scenario occurs all too frequently.

It is important that the child health professional who uses therapeutic hypnosis takes time to educate colleagues. This must be an ongoing process, such as the program we established to provide inservice education programs about clinical hypnosis at a children's hospital (Olness, 1977c). These programs were available not only to the pediatricians, nurses, house officers, and medical students but also to administrative, secretarial, and housekeeping personnel. House officers rotate frequently, but they are often the first physicians to make decisions about pain and anxiety management for children. It is important to teach them about therapeutic hypnosis not only for their patients but for self-hypnosis for themselves. The inherent stresses of being a house officer can be reduced by self-hypnosis practice. Sokel, Lansdown, and Kent (1990) developed a Pain and Symptom Management Team for the pediatric services on Great Ormond Street in London. They found a dramatic increase in referrals. Of the first 51 cases referred, 36 were taken on for therapeutic hypnosis. They note that, "It is essential to demystify clinical hypnosis in a hospital context, to convey to children and their parents, and often to colleagues, that we are harnessing a normal power" (Sokel et al., 1990).

In recent years, nurses in clinical practice settings and children's hospitals have become very active in promoting therapeutic hypnosis techniques, especially on postsurgical or chronic illness units. Valente (1991a) and Hobbie (1989) both described how nurses can apply clinical hypnosis. Valente (1991b) also detailed the myths, research, and effectiveness of therapeutic hypnosis as a strategy for managing cancer pain of school-age children. Pederson described the value of hypnosis and imagery for the pain and anxiety of cardiac catheterization in children (Pederson, 1995), with hospitalized children (Pederson & Harbaugh, 1995), and for children undergoing stem cell or bone marrow transplant procedures (Pederson & Parran, 1999). A nurse practitioner in Vermont, Linda Thomson has contributed substantially to the resources available to clinicians and families helping children with hypnosis through the creation of *Harry, the Hypno-potamus* (Thomson, 2005, 2009). She has conducted hypnosis workshops for nurses and pediatric nurse practitioners, spearheaded establishment of the American Board of Hypnosis in Nursing, and encouraged the presence and activity of nurses in the governance of the American Society of Clinical Hypnosis.

Regardless of whether a treatment is pharmacological or nonpharmacological, it benefits the child patient and increases efficiency if all members of the treatment team know something about that treatment.

## Parents

Traphagen (1959) found a preponderance of positive attitudes toward hypnosis among parents (65%), higher than she expected. We find positive attitudes among most parents of our prospective child therapeutic hypnosis patients. Some parents are interested to discover that they have unwittingly been using hypnotic-like techniques with their children; for example, Katie, 12 years old, frequently gagged or vomited when taking oral medication. Her mother spontaneously developed the idea of helping her child by describing in detail her favorite foods while the child swallowed her pills. When we pointed out the similarity to hypnosis, Katie quickly learned to use the favorite food imagery independently and easily resolved her problem with taking medication. Even when parents are at first reluctant, it is usually possible to help them shift to a more positive stance toward hypnosis. Gardner (1974b) described techniques designed to help parents who are reluctant about hypnosis to move from being obstacles to becoming allies in their children's treatment. The approach includes three basic steps: educational, observational, and experiential. Details of each of these steps follow:

> It is usually best to begin with a relatively didactic discussion with the parents, especially eliciting and responding to their specific questions and concerns. Hypnosis can be defined as basically a state of mind, usually combining relaxation with concentration on a desired point of focus so that other undesired thoughts or feelings then fade into the background. Such shifts of attention are easily demonstrated by asking the parents to focus on sounds which were not previously noticed such as the typing in the reception area or the soft hum of the air conditioner. The heightened attention which characterizes hypnosis is then described in the context of everyday events such as a mother's ability to waken to her infant's cry while sleeping through other louder but insignificant noises. [In answering other questions concerning hypnosis generally, information is available from the websites of the National Pediatric Hypnosis Training Institute (www.nphti.com) and the American Society of Clinical Hypnosis (www.asch.net).]
>
> This general discussion easily leads to the specific issue of why hypnosis may be appropriate for a particular child. Thus, the mother may be told that the goal is to help the child focus on comfort so that pain will ease, on feelings of well-being so that anxiety will diminish, or on pleasant hunger in order to counteract nausea and vomiting. A few basic principles of induction techniques, such as relaxation training and guided imagery, can then be explained, emphasizing the need to tailor the induction to the needs of each child, and providing some understanding of simple physiological and psychological principles that account for the success of the techniques. Throughout, the parents' specific questions are answered, and misconceptions are clarified including such things as the distinction between hypnosis and sleep and concerns about spontaneous hypnosis or greater susceptibility to charlatans. The goals are (a) to teach the parents that hypnosis can be described in simple, everyday terms without resorting to concepts suggesting magic or witchcraft and (b) to help the parents understand that hypnosis may be a specifically useful treatment modality for their child. This writer finds that, after this discussion, almost all parents are willing to let their children have a trial of hypnotherapy. For those who are not, the issue is not pushed any further.

If the parents become enthusiastic about the possible value of therapeutic hypnosis for the child, they have already accomplished a major step toward becoming a therapeutic hypnosis ally. Usually children look to their parents for guidance and assurance when facing new situations, and if the parents communicate a confident attitude toward hypnosis the child is much more likely to be trusting and cooperative.

For those parents who permit clinical hypnosis for their children, the second phase of parent training consists of having them observe their children in hypnosis. Observation is usually postponed, however – and especially in older children – until after the initial induction, since this is often the point of maximum concern for both the child and the clinician guiding the hypnosis regarding whether a state of hypnosis can be achieved and whether it will be effective for the problem at hand. This writer finds that having any third party present (e.g., parent, doctor, or nurse) increases the likelihood of anxiety about successful performance. This anxiety may then seriously interfere with success, since it draws attention away from the task and replaces desired relaxation with tension. However, occasionally the parents may be invited to observe the first session if the child is particularly anxious and wants his parents to stay with him.

When rapport is established between the therapist and the child, and when it is clear to both that the child can use hypnosis to alleviate his problem, the parent is then invited to observe a hypnotic session. Ideally this is done after the child has been taught self-hypnosis (easily mastered by most children 8 years of age or older), because then the parents see that the child can be in control both of induction (usually simple techniques such as eye-fixation, visual imagery, or reverse hand-levitation) and dehypnotizing. If biofeedback is used concurrently, parents can also see that their child is able to change physiologic responses while practicing self-hypnosis.

An important part of the observation session is to have the parent watch the therapist communicate with the child in hypnosis, requiring the child to give both nonverbal and verbal responses and then to transfer hypnotic rapport to the parents and have them also communicate verbally and non-verbally with the child. This exercise helps assure the parent that the child is in contact with his surroundings and in control of the hypnotic state as much as necessary. Parents who initially went along with the idea because of desperation or "blind faith" now have keener understanding and are able to be even more supportive, both in sessions with the therapist and when the child is asked to practice self-hypnosis for use with a chronic condition or for repeated painful procedures or unpleasant experiences where the therapist may not always be available.

Sometimes it is helpful to give parents the opportunity to experience hypnosis for themselves. This step further dispels the idea of hypnosis as magic, removes any remaining doubts and fears, and allows review of details not previously discussed. Often this occurs informally as a natural consequence of the observational phase. That is, the parents spontaneously report feelings of relaxation compatible with light hypnosis while watching their child in hypnosis. The dynamics of this phenomenon are not clear, though this writer has seen it with adults watching other adults as well as with adults watching children. Usually the observer is a "participant observer" in the sense of having warm, tender feelings for and/or identifications with the subject. There may also be an element of contagion of the trusting relationship between the subject and therapist. Once, when both parents observed a hypnotic session with a six-year-old nauseated girl, suggestions were given that she could feel quiet and a bit sleepy and that soon she would

> experience nice hungry feelings so that it would feel good to take fluids and medicine. Not only did the suggestions prove effective for the child, but the mother later reported that she became pleasantly sleepy, while the father said he developed marked hunger and went out for a snack! Both parents described their experience with amusement, commenting also that they were glad to know something of what their child experienced. Another parent, after experiencing a formal induction, reported that experiencing hypnosis herself really convinced her that a person in hypnosis is "awake and aware" and that this allowed her to feel more secure when she helped her son use self-hypnosis.

Since publishing her paper on parental attitudes, Gardner (1974b) continued the educational and observational steps of parent training but decreased the frequency of having parents actually experience formal hypnotic induction. Moreover, when parents did request formal hypnotic induction for themselves, Gardner asked that the child not be present, at least initially. This change developed when it became clear that some parents – even in brief hypnosis – might use the opportunity to experience grief or other feelings whose full expression might be inappropriate in front of the child.

The process and value of parental involvement have been wonderfully enhanced in recent years by the availability of books written for parents and children with the specific intention of teaching parents how to tell and utilize storytelling to facilitate hypnotic experiences, responsivity, and reduction or resolution of symptoms/conditions of various kinds. In addition to those noted earlier, other writers (Hudson, 2009; Reznick, 2009) have also recently published very user-friendly books accessible to therapists and parents alike to help children develop their innate imaginative skills to solve and resolve problems related to stress, illness, and discomfort.

## Situational Variables

Sometimes a child's physical or psychological condition may temporarily preclude the use of hypnosis. Such conditions include unconsciousness, anxiety, or pain to such an extreme degree that the child is unable to focus any attention on the clinician introducing therapeutic hypnosis, or at least in any way that we are able to detect, as well as extreme debilitation with an inability to move from a passive to an active posture in a therapeutic hypnosis relationship. Only rarely do time limitations preclude the effective use of hypnosis. Although concerns about time limitations often seem to be a preliminary or theoretical deterrent for therapists new to the use of hypnosis, we have been impressed repeatedly with how much can be accomplished in a very short period when circumstances seem suboptimal – for example, in an emergency situation when everyone, including the patient and perhaps the clinician, is markedly anxious.

## Conclusions

Gardner and Hinton (1980) reviewed correlates of hypnotic responsiveness in children. Considering the great diversity of possible correlates, they noted the lack of any serious attempt to ground the findings in the context of a cohesive theory. Even the comments of psychoanalytic writers have been limited in scope. In light of advances in the theoretical conceptualizations of hypnosis (e.g., Fromm, 1977; Fromm & Gardner, 1979; Fromm & Hurt, 1980), we anticipate that future research will more clearly identify correlates of childhood hypnotic responsiveness and evaluate their relative significance in a more orderly way.

## References


Ambrose, G. (1961). *Hypnotherapy with Children*, 2nd ed. London: Staples.

Ambrose, G. (1963). Hypnotherapy for children. In J.M. Schneck, Ed., *Hypnosis in Modern Medicine*, 3rd ed. Springfield, IL: Charles C Thomas.

Ambrose, G. (1968). Hypnosis in the treatment of children. *American Journal of Clinical Hypnosis, 11*, 1–5.

Boswell, L.K., Jr. (1962). Pediatric hypnosis. *British Journal of Medical Hypnotism, 13*, 4–11.

Bowers, P. & London, P. (1965). Developmental correlates of role-playing ability. *Child Development, 30*, 499–508.

Call, J.D. (1976). Children, parents, and hypnosis: a discussion. *International Journal of Clinical and Experimental Hypnosis, 24*, 149–155.

Cooper, L.M. & London, P. (1976). Children's hypnotic susceptibility, personality, and EEG patterns. *International Journal of Clinical and Experimental Hypnosis, 24*, 140–148.

Culbert, T.P., Reaney, J., & Kohen, D.P. (1994). Cyberphysiologic strategies in children: the biofeedback–hypnosis interface. *International Journal of Clinical and Experimental Hypnosis, 42(2)*, 97–117.

Dikel, W. & Olness, K. (1980). Self-hypnosis, biofeedback, and voluntary peripheral temperature control in children. *Pediatrics, 66*, 335–340.

Engstrom, D.R. (1976). Hypnotic susceptibility, EEC alpha, and self-regulation. In G.E. Schwartz & D. Shapiro, Eds., *Consciousness and Self-Regulation*, Vol. 1. New York: Plenum Press.

Erickson, M.H. (1958b). Pediatric hypnotherapy. *American Journal of Clinical Hypnosis, 1*, 25–29.

Frischholz, E.J. & Tryon, W.W. (1980). Hypnotizability in relation to the ability to learn thermal biofeedback. *American Journal of Clinical Hypnosis, 23*, 53–56.

Fromm, E. (1977). An ego-psychological theory of altered states of consciousness. *International Journal of Clinical and Experimental Hypnosis, 25*, 372–387.

Fromm, E. & Gardner, G.G. (1979). Ego psychology and hypnoanalysis: an integration of theory and technique. *Bulletin of the Menninger Clinic, 43*, 413–423.

Fromm, E. & Hurt, S.W. (1980). Ego-psychological parameters of hypnosis and altered states of consciousness. In G.D. Burrows & L. Dennerstein, Eds., *Handbook of Hypnosis and Psychosomatic Medicine* (pp. 13–27). New York: Elsevier/North-Holland Biomedical Press.

Gardner, G.G. (1974a). Hypnosis with children. *International Journal of Clinical and Experimental Hypnosis, 22*, 20–38.

Gardner, G.G. (1974b). Parents: obstacles or allies in child hypnotherapy? *American Journal of Clinical Hypnosis, 17*, 44–49.

Gardner, G.G. & Hinton, R.M. (1980). Hypnosis with children. In G.D. Burrows & L. Dennerstein, Eds., *Handbook of Hypnosis and Psychosomatic Medicine*. New York: Elsevier/North-Holland Biomedical Press.

Gould, R. (1972). *Child Studies Through Fantasy: Cognitive–Affective Patterns in Development*. New York: Quadrangle Books.

Hilgard, J.R. (1970). *Personality and Hypnosis: A Study of Imaginative Involvement*. Chicago, IL: University of Chicago Press.

Hilgard, E.R. (1971). Hypnosis and childlikeness. In J.P. Hill, Ed., *Minnesota Symposia on Child Psychology*, Vol. 5. Minneapolis, MN: Lund Press.

Hilgard, J.R. & Hilgard, E.R. (1962). Developmental-interactive aspects of hypnosis: some illustrative cases. *Genetic Psychology Monographs, 66*, 143–178.

Hobbie, C. (1989). Relaxation techniques for children and young people. *Journal of Pediatric Health Care, 3*, 83–87.

Hudson, L. (2009). *Scripts and Strategies in Hypnotherapy with Children: For Young People Aged 5 to 15*. Bethel, CT:Crown House Publishing.

Hunter, S.H., Russel, H.L., Russell, E.D., & Zimmerman, R.L. (1976). Control of fingertip temperature increases via biofeedback in learning-disabled and normal children. *Perceptual and Motor Skills, 43*, 743–755.

Jacobs, L. (1962). Hypnosis in clinical pediatrics. *New York State Journal of Medicine, 62*, 3781–3787.

Jacobs, L. & Jacobs, J. (1966). Hypnotizability of children as related to hemispheric reference and neurological organization. *American Journal of Clinical Hypnosis, 8*, 269–274.

King, N.J. & Montgomery, R.B. (1980). Biofeedback-induced control of human peripheral temperature: a critical review of the literature. *Psychological Bulletin*, *88*, 738–752.

Kohen, D.P. & Olness, K.N. (1993). Hypnotherapy with children. In J. Rhue, S.J. Lynn, & I. Kirsch, Eds., *Handbook of Clinical Hypnosis* (pp. 357–381). Washington, D.C.: American Psychological Association.

Kohen, D.P. & Ondich, S. (1992). Children's self-regulation of cardiovascular function with relaxation mental imagery (Self-Hypnosis): Report of a controlled study. *Paper presented at the 12th International Congress of Hypnosis, Jerusalem, Israel.*

Kosslyn, S.M., Margolis, J.A., Barrett, A.M., Goldknopf, E.J., & Daly, P.F. (1990). Age differences in imagery abilities. *Child Development*, *61*, 995–1010.

Krojanker, R.J. (1969). Human hypnosis, animal hypnotic states, and the induction of sleep in infants. *American Journal of Clinical Hypnosis*, *11*, 178–179.

Kuttner, L. (1988). Favorite stories: a hypnotic pain reduction technique for children in acute pain. *American Journal of Clinical Hypnosis*, *30(4)*, 289–295.

Kuttner, L. (1991). Helpful strategies in working with preschool children in pediatric practice. *Pediatric Annals*, 20(3), 120-127.

LeBaron, S. (1983). Fantasies of children and adolescents: implications for behavioral intervention in chronic illness. In D.R. Copeland, B. Pfefferbaum, & A. Storall, Eds., *The Mind of the Child Who Is Said to Be Sick.* Springfield, IL: Charles C Thomas.

LeBaron, S., Zeltzer, L., & Fanurik, D. (1988). Imaginative involvement and hypnotic susceptibility in childhood. *International Journal of Clinical and Experimental Hypnosis*, *36*, 284–295.

London, P. (1962). Hypnosis in children: an experimental approach. *International Journal of Clinical and Experimental Hypnosis*, *10*, 79–91.

London, P. (1963). *Children's Hypnotic Susceptibility Scale.* Palo Alto, CA: Consulting Psychologists Press.

London, P. (1965). Developmental experiments in hypnosis. *Journal of Projective Techniques and Personality Assessment*, *29*, 189–199.

London, P. (1966). Child hypnosis and personality. *American Journal of Clinical Hypnosis*, *8*, 161-168.

London, P. (1976). Kidding around with hypnosis. *International Journal of Clinical and Experimental Hypnosis*, *24*, 105–121.

London, P. & Madsen, C.H., Jr. (1968). Effect of role playing on hypnotic susceptibility in children. *Journal of Personality and Social Psychology*, *10*, 66–68.

Lynch, W.C., Hama, H., Kohn, S., & Miller, N.E. (1976). Instrumental control of peripheral vasomotor responses in children. *Psychophysiology*, *13*, 219–221.

Madsen, C.H., Jr. & London, P. (1966). Role playing and hypnotic susceptibility in children. *Journal of Personality and Social Psychology*, *3*, 13–19.

Morgan, A.H. (1973). The heritability of hypnotic susceptibility in twins. *Journal of Abnormal Psychology*, *82*, 55–61.

Morgan, A.H., Hilgard, E.R., & Davert, E.C. (1970). The heritability of hypnotic susceptibility of twins: a preliminary report. *Behavior Genetics*, *1*, 213–224.

Murphy, L. (1962). *The Widening World of Childhood: Paths toward Mastery.* New York: Basic Books.

Nowlis, D.P. (1969). The child rearing antecedents of hypnotic susceptibility and of naturally occurring hypnotic-like experience. *International Journal of Clinical and Experimental Hypnosis*, *17*, 109–120.

Olness, K. (1977c). In-service hypnosis education in a children's hospital. *American Journal of Clinical Hypnosis*, 20, 80-83.

Olness, K. & Conroy, M. (1985). A pilot study of voluntary control of transcutaneous $PO_2$ by children. *International Journal of Clinical and Experimental Hypnosis*, *33*, 1–5.

Olness, K. & Gardner, G.G. (1978). Some guidelines for uses of hypnotherapy in pediatrics. *Pediatrics*, *62*, 228–233.

Olness, K. & Singher, L. (1989). Five year follow-up of 61 children taught cyber-physiologic strategies as adjunct management in cancer. *Topics in Pediatrics*, 7, 2–6.

Olness, K., MacDonald, J., & Uden, D. (1987). A prospective study comparing self-hypnosis, propranolol, and placebo in management of juvenile migraine. *Pediatrics*, *79*, 593–597.

Pederson, C. (1995). Effect of imagery on children's pain and anxiety during cardiac catheterization. *Journal of Pediatric Nursing*, *10*, 365–374.

Pederson, C. & Harbaugh, B.L. (1995). Nurses' use of non-pharmacologic techniques with hospitalized children. *Issues in Comprehensive Pediatric Nursing, 18*, 91–109.

Pederson, C. & Parran, L. (1999). Pain and distress in adults and children undergoing peripheral blood stem cell or bone marrow transplant. *Oncology Nursing Forum, 3*, 575 582.

Plotnick, A.B., Payne, P.A., & O'Grady, D.J. (1991). Correlates of hypnotizability in children: absorption, vividness of imagery, and social desirability. *American Journal of Clinical Hypnosis, 34*, 51–58.

Reznick, C. (2009). *The Power of your Child's Imagination: How to Transform Stress and Anxiety into Joy and Success*. New York: Penguin Group.

Roberts, A.H., Schuler, J., Bacon, J.G., Zimmerman, R.L., & Patterson, R. (1975). Individual differences and autonomic control, absorption, and the unilateral control of skin temperature. *Journal of Abnormal Psychology, 84*, 272–279.

Sarbin, T.R. (1950). Contributions to role-taking theory. I. Hypnotic behavior. *Psychological Review, 57*, 225–270.

Shor, R.E. (1960). The frequency of naturally occurring "hypnotic-like" experiences in the normal college population. *International Journal of Clinical and Experimental Hypnosis, 8*, 151–163.

Shor, R.E. & Orne, E.C. (1962). *The Harvard Group Scale of Hypnotic Susceptibility, Form A*. Palo Alto, CA: Consulting Psychologists Press.

Shor, R.E., Orne, M.T., & O'Connell, D.N. (1962). Validation and cross-validation of a scale of self-reported personal experiences which predicts hypnotizability. *Journal of Psychology, 53*, 55–75.

Singer, J.L. (1973). *The Child's World of Make-Believe: Experimental Studies of Imaginative Play*. New York: Academic Press.

Singer, J.L. (1974). *Imagery and Daydream Methods in Psychotherapy and Behavior Modification*. New York: Academic Press.

Sokel, B.S., Lansdown, R., & Kent, A. (1990). The development of a hypnotherapy service for children. *Child Care and Health Development, 16*, 227–233.

Spanos, N.P., Lush, N.I., Smith, J.E., & deGroh, M.M. (1986). Effects of two hypnotic induction procedures on overt and subjective responses to two measures of hypnotic susceptibility. *Psychological Reports, 59*, 1227–1230.

Thomson, L. (2005). *Harry the Hypno-potamus: Metaphorical Tales for the Treatment of Children*. Bethel, CT: Crown House Publishing.

Thomson, L. (2009). *Harry the Hypno-potamus: More Metaphorical Tales for Pediatric Problems*. Bethel, CT: Crown House Publishing.

Traphagen, V. (1959). A survey of attitudes toward hypnotherapy with children. *American Journal of Clinical Hypnosis, 2*, 138–142.

Valente, S.M. (1991a). Clinical hypnosis with school-age children. *Archives of Psychiatric Nursing, 4*, 131–136.

Valente, S.M. (1991b). Using hypnosis with children for pain management. *Oncology Nursing Forum*, 18, 699–704.

Wechsler, D. (1949). *Wechsler Intelligence Scale for Children*. New York: Psychological Corporation.

Weitzenhoffer, A.M. & Hilgard, E.R. (1959). *Stanford Hypnotic Susceptibility Scale, Forms A and B*. Palo Alto, CA: Consulting Psychologists Press.

Zeltzer, L. & LeBaron, S. (1984). *Stanford Hypnotic Clinical Scale for Children – Revised (SHCS-C-R)*, unpublished scale.

# 5

# HYPNOTIC INVITATIONS FOR CHILDREN: TECHNIQUES, STRATEGIES, AND APPROACHES

## Techniques, Strategies, and Approaches

Children respond to a large number of hypnotic invitation/induction techniques, strategies, and approaches, each with countless variations. Any method of invitation to begin hypnosis may also be effectively utilized as a method of deepening or intensifying the hypnotic experience, and methods may be combined in almost any order. The choice of an appropriate invitation to begin for any given child depends on the needs and preferences of the child and on the experience and creativity of the therapist. Success is certain to be limited if a therapist is competent only in the use and application of one or two invitational (induction) approaches or techniques for children or attempts to utilize those suited for adults without providing or integrating modifications that may be necessary for child patients.

Any health specialist who undertakes invitation to hypnosis with children must first have considerable knowledge of child development and expertise in working with children in the context of his or her primary profession (e.g., pediatrics, child psychology, child psychiatry, pediatric social work, pediatric dentistry). One must also know something about the social and cultural backgrounds of child patients, their general likes and dislikes, and themes of interest related to books, television programs, current movies, music, "apps," and video and computer games. For individual patients, successful hypnosis invitations and beginnings are those that are often based on knowledge of the patient's particular likes and dislikes, comfort areas, language preferences, past experiences, and aspirations about the future. Sometimes unexpected or apparent "resistance" to one technique demands a rapid shift to another. In short, a child health clinician using hypnosis must first be a competent child therapist/clinician. The same requirements apply to researchers studying hypnotic phenomena in children.

Compared with adults, children are more likely to squirm and move about, open their eyes or refuse to close them, and make spontaneous comments during hypnosis invitations and, perhaps, even through the hypnotic procedure as well. Although these behaviors may seem at first experience to represent resistance, this is not usually or necessarily the case. In moving about or opening his or her eyes, most often the child is simply adapting the new hypnosis strategy to his or her own behavioral style, and the thoughtful clinician also adapts accordingly, reinforcing positively whatever behavior the child has reflected, thus creating a win–win experience, rather than an adversarial or problematic interaction. Many children have negative attitudes about going to

DOI: 10.4324/9781003243687-6

sleep or, having been told that a favorite pet has been put to sleep, equate being put to sleep with being put to death. For these reasons, we usually avoid such words as *sleepy*, *drowsy*, and *tired* in our inductions and in our hypnotic language in general. Likewise, because some children – especially 4- and 5-year-olds – resist closing their eyes and may even be frightened by the idea itself, we do not stress eye closure as being important to invitation or even continuation of hypnosis, although we sometimes tell children that they may be able to concentrate better when they close their eyes, or "See things more clearly in your inside mind." In all instances, of course, the choice remains theirs. We aim to be ever alert to adapting our language to the children's level of understanding, neither talking down to them nor using overly complex language.

The hypnosis invitation techniques that we will describe share characteristics of being permissive in nature, emphasizing children's involvement and control and encouraging their active participation in the process of experiencing and utilizing the hypnotic state. We avoid authoritarian methods widely used in the past, including avoiding phrases such as "You will … ," or "I want you to do … now," or "You won't be able to … ." Such methods, in which the clinician teaching and guiding the hypnosis uses a controlling or commanding manner, may indeed result in successful initiation of hypnosis in some children, although much less so now than in earlier times or in cultures in which children expect adults to be very strict and authoritarian.

When invitation to hypnosis is employed in the context of medical or psychological therapy, we believe that authoritarian methods and approaches are contraindicated, as they risk interfering with the evolution of a child's sense of mastery over the medical or psychological problems with which he or she is dealing or struggling. The use of challenges (e.g., "You will not be able to open your eyes no matter how hard you try") is especially to be avoided for these reasons, as such challenges risk the emergence of helplessness as opposed to the significant quality of empowerment that hypnosis offers. The purpose of therapy is always to increase the child's control of a desired feeling or behavior, and any invitation or suggestion that emphasizes loss of control can only inhibit therapeutic progress. We do not mean to imply that the clinician therapist must avoid any structuring of the situation or should dilute the patient's perception of him or her as a competent, helping person. We do, however, emphasize the distinction between being appropriately authoritative (as the clinician, guide, teacher, coach) and being authoritarian.

Although we shall describe several specific hypnosis invitation techniques, our list is by no means a complete or exhaustive compendium, nor is this chapter intended as a substitute for direct training with experts in the field. We suspect that many professionals who give up utilization of hypnosis do so because they never acquired a solid base of personal, experiential training. Appropriate avenues of training are discussed in the Introduction and in the chapter on Education for Clinicians (Chapter 22).

Although some children expect and benefit from relatively formalized invitational techniques, many respond equally well or better to a more simple, casual approach. In some cases, it may be sufficient to say, for example, "Just think about how you feel when you are building a house with LEGOs at home; just let yourself feel that way now." Or, it may be very effective to say, "Just pretend you're not here and that instead you're somewhere where you are very happy."

Erickson (1958b) was particularly aware that children frequently go into hypnosis without any formal technique or invitation/induction, and he taught that careful and sensitive observation by the hypnosis clinician would allow him or her to know what would best facilitate effective hypnosis and to "go with the child." This phenomenon can present problems to researchers who define hypnosis as whatever occurs following a precise or specific hypnotic technique or "induction"; however, the criteria for determining the presence or absence of hypnosis can only be based on patient or subject behaviors known to be characteristic of the state of hypnosis and not on behaviors of the person doing the invitation or guiding of a technique.

The choice of invitation techniques depends not only on patient variables but also on the style and preferences of the clinician/therapist. A clinician using hypnosis is not likely to be successful using a method with which he or she is uncomfortable. Moreover, child health clinicians using hypnosis should always be alert to the possible value of new methods along with inevitable changes in cultural trends such as norms for social behavior, child-rearing methods, and educational approaches.

New developments in science and the arts that shape children's interests and attitudes will also have relevance for hypnotic invitation approaches. It may turn out that some methods currently in general use will be outdated or inappropriate for children of future generations. We emphasize here, as well as in application sections that follow, the *importance of recognizing childhood as an ongoing, fluid, and dynamic state*. In this context, we must be mindful, therefore, that the maturing child patient who finds one or several hypnosis invitation strategies effective and pertinent to him- or herself now may have no use at all for those techniques 6–12 months from now as he or she moves into a new phase of development. Careful attention to our patients' developmental needs, therefore, will allow us to work closely with them to tailor hypnosis invitational strategies (and suggestions) that fit with their developmental as well as social-emotional needs. Some of the techniques we describe have been created by our child patients or by children in our families or their friends. For techniques in use for a long time, and with several variations, we have been unable to trace their originators, and we apologize to these unsung heroes.

In the course of any hypnosis beginning/invitation, we give positive feedback to the child's responses, and we communicate expectations of and for success by focusing on possibilities and by avoiding words such as "try" that imply that failure may be the outcome. Because we believe our patients will benefit most from hypnosis when they enjoy the invitation technique/process, we work in ways that are enjoyable to us as well, using humor liberally where appropriate and never taking ourselves too seriously. A concentrated focus on language uses and choices – both for introduction and invitation of hypnosis and throughout the hypnotherapeutic relationship – follows in Chapter 7 in Part II, as well as in the many case examples throughout the text.

## The Pre-Invitation Interview

Depending on the needs of the child, the pre-invitation interview may be quite brief or very extensive. In emergency situations, it may be deferred entirely. The interview usually includes discussion of the reasons for utilizing hypnosis in relation to a particular problem, review of the child's ideas about hypnosis, clarification of misconceptions, and full reply to questions. If details of the child's likes and dislikes, significant experiences, fears, hopes, and comfort areas have not already been ascertained, these areas are also discussed at this time. By being an astute observer, learning to pay attention to the subtleties and nuances of both verbal and nonverbal behaviors, the thoughtful clinician becomes aware that this pre-invitation interview in many ways represents the "introduction and invitation before the invitation" or the unofficial hypnosis before the hypnosis formally begins. This "finding the hypnosis in the encounter" (Sugarman, 1997/2007), which comes with ongoing skill development and experience with hypnosis with children, affords the clinician–child dyad the greatest opportunity for nurturing the success of the hypnosis experience.

## A Sample of Hypnotic Invitation (Induction) Techniques for Children

The following descriptions of these techniques consist of the actual words we might say to a child. Obviously, our own phrasing varies from child to child, as it does (and must) vary from one clinician/therapist to another. We emphasize again that these are samples and that variations are inevitable, as well as necessary and appropriate. We find that a questionnaire for families is helpful in learning about a child's interests, fears, and wishes and as such is helpful in guiding our selections of suggested imagery during the ongoing process of hypnosis.

## Visual (Multisensory) Imagery Techniques

### *Favorite Place*

"Think about a favorite place where you have been and where you like to be. It might be easier if you close your eyes, but you can leave them open if you like or leave them open until you close them, or until they close by themselves." For children who cannot think of a real favorite place, ask them to think of an imaginary one, such as "one you have always wanted to go to and will probably visit some day." It sometimes helps to ask children to tell the therapist their favorite place and several of their favorite or valued activities. The therapist can then enhance the imagery by adding specific details. Important information about the child is sometimes obtained, similar to the information obtained, for example, from psychological projective tests that elicit fantasy. When children offer more than one favorite place and indicate no preference, the therapist may enhance rapport by suggesting the one with which he or she is most familiar and thus able to talk most easily and comfortably about, thereby conveying a sense of comfort and confidence in turn to the child patient. The therapist may also suggest the situation that involves the patient most actively, especially if the goals of treatment include enhanced competence and active mastery of a problem. Sometimes mentioning several options of things the clinician knows the child enjoys may reinforce that the choice is theirs, e.g., "I don't know if you'll imagine about baking cookies with grandma, or riding your bike, or cuddling with your dog, or something else, but YOU will know because you are the boss of your imagination."

The imagery utilized in invitation of hypnosis need not be related at all to the problem: "See yourself, feel yourself in that favorite place that you have chosen or has popped into your imagination. Look around and see the shapes and colors, hear the sounds there. Let yourself really be there now … because you really are there in your imagining [or daydreaming or pretending]. It's good for everybody to be in a favorite place sometimes, a place where you like to be, a place where you like how you feel. You can feel those good feelings now. Take some time to enjoy it. When you feel as if you are really there – even partway there in your mind – let me know by lifting one finger to say yes." If the child looks troubled, the therapist should inquire directly as to the difficulty. A comment that not everyone likes to go to a favorite place will be reassuring, and then one can suggest a different method. Occasionally a child who successfully imagines a favorite place may then have an unexpected negative reaction – for example, sadness because a grandparent who also enjoyed that place has died. Depending on the goals of treatment, the therapist may choose either to shift to another method or to help the child explore the emotional reaction, in or out of the hypnotic state, depending on the individual circumstances.

Prior to the beginning of the hypnosis invitation, the child can be told that he or she can talk in hypnosis, especially if a hypnotic interview is part of the treatment plan. This can be presented easily as part of the clinician's demystification and education about hypnosis and is often a great relief to children (and parents) who, like many, have misconceptions about an all-powerful, controlling "hypnotist." It may be useful to tell a child before or during hypnosis that "even hearing yourself talking can help you help yourself be even more comfortable and to see things in your imagination more clearly." This kind of gentle challenge encourages and eases the child's ability, desire, and willingness to talk. One can add additional simple motivational suggestions to this, such as "When you talk and tell me what you are imagining about, then I can be an even better coach to help you help yourself." Such statements reinforce the cooperative nature of the therapeutic hypnosis relationship and as such are easily accepted and experienced by patients as facilitative.

## *Multiple Animals*

"Do you like animals? Good. Which do you like best? Fine. Just imagine that you can see yourself sitting in a very nice place with a puppy [or whatever animal the child has chosen]. It might help to close your eyes. Feel that puppy's soft fur [kinesthetic imagery] and see its color [visual imagery]. Now, just for fun, pretend it is another color or striped or polka-dotted. Let it be any way you like, and the puppy is happy, too. You can change the color anytime you choose because [this is the motivating portion of the suggestion] it's your imagination, and you are the boss of your imagination. And you can imagine a second puppy just like the first, the same colors, the same soft fur. Two puppies, and you can see yourself playing with them. Now, you may choose to make three puppies and change their color back to the first color or to another color. You can tell me about the puppies if you like."

## *Flower Garden*

"You said you like flowers. Just let yourself imagine being in a beautiful big flower garden with all your favorite flowers. You may have your favorite toy or stuffed animal with you. See the bright colors [visual imagery]. Smell the sweet smells [olfactory imagery]. If you like, you can touch the petals and feel how soft they are [kinesthetic imagery]. Imagine that it's all right for you to pick as many flowers as you want from this big flower garden. You can keep them for yourself. Or you can pick some for someone special. Feel your arms widening around a bigger and bigger bouquet until you have all you want. If you take them to a special person, you can see how happy that person looks when you give the flowers. And, you can feel happy, too!"

## *Favorite Activity*

The child answers the inquiry, "Tell me something you like to do." Or, one might begin by saying, "It says on this paper that your Mom and Dad wrote on the questionnaire that you like to do [name three or four things from questionnaire]; I wonder which is your very favorite?" Then, "Good, just imagine (or pretend) that you can see yourself doing that. Let yourself really enjoy it, and do it better than ever before." This method emphasizes the active participation mentioned in the favorite place technique. Some children actually engage in physical activity appropriate to the imagery, such as moving their fingers as if playing a piano or pretending to throw a ball or hold ski poles or bicycle handlebars.

## *Cloud Gazing*

"What are some colors you like? Good. Let yourself imagine some beautiful clouds in the sky and see them change into one of your favorite colors. Good. Now let them change into another color. Or perhaps several nice colors. The clouds may change shape too, as you continue to watch them. It will be interesting to see what they become. You can be part of those clouds, if you like, feeling very comfortable, very good." This technique may not be appropriate for a child who has been told that death means "going up to heaven to live with God." Use special caution if there has been a recent death of a family member, friend, or pet or if the child has an illness that may result in death.

### *Letter Watching*

"You have told me that you like to write. Let yourself see a blackboard, or a piece of paper with an A on it. Now watch the A turn into a B. Then, let the B turn into a C. See as many letters as you like. When you are feeling very comfortable, very good, let me know by lifting one finger (or by letting your head nod)." One can do the same with numbers. If the child looks troubled, consider the possibility that letters and numbers may have symbolic meaning – for example, letters as grades or numbers as ages. One may notice the occurrence of spontaneous age regression or age progression with the number or alphabet method, and this may or may not be desirable, depending on the purpose and therapeutic goals of the hypnotic experience.

### *Television or Movie Fantasy*

"You told me you like to watch TV and that your favorite program is … ." For children who name a particularly violent program as their favorite, some therapists prefer to inquire about other interests and use a different method. It is probably better to inquire casually for other interests than to ask the child for a less violent program, as the child may interpret the latter as a rejection or as a controlling statement. "Just imagine yourself getting ready to watch your favorite TV program. Where is the TV set you are watching? Good. Just get comfortable, and when you are ready turn on the set using the remote control. Feel yourself push the button of the remote and get to the right channel. Now you can see your favorite program. When the sound and the picture are just right for you, let me know by lifting one finger. Good. Just continue watching and listening, and feeling very comfortable, very good!" If the child is undergoing a medical treatment procedure, the therapist may give repeated suggestions for continued watching. If the therapist intends to give hypnotic or posthypnotic suggestions, these may often be interspersed in the context of the program. For example, if the child has "resisted" (refused?) taking oral medication, the therapist can suggest that the TV hero or heroine is happy to take medicine that will cure an illness. Or, the child can be asked to name a favorite food, then given the suggestion that the TV character is eating that food and wants to share it with the child. The medication is then hallucinated as the favorite food. Most children have no problem merging and immersing themselves into a TV program or a video.

The advent of remote controls and an awareness of multiple channels allows the clinician to use this TV or digital or YouTube imagery to move easily from hypnosis invitation into utilization and to solve problems. Thus, in going from invitation and beginning of hypnosis to utilization (or working on some specific area of the child's life), one could simply say, "Now switch to the [child's name] channel, where you see yourself in your mind – how you are now or how you want to be." This imagery also allows for a kind of safety valve in the event of an unpleasant experience in trance. As noted, the clinician may decide in some cases to focus on the sadness or some other unsuspected feeling that may appear abruptly, or he or she could simply invite the child to "just change the channel; you are the boss of your imagination."

We have seen desperately ill children accept oral medications in the context of these suggestions. In psychotherapeutic treatment, the therapist may use the TV technique to explore problem areas or to help the child toward constructive resolution. Similarly, this imagery may be used constructively to help a patient with changes he or she may wish to make as part of the therapeutic agreement. In the "split-screen" technique, one can visualize the old way or the problem on one video screen or on one-half of the video screen; on the other half, the patient can be instructed to "let the way you want it to be [i.e., the desired outcome] now come into view on the other screen [or other half of the screen]." Multiple variations can then be explored, such as inviting the child to visualize one image (the old one) getting smaller while the other gets bigger. Or, one might suggest one image gets dimmer and the other brighter, or one blows a fuse and the other is made out of invincible parts from outer space, and so forth.

As reflected in this example, in this and virtually all other hypnotic invitational strategies and techniques, there is really no sharp distinction between the beginning invitation of hypnosis and therapeutic work. Even when an invitation technique is used without any therapeutic suggestions, the child's experience of the invitation itself will be either therapeutic or countertherapeutic. The same is true, of course, for all aspects of the clinician–patient interaction in therapeutic hypnosis as well as in other forms of treatment.

## Auditory Imagery

### *Favorite Song*

"You said that you like to sing. Where do you like to do that best? Good. Imagine that you are there now, singing your favorite song. Sing the song through in your mind. Enjoy doing it very well, making just the sounds you like. When you have come to the end of the song, let me know by lifting one finger. Or, you can sing it again if you like and then let your finger lift." Note that "lifting one finger" is a conscious act, whereas "let your finger lift" is a hypnotic suggestion or request for dissociation and involuntary (ideomotor) movement. The patient may be asked to tap out the beat with one or more fingers. When the tapping ceases, the therapist knows the patient has ended the song.

### *Playing a Musical Instrument*

If the patient enjoys playing a musical instrument, the therapist can adapt the Favorite Song technique accordingly.

### *Listening to Music*

"You said you liked music. What kind of music do you like to listen to? Exactly what piece of music would you like to hear now? Good. Just imagine yourself hearing that very clearly now, as loud or soft as you like. You might want to turn it up … and then down … . You may imagine watching the musicians, too. You can let me know when the music has ended." For some children, actually listening to the music may be better than imagining it. We occasionally ask children to bring in a recording of the music, or we have brought one in ourselves (Gardner & Tarnow, 1980).

## Movement Imagery

### *Flying Blanket*

This method, invented by one of Karen Olness' children, should not be used if the patient is afraid of flying or of heights. "Imagine that you are going on a picnic, going with your favorite people to a special place for a picnic. You have your favorite things to eat and drink. You can see and smell and taste them. You can enjoy playing games with your family and friends. Then, when you are finished eating and drinking and playing games, you may see a blanket spread out there on the ground. It's your favorite color, smooth and soft. You may sit on it or lie on it. Pretend it's a flying blanket, and you are the pilot. You are in control. You can fly just a few inches above the ground, just above the grass or higher, even above the trees if you want. You're the pilot. You can go where you want and as fast or as slowly as you wish, just by thinking about it. You can land and visit your friends or you can land at the zoo or anywhere you like. You're the pilot, and you're in charge. You might fly by a tree and see birds in a nest. You can speed up and slow down. Enjoy going where you want. Take all the time you need to feel very comfortable. When you are ready, you can find a nice comfortable landing spot and land your flying blanket. When you have landed, let me know by lifting one finger." Therapeutically, one might also add, "When you are ready to learn more about how your inside mind can help your body or the way it can help with those problems that have been bothering you, then land your blanket."

### *Movement Imagery*

"Do you like to do things like ride a bicycle or ride a horse? Good. Which do you like best? Fine. Just get comfortable and imagine that you are doing that now. You are just where you want to be, and it's a perfect day. Imagine going exactly where you wish at the speed you wish. You are in control, and you can go wherever you like. Enjoy what you see. Enjoy the feeling. Enjoy being able to go at any speed you like. And each time you change speed or direction, let that be a signal to get even more comfortable than you were before. When you are very, very comfortable, you can gradually slow down. Find a good stopping or resting place and rest, very comfortably." For children who are frightened of passivity, it may be best to omit the suggestion to slow down and stop. Therapeutic suggestions may be given, of course, while the trip is in progress. Or, the end of the movement can be the signal for the therapeutic suggestions; for example, "When you are ready for me to tell you about the suggestion for dry beds [or control of that tic], you can gradually slow down and stop in a favorite place. When you are there, just let your yes finger lift. Then I'll know you're ready." This has the added advantage of emphasizing that the child is in control.

### *Sports Activity*

"You told me that you like to play football. Imagine yourself at the age you are now, or maybe older, playing on your favorite football team, wearing its uniform, playing the position you like. Let yourself get very comfortable as you imagine a game with your team winning. You are helping your team win. Feel your control as your muscles move the way you tell them, running, or throwing or catching or kicking. Enjoy being with the winning team, and continue until the game is won. Perhaps you'll hear the crowd cheering for you and your team. Let me know when the game is over by lifting one finger." This method may be especially suited for children for whom enhanced muscular control is a therapeutic goal, provided they do not have excessively negative attitudes about their sports ability.

### *Bouncing Ball*

"Sometimes it's fun to think of going wherever you want. Pretend you're a bouncing ball, maybe a big one, and you can be any color you want, even striped or with polka dots. It might be easier if you shut your eyes. Be that bouncing ball, and bounce wherever you want. Bounce, bounce, bounce. You can go wherever you wish. You can bounce up a tree and along a branch. You can bounce over your house or over the hospital. You can bounce along a path in the woods or on a sidewalk. If you like to swim, you can bounce and float, bounce and float. If anything is bothering you, you can let it bounce right off. Keep bouncing until you find the right place for you to stop, and when you've stopped let me know."

### *Playground Activity*

"I know you like to go to the playground and play on the swing and the slide. You can pretend you are there now. Imagine yourself getting on the swing and starting to swing back and forth. Just a little at first, then more, back and forth, just as fast or as slow you like, back and forth. Back and forth. Feeling very good. So easy. And when you are ready to go to the slide, just let the swing slow down and imagine yourself at the top of a nice, long, smooth slide, a slide that is just right for you. As you go down that slide, you can feel more and more comfortable. Feel your body going gently down and down. So smooth. So easy. Down and down. When you reach the bottom, you may find something you like very much. So comfortable. When you reach the bottom, you can just enjoy what you find there. Lift one finger when you get to the bottom. If you like, you can tell me what you find there, or you can tell me later, or you can keep it private."

### *Be a Snowman [Snowgirl] → Be a Tree*

"Just be a beautiful frozen snowman [snowgirl]. That's great, what a nice-looking snowman [snowgirl]. Now Mr. [Ms.] Snowman, it's the end of winter, and the sun is going to come out, and it's getting quite warm." Note that most children will begin to melt from the top down without any help. Most of the time it may help to have them do it in slow motion. "That's right, so melty until you get all the way to the ground and become a beautiful puddle in the springtime, and now, with the new spring, the seeds in the ground are going to use that water and start to grow now into a tree." Note that most children do not need any further verbal or physical cue to start getting up. "A beautiful, big, strong tree with roots deep into the ground, big, beautiful branches this way and that, with beautiful leaves and maybe even lots of fruit. Now the winds of spring come and begin to blow, and the tree sways this way and that, but the tree is so strong and its roots are so deep that it stays up, comfortable and safe."

## Storytelling Techniques

With young children or those who are too anxious to participate much in other imagery techniques, the clinician/therapist may decide to make up a story suited to the child's needs and interests. This technique may be especially useful with small children who are undergoing painful or frightening medical procedures. The story may be an entirely new fantasy production or it may be a variation of a TV program or other theme with which the child is familiar. The therapist may take full responsibility for the story or may ask the child to contribute ideas to the extent that he or she is able. This method provides an opportunity for the therapist to engage the child in humorous fantasy, a good antidote for anxiety.

The clinician might begin by telling a familiar story and then substitute doctors, nurses, or family members for the original characters. Most young children delight in these antics, although a few will of course insist that the story be told the "right way." Although some might consider storytelling a distraction technique rather than a storytelling technique, we do not see these as mutually exclusive, and we have seen narrowed focus of attention and altered sensation, which typically characterize the hypnotic state. Of course, the therapist can also intersperse into the story suggestions for comfort, analgesia, and calm.

Just as these techniques may function as invitational strategies for younger children, so may storytelling play an important role in the formulation of therapeutic hypnosis suggestions for all age groups and for a wide variety of problems as described in later chapters. We do not offer any examples here, as this method is almost entirely a function of the therapist's own creativity and ingenuity in the context of individual child patients and their own personal lives and stories.

## Ideomotor Techniques

These methods are distinguished from movement imagery techniques because the latter do not necessarily involve any actual or conscious intentional movement by the child, although movement may occur. Ideomotor techniques ask the child to focus mentally on the *idea of a particular* movement and then to *let the movement occur* without conscious muscle activity. Such methods are especially valuable when the therapist wishes to communicate the idea that the child can gain increased control over pain and other physical responses that previously seemed beyond control. They may also facilitate the idea that one's attitudes can affect the healing process and that willingness or openness to change can replace complete passivity in treatment. These methods are most often suited for children of at least school age, but sometimes younger children may benefit.

## Hands Moving Together

"Hold your arms straight out in front of you, your palms facing each other, about a foot apart. Good. Now imagine two powerful magnets, one in each palm. You know how magnets attract each other. Just think about those two very strong magnets, and you may notice that your hands begin to move closer together all by themselves, without you doing anything, Don't help your hands … just notice. Good. Notice that the closer the magnets are together, the stronger they pull. And the stronger they pull, the closer your hands move together. Don't help your hands; see what they'll do all by themselves. Soon they will touch. When that happens, just let go of those imaginary magnets, let your hands and arms drift down to a comfortable position, take one deep breath and let yourself relax all over."

## Hand Levitation

"Let your hand and arm just rest comfortably on the arm of the chair. Notice and feel the texture of the fabric beneath your fingers. Now imagine that there is a string tied around your wrist and that big, bright helium-filled balloons are tied to the other end of the string, the kind of balloons that float up all by themselves. Lots of balloons, your favorite colors, just floating, so light, so easy. Effortless. As you focus on the lightness of those balloons, you may notice how that hand begins to feel light, too." (Note the shift from "your hand" to "that hand" in order to facilitate dissociation.) "Soon one of the fingers may begin to feel especially light. One of the fingers may begin to lift up." Notice carefully which finger moves and comment accordingly; for example, "Good, I see that finger moving, I wonder what will move next. Yes. Good. Now another finger is moving. Now the whole hand. Just focus on the balloons and on the feeling of lightness in that hand. And the higher it goes, the lighter it can feel, and the lighter it feels, the higher it goes. Just floating up all by itself. Drifting higher and lighter and higher and lighter. Now imagine a soft breeze. That hand may float over toward your lap, or it may float even higher, or it may just stay where it is now. Very comfortable, very relaxed all over. You can just let that hand [or arm] float, or, if you choose, you can let the string loosen and the balloons float away and let that hand slowly drift back down to a comfortable resting place, because it's fun and because it feels good to do. So easy. Just effortless." If the child seems to be having difficulty, the therapist can first induce a hand or an arm catalepsy and then suggest further movement.

## Arm Lowering

"Stretch one arm out straight in front of you with the palm of your hand facing up." Assist the child as necessary. "Good. Now imagine that I am putting a dictionary on that hand." For young children the image of a large rock might be preferable. "You may notice that it begins to feel pretty heavy. Now, imagine a second dictionary [rock] on top of the first one. That arm can feel even heavier. Soon it will want to drift down. When it feels heavy, just let it drift down. Heavier and heavier, down and down. I can see it moving down now. Good. Just let that happen." As with most invitational techniques, timing and especially *pacing and leading* are essential to success. The therapist can add dictionaries as needed but should be careful to comment on actual movement that occurs. For the few children who seem to resist this technique, the therapist can shift to another kinesthetic strategy such as arm rigidity or arm catalepsy.

## Finger Lowering

This method appeals to young children and may also be used with older children for whom arm lowering may be difficult, perhaps because of physical debilitation. The therapist helps the child rest the little finger on the bed or arm of the chair, leaving the other fingers extended in the air. "Pretend that this little finger is having a nice rest or nap on the arm of the chair. The other fingers would like to rest or nap, too. Watch them. Soon they will want to drift down and down … until they are resting, too. I wonder which finger will drift down first. Look, that one is resting now. When they are all resting, you can feel very comfortable and rested all over too. You can close your eyes if you like, or leave them open until they close all by themselves, rested. More and more comfortable."

## Arm Rigidity

"Stretch one arm straight out to the side and make a tight fist. Imagine that the arm is very strong, just like the straight strong branch on a tree. Stronger and stronger. So strong that I cannot push it down. I cannot bend it. That arm is very powerful. It can be as strong and powerful as it wants, even as powerful as [fill in the name of the child's favorite female or male superhero]." Note how easily this method can lead into ego-strengthening suggestions.

## Mighty Oak Tree

This method is especially useful in groups but is also appealing to young children who do not naturally or easily sit still. It also serves as a wonderful method for modeling or teaching parents that children can experience and learn to utilize hypnosis without having to insist that they sit still. "Stand up, tall and straight as a strong oak tree. That's good. Let your arms be branches and stretch toward the sky. Your feet are roots that go down through the floor. Feel how strong you are! Very strong. You can't be moved. Feel the sun and air and rain come in through your branches to make you even stronger. Feel those strong tough roots hold you even while the wind blows through your leaves. When you're ready, when you feel like a powerful oak tree, I'll try to lift you."

## Arm Catalepsy

"Is it okay with you if I pick up this hand? Good. Just let it relax. Let me do the work." If the child cooperates by raising the hand and arm, indicate that such conscious cooperation is not necessary and repeat until there is no conscious cooperation. This is usually accomplished easily by saying something – for example, "Thank you, but just let your arm do it by itself; you don't have to help your arm. Good. Just let the hand rest. Let me do the work of lifting it. Fine. Now look at that hand as though it were part of a sculpture, just floating there by itself. Just imagine it floating there all by itself." The therapist gradually loosens hold of the hand, sensing when the catalepsy has been achieved. "Good. That hand is floating by itself now. Now just raise the other hand and notice the difference. Now you can begin to understand how your strong unconscious, inside mind can help you do what you want."

## Progressive Relaxation Techniques

These methods are essentially the same for children as for adults. They are often used as invitational beginnings of hypnosis with adolescents and sometimes with younger children who have medical problems that can benefit by deliberate programming of physiological relaxation (e.g., the child with leg muscle spasm associated with a fractured femur). The main difference in response between children and adults is that children often respond very quickly with total body relaxation. The therapist must observe the rate of response and through *careful pacing and leading* be ready to terminate the longer invitation with a simple suggestion for complete relaxation. Lengthy details about specific muscle groups may be necessary for some children, whereas others will experience boredom that can then interfere with response to further suggestions.

## Following Breathing

"Focus your eyes easily on some point on your lap or anywhere you like, and pay attention to each time you breathe out. Notice what happens to your shoulders automatically while you breathe out ... they go down, don't they? Good. That's the mind and body working together all the time; even without thinking about it, every time we breathe out we relax some automatically. That feeling is relaxation. When you breathe out you loosen your chest muscles. Each of us does that about 10 or 12 times each minute. Pay attention to breathing out, and each time extend your own relaxation feeling a little further ... past your chest and into your tummy muscles. Next time you breathe out, let the comfortable feeling move down into your hips and your upper leg muscles. Relax your lower leg muscles now and feel a flow of comfort, a loosening relaxation feeling from your chest muscles down to your ankles, your feet, and your toes. Go at your own pace and your own speed. When you're ready, focus on your lower back muscles, and let them feel very comfortable. Loosen your upper back muscles. And now let a flow of relaxation spread past those shoulders that were already relaxing, down into your upper arms, gradually past your elbows and into your lower arm muscles, into the small muscles of your wrists, hands, and even the little muscles of the fingers. When you're ready, allow your neck muscles to become comfortable more than they were already. Loosen them but just the right amount to keep your head very comfortable. Let the flow of relaxation move into your cheek muscles, your forehead, around your eyes, even to the tiny muscles of your head and scalp, and even into your hair muscles. When you're nice and comfortable all over, please give me a signal by nodding your head or raising a finger. You can tell me if there is any part of your body that doesn't seem ready to be comfortable yet, and we can do some other things so that you can be even more comfortable all over." (See also "The '3 and 6' Hypnotic Induction Technique for Children and Adolescents") (Kohen, 2017).

## Teddy Bear

This method is especially useful for young children for whom sleep is desirable, such as in pre- or postoperative situations, but for whom direct suggestion for sleep might produce resistance. A doll or stuffed animal might be substituted according to the child's preference. "What does your teddy bear do when he is sleepy? Hold him the way he likes to be held. Let his head get very comfortable. Maybe you should pat him gently … so gently. That's good. Is he getting sleepy? Let his arms get cozy and comfortable. Don't forget his tummy … comfortable and sleepy. Let his feet get comfortable. Pretty soon now the whole teddy bear will be sleepy. Comfortable, drowsy, dozy, and cozy. You can rock him if you like … maybe even sing him a nice quiet song. So comfortable. So nice. Such a good feeling. So easy. So quiet. So nice of you to help him [her] this way."

## Balancing Muscles

"Sit forward, drop hands to your sides, and move your feet out and spread them a little apart from each other on the floor. Move your body forward until you feel your abdominal muscles pull, then move back until your back pulls. Do this until you find a balanced, neutral position for your trunk. Do the same with your head. Move a little forward, a little back until it feels right. Imagine a thread from the ceiling to your head. Think of your head stretched up a little. Hold the position easily for as long as you wish, then think of the thread being cut, and your head bending forward, very relaxed and comfortable throughout."

## Floppy Raggedy Ann or Andy

"Pretend that you are Raggedy Ann [Andy], floppy all over, so loose and comfortable. Let's be like Raggedy Ann and feel floppy. Let me check this arm. Good. See how it flops down when I pick it up? Just like Raggedy Ann [Andy]. Now let me check the other arm. Good. That's floppy, too. Now let yourself feel floppy all over, loose all over, and very comfortable all over; you can be floppy Raggedy [name]."

## Eye Fixation Techniques

### *Coin Technique*

Present a coin and ask the child to hold it between the thumb and first finger. For some children, attention is heightened by first drawing a smiling face with a colored marking pen on their thumbnail. Younger children often prefer to have their favorite stuffed animal hold the coin, sometimes in a paw, sometimes under a nose. Whether they fix their eyes on the coin held by themselves or by the stuffed animal is immaterial. "Just look at that smiling face on the thumb that's holding the coin [or just look at that coin] real easy. That's good. After a while the fingers [or paw] will begin to get a little tired of holding it, and after a while the coin can slip down to the floor [or sofa or bed]. It will be safe there. You can get it later. When it falls, that is your signal to yourself to just let those eyes close by themselves. That's right."

### *Looking at Point on Hand*

"Move around until you have a comfortable position and let your eyes look down, easily, at a point on your hands or fingers, on your ring, or on a painted nail or some other spot. Just hold your eyes there easily while you take five … long … deep … comfortable breaths. After the fifth breath, or even sooner if you choose, let your eyes close easily and comfortably."

### *Biofeedback*

Children as young as 3 or 4 years are intrigued by watching changing numbers on a thermal biofeedback monitor and have a remarkably long attention span for the machine. Some children may simply be asked just to watch the numbers change. This invitation strategy combines simple eye fixation with absorption and fascination with the changing colors and numbers. In addition, some children may be encouraged to change finger temperature by specifically thinking about hot or cold. This process emphasizes bodily control and may be a good introduction to related therapeutic suggestions; for example, "This machine tells you how warm or cold your fingers are. Look at the numbers [invitation for eye fixation]. When they go up, that means your fingers are warmer. When they go down, that means your fingers are cooler [education]. Sometimes you can make the numbers change just by thinking about your fingers being warm or cool [hypnotic suggestion about mind–body connections]. I wonder which way the numbers will go for you. Good. The number went up. Your fingers are warm and comfortable. Look. The number has changed again. Just watch the numbers and feel more and more comfortable [definitive link between visual biofeedback – 'Look' – and the hypnotic suggestion to feel more comfortable]." Computer game biofeedback, used in our programs, is very appealing to many children and is becoming increasingly useful in the therapeutic approach to a variety of pediatric and adolescent biobehavioral problems. Computer-based biofeedback technology now permits easy access to recording and displaying a wide variety of physiological parameters, including blood pressure, pulse, respiratory rate, electrodermal activity (galvanic skin response), muscle tension (EMG), and (peripheral) temperature, which are fed back to the child patient through visual or auditory displays. The liberal use of colors and the implementation of increasingly creative, attractive games and scenarios tap into the child and adolescent's sense of adventure, challenge, and desire for active participation. Linked to either direct or indirect measurement of their "problem," such biofeedback opportunities provide a natural connection to hypnotic inductions and hypnotherapeutic strategies. Culbert, Reaney, and Kohen (1994) noted that individual patient problems suggest a need for varying degrees of integration of biofeedback and hypnosis; as discussed in detail in Chapter 16, our belief is that there is a hypnosis invitation component for all biofeedback. These two cyber-physiologic (self-regulatory) methodologies may thus be combined creatively in the best interest of the patient and his or her individual problems. Computer games for these purposes are now being displayed prominently in some museums around the United States, and varying forms are now described on the internet and available for home use. Many children continue to be delighted and intrigued with watching simple BioBands® or Biodots® applied to their fingers; these change color as temperature changes, and children can use these at home to reinforce their learning.

## Distraction and Utilization Techniques

These methods, based on techniques developed by Erickson (1959), are especially helpful with children who are frightened or in severe pain. They attract attention often by a seeming lack of logic, shifting focus from a negative to a positive aspect of the situation. Once the therapist can get the child's attention, the trance of hypnosis often may occur spontaneously, and therapeutic suggestions may be easily accepted. The success of these techniques is chiefly a function of the therapist's creativity. Here are a few examples:

> "It hurts, and it's going to hurt a while longer. It will probably keep right on hurting until it stops." (The child hears "it stops.") "I wonder if it will stop hurting in 5 minutes or 7 minutes or 30 seconds or right now?"
>
> "Your right hand is hurt. Let's be sure the left hand is not also hurt. Does it hurt here … or here … or here?"
>
> "Those are pretty sparkling tears. Can you cry some more of them? I wonder which eye will have more tears."
>
> "What's that dog in the corner doing?"
>
> "What color is the air today?"
>
> "Listen to that scream. You certainly have strong lungs. Now scream a few more times, and then we'll count in a whisper. One, two, three … you're good at whispering. We'll count when you scream, and we'll count when you whisper … four … five … ."

## Using Modern Technology: Technology-Aided Induction Techniques

### *Videotapes, Digital Video Recordings on Computers, Smartphones*

Young children who are shy or hesitant may benefit by watching a video of a child of similar age responding to an invitation to hypnosis as described above. These often are very valuable in pre-hypnosis conversations with children and families to demystify the forthcoming hypnosis invitation experience expected to be of help for the child. They also serve to remove misconceptions as well as to clarify modern mythology about what hypnosis is and is not. With the increased prevalence of home and school video cameras, and the now almost ubiquitous cellphone cameras, many children are camera eager rather than camera shy. Video recording a given hypnotic experience sometimes serves to facilitate a child's interest, concentration, and absorption. Such a video recording might also be used as a form of personal (video and audio) biofeedback in later, ongoing therapeutic work with a child – for example, to show the child through a previous video how he or she looked, how well he or she was relaxing, how pain free he or she was during hypnosis.

### *Smartphone Recording*

For some children who have difficulty learning to go into hypnosis without the therapist present, invitational strategies/techniques may be recorded on audio recording. Smartphones or computers (as an MP4) for use at home, in a hospital room, or even in the nurse's office at school. We have a strong preference, however, that children achieve full independence in using hypnosis for their own benefit, rather than becoming dependent on our audio-recorded hypnosis invitation/ therapeutic suggestions. Although we acknowledge and wish to promote the value of personally prepared audio recording for rehearsal reinforcement and review, in the interest of avoiding dependence we most often prefer to wait until a child has demonstrated comfort and facility with self-hypnosis before offering to prepare a personalized recording. Once a child has learned hypnosis and upon one or more return visits has demonstrated through discussion and self-initiation of hypnosis that he or she has begun to integrate self-hypnosis into his or her life, then we may offer to prepare a recording for home use.

A typical approach might sound like this: "Now that you know how to do this for yourself, I know that sometimes there must be times when one part of you knows that you probably should practice your RMI [relaxation, mental imagery, self-hypnosis], while another part of you is too tired, or bored, or just doesn't feel like it. So, I was thinking that maybe what we could do is today, when we practice in a couple of minutes, maybe I'll just record what I say, and then if it comes out good you can have a copy of it, and it will be like having the coach at home. Then, sometimes if you know you should practice and don't feel like it, that would be a good time to listen to the recording, and it will be easier to just listen the way you do when you're here. What do you think?" The vast majority of children and teenagers like this idea and are eager and thrilled to have the recording e.g., available to them at home on their smartphone, I-pad, computer, etc., which they then use in widely disparate ways. Many immediately import the recording to their iPod® or other mp3 player or to their home computer or their own smartphone. Occasionally, however, the child experiences the offer of a recording as something of an insult to his or her ability to do this for him- or herself and refuses, saying "Naw, I don't need it, thanks anyway."

The availability of portable, personal playback units such as smartphones and I-pads has been a boon, especially for chronically ill children. Their use during procedures may allow for and promote rapid induction of hypnosis when the child's favorite music is played or a specific tape is used with instructions for entering and maintaining the hypnotic state.

When a recording is requested by a child or family, the clinician therapist should ask for recommendations from the child regarding what should be placed on the recording. Each recording should be tailored to the child's particular needs. Some children like to dictate their own induction onto the recording, thus taking a major step toward mastery. The child should be told that the recording is for his or her use only and is not to be played for other children. We have not seen children abuse recorded hypnosis invitations or therapy when the therapist explains that the recording would probably not be helpful to other children. In the interest of promoting mastery and autonomy, we usually urge parents to not listen to the child's recording unless and until the child invites them to share the experience. We often present this to the parents by pointing out in the child's presence that although *we* don't mind if the child shares the tape with the parents, that the parents don't mind (we hope!) if the child decides to keep it private (at least for a while).

### Telephone

As long as the patient and therapist are well known to one another, we have found that children respond easily to hypnosis invitation rehearsal, review, and reinforcement by telephone, e-mail, and/or TeleHealth platforms (such as ZOOM) which have become popular and as sometimes mandatory substitutes for in-person clinician visits during this time of the Coronavirus Pandemic. Sometimes distance precludes a face-to-face visit or the therapist is not immediately available when some unexpected special circumstance arises in which immediate reinforcement of hypnotic suggestions is advisable. A burned child, for example, may suddenly be faced with an unexpected procedure or may otherwise experience intense pain and be unable to use techniques of self-hypnosis. Although privacy and quiet are desirable, we have used telephone hypnosis invitations and reinforcements in a busy intensive care unit where as many as a dozen adults were working with our patients and others. In long-term follow-up of children with habit problems, Olness (1976) has children telephone the office on a regular basis. Many selected children also call or e-mail us with follow-up reports after frequent office visits are no longer necessary. In addition to updating progress, during these conversations the patient also verbally reviews self-hypnosis exercises, and the therapist reinforces suggestions. Obviously, it is important that the patient be able to use self-hypnosis invitations and self-hypnosis suggestions that do not require the therapist's actual presence. After the patient has told the therapist about the current situation, the therapist can begin the hypnosis. In selected situations, especially with pre-school children and hospitalized or immobilized patients, parents may help by holding the telephone receiver near the child's ear and mouth.

## Group Hypnosis Experiences

Simultaneous hypnosis invitation with several children in a group has been reported to be successful, particularly with children who have chronic illnesses such as hemophilia (LaBaw, 1975), or asthma (Kohen & Wynne, 1988), or leukemia or other type of cancer (Olness & Singher, 1989). This method may be especially useful with very young children, who often feel more comfortable in groups and can capitalize on their natural tendencies to imitate their peers. Sometimes parents also enjoy desired relaxation and confidence when they are given the opportunity to participate with their children in group exercises. They may also enjoy sharing the benefits of learning self-hypnosis to reinforce these general goals. The therapist may choose to have all participants use the same invitational hypnosis suggestions, such as favorite place imagery, the coin technique, or storytelling, a particular favorite with preschool children. At other times, and especially if the children in the group differ widely in age, the therapist may use a patient's-choice of [self] invitation in which each patient uses a self-hypnotic technique most beneficial (for themselves) in the past. During this time the therapist may choose to purposely remain silent, play music, address general comments to the group, or intersperse particular statements directed to specific individuals or to the whole group. When the therapist makes therapeutic hypnosis suggestions, these may be addressed to the group as a whole or to individual members. Rivalry can be eliminated or minimized in such a setting when each member receives a brief personalized comment or suggestion during the group hypnosis.

In group hypnosis experiences, some children – especially the younger ones – may choose to have their eyes open, at least at the beginning, so they can observe and imitate their peers. For most children, the therapist may comment that distraction will be lessened and concentration heightened if they close their eyes at the outset, perhaps opening them briefly from time to time as needed.

## Arousal: Ending the Hypnotic Experience

When choosing a method of terminating a hypnosis trance experience, the clinician takes into account the child patient's need for structure and (normal) tendency to resist finishing the experience for the moment. Compared with adults, children usually need less formality and ritual. If structure appears to be helpful or important for a particular child, the therapist may count or ask patients to count to a certain number. Or, children may count silently, using suggestions that they will open their eyes at some point in the counting and feel fully alert, aware, and refreshed by the end of the count.

If a less structured approach seems best, as it commonly does, the therapist might say, "Enjoy that experience [or scene or place or game] for a little while longer, and then, when you're ready, slowly, comfortably, easily open your eyes and return to your usual way of being, and your usual regular self." For an older child or teenager, one might address him or her as one might an adult, noting, "When you're ready, slowly, comfortably, easily open your eyes and return to your usual state of consciousness and alertness." For a younger child: "Do that a little longer, and when you're ready go back [or return] to what you were doing before we began this practice." For all age groups, it is useful to combine the invitation to complete the experience with acknowledgment of the difference and value of the hypnotic state as compared to the nonhypnotic state by saying, "... and be sure to bring your good and relaxed feelings with you when you come back here." If the child is in pain or distress before the hypnosis invitation experience, the therapist needs to add some clarification, such as "We can do this with you lying in your bed with your teddy bear, and you can keep all the comfortable nice feelings you have now." Some children may be told to enjoy the hypnotic state "for as long as you like," but this phrase should be avoided with children who might use it to extend the session beyond appropriate limits or otherwise seek to manipulate the therapist. Occasionally, a child in a group hypnosis session may compete with peers by resisting arousal/alerting from the trance. The therapist can usually solve the problem with a casual remark such as, "I wonder who will be the first one to be able to get fully alert again." Rarely, a direct comment to the child may be in order.

Consistent with our usual avoidance of the terms *asleep*, *sleepy*, *tired*, or *drowsy*, we also avoid instructing the patient to *wake up* from the trance experience. However, when doing especially an initial hypnosis invitation with a child for whom it would be appropriate to drift from the state of hypnosis to the state of sleep without intermediate arousal, we would say, "Now, if you wish, you can just drift off to sleep. When you wake up, you can feel fully refreshed and alert. When you wake up, you will no longer be in hypnosis; you can be in your usual state of awareness and give yourself an inside message to enjoy the rest of the day."

## Self-Reinforcement Using Patient-Recorded Digital Audio Recording

It is helpful to some children to make recordings of themselves dictating the self-hypnosis exercise. This is done after several sessions with their hypnosis clinician. When they are practicing at home, some children do far better when they actually hear themselves speaking on the audio recording player, smartphone, I-pad than when they try to concentrate on the exercise by memory. It is important that the therapist also hears the recording at some point in order to make sure that appropriate suggestions are recalled and given. Aronson (1986) has reported the use of the technique with a 15-year-old adolescent. Sometimes older children and teenagers may benefit from writing a script for what they want their recording to say, occasionally brainstorming and reviewing it with the clinician and then preparing it for themselves.

## Hypnosis Invitation Techniques for Different Ages

Children of different ages often prefer different hypnosis invitation techniques. Although we can group techniques roughly according to the age groups for which they are most often appropriate, there are no hard and fast rules, especially in cases where levels of cognitive or social-emotional development are at variance with expectations based on chronological age. Immature adolescents may do well with techniques that normally would appeal to younger children. Likewise, some young children succeed best with methods that appeal to older age groups, especially techniques

**TABLE 5.1** Induction Techniques by Age

| *Preverbal (0–2 years)* | *Early Verbal (2–4 years)* | *Preschool and Early School (4–6 years)* | *Middle Childhood (7–11 years)* | *Adolescence (12–18 years)* |
|---|---|---|---|---|
| Tactile stimulation such as stroking or patting | Storytelling | Favorite place | Favorite place | Favorite place |
| Kinesthetic stimulation such as rocking or moving an arm back and forth | Pop-up books | Storytelling (alone or in a group) | Favorite activity | Favorite activity |
| Auditory stimulation such as music or any whirring sound (e.g., hairdryer, electric shaver, vacuum cleaner placed out of reach of the child) | Favorite activity | Pop-up books | Blowing breath out | Sports activity |
| Visual stimulation such as mobiles or other objects that change shape, color, or position | Stereoscopic viewer | Playground activity | Cloud gazing | Arm catalepsy |
| Holding a doll or stuffed animal | Blowing bubbles | Stereoscopic viewer | Flying blanket | Following breathing |
| | Speaking to the child through a doll or stuffed animal (e.g., floppy Raggedy Ann or Andy or a teddy bear) | Blowing breath out | Videogames (actual or imagined) | Videogames (actual or imagined) |
| | Watching induction or self on videotape | Multiple animals | Coin watching | Computer games (actual or imagined) |
| | | Flower garden | Riding a bike | Fantasy games (e.g., Dungeons and Dragons) |
| | | Mighty oak tree | Arm lowering | Eye fixation on hand |
| | | Coin watching | Favorite music | Driving a car |
| | | Letter watching | Listening to self on tape | Playing or hearing music |
| | | Television fantasy | Fixation at point on hand | Hand levitation |
| | | Videotape | Hands (fingers) moving together as magnets | Hands (fingers) moving together as magnets |
| | | Bouncing ball | Arm rigidity | |
| | | Thermal (and other) biofeedback | | |
| | | Finger lowering | | |

they know are used by older siblings or parents. As usual, we remain flexible and let the patient be the guide, tailoring techniques to the individual and developmental needs of a given child. In Table 5.1, we have included methods that need no description and therefore have not been discussed previously.

## Modifications for Children with Special Problems

It is especially important that the therapist working with children who have various disabilities be familiar with a variety of invitational approaches, strategies, and techniques and be capable of creative modification to suit and accommodate to special circumstances and needs.

## Physical Disabilities

Therapeutic hypnosis invitation can be successful with children who are at bedrest or who have motor limitations, verbal dysfluencies, blindness, or deafness. Even delirious or comatose children may respond (D.M. Markowitz, pers. comm.). In general, the therapist chooses a method in which the disability itself is not involved or appropriately modifies a method while taking account of the problem. For example, in the case of a child who is deaf, it may be necessary to agree on written suggestions or enlist the aid of someone fluent in sign language. In so doing it is obviously critical to provide education about hypnosis for, and spend time developing rapport with, the individuals who will be doing the signing in order to maximize therapeutic hypnosis communication and success (Kohen, Mann-Rinehart, Schmitz, & Wills, 1998). Korn and Johnson (1978) reported using therapeutic hypnosis to facilitate rehabilitation of a 16-year-old girl with significant brain damage. The patient was comatose when the therapists first began making suggestions for invitation of hypnosis. She responded to specific imagery designed to help her recapture her ability to swallow, to move extremities, to dress herself ("Imagine yourself dressing a life-sized doll"), and to speak. Over a period of weeks, this patient became alert and regained autonomic reflex responses, motor skills, and speech.

## Intellectual Disabilities and Developmental Delay

Hypnosis invitation with developmentally delayed children and adolescents must take into account the mental age of the patient. The therapist can then proceed to some extent as if the child's chronological age were the same as his or her mental age. As development in children with delays may be very uneven, and social skills may sometimes be far more advanced than cognitive skills, it will be particularly important for the clinician not only to have developed a careful rapport with the child but also to have a clear understanding of the child's level of ability and disability. We have had successful experiences children with mild intellectual disabilities (e.g., IQs 50–70) and with young adults who are developmentally childlike. Children with more severe delays or retardation usually respond poorly or not at all to invitation to hypnosis. Such patients do not seem capable of necessary levels of ability to relate to the therapist, of focusing attention selectively, and of following instructions. Even if they do respond to an invitation to hypnosis process, they usually do not benefit from therapeutic hypnosis suggestions, probably because of limited conceptualization, memory, and language skills.

## Learning Differences

As much as possible, the therapist must understand the specific areas of disability in order to modify invitation and therapeutic hypnosis accordingly. Many children with learning differences and difficulties may also have difficulties with associated inattention, impulsivity, distractibility, and a variety of behavioral problems, some of which may be secondary to their learning problems, and some of which may be part of an overall problem such as attention-deficit disorder (with or without hyperactivity). Increasingly, clinicians and educators who work with children with learning difficulties are utilizing creative approaches such as various forms of hypnosis-like self-regulation (e.g., imagery or biofeedback) to maximizing learning.

## Abused Children

Prior to the consideration of therapeutic hypnosis for a child or teenager who has been abused, the clinician must ensure that the young person is safe; that thorough medical, psychological, and family assessments have been conducted; and that care for all involved is ongoing. Recognition of the powerful and potentially far-reaching impact of physical or sexual abuse will remind clinicians to think carefully about the principles of forming relationships and the critical aspects of developing rapport with abuse victims. In doing so, we will recognize the (potential) vulnerability of abuse victims and will be more effective in becoming part of the solution rather than part of the problem.

Children and adolescents who have been the victims of physical or sexual abuse may be best understood to have experienced some degree of posttraumatic stress disorder (PTSD). Friedrich (1991) suggested that a hypnotic state is induced or occurs at the time of abuse, similar perhaps to the "negative" trance phenomenon experienced by children or adults in emergency situations (see Chapters 8 and 13), during natural disasters (such as floods, tornadoes, or earthquakes), or by victims and refugees of wars. Because of our awareness of this vulnerability, we encourage clinicians to proceed with caution even in initial history taking and rapport development and to be alert to the reappearance of spontaneous hypnotic states (e.g., especially dissociation) for their potential diagnostic and therapeutic value. In his work with abused children, Friedrich (1991) emphasized that hypnosis may be used therapeutically for symptom stabilization and removal, for controlled uncovering of the traumatic events through regression, and toward integration with the goal of facilitating mastery and a return to optimal pre-trauma functioning. As we have noted for many clinical situations, Friedrich (1991) emphasized "joining" with the child victim and suggested that by listening carefully and through the use of his or her own language the clinician can more easily help the child victim hypnotically to begin to understand and reframe his or her traumatic experience to facilitate positive rather than maladaptation.

Rhue and Lynn (1991, 1993) described the application and value of storytelling as a therapeutic hypnosis strategy for treatment of sexually abused children. They, too, emphasized the importance of therapeutic rapport and describe collaborative storytelling (1993) with a major beginning focus being the identification of a "safe context" and "building a safe haven, a favorite place," in which ongoing therapeutic hypnosis can proceed.

Clinicians who work with victims of abuse or other trauma are encouraged to review Friedrich's (1991) and Rhue and Lynn's (1991, 1993) detailed case reports for more specific information and the description of various thoughtful, creative, and successful hypnotic strategies. (See also Chapter 8 for more extensive discussion of therapeutic hypnosis and PTSD.)

## Autism Spectrum Disorder (ASD) and Severely Disturbed Children

Gardner and Tarnow (1980) provided a case report regarding the use of therapeutic hypnosis with an adolescent with mild ASD. Efforts to use traditional approaches to therapeutic hypnosis were met with minimal responses. Listening to a favorite piece of music proved to be successful initiation of hypnosis, during which this patient responded with spontaneous eye closure, neck and jaw relaxation, and hand catalepsy. Severely autistic children who have little capacity for interpersonal relationships are not likely to respond to more "traditional" hypnosis invitations (see also Chapter 9). Olness has found the use of eye fixation on a biofeedback monitor to be a successful initiation method for some severely disturbed children. As they watch the shapes, lines, or numbers change, appropriate suggestions are made regarding their ability to concentrate, to control their body, and to do positive things for themselves. Kohen has noted that many youths with mild ASD engage easily and with curiosity with, and are highly responsive to, biofeedback and especially portable devices such as the emWave Personal Stress Reliever® (www.heartmath.com) (see also Chapter 9). As with any child, such approaches must be individualized to the unique needs, likes and dislikes, and style of each child. It seems reasonable that children with severe ego deficits might respond best to induction techniques that are adaptations of soothing, comforting, nonverbal methods similar to those recommended for use with young children.

## Terminally Ill Children and Adolescents

It is very important that invitation to and initiation of hypnosis with terminally ill children and adolescents enhances their sense of mastery. It should be clear to such patients (and their families) that they are involved in treatment planning from the beginning and that the methods chosen are their own. Whenever possible, clinical consultation for possible hypnosis with young people who are dying should take place well before their final hours. Unfortunately, that does not commonly happen. Many of these patients are weak and sometimes affected by sedatives and pain medications when we meet them. If possible, the timing of initiation/invitation of therapeutic hypnosis should be the maximum possible number of hours after the last sedative or pain medication. Sometimes, however, even a heavily sedated child will respond. For these patients, reinforcement via audio recording may be helpful so they may choose to listen whenever and as often as they choose and are able. Parental assistance and telephone reinforcement from the therapist are necessary more often than in those with self-limited or non-life-threatening problems (see also Chapter 15).

## Teaching Self-Hypnosis

It is almost always useful and important to teach children self-hypnosis, particularly when problems relate to recurrent difficulties or discomfort, or to undesirable habits. This subject has been discussed in the literature both separately (Gardner, 1981) and in the context of treatment of specific pediatric problems such as hemophilia (LaBaw, 1975), functional megacolon (Olness, 1976), or habits (Kohen, 1991). For children who practice self-hypnosis, the advantages are twofold: (1) their sense of control and mastery is acknowledged, and (2) desired behavior is more frequently reinforced by repetition of appropriate imagery exercises.

Gardner (1981) noted that brief didactic teaching concerning the abuse of self-hypnosis is usually sufficient to prevent children from giving demonstrations to their friends or acting as well-meaning but untrained "hypnotherapists." The risk of abuse is higher in children with poor judgment or poor impulse control or children with sociopathic tendencies; teaching self-hypnosis as such is usually contraindicated in such cases. Using these guidelines, we have not known any of our patients to abuse their self-hypnotic skills.

We find that the major problem with teaching children self-hypnosis is ensuring that they actually do practice the exercises on a prescribed daily basis. In one study (Kohen, Colwell, Heimel, & Olness, 1984), some children reported becoming bored with the prescribed practice, or "forgot" to do it. Even with cooperative parents, an excellent response to therapeutic hypnosis, and office or telephone reinforcement from the therapist, relatively few children continue self-hypnosis practice beyond a few months. This is particularly so if they have had success in resolving their problem. Some children resist the recommendation of using self-hypnosis. Factors producing this sort of resistance include inadequate motivation to solve the problem, the age and developmental level of the child, transference to the therapist, fear that therapy visits will cease if the child uses hypnosis independently, and parental interference. It is usually possible to deal successfully with resistance to using self-hypnosis. In the case of very young children, we prepare a personal recording for the child or involve a parent in the practice, striving to make the process both creative and fun, as well as successful. The involvement of the parent serves a dual purpose, as the parents of children with chronic illness benefit from acknowledgment by healthcare providers that they are able to contribute in some way to the therapeutic process.

Children who resist self-hypnosis because of fear that therapy visits will cease can be specifically reassured that this will not occur. The therapist can also make phone calls for a time in order to effect a smooth termination in cases where cessation of therapy is, in fact, appropriate and desirable. We have also found that writing letters or e-mails to the patient after or as part of the ongoing termination or separation process can have a positive effect on encouraging regular self-hypnosis practice.

Some children resist self-hypnosis as a reaction against parental interference, sometimes well-intentioned and sometimes not. The problem is especially likely to arise in the case of children with enuresis (Kohen et al., 1984), probably because wet beds can be especially vexing to parents and can trigger their anger and frustration more easily than other problems such as pain or anxiety.

Jacobs (1962) reported a case history of a 6-year-old girl suffering from enuresis. The child believed that her parents didn't love her. When the child was in a hypnotic trance, suggestions were given that she would learn a signal when her bladder was full and that her parents loved her whether or not she was wet. At first, she did very well. The mother was instructed that each night she put the child to bed she should hold her and kiss her, tell her what a good girl she was, tell her how much the family loved her, and how easy it would be to remember the signal, thus reinforcing the therapist's suggestions. After family financial setbacks, the mother subsequently became distraught, shouted at the child, and spanked her, and the patient experienced a relapse. After discussion with the therapist, the previous suggestions were reinforced, and the patient had no further problems. It is important to remember that unpleasant habits and behavior patterns in children commonly induce unpleasant habit reaction patterns in family members, and therapists must consider those patterns when developing a treatment plan that is tailored to a particular child in the context of his or her family.

We specifically request that parents not remind children who have habit problems to practice self-hypnosis, often suggesting more positive ways for them to give attention. We tell children in the presence of the parent that their parents are not to remind them. We then focus in detail with the child concerning how best to remember to practice. Possibilities include putting a sign on the door, tying a string around the toothbrush, putting a note beside the dinner plate, or tying a sign around the neck of a favorite stuffed animal. The goals, of course, are to engage the parent to agree with and acknowledge the child's decision and to shift a negative frame of mind (about this problem) to a positive one for child and family alike. Following this, the parent is asked to leave, and the therapist works with the child alone.

It also seems useful to agree on the place where the child will practice self-hypnosis and to allow for trips out of town or overnight visits to friends. In general, we ask that the child practice in a sitting position (because it is too easy to fall asleep if one practices imagery and relaxation in the recumbent position!) in his or her room. Occasionally, and in consultation with the parent, the therapist and child might decide on a particular chair in the study or living room. The chosen place should be quiet. The child should usually practice alone, although we know of children who successfully practice during rest periods or other breaks during their school day.

When desired therapeutic objectives are being accomplished and frequent office visits are not necessary, we recommend that the child call or write to the therapist on a regularly scheduled basis. The child is then asked to verbalize the self-hypnosis exercise over the phone, and the therapist reinforces where necessary. It is also essential to arrange for a time to terminate self-hypnosis exercises – for example, 1 month after all beds are dry. This implies that the therapist expects success and that the patient is motivated to continue. Occasionally, a child will become bored with a certain image in the induction, and suggestions can be provided for change.

Gardner (1981) described a three-step method for teaching children self-hypnosis, easily accomplished in one session. For a historical perspective the reader may be interested in this method:

1. The therapist uses various invitation and intensification methods, usually emphasizing imagery and ideomotor techniques. The latter are especially useful for children who want some outward and visible sign that hypnosis has been achieved. After allowing time for enjoyment of the imagery, the therapist asks the child to count silently up to five, eyes opening at three, fully alert at five. The therapist comments that the child now knows how to come out of hypnosis and return to the alert state without help. Rapid alerting in emergencies may also be discussed.

2. Therapist and patient discuss which of the invitation/initiation techniques employed in step 1 were most helpful and agree to discard the rest. The child is then asked to describe to the therapist in detail the techniques chosen for induction, to feel the same good feelings, and to go into hypnosis easily and naturally as the description proceeds. The therapist may add details if the child's wording is too general. After another pause and a reassuring comment, the therapist asks the child to return to the normal alert state. Problems are discussed as necessary.
3. This is the same as step 2 except that the child is asked to recall and to decide to experience the (self) invitation silently. Neither child nor therapist speaks. The child nods when trance is achieved. After another pause, the child returns again to the usual state of alertness. Any remaining problems or questions are then discussed. The child is then ready for full independent use of self-hypnosis.

Alternatively, one of us (DPK) invariably teaches self-hypnosis during each patient's first hypnotic experience, with incorporation of Ericksonian-like expectancy suggestions and liberal use of ego-strengthening and future-oriented suggestions. Following induction and intensification (deepening) of hypnosis, and whatever therapeutic utilization suggestions may be offered during the first hypnotic experience, suggestions for and training in self-hypnosis are provided along with posthypnotic suggestions before the end of the experience (see also Chapter 17):

> Before you come to the end of what you have learned so well today, be sure to congratulate yourself for how well you've done, and be proud of how your brain and body are learning to talk to each other so well. It's nice before you finish to remind yourself of what you did to help give yourself the good feelings you have now, so that when you practice this one or two or three times each day for 10 or 15 minutes, you'll know exactly how to do it. So, just picture in your mind where you might sit at home when you practice, and then see yourself doing the fingers-together game [or whatever induction was used] to start off your self-hypnosis [or self-relaxation and imagination or whatever words are being used]. Great … now notice that as your eyes close and you start to get comfortable that you can imagine about anything you want … perhaps it will be about playing soccer or [add choices of several of child's favorite activities] … and you can notice everything about it … and when you practice this at home in this same way, you'll be able to notice just as you have today and now the way your muscles relax as you breathe out. And you can allow the relaxation feeling to move down your body all the way … that's right … and then, just like today, as soon as the relaxation has gotten all the way to your head [or toes], then you can let your head nod [or your finger lift], and that will be the signal to yourself that you are as comfortable as you want to be for that practice time. And then, before you finish practicing, make sure you give your mind and body any directions or new ideas you want them to have [substitute here any therapeutic hypnotic suggestions specific to the child and his or her problems]. And the last thing that you need to know when you practice at home and here is that if you happen to be practicing at bedtime, you don't have to even finish, you can just let your self-hypnosis practice finish by falling asleep. And if you happen to be practicing at some other time, then when you're finished, you'll be done, and you can open your eyes and bring your good feelings back with you.

## Hypnotic Invitations with Other Names

We have noted that there are still uncertainties about what hypnosis is and what should be the correct definition. In spite of documentation of the therapeutic benefits of hypnosis for many problems, there remains a public suspicion that it is dangerous or ineffective or silly. Unfortunately, hypnosis appears as entertainment on television, in schools, on social media, and other public venues.

Throughout this book we note the similarities among hypnosis and other self-regulation training, including biofeedback, relaxation response training, guided imagery, mind-body therapy, mindfulness, mindfulness meditation, autogenic training, CBT, progressive relaxation, Integrated Mental Training, Koru mindfulness training, visualization, and dozens of variations sold on the internet. What is the generic piece among all of these strategies, tools, and programs? Each intends in some way to help increase the capacity to self-regulate some part of human mind-body connections.

Depending on the individual differences and preferences in children and adolescents the child health professional might offer a ritualistic invitation such as progressive relaxation or a focus on breathing or, rather, conversational hypnosis. The child health professional must take time to establish meaningful rapport and emphasize that this tool belongs to the child or adolescent. Offering guided imagery could be risky; the child may not appreciate the image offered. Offering a focus on breathing may be of no interest to a young child.

## Conclusions

Hypnotic invitation/initiation is usually a pleasant and creative experience both for child patients and for their therapists. Techniques can be modified to suit children of different ages or with special problems such as physical disability. Most children readily learn self-hypnosis and can benefit from this additional skill. It is important to consider learning styles and family and cultural differences for an individual child before deciding which hypnotic technique is most apt to be suitable for that child. The choice of specific [self] initiation/invitation techniques is based on the therapist's ingenuity as well as on the child's needs, preferences, and abilities. Although such choices are now based on clinical judgment, future research may show that some problems or some children respond better to one technique than to another. To date, such studies have not been reported.

## References

Aronson, D.M. (1986). The adolescent as hypnotist: hypnosis and self-hypnosis with adolescent psychiatric inpatients. *American Journal of Clinical Hypnosis, 28*, 163–169.

Culbert, T.P., Reaney, J., & Kohen, D.P. (1994). Cyberphysiologic strategies in children: the biofeedback–hypnosis interface. *International Journal of Clinical and Experimental Hypnosis, 42*(2), 97–117.

Erickson, M.H. (1958b). Pediatric hypnotherapy. *American Journal of Clinical Hypnosis*, 1, 25-29.

Erickson, M.H. (1959). Further techniques of hypnosis: utilization techniques. *American Journal of Clinical Hypnosis, 2*, 3–21.

Friedrich, W.N. (1991). Hypnotherapy with traumatized children. *International Journal of Clinical and Experimental Hypnosis, 39*(2), 67–81.

Gardner, G.G. (1981). Teaching self-hypnosis to children. *International Journal of Clinical and Experimental Hypnosis, 29*, 300–312.

Gardner, G.G. & Tarnow, J.D. (1980). Adjunctive hypnotherapy with an autistic boy. *American Journal of Clinical Hypnosis, 22*, 173–179.

Jacobs, L. (1962). Hypnosis in clinical pediatrics. *New York State Journal of Medicine, 62*, 3781–3787.

Kohen, D.P. (1991). Applications of relaxation/mental imagery (self-hypnosis) for habit problems. *Pediatric Annals, 20*(3), 136–144.

Kohen, D.P. (2017). The '3 and 6' Hypnotic Induction Technique for Children and Adolescents Chapter 8, pp 145-160. In M.P. Jensen Ed. *(2017) The Art and Practice of Hypnotic Induction – Favorite Methods of Master Clinicians*. Kirkland, WA: Denny Creek Press. 98033.

Kohen, D.P., Colwell, S.O., Heimel, A., & Olness, K.N. (1984). The use of relaxation/mental imagery (self-hypnosis) in the management of 505 pediatric behavioral encounters. *Journal of Developmental and Behavioral Pediatrics*, *5*(1), 21–25.

Kohen, D.P., Mann-Rinehart, P., Schmitz, D., & Wills, L. (1998). Using hypnosis to help deaf children help themselves: report of two cases. *American Journal of Clinical Hypnosis*, *40*, 288–296.

Kohen, D.P. & Wynne, E. (1988). A Preschool Family Asthma Education Program: Uses of Storytelling, Imagery, and Relaxation, paper presented at the 11th International Congress of Hypnosis and Psychosomatic Medicine, The Hague, The Netherlands.

Korn, E.R. & Johnson, K. (1978). Hypnosis and Imagery in Rehabilitation of a Brain Damaged Patient, paper presented at the annual meeting of the American Society of Clinical Hypnosis, St. Louis, MO.

LaBaw, W.L. (1975). Autohypnosis in hemophilia. *Haematologia*, *9*, 103–110.

Olness, K. (1976). Autohypnosis in functional megacolon in children. *American Journal of Clinical Hypnosis*, *19*, 28–32.

Olness, K. & Singher, L. (1989). Five year follow-up of 61 children taught cyber-physiologic strategies as adjunct management in cancer. *Topics in Pediatrics*, 7, 2–6.

Rhue, J.W. & Lynn, S.J. (1991). Storytelling, hypnosis and the treatment of sexually abused children. *International Journal of Clinical and Experimental Hypnosis*, *39*(4), 198–214.

Rhue, J.W. & Lynn, S.J. (1993). Hypnosis and storytelling in the treatment of child sexual abuse: strategies and procedures. In J.W. Rhue, S.J. Lynn, & I. Kirsch, Eds., *Handbook of Clinical Hypnosis* (pp. 455–478). Washington, D.C.: American Psychological Association.

Sugarman, L.I. (1997/2007). *Hypnosis in Pediatric Practice: imaginative Medicine in Action (video and instructional manual)*. Bethel, CT:Crown House Publishing.

# PART II

# Therapeutic Applications of Hypnosis with Children

# 6

# GENERAL PRINCIPLES OF THERAPEUTIC APPLICATIONS OF CHILD HYPNOSIS

## Introduction

We will now review techniques and results of hypnosis for a wide range of childhood problems. Most published accounts of hypnosis and hypnotherapy for specific childhood problems include some general comments concerning principles, indications, contraindications, and pitfalls of this therapeutic modality. A few papers (Call, 1976; Erickson, 1959; Kaffman, 1968; Olness & Kohen, 1984; Williams & Singh, 1976; Wright, 1960; Wright & Wright, 1987) have focused directly on basic issues. To avoid repetition in succeeding chapters, we devote this chapter to a discussion of general principles of therapeutic child hypnosis. Some of our thoughts are shared by most people in the field, whereas others will provoke varying degrees of controversy.

## Definition and Boundaries of Hypnotherapy (Therapeutic Hypnosis)

Hypnosis and hypnotherapy are two different entities. Over the decade since our fourth edition we and others researching, writing, and teaching pediatric hypnosis to colleagues, patients, and families have come to preferentially use the word Hypnosis to describe both the phenomenology and the therapeutic application and utilization of hypnosis. That has led us to the retitling of this edition as Hypnosis with Children.

Hypnosis is an altered/alternative state of awareness that may have certain temporary beneficial effects, such as tension reduction, but it is not in itself designed for that purpose. What has been called "Hypnotherapy" is a treatment modality with specific therapeutic goals and specific techniques utilized *while* the patient is in the state of hypnosis. We also distinguish between a hypnotist and a hypnotherapist, for these terms are often confused in the context of clinical work. A hypnotist – often found listed in the classified advertisements of newspapers or in the yellow pages of the telephone directory under "Hypnotists" – may be a person with limited education whose only skill is the use of hypnosis and who often accepts nearly everyone for treatment. Although such people may get some good results – otherwise they could not stay in business – they may engage in indiscriminate use of their one skill, sometimes with unfortunate results. In our experience most who refer to themselves as "Hypnotists" are generally not health care professionals.

A hypnotherapist is, first of all, a therapist. A child hypnotherapist has advanced training in one of the child health professions and uses hypnosis, or so-called hypnotherapeutic techniques (to which we

DOI: 10.4324/9781003243687-8

now refer as therapeutic hypnosis) as part of a comprehensive approach to the diagnosis and treatment of certain disorders. In this context, it is a good rule of thumb that one should NEVER attempt to treat a problem with hypnosis or hypnotherapy unless one is also competent to assess and manage the problem without hypnosis and/or recommend other therapists if appropriate. When parents ask us about hypnotists, we do our best to educate them with regard to these distinctions.

We believe that the practice of clinical therapeutic hypnosis with children should be limited to health professionals who typically assume primary responsibility for treating children's problems, including, for example, child psychologists, pediatric social workers, psychiatrists, dentists, pediatricians, pediatric nurse practitioners and clinical nurse specialists, child life specialists, and other specialty and sub-specialty physicians and surgeons who work with children. Other appropriate child health specialists who might well incorporate and integrate hypnosis or hypnotic strategies in their therapeutic work include pediatric occupational therapists, pediatric physical therapists, speech pathologists, and nurse anesthetists. Furthermore, these professionals should appropriately limit their hypnosis work to their own areas of competence. This does not mean that a psychologist should never treat pain with hypnosis. It does mean, however, that the psychologist who does so is also competent to treat pain with other methods (e.g., supportive psychotherapy or biofeedback).

Increasingly, nurses, physical therapists, speech pathologists, and other child health specialists utilize hypnosis in the context of their specialty practice, either in the context of a multidisciplinary team or practice or in an independent private practice. If their practice is performed under the supervision or responsibility of a physician, dentist, or psychologist, then their use of therapeutic hypnosis should also be conducted under the direct supervision of a health professional with appropriate training and competency in the use of therapeutic clinical hypnosis with children.

## Goals of Therapeutic Hypnosis

People who come to us requesting hypnosis begin by saying, "I have a problem." Often they really mean to say, "A problem has me." That is, they perceive themselves as having been rendered passive and helpless, the victim of a situation over which they have virtually no control. Often, previous therapeutic efforts either have been of limited value or have contributed to the patient's passive-dependent stance by forcing continued reliance on external powers such as machines and medication.

The goal of hypnosis is always to teach the patient an attitude of hope in the context of mastery. The patient learns to be an active participant on his or her own behalf, to focus on creating a solution rather than on enduring a problem, and to discover and use resources for inner control as much as possible. The goal of mastery does not mean that the patient necessarily turns away from external aid, although this may sometimes be possible. An anxious child may no longer need tranquilizers; a child with asthma may no longer need a nebulizer. However, the child successfully using [self] hypnosis may continue to require external help, albeit now in a different psychological context. Thus, a child in renal failure may continue regular dialysis but has less anxiety and depression, is more motivated to participate in treatment, and is more cooperative with necessary dietary restrictions. Because the child is now cooperative with the diet, the need for dialysis is reduced, and the child may perceive the machine as a useful aid rather than as an external imposition.

The so-called First Law of Hypnosis emphasizes that the patient must be able to define or perceive a desired therapeutic outcome. It is essential that the therapist also keep this in mind. Sometimes, the outcome desired by the parents or therapist is not the same as that desired by the child. This can be explored in various ways with children – for example, "We've been talking for a while. Am I right in understanding that what you want is to have all of your beds dry in the morning?" Or, during the first hypnotic invitation the therapist can ask the child to indicate which finger represents "yes," which represents "no," and which represents "I don't know." Then, when the child appears very comfortable, the clinician can say, "I'll ask some questions that you can answer with your fingers. Do you like chocolate ice cream? Do you like to go to bed at night? Do you like the color blue? Would you like to have dry beds at night? Do you like to eat pizza?" Occasionally, the ideomotor response will be "no," and this is an indication that further work must be done before teaching the child self-hypnosis. It is also important in structuring suggestions to include *future programming* – for example, "Think of something you're looking forward to next summer. You needn't tell me what it is. Imagine that it's next summer, and you are enjoying what you're doing, just as if you were really there. And, while you are enjoying it, you can also enjoy thinking how nice it is that your beds are all dry because of your work, because you have become the boss of your bladder – and then you can continue to imagine you're enjoying what you are looking forward to next summer."

### Recognizing Developmental Issues

That a child is not an adult seems obvious, but it is a fact sometimes overlooked in hypnosis. If a child patient is to achieve the goal of mastery through successful response to hypnotic invitation and therapeutic techniques, language must be adapted to the level and interests of that child, being neither too complex nor too simple and patronizing. As in any therapy, the clinician teaching and guiding hypnosis must take into account the child's perceptual and conceptual skills with respect to problems and possible solutions. For this reason, it is often best to let the child select some of the details of imagery used in therapeutic hypnotic suggestions. The therapists might say, "Think of a way you can feel safe," and then follow the child's lead instead of suggesting a particular plan. If the child patient is seen at different points over a period of time, it is important to remember that techniques that were appealing and helpful at one age may have no value or even be aversive at a later age. The degree to which children mix reality and fantasy is often a cause of fears and other problems, but this developmental tendency can become an advantage in doing hypnosis work. The child may respond particularly well, for example, to imagery techniques such as rehearsal in fantasy, experiencing a new behavior first in hypnotic imagery and then quickly becoming able to make the transition to incorporating that behavior in reality situations.

### Misinformation about Hypnosis and Clinical Therapeutic Hypnosis

Unfortunately, many children have developed misconceptions about hypnosis before they come to a medical office for therapeutic clinical hypnosis. This may come from television programs, movies, books, or friends. In the children's book *A Dinosaur's Story: The Wildest Show on Earth* (Hughes, 1993), two children are hypnotized by Professor Screweyes to join his Eccentric Circus. Such a story is frightening to many children. It is important that clinicians learning and utilizing hypnosis learn what the child's perceptions about hypnosis are, to explain hypnosis in the appropriate language, and to emphasize that the therapist will teach the child a skill that belongs to the child and over which the child has control.

### Parental Involvement

In some instances, particularly when the parent has been overprotective or when the child needs greater autonomy, it is best to minimize the parental role in hypnosis. The parents may be asked specifically to refrain from reminding the child to practice self-hypnosis and to allow the child privacy during practice sessions. The clinician therapist gives the parent a general explanation of the treatment program. The following vignette is an example of this approach.

Hugh N., age 7 years, suffered from severe asthma. Finding self-hypnosis very helpful, he became able to participate more fully in school and in sports and was especially proud of being able to help himself and not always have to rely on his parents for medication. Soon after therapeutic hypnosis began, his mother said to the therapist, "When Hugh begins to wheeze, he goes to his room and closes the door. After about 5 minutes, he comes out, and he's not wheezing, and I don't know what he does in there!" The therapist answered, "I know what I asked him to do, but I don't know what he really does in there, either. What is important is that Hugh is better." The mother continued to allow her son the privacy and independence he needed.

In some cases, the child may need the parent's presence either in the therapist's office or during the use of self-hypnosis in order to help focus on hypnotic suggestions or to provide reassurance. Ellen L., an adolescent girl, had difficulty sleeping because of chronic, progressive pain with associated anxiety. Although she learned self-hypnosis, the severity of her pain sometimes interfered with her ability to concentrate on hypnotic suggestions. Her mother willingly served as a surrogate therapist when needed, with the results that both the mother and Ellen got more sleep and felt more hopeful about Ellen's condition.

Most parents abide by the therapist's recommendations concerning the degree of their involvement. A few parents consciously or unconsciously sabotage the therapy. This seems to occur most often when the child is not improving at the speed at which the parent would have hoped or would prefer, or when parents have the mistaken idea that they are in charge of the child's self-hypnosis practice. Thus, sometimes a parent, albeit well-intentioned, will insist that the child "go practice self-hypnosis and relaxing, right now!" much as they might insist that the garbage be taken out or that it is now time for piano practice or homework. This usually comes to our attention as clinicians when the child is not improving, when progress seems to plateau, or when the parent complains that "it's not working." A careful review of the history will commonly reveal parental over-involvement or misconception and will lead to a thoughtful conversation (or more, as needed) regarding the child's normal developmental and maturational needs, the significance of their belief in ownership of the self-hypnosis, and ways that the parent can and perhaps even should be involved that do not risk sabotaging a positive outcome.

Sometimes careful assessment points to the need for the parents or other family members to be involved, not just to support the child but as full participants in family therapy, with or without hypnosis. Just as in child psychotherapy, parents of children presenting for hypnosis may focus the pathology on the child when they also need help. If the parents refuse to participate in therapy, sometimes it is possible to make at least partial gains with the child alone. In such cases, the parents may be willing to be seen every few weeks for counseling or for a review of the current home situation. We prefer this "half-measure" approach to that of no therapy for the child. Sometimes the parents' trust will eventually increase to the point that they enter therapy. At the least, it may be possible to teach the child more effective ways of coping in the family situation. We realize, however, that this therapeutic strategy may reinforce the parents' conviction that the locus of the problem is in the child, making the parents even more resistant to treatment for themselves. There is the added risk, if therapeutic hypnosis with the child is successful, that the parents may then find another target for the pathology, perhaps another child or even the marital relationship itself.

## Types of Therapeutic Approaches with Hypnosis

To say that a child is using therapeutic clinical hypnosis really tells us very little by itself except that hypnosis is being employed somehow in the treatment program. Therapeutic hypnosis refers to the use of a variety of hypnotic techniques in the context of some form of psychotherapy, using that term in its broadest sense. Thus, therapeutic hypnosis may be employed in the context of relationship or supportive therapy, behavior modification, psychoanalysis and dynamic therapies, gestalt therapy, or cognitive behavioral therapy. Some therapeutic hypnosis methods are common across several psychotherapeutic approaches, whereas others have more limited application; for example, hypnotic relaxation is used to facilitate progress both in analytically oriented therapy and in behavior modification. Hypnotically induced dreaming, on the other hand, might be employed in the analytic approach but probably not in a behavior modification program.

The specific therapeutic hypnosis techniques used with a particular patient are derived from the nature of the presenting problem, the patient's goal, other patient characteristics, the therapist's theoretical orientation, and certain situational factors such as the amount of time available for treatment. The numerous possible therapeutic hypnosis techniques have many variations. Specific examples will be described in Chapters 7 through 15. At this point, we simply divide therapeutic hypnosis methods into three broad categories.

### *Supportive, Ego-Enhancing Methods*

The chief goal here is to help the child feel more worthy, more capable of dealing effectively with problems and challenges, and more able to contribute to his or her own well-being and to be in control of circumstances both internal and external. Patients who fear necessary surgery, who experience pervasive anxiety, or who manifest borderline or psychotic behavior often derive special benefits from supportive techniques. These methods may also be used prospectively in the course of routine pediatric care – for example, "I will look forward to your telling me about the fun things you do in kindergarten" or "Your muscles feel strong. I think you can use them to learn to ride your new bike." Such supportive phrases may be applied appropriately in emergency situations such as when a child arrives in the emergency room with a laceration.

### *Symptom-Oriented Methods*

Here the therapeutic effort is directed at removing, altering, or alleviating specific symptoms, either physical or emotional in nature. Difficulties associated with phobias, pain control, and habit control, among many others, often respond to symptom-oriented approaches, especially if the patient is highly motivated to be rid of the symptom. These symptom-oriented approaches are contraindicated if the symptom serves as a major defensive purpose such as to protect the patient from severe underlying depression or the outbreak of psychosis.

### *Dynamic, Insight-Oriented Methods*

Again the goals are symptom relief and ego strengthening, but now special methods are employed to help the patient understand issues that create and maintain problems, gain insight into and work through underlying conflicts, and achieve a more extensive shift toward personality maturation in broad cognitive, affective, and social spheres. Generally speaking, supportive and symptom-oriented methods are most often used with children, and dynamic methods are used to a somewhat lesser extent. For some child patients, therapeutic hypnosis includes a combination of all three of these approaches.

### *Indications for Therapeutic Clinical Hypnosis*

Because the rest of this fifth edition is devoted to a detailed review of situations in which children can benefit from therapeutic clinical hypnosis, we limit this section to a few general comments. It is generally accepted that clinical hypnosis as a therapeutic modality is underutilized in the treatment of children. Moreover, clinical hypnosis is too often considered as a last resort, despite the fact that it might have several advantages over other – even previously considered "standard" treatment modalities or "treatments of choice." These advantages include frequent appeal to and acceptance by the child patient, few risks and side effects, frequent rapid response to treatment, and the fact that therapeutic hypnosis fosters attitudes of independence and mastery in coping with problems. A child can be considered a suitable candidate for clinical hypnosis if: (1) the child is responsive to invitation to hypnosis methods, (2) the problem is known to be treatable by therapeutic clinical hypnosis, (3) the child can relate positively to the clinicians/therapists, (4) the child has at least minimal motivation to solve the problem and is willing to do self-hypnosis practice, (5) the parents or other responsible adults agree to the treatment plan, and (6) the use of clinical hypnosis for the problem at hand would not harm the patient.

## Contraindications

As child therapeutic clinical hypnosis achieves continued increasing acceptance by health professionals and the general public, the problem of underutilization gives way to excessive enthusiasm and sometimes inappropriate utilization. Parents and other well-meaning adults sometimes put great pressure on us to use clinical hypnosis as rapidly and forcefully as possible with child patients so as to eliminate troublesome symptoms. Children, too, sometimes make inappropriate demands for clinical hypnosis. It is incumbent on us to resist this pressure.

We also occasionally see excessive enthusiasm about therapeutic clinical hypnosis in some health professionals who have just begun training in this subspecialty and have been exposed to accounts of dramatic cures. Sometimes these professionals think of their patients with the most difficult problems and conclude that clinical hypnosis is bound to be the answer to their unsolved problems. While occasionally this is true; more often it is not. In detailed discussion of such cases, we tend to find either that the therapist has underestimated the patient's degree of pathology or that the therapist has problems with a counter-transferential need to be all things to all people. In such cases, we try to educate professionals toward more rational use of therapeutic clinical hypnosis.

The situations in which we believe hypnosis is absolutely contraindicated may be categorized as follows:

Granting the request could lead to physical endangerment for the patient.
Granting the request could aggravate existing emotional problems or create new ones.
The request is simply to "have fun" experimenting with hypnosis.
The problem is more effectively treated by some method other than hypnosis.
The diagnosis is incorrect, and the real problem should be treated some other way.

There are also some relative contraindications for hypnosis, usually based on inappropriate timing of the referral. In these situations, granting the request for immediate therapeutic clinical hypnosis treatment would involve overlooking a significant medical problem, overwhelming the patient's ego, or trying to impose change on an unmotivated child. In such situations, clinical hypnosis may be appropriate if utilized at a later time or in a manner different from what the patient or parent demands.

### Absolute Contraindication: Risking Physical Endangerment

Eddie Y., a 15-year-old, admitted with some embarrassment that although he enjoyed playing football he became frightened when he was rushed by larger players. Convinced that anxiety impaired his running and passing skills, he asked, "Could you hypnotize me so that I couldn't see these big guys, and then I wouldn't be afraid?" Eddie was told that it might be possible for him to experience such a hypnotic negative hallucination, but that it was most inadvisable since he couldn't dodge players if he couldn't see them. He quickly understood that he would not only endanger himself by such use of hypnosis but would also quickly become a detriment to the team. He also agreed with the idea that a mild degree of anxiety can be appropriate and even beneficial to his performance. Reconsidering, he concluded that his anxiety was within normal limits. He felt assured that he could seek more appropriate kinds of treatment, with or without hypnotherapy, if ever his anxiety truly reached irrational and maladaptive proportions. He continued playing football without further difficulty.

### Absolute Contraindication: Risking Aggravation of Emotional Problems

Cynthia N., an angry and depressed adolescent girl, telephoned the therapist to report a very unhappy experience with a boyfriend and requested one or two sessions of clinical hypnosis for the sole purpose of developing amnesia for her entire relationship with him. The therapist explained that it was unlikely that she could achieve and maintain such an extensive amnesia; that clinical hypnosis could not produce such magic cures. Even if she could accomplish this goal, however, it was inadvisable because she might then develop much more serious emotional difficulties. For example, instead of learning skills for coping with this circumscribed problem, she might achieve only partial repression and then develop a maladaptive reaction such as general depression or anxiety, perhaps leading to deeper problems in relating to men. The therapist suggested a longer course of psychotherapy that might include therapeutic clinical hypnosis, but not for the purpose of creating amnesia. Cynthia refused and insisted that she would continue her search until she found someone who would grant her request. We have no follow-up on this girl.

### Absolute Contraindication: Hypnosis for Fun

Walter B., an adolescent boy who had recently met the therapist socially, asked to be hypnotized "just for fun." The therapist denied the request and explained why hypnosis should be limited to research and therapeutic situations. Walter agreed with the decision after he understood that hypnosis is an altered state of consciousness in which he might have unexpected emotional reactions that could not and should not be treated in a brief social encounter. He was impressed by a few vignettes of professionals participating in hypnotic invitations as part of hypnosis workshops. Although the hypnotic suggestion was simply to recall and enjoy a pleasant experience, two persons developed unexpected grief reactions, and a third developed a mild paranoid reaction. Though such reactions are rare, they are unfortunate. Walter saw that one might choose to risk such a reaction as a participant in a hypnosis workshop or as a subject in a research study, but that there was no sense in taking such a risk when the only goal was "to have fun."

### Absolute Contraindication: Clinical Hypnosis Considered Not the Most Effective Treatment

Bobby A.'s mother sought clinical hypnosis for her 5-year-old son to help him overcome an extreme fear of dogs. He refused to play outdoors for fear of meeting a dog, and his little sister was now beginning to share his fear. In an initial interview, Bobby demonstrated little fear when talking about dogs and cheerfully joined the therapist in playing with toy dogs. Further discussion with the mother soon revealed that it was really she who had a moderate fear of dogs and that Bobby was basically doing what she expected him to do, although he did have a mild degree of fear. The therapist counseled the mother, who achieved rapid fear reduction. As a further means of helping her family move from inappropriate fear to adaptive enjoyment of dogs, she agreed to buy a puppy. A week later, the dog joined with the therapist, the mother, and her two children in a playful visit on the lawn outside the therapist's office. Bobby and his little sister easily resolved their fear, and the boy proudly took charge of feeding his new pet.

### *Absolute Contraindication: Request for Hypnotherapy Based on Misdiagnosis*

Tim, R., a 6-year-old, had trouble paying attention in school and failed to follow the teacher's instructions, although he had at least average intelligence. When his mother requested that Tim have therapeutic hypnosis for his "behavior problem," the therapist insisted on taking a careful history. She learned that Tim had had recurrent middle-ear infections and that his failure to pay attention was chiefly related to a previously undetected hearing loss. When Tim was treated for his medical problem, his "behavior problem" disappeared.

### *Relative Contraindication: Immediate Medical or Surgical Treatment Takes Precedence over Therapeutic Hypnosis*

Anne C., a 10-year-old, had a long history of complaints of vague abdominal pain associated with reluctance to go to school. One day, when the complaints became particularly severe, the mother requested therapeutic clinical hypnosis for Anne. The therapist insisted on a physical examination that resulted in a diagnosis of acute appendicitis and immediate surgery. Following Anne's recovery from surgery, the therapist re-evaluated her, and she successfully used self-hypnosis to resolve a relatively mild school avoidance problem.

The frequency of occurrence of such cases, in which the children referred for therapeutic hypnosis were proved later to have biological bases for their symptoms, inspired a survey by Olness and Libbey (1987). Of the 200 children surveyed, 39 had unrecognized biological bases for their symptoms; within this overall group, 80 had been referred specifically for clinical hypnosis and 20 of these had previously unrecognized organic conditions that explained their symptoms. Within this group of 20 patients, the average duration of symptoms prior to diagnosis was 18 months. All had been seen by physicians within 1 year before their referral to the clinic. Eleven had been in psychotherapy for periods ranging from 3 to 30 months; of these, two had been hospitalized for 6–12 months in inpatient units. Each child had a complete remission of the presenting symptoms with treatment of the underlying disease. Although it is important to recognize the psychological or behavioral aspects of many illnesses, it is also important to recognize a biological base for certain behavioral symptoms.

### *Relative Contraindication: Another Form of Psychotherapeutic Management Takes Precedence*

Larry W., age 14 years, was hospitalized because of total body weakness and rapidly developing inability to walk. Finding no organic basis for the problem, the physician made a diagnosis of conversion reaction and requested therapeutic clinical hypnosis. In psychodiagnostics interviews, it became clear that Larry's symptoms served as defense against psychosis. After consulting with the physician, the therapist refused clinical hypnosis for symptom relief and urged the parents to admit their son to an inpatient psychiatric program for intensive treatment. The parents denied that their son could have such a serious psychological problem, and they took him home. Follow-up about 1 year later revealed that the patient had indeed developed a frank psychosis. It is possible that, at some point in the course of intensive inpatient psychotherapy therapeutic clinical hypnosis might have been a useful adjunct, but its use for abrupt symptom removal was clearly contraindicated.

### *Relative Contraindication: The Symptom Provides Significant Secondary Gain for the Child*

Erickson (1991) described a teenage girl who was able to use hypnosis quite well to control the pain of her sickle cell disease; however, after several months, when she was hospitalized for crisis pain and the therapist came to see her, she refused hypnoanalgesia on the first day although she was in pain. The therapist stayed with her for half an hour, talking with her. On the second hospital day, she was willing to use her self-hypnosis skills. After several hospitalizations during which she demonstrated the same pattern, she was able to explain that everyone avoided her when she was in pain. Her therapist was the only person who was willing to be with her when she was in pain; therefore, she rejected helping herself because the presence of a sympathetic human being was more important than pain reduction.

## Conclusions

This brief review of general principles is intended to provide a framework in which to consider management of the clinical problems presented in succeeding chapters. The following clinical material includes techniques that were utilized and why, what suggestions were given, and how the results were interpreted. We take the position that as long as a given therapeutic hypnotic approach has not been shown clearly to be ineffective, there may be at least some features of it useful to child health clinicians utilizing hypnosis with their patients. We maintain this position even when we are critical of the claims made for positive results, departing from it only when it appears obvious that the use of clinical hypnosis had no relationship to the results obtained. Given the scope and complexity of problems to be discussed, we have sometimes had to be arbitrary about including a particular problem in one chapter rather than another.

## References

Call, J.D. (1976). Children, parents, and hypnosis: a discussion. *International Journal of Clinical and Experimental Hypnosis*, *24*, 149–155.

Erickson, C.J. (1991). Applications of cyberphysiologic techniques in pain management. *Pediatric Annals*, *20*, 145–156.

Erickson, M.H. (1959). Further techniques of hypnosis: utilization techniques. *American Journal of Clinical Hypnosis*, *2*, 3–21.

Hughes, F. (1993). *The Wildest Show on Earth, Adapted from a Screenplay by John Patrick Shanley Based on the Book by Hudson Talbott.* New York: Grosset & Dunlap.

Kaffman, M. (1968). Hypnosis as an adjunct to psychotherapy in child psychiatry. *Archives of General Psychiatry*, *18*, 725–738.

Olness, K. & Kohen, D.P. (1984). Suggestion and hypnotherapy in pediatric practice, Parts I and II. In C.L. Tishler & M.T. Plaisted, Eds., *Peelings and Their Medical Significance* (pp. 13–20, 26). Columbus, OH: Ross Laboratories.

Olness, K. & Libbey, P. (1987). Unrecognized biologic bases of behavioral symptoms in patients referred for hypnotherapy. *American Journal of Clinical Hypnosis, 30*, 1–8.

Williams, D.T. & Singh, M. (1976). Hypnosis as a facilitating therapeutic adjunct in child psychiatry. *Journal of the American Academy of Child Psychiatry, 15*, 326–342.

Wright, M.E. (1960). Hypnosis and child therapy. *American Journal of Clinical Hypnosis, 2*, 197–205.

Wright, M.E. & Wright, B.A. (1987). *Clinical Practice of Hypnotherapy*. New York: Guilford Press.

# 7

# FACILITATING EFFECTIVE INTERPERSONAL RELATIONSHIPS WITH HYPNOSIS – LANGUAGE FOR CLINICIANS AND PARENTS

## Introduction

> Therapy happens within language and language is what therapists and clients use to do therapy. … If therapy *is* conversation, then conversation *is* therapy. … The idea that doing therapy can be seen as a conversation points to and reminds us of the interactional aspects of the endeavor, something that is quite easy to neglect.
>
> *(de Shazer, 1994, p. 4)*

So, we must talk so people can listen and understand, and we must listen so that what we say next makes sense and has a goodness of fit with the person with whom we are having a therapeutic conversation. Years ago, a Rabbi friend was speaking at a first-ever bioethics conference in our community. He enjoined the audience, "Physicians, guard thy words carefully," a modernization of a quote from the *Ethics of the Fathers* (*Pirkei Avot* 1:11; Neusner, 1983 pp. 31, 1–11), which says, "Sages, be careful with your words." He was implicitly sensitive to the reality that when doctors talk, patients listen carefully. And so it is that we must think before we speak, *because* people – and especially children who are in distress and come to us for help – are listening carefully. Indeed, they are in, if you will, a spontaneous hypnotic state, narrowly focused, listening carefully, and attending to precisely what we say and how we say it. Therefore, we must be thoughtful and cautious about what we say and how we say it.

### *Introducing Hypnosis to Children and Families*

How one introduces hypnosis to a child and his or her family really depends on how they happened to come to the clinician. Were they referred for help by someone else familiar with and satisfied or happy with the clinician? Did the referring clinician (or school or friend) offer the family the positive expectation that "s/he will help you" without any mention of anything like hypnosis, preferring instead to mention such integrative techniques as biofeedback, either because the referring clinician really thinks you will do biofeedback or, more likely, because the clinician knows that you use hypnosis and is him or herself sufficiently unfamiliar with or afraid of using the word *hypnosis*.

What if the family brings up hypnosis as opposed to the clinician bringing it up? Though clinicians have varying personal styles, it is often much more valuable and rapport facilitating to

DOI: 10.4324/9781003243687-9

bounce questions back to children and families before offering one's own answer. Thus, when a child or parent says, for example, "Our doctor said we should come here for hypnosis" or "She said that you would hypnotize me!," I am likely to respond by asking in turn, "Well, what did you think of your doctor saying that?" I might then add, "What *is* hypnosis anyway? I know you may not know for sure, but what have you heard? How do they show it on TV or in the movies?" This sort of dialogue not only will likely convey the message that you are interested in them as a person as well as interested in their ideas, but will also communicate that you are open to discussion and that you will in turn offer your perspective and response to the same question. This allows for demystification of whatever misconceptions they may well have about hypnosis, especially as it is often misrepresented in the media. It allows the natural opportunity to educate the family that: (1) one can understand that all hypnosis is self-hypnosis; (2) amnesia does not usually happen after hypnosis but amnesia can be taught if it is important in a given situation; (3) people cannot be made to do things against their will (e.g., barking like a dog or walking like a chicken as often shown in cartoons); and (4) most people have been in a state of hypnosis without realizing it, because it is really the same feeling we have when we are daydreaming, pretending, or imagining.

## *History Taking*

Most sensitive, thoughtful clinicians who take hypnosis workshops discover very quickly that they have really been doing hypnosis kinds of things right along without really knowing that they were, and *when* they take a clinical hypnosis workshop they *then* begin to discover the nuances of language we have been discussing here, and nomenclature, and framework within which to build skills and cultivate further success on behalf of their patients. Prior to learning hypnosis work I used to practice medicine by introducing myself and immediately launching into what I was taught to do – take the history ("getting down to business"), identify the *problem*, and explore all aspects of the problem, much as a good detective would. That model served well for a while, until it became stereotypical, stale, boring. The "because" part of it got old and stale, likely because it lost its uniqueness, its individuality, its human-ness. *When*, however, we allow *rapport* to drive our history taking, *then* we really learn about who this person is, the reasons for which they have come to see us, and, ultimately, the best ways to help them. Consider viewing history taking as rapport-building that is future (not just past) oriented, strength-based, change-based (vs. stuck), and positively expectant.

A continuing dialogue about what hypnosis is and is not may easily evolve by talking about naturally occurring hypnotic phenomena. This is often easily accomplished by explaining that there are really two kinds of hypnosis or hypnotic behaviors: those that occur spontaneously every day and those that we induce/invite or create or develop on purpose with the goal and intention of using the state of hypnosis to help relieve discomfort, reduce a habit, or solve a problem of some kind. It is often very useful and effective to explain, for example, "Did you know that it's probably true that you've been in hypnosis without knowing that it was hypnosis?" I offer the child a description of the common scenario of their parent dropping them off at a birthday party at 5 p.m., saying they'll see them after the party at 8 p.m. When the parent comes to pick up the child later and says it's time to go home, that 3 hours have passed, the child may well protest by claiming "3 hours? No way! I just got here!" We even have a phrase for that: "Time flies when you're having fun." Time distortion of the opposite nature may occur when we are waiting in a surgical waiting room while our family member goes in for an operation. They may go into surgery at 1 p.m., and commonly we may experience pacing around the waiting room for what seems like an hour only to look at the clock and see that perhaps is only 1:15 pm and only

15 minutes have passed. These are examples of the everyday hypnotic phenomena of time regression and time progression.

In analogous fashion, it is easy – and perhaps really important in many cases – to describe for children and families other natural hypnotic phenomena. Examples may include the child who falls off his bicycle and skins his knee a block or two away from home, picks himself up, and rides back home, not crying until seeing his mother. Did he not feel pain or did he suppress his discomfort until he got home? Upon arriving home, when he cries and the scraped, bloody-skinned knee is cleansed and dried, his discomfort abates when his mother kisses the "boo-boo." This, of course, represents the spontaneous phenomenon of modulation of discomfort, in which the child (through the parent's comforting action and positive expectation) perceives a difference, and the skinned knee simply does not hurt the same way it did before (see further details in Chapters 12 and 14).

Appropriate debate centers on whether clinicians utilizing hypnosis (Sugarman & Kohen, 2007) should do so by *being hypnotic* (i.e., using hypnotic language) and facilitating change through our language and the way we help children learn about change (e.g., about mind–body relationships). For example, as rapport is developing and a comfortable relationship is emerging, I sometimes will notice a child or teenager take a deep sigh in the midst of our conversation. It is always appropriate for a clinician to make a mental note of such a behavior and wonder about its meaning, its importance. It is sometimes advisable to initiate a dialogue about this so-called *teachable moment* with the child:

Clinician: "Wow … that was GREAT what you just did!"
Child (often not consciously aware of what he did): "What did I do?"
Clinician: "Right, what *did* you *do*?"
Child: "I don't know."
Clinician: "Yes, you do. You took a deep breath, right?"

OR

Clinician (taking a deep breath): "You did this."
Child (perhaps a little confused, as in "so what?"): "Yeah, I guess so."
Clinician: "Do you know what that's called? It's a *sigh*, right?"
Child: "Right."
Clinician: "Do you know why we do it?"

Note the use of *we*, not *you*. This universalizes the discussion and takes the focus away from the child, allowing them to engage, focus, and learn more from the discussion.

Clinician: Well, we do it to get relief, to express an emotion, like relief, frustration, anger, comfort … like when someone finally stops yelling at us, or when we jump back on the curb because a car came close to us while we were crossing the street … like "*whew*!"
Child: "Yeah, I get it."
Clinician: "And what *happens* when we breathe out? We relax … right? Just notice that and do another deep breath now. Watch what happens to your shoulders. They go down, don't they? That is the mind talking to the body, isn't it?"

In hypnotic suggestion language this is referred to as a *truism*; it is what it is, and most children and families find it appropriately interesting. It is easy to give people other examples of how the mind and body talk to each other all the time. Ask each person in the room, for example, if they fall out of bed at night. They (usually) will answer that they do not. Ask if they stay in one spot all night or if they move around. They will answer that they move. Finally, ask why they don't fall when they get to the edge of the bed. Many children get it immediately and explain that, even though they are asleep, *the brain knows where the body is* and directs the body to either move and not fall or to wake up.

Although it obviously will be more important with some patients and families than others, this type of pre-hypnosis conversation goes a long way toward helping them learn that they really already do know a lot about mind–body communication and about self-regulation. This is important because when we go on later to offer suggestions, ideas, and teaching about how the mind can help the body with the child's particular problem, they will realize, because the seed has been planted with this conversation (we are, after all, gardeners!), that they already *know* how to have their mind (or "inside brain," "subconscious mind," etc.) talk to their body about, for example, not falling out of bed, not peeing in your pants in the daytime even when you have to go real bad, or not having to think before walking or throwing a ball or signing your name.

### *Ego Strengthening*

Ego strengthening is always okay in the service of problem resolution, mastery, and empowerment. Ego-strengthen whenever possible – before, during, and after hypnosis. Emphasize confidence, competence, comfort, pride, joy, satisfaction, peace, and serenity. Words such as *comfortable*, *easily*, *effortlessly*, *relaxed*, *slowly*, and *gradually* are just examples of the many, many accessible, positive words.

### *Elements of Therapeutic Communication*

What *are* the elements of effective therapeutic communication in hypnosis and therapeutic hypnosis work? The main ingredients of effective clinical hypnosis are expectations (the child's expectations, the parents' expectations, *and* our expectations) and motivation – again, not only the child's motivation (e.g., to feel better, improve, solve a problem) but also the parent's motivation and ours as the clinician providing the teaching, vehicle, and potential for transformation through that which we call hypnosis.

As we have noted earlier, what goes on in the mind of children during hypnosis is best understood by them as equivalent to, or at least analogous to, what they experience when they pretend, daydream, or use their imagination. Accordingly, if we want to know what a child's imagery (hypnotic experience) is, we have to ask that child, and we have to listen carefully to the response. Of course, all children who like to go to the beach do not have the same imaginative experience about the beach, and certainly not necessarily what *we* experience at the beach in our internal, imaginative experience. Some may see or feel themselves making sand castles, others swimming in the lake or ocean, others steadfastly avoiding the water but loving to lay on a beach blanket. This is all by way of reminding us, as we will return to often in this text, that even the very first time that a child experiences an "official" or formalized hypnotic invitation and "trance" with us in the office, *nothing happens unless the child wants it to*. The child wanting it to happen and the clinician facilitating it MUST and therefore will be based on a foundation of thoughtful and sensitive building of *rapport*, careful solicitation of the evolution of the child's *history*, and ongoing attention to taking *notice* – paying attention to everything that the patient says and does (or doesn't say and do) during the course of our interaction and connection.

Nothing is more important than the effective development of rapport and the gathering of the patient's history of our interaction in the context of that rapport and noticing the "how" as well as the "what" of their communication. As Milton Erickson said:

> When patients come into my office, I greet them with a blank mind and I look them over to see who and what and why they are without taking anything for granted.
>
> *(Haley, 1985, p. 114)*

This should indeed be our goal and starting point with each next encounter. It is our belief that all children (who have a reason) can learn to do hypnosis because they already know how, they just don't know (consciously) that they know. Although what happens in therapeutic hypnosis is ultimately up to the patient, as clinicians we nonetheless have the significant responsibility and obligation to help them learn how to best help themselves. Toward this end, there are some very important guidelines for what works best in language and what does not.

*Caution*: How we talk reflects how we think, what we believe, how we feel, how we act/behave, how we teach, and what we come to expect.

For the duration of this chapter we comment on specific uses of phrases, words, and construction of language that are facilitative of effective hypnosis, and we make suggestions about what to avoid, and the reasons. After we have made a big deal about how certain words may not be allowed or welcome in my office (such as *try* or *attack*; see further discussion below), we explain why to the child and family in much the same way as noted above: "The reason I make such a big deal out of some words is because how we talk is how we *think*. And, how we think is how we *feel*. And, how we feel is how we *act*. So, if we don't like or want how we act [such as being in pain, having a habit, being nervous or worried or sad] then it works better to **start by changing how we talk** *because* that will get us *thinking* differently, and thinking differently helps us get to *feeling* differently and, therefore, *acting* differently."

Because our young patients are listening carefully, particularly but not only when formally or "officially" in hypnosis, we must speak carefully, especially when constructing what we say and how we say it during invitation to hypnosis and utilization (suggestions). In the context of teaching children what we are going to do when we do hypnosis (e.g., "in a few moments") it is often useful to approach this in a way analogous to how we all learned to approach writing a paper or giving an oral presentation. Thus, say what we're going to do (and how), then do it, and then review what we did. Often, we will say to the child something like: "Here's what we'll do in learning about and doing hypnosis. First, you sit there and I'll sit here." This is concrete, sets the tone for safety, begins to describe the "how," and dispels myths about what might happen if the patient trusts enough to in fact close his/her eyes.

"Next, I'll show you how to start hypnosis and then we'll do it. Then I'll just (saying 'just' highlights an important approach in hypnosis, i.e. the use of *implication within our language construction*. The word 'just' implies that what follows is *'easy')* talk with you about making the hypnosis feeling even better than it already is. I'll probably say something about relaxing your body and how to do that from head to toe or toes to head, and I'll also talk about imagination, like daydreaming that you're somewhere doing something you like, maybe playing football or video games or visiting your cousins like you told me you like to do. Then I'll say something about how to *use* this good feeling of being in hypnosis to give messages or instructions to your mind and body about [whatever the problem is] and how to help that get better; or, how to program that computer we call the brain to help relieve the [whatever the problem is]. Then, before we finish, I'll teach you how to **do** *self*-hypnosis so it will be even easier than you thought *when* you practice and *do this for yourself* at home. And, finally, when we're finished, we can talk about what it was like, how it felt, what you liked *best*, and any questions that come up. How does that sound so far?"

The words in this example are carefully selected and emphasis is placed particularly to represent what indeed are the "hypnosis before the hypnosis" and the "invitation before the invitation." I'm sure you noticed the various so-called embedded suggestions within the preceding explanation of "what *will* happen." One example of an embedded suggestion is the casual mention of the re-framing of thinking of one's brain as analogous to a computer than can be programmed with hypnosis. This foregoing explanation might also be called the "pre-invitation" or "pre-hypnosis" conversation that sets the tone for what will follow. Just as setting the supper table prepares one for and complements the meal to follow, so has "setting the table" become a phrase that appropriately is used to help prepare for what is coming next. Because the child has already been busy concentrating on the therapist and *vice versa*, and rapport has begun to be established in this context, one can easily see that the pre-invitation conversation has indeed a hypnotic quality about it. It conveys positive expectations. It provides future projections about what will happen and how, and it offers posthypnotic suggestions and implications about what will or could happen later (e.g., *when* you practice this at home).

One might also add something like: "As I'm talking during the hypnosis, if I accidentally say something that is not useful to you, let your inside mind just change it. You can do that by just ignoring it, or by changing a word or words like you would change a radio or TV station, or in some other way. What is *important* is how your inside thinking allows my words to become your own words [why?] *so that you can help yourself the most.*" As you learn and improve (please note the hypnotic suggestion!), use other people's words and phrases and *make them your own. When* you do that, your authenticity and genuineness will come through.

As we think about how we talk with children and families, it is essential to understand what we are and what we are not (i.e., how we define ourselves). We believe that we are clinicians who are utilizing, applying, and teaching hypnosis to promote well-being and to help work on or solve a problem. We are *not* "hypnotists." Though we have previously used the word *hypnotherapist* for convenience in prior editions of this text, we have carefully eliminated the vast majority of usage of the word "hypnotherapy." After all, we are *not* hypnotherapists (although we do therapy with the use of hypnosis) any more than we are penicillinologists. We *are* clinicians who use and teach hypnosis within therapy as treatment strategies and techniques. We are guides, coaches, teachers, and facilitators.

Everything that we do and say and how we do it should convey assurance that we know what we are doing, have experience, and are both competent and confident that we can help them. We should believe and honor our young patients and their families. In a variety of ways, we seek to *evoke curiosity because people who are curious listen carefully and pay close attention to what is being said.* This can be done in any number of ways. I (DPK) begin when I greet someone for the first time in the waiting room. Not knowing who the patient is, I announce that "I'm looking for someone named Debbie." Debbie will always identify herself. If she is 5 years old, she will perhaps hide behind her mother or father's chair and peek around the corner. If she is 9 or 10, she is developmentally likely to extend her hand and make eye contact; if she doesn't, then there is always a reason why … perhaps anxiety? If Debbie is a teenager, perhaps she will sit still, wave, and roll her eyes as adolescents commonly, but not always, do. And, perhaps she will say, as adolescents in the 21st century are wont to say, the somewhat disdainful word "Whatever … .!" In this way I can learn a lot about the child who is soon to be my patient. Then, continuing to evoke curiosity, I introduce myself to the child first (not to the parents) and I ask who these people are who have accompanied the child. Generally, children find this amusing or, if not, certainly curious. The child might answer, "These are my parents" or "They are my mom and dad." I ask them to please introduce me to their parents. I do this to find out *if* they can do so and *how*, and I also notice how the child responds. It is always interesting to discover which child says "This is Mom and this is Dad," prompting me to say "but I can't call them Mom and Dad 'cause they're not my Mom and Dad … do they have *names?!*" This intentional use of both young child concreteness and some (hopefully!) humor are designed to continue to evoke curiosity and to offer the unspoken message "It's okay to have fun at the Doctor's office." However they react/respond (or not) continues to give me information about who they are, and how they understand.

I then invite them to come into my office. I hold the door so the child can walk ahead and I tell the parents to "follow Debbie because she knows where she's going," although Debbie in fact does *not* know where she is going as she has never been there before. Before Debbie can protest, from behind I offer information such as "straight ahead and turn into the first office on the left." I learn quickly then if the child can hear (!) and if she knows left from right.

When initiating the conversation – and continuing to develop our rapport and to evoke curiosity – I turn my attention almost universally first to the child by asking, "How come you came over here?" Assuming that I am paying attention and listening (!) their response is always instructive. Often, children respond with a shrug of their shoulders or verbally say "I don't know" when in fact it is usually the case (though not always) that their parents have indeed discussed something about the appointment with them. Children might seek to defer to their parents nonverbally by turning to them with a pleading look or by saying "Mom?" or by saying to me "I don't know, ask them." Not only do I learn more from their responses, but it also affords me the opportunity to continue to develop rapport by explaining simply that, "I'm asking you *because* you're the child and I'm a doctor for children, so children *get to go FIRST in my office* [= it's a privilege!]. I promise I'm not going to leave your mom and dad out; they just get to go second." Most parents don't mind, and most children "get it."

Of the multiple levels of meaning that this and most verbal communication has, one of my intentions is to convey the idea that "*you* are *important* in this office and I *believe* what you say. I *trust* what you say." This is essential to driving our *rapport* in a positive direction. If the topic for discussion (i.e., the presenting complaint or concern) is difficult to talk about, such as anxiety, or embarrassing, such as wetting the bed or thumb-sucking, the child may still not wish to talk right away. In such situations, it may become strategically and emotionally easier to switch to something much easier for them to talk about, with the intention to return to the presenting complaint a bit later after rapport, comfort, and safety have become more established. That occasion may be only 10 minutes later or a half-hour later, or it may not be until the second or later visit. When this occurs I often seek to empower the child further by saying something like: "Would it be better to talk about something easier to talk about?" The child typically nods or says yes, and I then ask about traditionally safer subjects, such as family, school, or favorite activities, books, "apps," games, or television shows.

## *Words to Use and Words to Avoid*

### *When … Then*

Both in the "hypnosis before the hypnosis" and in the therapeutic hypnosis itself, it is far preferable to use *when* than *if*. "*If* you can learn hypnosis" introduces the possibility that it may not occur, whereas "*when* you learn hypnosis" implies that it will in fact occur, without predicting at all when or even how that may take place. *When* we program ourselves to remember that a *when* clause can be even more effective when followed by a *then* phrase, *then* we will be that much more effective in generating positive outcomes. "*If* you can feel your muscles relax in your shoulders" is a somewhat of a challenge to the patient. A better alternative is "*When* the muscles in your shoulders relax, *then* you can let the relaxation move further down into your arms and hands" or "*When* the muscles in your shoulders relax, *then* you'll be very proud of yourself and the way you can create comfort for yourself *when* you need it." The difference is obvious i.e., the *when* … *then* construction is real permission and an invitation to learn and assume control. Leslie, Lemke, and Damis have emphasized the use of " when" and language uses to create positive expectancy in their recent publication regarding hypnosis and hypnotic language in helping children who have experienced trauma (Leslie, Lemke, & Damis, 2021).

### *You vs. I*

It is preferable to use "*You* may wish to … " rather than "*I* want you to … ." The latter is control oriented and authoritarian. Most children find "I want you to … " to be all too familiar, as they hear it in the context of parents or teachers or other adults telling them what to do – for example, "I want you to turn around and face the front of the room," "I want you to leave the dog alone and finish your supper," "I want you to make your bed and get ready for school," or "I want you to put on your pajamas and brush your teeth."

### *Will vs. May*

Instead of "You *will* relax your body [feel less pain, be less anxious]," it is preferable to consider saying "You *may*, *when* you're ready, let yourself relax [feel more comfort, notice less worry]." Note here also the switch to permissive suggestion in the form of "let" yourself relax and the change from negative words to less negative or more positive ones: "feel more comfort" rather than "feel less pain," "notice less worry" rather than "be less anxious."

### *Try*

Consider abandoning or at least avoiding the use of the word "*try*." Why? *Try* implies failure. The saying "If at first you don't succeed, try, try again!" is seemingly a formula for failure. In *Star Wars Episode V: The Empire Strikes Back*, Yoda, the Jedi Master, said, "Do or do not; there is no try." And, it is not surprising that the advertising logo for Nike® has always been "Just *do* it," certainly not "Just *try* it."

### *Reading Minds*

During hypnosis, do not describe events that are not happening or which you really do not know to be true. Clinicians are commonly apt to think and say something like "you are feeling relaxed now" when they don't really know that, and what they may really only know is that the child looks or seems relaxed. Because *relaxed* describes both affect or emotional state and physical muscle relaxation, it is really only okay to make the verbal observation of "you are feeling relaxed now" when the therapist has already asked the patient in hypnosis "How are you feeling?" or "Let me know, please, *when* you are beginning to notice the relaxation." Otherwise, there is the risk that subjects (especially with their eyes closed) may become confused and think that the therapist is reading their mind.

### *"-ic" Words*

We should avoid using "-ic" words. Because people, children especially, are *not* their illness, we should avoid adjectival words that imply this. Thus, a child with asthma is *not* an asthmatic.

Having epilepsy does not make one an epileptic, and having diabetes does not mean one is a diabetic – similarly for the use of cystic (cystic fibrosis), leukemic (leukemia), and sickler (sickle cell disease). Importantly, someone who has been identified/diagnosed as being on the Autism Spectrum should not be called "Autistic," but more appropriately as being "on the spectrum" or having been characterized as having an Autism Spectrum Disorder.

### *Time*

References to time are better when offered vaguely than specifically, particularly as people in hypnosis are very literal and concrete, and time distortion is a common hypnotic phenomenon that occurs spontaneously. Time progression occurs when 1 hour seems like 4 hours (e.g., to promote or prolong comfort), and time regression occurs when an hour "flies by" as though it lasted only a minute (e.g., to hasten the experience of an otherwise uncomfortable procedure). Thus, suggesting "when we are finished in a few *moments*" is preferable to "when we are finished in 3 *minutes*."

### *"Yet" and "just"*

Often a single word may introduce a dramatic change in expectation and with it a substantive alteration of a negative demeanor … i.e., a shift from despair, sadness, ongoing worry, to one of hopefulness and positive expectancy. A common example can be found in talking with a child who has had nocturnal enuresis and is just beginning to learn how to become dry at night. The child returns for a second or third follow-up visit and at the outset seems to be "down in the dumps." When asked how things have been – or if s/he has their calendar (recording dry beds), s/he may appear sad, quiet, and avoid eye contact before ultimately saying "I didn't get any dry beds." The clinicians' simple, firm declarative response of "YET!" often changes the mood abruptly and may evoke confusion resulting in "What?" The clinician can amplify the positive response with "You didn't have any DRY BEDS YET, I wonder WHEN that will start to happen very soon. After all, this is JUST your 2nd (or 3rd or??) visit." The shift in the child's demeanor is often dramatic and "just" the beginning of a series of further positive expectations to follow.

### *Silence*

What should clinicians say or do when they don't know what to say next? Because listening is a cultivatable skill, it is often right and best to just wait and say nothing, waiting and watching to see and hear what *happens* next. Silence is, after all, a great motivator. If we run out of things to say in the moment, it is often best to wait for a clue of some kind, verbal or otherwise. It is interesting in this context to note that a simple rearrangement of the letters of the word *silent* spells the word *listen*! While waiting or thinking about what to say next, one might offer the patient who is in a comfortable state of hypnosis simple reinforcing, so-called ego-strengthening suggestions or compliments such as "That's right," "Great!," "You're doing this right," or "Very nice."

## *Negative Patient Reaction*

What should the clinician *say* when the patient reacts negatively? If the patient appears to be uncomfortable or speaks uncomfortably, it is essential, of course, to honor that, to learn more about it, and to help. The clinician who has inadvertently said something incorrect or inadvisable should own it and fix it (e.g., "What I meant to say was … "). If the patient is upset or tearful, one could ask, "What's happening right now in your mind? You can stay in your hypnosis and tell me so I can help *or* you can slowly, gradually return to your usual alertness and *then* we can talk about it together." Another alternative would be to say, "You can notice that feeling of sadness [anger, etc.] as long as you need to, then notice it start to go away, learn whatever was important to learn from it, and *then* shift your attention to something else more comfortable. That's right … and let me know when you have done that. Great!"

### *Remember the "Because"*

In the formulation of hypnotic suggestions it is essential to remember the "because"; that is, people really do better when they have a reason to *do* the suggestion that we have offered. Thus, it might sound fine to say, "Allow yourself to relax down to your toes," but it works better to say, "Allow yourself to relax down to your toes *because* relaxing feels good" or " … *because* as you do that you realize you are in control of your relaxing" or " … *because* when you do, then you can move on to learning more about how self-hypnosis can help you help yourself with your [problem]."

### *Trance Termination*

Trance termination should not be abrupt, but, like the rest of the hypnotic experience, should be paced to the individual session and needs of the individual child in the moment. Some children may be invited to "count slowly to yourself from 1 to 5 or 5 down to 1 or 10 down to 1 or 1 up to 10 *or* whatever is comfortable for you; and in your own way slowly and gradually return to your usual state of alertness along the way. And be sure to bring your good feelings with you." Other clinicians prefer to be even less prescriptive than counting and might say, for example, "Before we are finished in a few moments, remind yourself what you learned [when teaching self-hypnosis]" and then, "When you're ready, bring yourself back to the room, and when you're finished, you'll be done."

### *Re-Alerting*

As noted earlier, we should not refer to re-alerting as *waking up*, as hypnosis is not sleep. To be sure, hypnosis may be effectively utilized to facilitate relaxation and falling asleep (see Chapters 8 and 13), but it is not sleep, so we don't wake up from it. The state of hypnosis is not at all like sleep electroencephalographically.

Some simple examples of hypnotic language that have become part of our everyday communication with children include the use of re-framing, mixture of tenses, and changing a response set from a "no" set to a "yes" set:

> A child working on the problem of migraine headaches returns to the office for follow-up. He is forlorn and says, "I still have headaches. didn't get rid of them." One potential clinician response would be a direct, simple statement: " … yet." If this has to be explained or discussed, the clinician can say, "You didn't get rid of all your headaches … . *yet*, but you *will* because you are learning how, and are already reducing them, right?" Do not focus on sadness or on past; only focus on that it has not happened *yet*, which equals it *will* happen in the future – a positive expectancy, a "yes" set.

A child in the office with a stomachache says, "It really hurts!" One potential clinician response would be "I know, and it will keep right on hurting until it *stops*." The patient hears your belief that you acknowledge the discomfort *now* and that it *will* indeed *stop*. The clinician can add, for example, "I wonder what you can *do* to have it not bother you until it stops altogether? What do you *do already* to help yourself?" This honors the patient's competency and ability to grow all in one statement.

## Conclusion

With practice and experience, most clinicians utilizing hypnosis discover that so-called hypnotic language and hypnotic ways of talking, creating positive expectations, and offering re-framing toward resolution of problems become part of everyday communication with our patients, and not reserved for only when they are in a formal, or invited, hypnotic state. Awareness of this and cultivation of it allow us to be that much more therapeutic with our patients most, if not all, of the time. The ability to do this, like the refining of any skill, comes with practice and experience.

Additional examples [1] of how to talk and what to say when, how, and why are provided in the many case illustrations that follow in subsequent chapters.

## Note

1 Additionally readers may also wish to consult recent publications that include a variety of case examples of the utilization of the language of hypnosis with children and adolescents:

- Kohen, D.P. & Kaiser, P. (2014). Clinical hypnosis with children and adolescents what? Why? How?: Origins, applications, and efficacy. *Children, 1, 74–98; doi: 10.3390/children1020074*
- Friedrichsdorf, S.J., Kohen, D.P. (2018). Integration of hypnosis into pediatric palliative care. *Annals of Palliative Medicine. Doi: 10.21037/apm.2017.05.02*
- Kaiser, P., Kohen, D.P., Brown, M.L., Kajander, R.L., Barnes, A.J. (2018). Integrating pediatric hypnosis with complementary modalities: Clinical perspectives on personalized treatment. *Children, 5, 108; doi: 10.3390/children5080108*

## References

de Shazer, S. (1994). *Words Were Originally Magic*. New York: W.W. Norton.

Haley, J., Ed. (1985). *Conversations with Milton H. Erickson*, Vol. 1. Rockville, MD: Triangle Press.

Larkin, D.M. (2014). Principles of therapeutic suggestions (part I) and clinical applications of therapeutic suggestions (part II). *Explore,* 10(6), 380–388.

Leslie, T., Lemke, W., & Damis, L.F. (2021). The relevance of being hypnotic in addressing trauma in children across settings. *American Journal of Clinical Hypnosis*, *63*(2), 128–138.

Neusner, J. (1983). *Torah from Our Sages – Pirke Avot (Ethics of the Fathers) – A New American Translation and Explanation*. New York, NY: Rossell Books.

Sawni, A. & Breuner, C.C. (2017). Clinical Hypnosis, an effective mind-body modality for adolescent with behavioral and physical complaints. *Children, 4(4), 19 Special Issue Mind-Body Medicine in Children and Adolescents*. 10.3390.children4040019

Sugarman, L.I. & Kohen, D.P. (2007). Integrating hypnosis into acute care settings. In W.C. Wester & L.I. Sugarman, Eds., *Therapeutic Hypnosis With Children and Adolescents* (pp. 301–332). Bethel, CT: Crown House Publishing.

# 8

# HYPNOSIS FOR PSYCHOLOGICAL DISORDERS

## Introduction

Hypnosis is not a therapy in itself. When it is combined with various forms of medical and psychological treatment, it becomes hypnotherapy.

In this chapter, we refer to the use of hypnosis in the context of psychotherapy, omitting treatment of habit disorders and learning problems. Although there are fewer reports of child hypnosis for primary psychological problems than for medical and surgical problems, there has been an increase in both clinical research and evidence-based, randomized controlled studies of hypnosis for anxiety, depression, and other psychological problems (e.g., Catani, Kohiladevy, Ruf et al., 2009; Gordon, Staples, Blyta, Bytyqi, & Wilson, 2008; Nikulina et al., 2008; Shooshtary, Panaghi, & Moghadam, 2008; Zaider, & Heimberg, 2003). These have included several *Cochrane Database Systematic Reviews*, including one on cognitive behavioral therapy (CBT) for anxiety disorders in children and adolescents (James, Soler, & Weatherall, 2006) and one on behavioral and CBT for obsessive–compulsive disorder (OCD) in children and adolescents (O'Kearney, Anstey, & von Sanden, 2006). The difference may be related to the greater frequency of positive attitudes toward hypnosis expressed by pediatricians and pediatric nurses as compared with child psychologists and psychiatrists (Gardner, 1976a). Yet, interest and acceptance of hypnosis in psychotherapy is growing, as evidenced by Division 30 of the American Psychological Association, the hypnotherapy section; by the substantial increase in clinical reports and controlled research studies; and by a recent comprehensive review of the broad applications and value of hypnosis in child psychiatry (Huynh, Vandvik, & Diseth, 2008). We hope that our review of this area will stimulate further use of psychological hypnotherapy by illustrating not only its substantial advantages and clinical applications but also the growing research support for what is an increasingly clinically efficacious and evidence-based practice. Cautions and contraindications have been discussed in Chapter 6 (General Principles) and are also reviewed well in the major text *Handbook of Clinical Hypnosis* (Rhue, Lynn, & Kirsch, 1993).

## Advantages of Psychological Hypnosis

Williams (1979) commented on the essential value of psychological hypnotherapy: "Hypnosis can accelerate and augment the impact of psychotherapeutic intervention. … The increased

DOI: 10.4324/9781003243687-10

therapeutic leverage afforded by hypnosis can often facilitate both the conversion of insight into action and the more rapid relief of disabling symptoms" (p. 108). We believe that children in hypnosis are more able to accept the therapist's interpretations and to utilize their own capacities for achieving insight into conflicts and other dynamic issues. Increased readiness for insight follows from the combination of heightened ego receptivity and ego activity, intensified transference, and focused attention that typically characterize the hypnotic state and the hypnotherapeutic relationship. Moreover, the emphasis on mastery that underlies contemporary permissive hypnotherapy further enhances children's motivation to solve their problems, for they are taught that the solution truly belongs to them and not to anyone else (Fromm & Gardner, 1979).

The chief difference between hypnosis for children and for adults is that child therapists are less likely to use hypnotic techniques with the intention of purposely eliciting intense emotional abreactions (Williams, 1979). Specific hypnotherapeutic techniques vary with the age of the child, the nature of the problem, and the therapist's theoretical orientation. The techniques described below are not an exhaustive inventory, but rather a sample based on available clinical material.

In presenting clinical data, we are aware of the problem of diagnostic nomenclature, an area in which the very nature of child development makes for greater disagreement among child therapists than among those working with adults. Changing trends in the meaning and use of diagnostic labels further complicate the issue. In general, we have retained diagnostic labels contained in published reports or as they were used when we treated those patients described. In grouping cases, we have usually followed the guidelines of the American Psychiatric Association's (2013) *Diagnostic and Statistical Manual of Mental Disorders* (DSM-V-TR).

## Risks of Psychological Hypnosis

With respect to subsequent discussion of behavior disorders, anxiety disorders, sleep disorders, or somatoform disorders, we strongly emphasize the importance of careful diagnostic procedures. In a retrospective review of 200 children referred to a behavioral pediatrics clinic, a subset of 80 patients had been referred specifically for hypnosis. Overall, 39 of the 200 children (19.5%) had unrecognized biological bases for their symptoms; within the subset, 20 (25%) had previously unrecognized organic conditions that explained their symptoms. Each of these children had a complete remission of presenting symptoms with treatment of the underlying disease. Examples included children with a presenting symptom of anxiety who proved to have hyperthyroidism or those with cyclic vomiting who had a genetic enzymatic defect. It is essential that child therapists keep in mind the possibility of such biological bases for presenting symptoms (Olness & Libbey, 1987). We encourage clinicians not only to rely strongly upon comprehensive history taking, rapport, and intuition but also to consider appropriate screening tools to support and assist in the diagnosis of psycho-emotional disorders in children. Though there are many such screening tools, those which we have found very useful include the Achenbach Child Behavior Checklist (CBCL) and its related Teacher form and Youth Self Report (Achenbach, 1991), the Behavior Assessment System for Children (BASC) (Reynolds & Kamphaus, 2002), the Child Depression Inventory (Kovacs, 1992), the Strength and Difficulties Questionnaire (http://www.sdqinto.com), Parents Evaluation of Developmental Status (PEDS) (http://www.pedstest.com), and the UCLA PTSD Reaction Index for Children and Adolescents (PTSD-R) (Steinberg, 2004).

## Behavior Disorders

The problems in this group are manifested by children of all ages and are essentially characterized by impulsive or aggressive infringement on the basic rights of others or violation of major societal rules.

Examples include destructive behavior, rebellion at home or at school, poor self-control, and tantrum behavior. Hypnosis is rarely utilized early in the treatment of such problems. Psychotherapists often use behavior modification as a first approach, although insight therapy may also be employed.

Although hypnosis has often been the last resort in treating primary behavior disorders, reports describing its value tend to be positive provided that the patient experiences distress and therefore is motivated to achieve change and that the parents are willing to cooperate in the treatment program. Younger children often respond better than older ones. By the time the behavior problem has crystallized into character pathology, manifested by ego syntonicity and minimal anxiety, then treatment by any method becomes exceedingly difficult if not impossible (Crasilneck & Hall, 1985; Mellor, 1960; Solovey & Milechnin, 1955).

Much research has elucidated the neurochemistry and neurophysiology of neurotransmitters and how they are involved in the regulation of major behavioral systems; for example, norepinephrine, dopamine, and serotonin are significant in the regulation of an individual's behavior with the external environment (Rogeness, Javors, & Pliszka, 1992). A behavioral facilitatory system (BFS) and a behavioral inhibitory system (BIS) were described by Gray (1987). The BFS, controlled by the mesolimbic dopaminergic system, is activated primarily by environmental stimuli that are appealing, such as a plate of cookies on the table, and it is unrestrained by internal systems. The BIS, controlled by the septohippocampal system, can inhibit the BFS. Children with a strong BFS relative to the BIS would internalize poorly and be much more dependent on environmental controls (such as a parent in the vicinity), have less insight into reasons for punishment, and be more likely to blame others for their behavior. Several behavioral disorders of children may be secondary to dysregulation of neurotransmitter systems that impact the BFS or BIS.

Lembke has described a new problem for children related to dopamine release association with video games. Noting that pleasure and pain are processed in the same parts of the brain and that the brain tries to maintain homeostasis, the release of dopamine reduces the number of dopamine receptors. This eventually leads to a feeling of depression. If video games are played many hours a day, it becomes necessary to repeat this in order to feel normal. The person who plays excessively becomes addicted (Lembke, 2021).

Kagan (1994) noted that children with behavioral inhibition had increased urinary norepinephrine and increased heart rate. He also noted a striking persistence of personality types in following children from 2 to 13 years. Although the intrinsic personality types and behavior were modified somewhat by parenting styles, Kagan also noted evidence that differences in behavior and physiology reflect differences in thresholds of responsiveness in the limbic system. We know that the limbic system is a mediator of short-term memory (i.e., mental images to be stored) and connects many different systems involved in perceiving threats and responding to stress. One can speculate that deliberate changes in mental images, as occurs in hypnosis, may be mediated in the limbic system. Behavioral inhibition in children has been associated with major depression and panic disorders. Children with conduct disorders have been found to have decreased noradrenergic activity and decreased serotonergic function. Although research has developed medications to normalize these neurotransmitters, we speculate that, with increased precision in understanding the neurotransmitter abnormalities' relationship to chronobiological or nutritional or activity factors, it may be possible to combine hypnosis with biofeedback of relevant physiological responses for more predictable treatment of conduct disorders.

## Assessment of Learning Styles

It is important that the child health professional consider the possibility that learning disabilities are contributing to the presenting symptom and to modify therapeutic approaches accordingly.

A study by Gualtieri, Koriath, Van Bourgondien, and Saleeby (1983) examined a survey of 40 consecutive admissions to a child psychiatry inpatient service, in which at least half of the patients had moderate to severe language disorders. Routine intelligence testing did not discern most of the disorders. This was especially true in the areas of auditory analysis, memory, or integration, rather than in the more general test areas covering expressive or receptive language. Children with the former types of disorders demonstrated peculiar responses to instructions, compensatory talkativeness, and tantrums. They often did not understand or respond to verbal instructions. Awareness of their limitations led therapists to simplify language and use pictorial charts, drawings, and other nonverbal approaches. There were marked improvements in the progress of these children when therapy was adapted to their language disorders. Studies also note that learning disabilities are more apt to be missed in high-IQ children (Faigel, 1983). Although learning deficits are obvious with respect to some conditions such as pervasive developmental disorders, they may not be obvious in bright children who present with a variety of behavioral problems. Grynkewich (1994) has documented that mental imagery strategies, including hypnosis, may be adapted to improve school performance in children with significant learning disabilities.

## Behavior Disorders in Young Children

Behavior problems in preadolescent children are sometimes described as tension discharge disorders, commonly a reaction against inconsistent parenting, family strife, or inability to adjust at school. Genetic or physical problems such as the fragile X syndrome may have disruptive behaviors as part of their clinical presentation. Very often the behavior disorder represents an immature and maladaptive defense against anxiety and low self-esteem. The therapeutic task is to provide a context in which the child can cope more adaptively. Hypnotic relaxation and the intensity of the transference to a benign therapist may provide such a context when other methods fail or even provide a primary therapeutic modality.

Williams and Singh (1976) reported briefly on the case of a 10-year-old boy who presented a 3-year history of temper tantrums. He had not responded to previous therapeutic efforts, including medication, psychotherapy, and behavior modification. After three sessions of weekly hypnosis marked abatement of the temper tantrums was observed. Specific hypnotic techniques with this child were not described. Over the next 19 months, he maintained his gains in individual and family therapy, together with medication and special class placement. He also used self-hypnosis successfully at times of stress. We can assume that the parents willingly involved themselves in the treatment and that negative reactions to the tantrums from peers and family enhanced the child's motivation. This case is an example of the way in which hypnosis seems to provide the added impetus necessary for change to occur.

Two single case reports (Erickson, 1962; Lazar & Jedliczka, 1979) describe treatment without any formal hypnotic invitation (induction), emphasizing hypnosis utilization techniques, especially "prescribing the symptom." Both cases concerned "uncontrollable" children who in fact did control their environments, albeit maladaptively, and who then learned ways of more adaptive control. Erickson's (1962) patient was an 8-year-old boy who became progressively defiant and destructive following his mother's divorce. Her disciplinary efforts served mainly to further the power struggle in which the child invariably proved himself the stronger. At the same time, he unconsciously communicated his need to know that he was not all powerful and that there was a secure reality in which he could thrive. Erickson worked first with the mother, using double-bind techniques to enlist her cooperation to prove absolutely to her son that she was more powerful than he. Several months later, when the symptoms recurred, Erickson worked directly with the boy, establishing his own authority by challenging the child to live up to his boast that he could stomp the floor or stand still for extremely long periods. This maneuver shifted the child's focus of attention so as to permit him to benefit from reality confrontation, with resultant positive behavior change. Follow-up after 2 years indicated that the gains were maintained.

Lazar and Jedliczka (1979) described a single session of hypnosis with a boy who had moderate intellectual disabilities and cerebral palsy. His behavior problems included ignoring his mother, making himself late for school, using unacceptable language, and deliberately waking his parents by coughing at night. The child and his mother agreed that he was a "cripple." As a result, she never disciplined him, and he used disruptive behavior as a means of gaining some sense of control and probably also as a way of asking for appropriate external control. The therapist used several hypnotic techniques, including prescribing the symptom, confusion, and double bind, in order to help the boy alter his perception of the value of his behavior. She asked him to spend a certain time each day saying bad words, and she asked him to choose which nights he would cough. In this way, she neutralized the pleasure of the bad language and subtly suggested that the patient would also choose nights when he would not cough. Similarly, she devalued his misbehavior in her office, either by ignoring it or by asking him to increase it until he stopped from fatigue and boredom. At the same time, she gave the mother very specific suggestions as to how to demonstrate parental control to the boy.

Both mother and therapist deemphasized the identification of the boy as handicapped and focused instead on the fact that he could experience mastery in his own development and enjoy more positive experiences with others. The child's behavior problems virtually disappeared in one week, and follow-up 20 months later revealed no recurrence. Though some might argue that neither of these cases really involved the use of hypnosis, we consider them both examples of the breadth of conversational hypnotic approaches to which children can respond, especially since hypnosis can occur without any formal invitation, induction, or even a mention.

The following case is an example of our work with young children who have behavior disorders. Ray, a 10-year-old adopted boy, was seen for hypnosis regarding frequent temper outbursts that occurred both at home and at school. These were triggered by seemingly minor frustrations, such as being unable to accomplish a task, being denied a privilege, being asked to go to bed (at normal bedtime). His mother perceived him as being easily frustrated and having a short attention span, although he did well academically in school. The patient had been adopted in infancy. When he was 4 years old, his parents adopted two biological sisters, ages 3 and 6 years. The patient subsequently manifested frequent jealousy of his adopted sisters. He had been examined by his pediatrician and a neurologist and had been receiving psychotherapy for several months without noticeable improvement.

At the time of the first visit for hypnosis, Ray appeared angry and embarrassed. The therapist first demonstrated peripheral temperature biofeedback and gave him the opportunity to raise his fingertip temperature which he did successfully on the first attempt. The therapist explained that he had accomplished this because of his own control, just as he had developed controls in many performance areas such as body control when he performed on athletic teams. He was then taught a simple breathing relaxation hypnotic induction and was asked to practice this daily. He was also asked to organize practice sessions for the entire family during which they would review relaxation exercises from *The Centering Book* (Hendricks & Wills, 1975).

Because of illness in the patient, the second visit did not occur for 3 weeks; however, telephone follow-up revealed that Ray seemed much more confident and happy and that the family was practicing self-hypnosis at home. He said he had had no tantrums in school and only a few at home. During the second visit, after introduction of and invitation to hypnosis, he was taught a jettison technique for ridding himself of things that bothered him, a method to replace the tantrums. During the third visit, the parents reported a marked reduction in Ray's tantrums.

The session was audio recorded, and Ray took the audiotape home for review three times weekly. Telephone follow-up 1 month later confirmed that he "has pretty much quit temper tantrums." The mother said that, other than fidgeting in church services, he was doing well and feeling much better about himself. In the case of young children with behavior disorders, some therapists prefer to work primarily with the parents. Petty (1976) used this approach with the mothers of two children, a 4-year-old girl and a 5-year-old boy, both with severe tantrum behavior. Both mothers were initially instructed to ignore the tantrums but simply could not do so. Petty then utilized hypnotic relaxation and desensitization techniques. The mothers developed hypnotic images of past tantrums without feeling anxious or disturbed, then repeated the procedure with an imaginary future tantrum. In the first case, the tantrums abated after 3 months; improvement continued during the following year. In the second case, follow-up after 1 month also revealed a marked decrease in tantrum behavior. Petty concluded that, as a result of the mothers' changed attitudes and responses, the children's tantrums lost their reinforcing value and extinguished. It is important that therapists be aware that tantrum behavior beyond the first few years may reflect brain injury with problems in self-modulation. Older children who have prolonged tantrums that do not respond to a brief period of intervention may need further diagnostic evaluation.

## Behavior Disorders in Adolescents

Kaffman (1968) described a 14-year-old boy on a kibbutz who displayed a 4-year history of poor self-control and marked antisocial behavior, including lying, stealing, property damage, and physical attacks on other children. Both the referring therapist and the boy's teacher had recommended residential treatment. Although the boy had refused to cooperate with earlier psychotherapy lasting 2 years, he now quickly accepted the suggestion of a 10-session trial of hypnosis, with the knowledge that the decision for residential treatment would be temporarily postponed. According to Kaffman, "Hypnotic suggestions included the strengthening of his will to be and behave like other children, emphasis on his own responsibility and capacity to achieve this aim in the area of school, work, and social interaction, together with increased motivation to cooperate in treatment" (p. 733). From that day forward, the boy's behavior problems ceased. He completed the ten therapeutic hypnosis sessions and continued in psychotherapy every 2–4 weeks. At the end of 2 and ½ years, he had maintained his gains, described by the author as "remarkable." Although the behavior change indeed may have resulted from the introduction of hypnosis, we wonder about the effect of the serious threat of residential treatment. This is a case in which a 5–10-year follow-up would be helpful to determine whether the boy really wanted to change his behavior or merely wanted to avoid the "punishment" of residential treatment. In the latter instance, we might expect eventual return of antisocial behavior. On the other hand, the hypnosis may have given him confidence that he could change his behavior.

The question of patient motivation arises for similar reasons in Mellor's (1960) series of 14 cases of juvenile offenders, all of whom had been in a juvenile detention center. Their agreement to learn self-hypnosis was part of the requirement for probation. The patients, ages 13–17 years, included 2 girls and 12 boys. The average total treatment lasted 6 hours, with successful results in 13 of 14 cases. Follow-up ranged from 7 to 17 months, with 4-year follow-up in one case. The one treatment failure was a narcotics addict who showed no motivation for behavior change after five sessions.

Mellor's technique consisted of using ideomotor finger signaling to help the patients get at underlying emotional tensions and to elicit confidence that they could acquire more appropriate behavior patterns. Mellor believed that this technique facilitated regression, recall, and reorientation of thoughts and feelings. Because the patients were in a light to medium trance, they experienced rapid integration and soon developed insight and took responsibility for overcoming their problems. They moved from the ego passivity that often accompanies impulsive behavior to ego activity and true self-control. These results are certainly impressive and the relatively short-term follow-up encouraging. But, given the adolescents' histories, one would need a 5–10-year follow-up to be able to judge more clearly the value of the treatment. As with Kaffman's (1968) patient, we have to wonder whether the motivation for treatment was based chiefly on a desire for change or on a wish to avoid the punishment of incarceration. Also, the concept that a therapist can judge depth of trance or maintain a certain depth is in question. Based on developmental issues raised at the beginning of this section, we are more confident of the validity of the positive reports of young children with behavior disorders than of those concerning adolescents.

Goldbeck and Schmid (2003) studied the effectiveness of autogenic relaxation training for children and adolescents with behavioral and emotional problems. Fifty children (mean age, 10.2 years; range, 6–15 years) in Southern Germany were part of this group intervention. Fifteen were randomly assigned to a waiting list control group. The experimental group of children "with mild to moderate behavioral and/or emotional problems" were taught autogenic relaxation, which the authors describe as "an auto-hypnotic relaxation method," noting its widespread use in German-speaking countries and its use as a method to enhance effective coping with stress in healthy populations and as a basic psychotherapy. The study investigated the hypotheses that autogenic training reduces multiple internalized and externalized symptoms as reported by parents on the CBCL (Achenbach, 1991), that it reduces a broad spectrum of somatic complaints as reported by children and adolescents, and that it reduces the degree of stress as perceived in specific questions and as reported by a standardized stress questionnaire.

All parents reported behavioral problems or somatic complaints in their children, although only 14% had sought treatment (psychotherapy or medication) before participating in the study. The main problems described by parents were recurrent headache (46%), sleep problems (36%), attention problems (32%), hyperactivity (30%), recurrent abdominal pain (18%), and nervousness (14%). Most parents reported multiple problems in their children, and 90% had chronic symptoms of over 6 months duration. After baseline scales (including the CBCL and a self-report subjective complaint scale for children) were obtained, autogenic training was provided in groups of 9–12 per group, ages 6–11 or 11–15; eight sessions were provided for 30 minutes each, once a week. Relaxation units of 10 minutes each were embedded in a child-centered framework of play and conversation, and the six basic exercises of autogenic training were taught; children were encouraged to practice one or two times per day at home between training sessions.

At the beginning of the study, before autogenic training was begun, there were no significant differences in symptoms between the experimental group and the wait-list control group. Following training, the experimental (hypnosis, autogenic training) group showed a statistically significant decrease of behavioral and emotional symptoms and a significant decrease in self-reported stress and overall somatic complaints compared to the control group, confirming the hypotheses of the study. In their discussion of the results, the authors noted two ingredients that we agree are very significant in the clinical efficacy of training in self-regulation such as autogenic training/self-hypnosis: (1) the value of parental support and praise (e.g., for their children's home practice of newly learned skills), and (2) the intrinsic importance of daily practice of newly acquired skills in order to build competence and confidence. In addition, the treatment process enhanced the sense of personal control and competency for each participant.

## Anxiety Disorders

Generalized anxiety disorder, separation anxiety disorder, and social anxiety disorder (social phobia) affect between 6 and 20% of children and adolescents (Costello, Egger, & Angold, 2004; Emslie, 2008). This category includes children consciously aware of and distressed by excessive anxiety, as manifested by phobic reactions, posttraumatic stress disorders (PTSD), panic disorder, misophonia (see details in chapter on Habit Disorders also), sleep disorders (e.g., sleep onset insomnia), or social anxiety disorder (Kellerman, 1981). Several studies, including systematic reviews by the Cochrane Collaboration (James et al., 2006; O'Kearney, Anstey, & von Sanden, 2007), have evaluated the efficacy of behavioral or CBT for several different forms of anxiety disorders. Sometimes CBT programs describe a required component of "relaxation training" (James et al., 2006) and often include descriptions of relaxation imagery practice. These are probably the equivalent of hypnosis. Accordingly, we briefly discuss the outcome of these reviews as part of the growing evidence-based support for hypnosis in anxiety problems.

James et al. (2006) identified 13 randomized controlled trials of CBT versus waiting list or attention controls in children over 6 years of age with a diagnosis of anxiety. Excluded from consideration were any studies that included simple phobias, OCD, or PTSD. For consideration in the Cochrane Review, a study had to conform to principles of CBT with the use of a protocol and comprising at least eight sessions. Thirteen studies with a total of 498 subjects and 311 controls met these criteria. Analyses showed a remission of anxiety response rate of 56% for the CBT groups as compared to 28.2% remission of any anxiety diagnosis in the control group. Various anxiety scales were used to assess symptoms in the different studies, and all were considered to be reasonably reliable and valid measures. In general, there was poor agreement between parent and child reporting of anxiety symptoms, so child self-report ratings were preferred when the meta-analysis was conducted. Although there was no apparent effort to tease apart the varying elements of CBT to discern what elements might be most operative in facilitating the positive response of anxiolysis, the authors do question whether cognitive elements of CBT are a necessary part of a psychological treatment package, rather than a pure behavioral treatment, particularly since some studies have shown behavioral treatments (alone) to be effective for different forms of anxiety (James et al., 2006; Masia, Klein, Storch, & Corda, 2001).

This report supplements and reinforces the earlier review by Ollendick and King (1998) of empirically supported treatments for children with anxiety disorders and phobias. As in later studies, Ollendick and King described CBT as by definition including elements which are clearly hypnosis, such as the use and training or reinforcement of imagination skills and relaxation training.

A study in 2008 (Walkup et al., 2008) compared CBT, sertraline, or a combination in childhood anxiety. In this randomized, controlled trial, 488 children from 7 to 17 years old who were diagnosed with separation anxiety disorder, generalized anxiety disorder, or social phobia were assigned to receive 14 sessions of CBT, sertraline alone, CBT + sertraline, or a placebo drug for 12 weeks. Ratings of severity and impairment were conducted at baseline, and at weeks 4, 8, and 12. Results were described in terms of percentages of children rated as very much or much improved on the Clinician Global Impression Improvement scale: 80.7% for the combination of sertraline and CBT ($p < 0.001$), 59.7% for CBT alone ($p < 0.001$), 54.9% for sertraline alone ($p < 0.001$), and 23.7% for placebo. All therapies were superior to placebo, and the combination of CBT and sertraline was superior to either treatment alone (Walkup et al., 2008). As with the Cochrane Review described earlier, this study supports and reinforces our long-observed clinical experience and perspective on the value of self-regulation training via self-hypnosis. While reinforcing that self-regulation/self-hypnosis training is effective, in some situations patients benefit from a combination of self-hypnosis, other behavioral treatments, and medication. As such, hypnosis should be understood as a significant option – but not necessarily the *only* option – in a clinician's toolkit for children with anxiety.

In addition to these randomized controlled studies, over the last decade many clinical reports have continued to inform and enhance our knowledge about the breadth and extent of successful and creative applications of hypnosis for young people experiencing various forms of anxiety problems (Aviv, 2006; Emslie, 2008; O'Kearney et al., 2006; Roberts, 1998; Zaider & Heimberg, 2003). We review some of the most interesting and significant such contributions here.

Kendall (1994) conducted the first randomized controlled trial of CBT for children with anxiety disorder. Of the 47 children (9–13 years old), 9 had a diagnosis of avoidant disorder. The 16-week intervention combined educational, cognitive, and exposure-oriented techniques but clearly included hypnotherapeutic components in the form of role-playing and relaxation training. Posttreatment, 64% of treated cases no longer met criteria for an anxiety disorder. Kendall's replication of this work included 9 children with anxiety disorders, also 9 to 13 years old (Kendall et al., 1997), and at the end of the 16-week treatment over 50% of participants no longer met criteria for anxiety disorder as compared to only 2 children in the waiting list control group.

Esch and associates (Esch, Fricchione, & Stefano, 2003) described the value of various mind–body interventions, including relaxation training, in reducing anxiety as well as helping with related problems of insomnia, recurrent headaches, etc. Deckro and colleagues (2002) examined the effect of a 6-week mind–body intervention (including relaxation response training and cognitive behavioral skills) in 128 college students. Significantly greater reductions in anxiety, perceived stress, and psychological distress were found in the experimental group (63) compared to the wait-list control group (65). Kaiser (2014) noted that anxious and fearful children and teens need help in reducing exaggerated psychophysiological stress reactivity. This article included a case that described hypnotic techniques aimed at teaching children more accurate discrimination with respect to danger and ways to increase self-regulation.

## Social Anxiety Disorder (Social Phobia)

For both temperamental and psychodynamic reasons, some children and adolescents feel especially insecure in social situations outside the immediate family. Many of these youngsters learn adaptive social skills as a result of participation in preschool groups, with the support of parents, teachers, and other helping adults. Some, however, continue to be generally shy and withdrawn, and their difficulties may become pronounced when there is additional social stress such as occurs with a move to a new neighborhood or a change of schools. Although long-term psychotherapy may be indicated, sometimes brief supportive hypnosis can help these children use their strengths to overcome the problem. The following case example illustrates the possible value of this.

Diana, age 15 years, came into the office with her mother to request help in overcoming shyness that had become incapacitating in school and in social situations. The patient described herself as always having been introverted, especially when compared to three older siblings, but this had become more of a problem at age 13 when she entered junior high school. Previously, she had attended parochial school and had known the same classmates for 6 years. In the new junior high school, she found herself unable to stand up in class and recite or raise her hand to answer questions. She preferred accepting failing grades to giving oral presentations. In the therapist's office, she also expressed her reluctance to initiate friendships except with her siblings and said that she engaged in social activities only when with her older sister and two older brothers.

Diana was a strikingly beautiful, well-groomed adolescent. According to her mother, she had been a good student until entering junior high school. She got along well with her parents, siblings, other relatives, and a few girlfriends. Her mother volunteered that, although she accompanied her daughter for the first visit, she would encourage her daughter to come alone on subsequent visits. This and other comments suggested that the mother truly wanted her child to achieve greater independence and social participation. There was no evidence of significant family pathology.

Diana was seen three times to learn and practice hypnosis. In the first interview, it became apparent that she was interested in becoming a model, perhaps a counterphobic reaction but still one that could be used to her advantage. She was invited to learn hypnosis with eye fixation and progressive relaxation. Diana was asked to imagine herself feeling comfortable as a model. She was asked to practice self-hypnosis twice daily, using ego-strengthening imagery. When seen 2 weeks later, Diana reported that she was feeling more comfortable in social situations and had been able to recite in class. During this visit, she was asked to regress to a past experience that had been pleasant and represented success to her. She was asked to squeeze her right fist to make the recollection of positive, happy feelings more vivid. When she did this, the therapist asked her to let herself be aware of something that might be bothering her, to consider whether or not she could let go of this, and then to imagine sending it off on a plane or freight train. She was told that she could repeat this imagery in her self-hypnosis exercises at home if she wished.

On the third visit, 6 weeks later, Diana reported proudly that she had had her first date, she was comfortable in the classroom, and she was now practicing self-hypnosis once daily. While Diana was in a hypnotic state, the therapist asked her to imagine herself on a stage, performing in front of people whom she liked and feeling good about herself. She was followed by telephone and continued to do well at 6-month follow-up.

## Phobic Reactions

In general, it has been believed and taught that the longer a child has had a phobia, the more difficult it is to resolve. Parents and other well-meaning adults often insist that a child will soon "outgrow" his or her fears. Although sometimes this is true, often, however, the child develops a series of avoidance strategies in order to avoid the feared situation. Parents may reinforce and even encourage such avoidant behavior, thereby unwittingly communicating to the child that the fear is valid and depriving the child of opportunities for corrective experiences and mastery. As the avoidance strategies become more complex, with increasing involvement of parents and siblings, the problem may evolve into a *folie a famille*. Given the ease of resolving recently developed phobias, early intervention makes much more sense than the approach of hoping the child will outgrow them (Gardner, 1978b).

When hypnosis is offered in the treatment of phobias, our most common approach is based on desensitization, advanced and enhanced with hypnotic elements that are similar to the method used in behavior modification (Schowalter, 1994). In a state of hypnotic relaxation, children develop images in which they experience safety and mastery. They then develop a series of images related to the feared event, maintaining the feeling of mastery as they visualize each image. The therapist then gives posthypnotic suggestions that they can increasingly experience the same feelings of mastery in related reality situations. Sometimes the hypnosis sessions include *in vivo* desensitization such as when there is a needle phobia. Research has suggested that these active participation techniques are as good as the use of imagery alone and may, in some instances, be more effective (Hatzenbuehler & Schroeder, 1978). Symptom substitution is rare.

Ambrose (1968) described another method (a jettison technique) for helping children cope effectively with anxiety. In a hypnotic state, the child is asked to make a fist and then "is told that he has all his fears and problems clasped in his fist. On the count of three he will open his fist and all his anxieties will disappear into thin air and he will feel happy, confident, etc." (p. 3). As in the desensitization method, the emphasis here is on mastery. Ambrose further stated that, especially in the case of deep-seated phobias, dynamically oriented therapy – with or without hypnosis – is necessary for lasting results. We believe that analytic work may be necessary more often with Ambrose's brief, almost magical method than with the desensitization techniques in which the child can easily see the connection between therapeutic method and problem resolution; however, we have no data comparing the relative efficacy of the two methods.

## School Avoidance

As in all therapeutic approaches to school refusal (previously known as school avoidance or school phobia), the child health professional must first explore and understand the underlying dynamics, a task often accomplished quite rapidly. Although the problem is usually connected to separation anxiety about leaving their parents rather than a fear of school *per se*, these are of course not mutually exclusive, and there may be other precipitating factors (Schowalter, 1994). Crasilneck and Hall (1985) described a 7-year-old boy whose mother had impressed on him that he should "do what he was told" in school. When older children on the school playground threatened to pull his pants down, his fantasized participation and its attendant anxiety led to refusal to go to school. In another case, a young child's fear of school turned out really to be fear of the school station wagon, which reminded him of an ambulance and associated fear of sickness. In both cases, assurance and clarification in both the usual state of awareness and in hypnosis produced rapid symptom relief and return to school. Crasilneck and Hall further noted the importance of parent counseling in such cases to avoid parental behavior that either reinforces the fear by excessive comfort or is overly critical.

Lawlor (1976) described three cases of school avoidance, two of which included hypnosis as well as parent counseling and environmental manipulation. In both cases – a 5-year-old boy and a 4-year-old girl – the purpose in teaching hypnosis was to interview the child in a relaxed state to gain information about the dynamics of the problem. The first child readily verbalized feelings of hostility and destructive wishes toward his parents and siblings, with concurrent fears of abandonment. After reassurance from the therapist and the mother, the boy soon made a satisfactory school adjustment. In the second case, the situation was more complicated, including the mother's suicide shortly before the onset of phobic symptoms. Hypnotic interview revealed that the child blamed herself for her mother's death, feared her own death, and hoped to reunite with mother by staying home. She was placed with an aunt and uncle. The security of her new home combined with therapeutic reassurance to facilitate a good adjustment in her new school. In both of these cases, it is not clear whether the clarification of dynamics and therapeutic reassurance might have been equally successful without hypnosis. There were no previous attempts at psychotherapeutic intervention. In our own practices, we find rapid success with young school-avoidant children using play therapy, nonhypnotic interviews, and parent counseling. It is probably reasonable to conclude that hypnosis is at least as useful alone or in combination with more traditional methods of treating school avoidance in young children.

The value of hypnosis in helping older children with the anxiety associated with school avoidance has been described in several reports (Aviv, 2006; Roberts, 1998). Roberts described the case of a 14-year-old adolescent female, J., who presented with a long history of difficulty attending school, beginning as early as third grade, intensifying in fifth and sixth grade, and again so much so in eighth grade that her attendance decreased to 25%. Throughout these years, the family sought and participated in a variety of behavioral interventions from guidance clinics and school and private psychologists, most of which seemed to work briefly before relapses later in the same or subsequent school year. Quite typically, J. was described as having very intense difficulty separating from her mother at school, with tension and crying. In seventh grade, yet another school change was made and she seemed to be improved, but in eighth grade she was extremely distressed when attempting to go to school, complained of stomachaches and experiencing panic attacks, and had only 25% school attendance. In ninth grade, she had only 3% attendance in the first 2 and ½ months of school. She was referred to a psychologist for help with her attendance and separation anxiety, to address her need for confidence building, and to help cope with panic attacks. J.'s panic attack the morning of the scheduled first visit precluded her attendance and the psychologist met with the parents to review the history and agree upon a plan of phased return to class along with training in strategies for coping with panic via relaxation techniques.

During the first session, J. spoke openly about her history of panic, how it was always worse on Mondays, and about her motivation to go to school full time and not experience these feelings. When J. was encouraged to discuss favorite activities, she did so readily; she said that she liked animals and had recently gotten a new puppy. The puppy was "used as a metaphor to give positive suggestions about successful early learning experiences, separation and independence, using the idea of a healthy puppy growing up, being weaned, leaving its mother for a family that will adore it, learning its name, being house-trained, and learning to walk, to heel, and all the other tricks and routines of life at home and outside" (Roberts, 1998). The first official hypnosis experience followed with suggestions for deep breathing and relaxation followed by imagining getting into the car and going to school. The intention to access negative feelings was accomplished, as she complained of feeling sick to her stomach and alerted. Fractionation followed, with an invitation to go back into trance and imagine something that made her feel great, relaxed, happy, and confident. After reinforcement, she was given the suggestion to return to trance and imagine she was now ready to get in the car and go to school the following Monday. An anchor of the car door closing was provided, followed by the suggestion to recreate the resourceful, positive imagery while continuing comfort, confidence, and relaxation. Homework was given to notice any new changes and new learning accomplished by her puppy in the intervening week.

At the next visit, J.'s mother reported that the interim Monday, despite her not feeling well, had been J.'s best Monday in 4 months. The visit with J. focused upon ego-strengthening compliments for her success and reinforcement with planning to extend the school day to include afternoons as well as mornings. She was taught self-hypnosis with progressive relaxation and metaphors for anxiety reduction and confidence. Her school attendance rose from 67% to 90% in response to self-hypnosis training. When discussing J.'s success, the author noted that he believed improvement could be attributed to her motivation to change and replace unwanted behavior patterns and to the provision of self-hypnosis techniques which, when practiced regularly, empowered her to achieve the changes and substantial improvement that followed.

Aviv (2006) reported on the use of "telehypnosis" in the treatment of adolescent school avoidance. In this case series of 12 adolescents (8 boys and 4 girls, ages 12–15 years), the duration of absence prior to therapy was an average of 65 weeks of missed school, with a range of 24–120 weeks. Three had been absent less than 40 weeks, and the majority had missed more than 60 weeks. Follow-up after treatment showed that more than a year later, 8 of 12 (67%) had maintained full-time attendance, three had maintained partial improvement, and only one had not improved. Treatment involved between six and ten in-person visits for therapy, which included "hypnosis, relaxation, breathing training, guided imagery with suggestions for confidence building, anxiety reduction and positive reframing of negative associations" (Aviv, 2006). Uniquely, the author provided the teenagers each with the opportunity for cellphone access to him for telephone reinforcement of hypnosis as needed in the morning at the most critical and challenging time in anticipation of getting and going to school. Preparatory to this, hypnotic suggestions were offered for "cueing," such that the sound of the therapist's voice on the phone would help them to quickly go into their self-hypnosis, access their favorite place imagery ("area of comfort"), and recreate the comfort and confidence required to proceed with getting to school. During the phone conversations, which lasted 5–15 minutes, individual guided imagery reinforcement was provided. As agreed during individual face-to-face therapy sessions, the adolescents only called when their anxiety had reached a level of 5 or higher on the 1–10 point anxiety scale, with 10 being the worst anxiety. During the first 2 weeks of return to school after therapy, 8 of 12 initiated cellphone contact with the therapist while getting ready for school; 65% of the calls were made from home during early morning, 20% were made en route on the school bus, and 15% were made after the patient had arrived at school. Collaboration with and cooperation of school counselors and teachers facilitated the ability of the students to have the hypnosis-reinforcing phone conversations with the therapist.

## Needle Phobia

Needle phobia is common among both adults and children. In children, the fear of being poked or stuck with a needle produces violent reactions such as tantrums, vomiting, struggling enough to require restraint for the injection, and physical assaults on the person doing the procedure. We believe that the development of severe needle phobia can be avoided by anticipatory training in the outpatient clinic, the dentist's office, or on the hospital ward. Jody Thomas, child psychologist, has developed an appealing series of video programs to help children learn to cope with injections or pokes (Thomas, 2019).

Because injections usually are portrayed as though they cannot be postponed, requests for help from colleagues are often characterized as urgent. In some of these situations, we believe that we have the opportunity – sometimes perhaps at some political or organizational risk – to help everyone involved hypnotically by restructuring the crisis mode of the moment, perhaps defusing what really is not a "we have to do this injection *right now*" and planning a more thoughtful, preventive, positive coping experience for a bit later. Sometimes, however, as in the emergency room (see also chapter on Surgery and Emergencies), circumstances demand we must work as rapidly as possible.

Approaches depend on the age of the patients, their developmental stage, past behaviors during injections, and the therapist's creativity. We reported treatment of a 7-year-old boy who required repeated intravenous infusions of plasma in the treatment of Bruton's agammaglobulinemia (Olness & Gardner, 1978). He responded with hysterical outbursts and had to be restrained by six people. The treatment was as follows:

> It was explained to the patient that his unique imaginative ability, better than that of many adults, could help him learn a method to "turn off his pain switches." When he learned the method, he could then turn off these switches prior to his injections and it would no longer be necessary for him to feel uncomfortable or upset. The patient was taught a standard method of relaxation, visual imagery exercises, and the switch-off technique. During the first visit he demonstrated immediate ability to tolerate pin pricks in his self-anesthetized hands and arms. Subsequently, he joined a group of boys with hemophilia who met regularly for review sessions. The next visit for gammaglobulin, which occurred three weeks after his initial visit to our hospital, was calm. He proudly hypnotically turned off his switches and held out his arm for the injection. He has been followed for one year with no further difficulties, and one nurse now starts the intravenous infusion. (pp. 230–231)

Another patient was a husky, 17-year-old adolescent boy with a needle phobia of many years duration; he was being treated for meningitis with a 6-week course of continuous intravenous (IV) antibiotics. Each time the IV had to be restarted, he became hysterical and had to be restrained by several people. When offered hypnosis to overcome his phobic response, he responded enthusiastically. The treatment consisted of asking the patient to focus on pleasant mental imagery and following with *in vivo* desensitization, beginning with a small tuberculin needle in his forearm, then increasing the size of the needle, and later injecting him with normal saline. Instead of suggesting anesthesia, the patient was told in hypnosis to recall feelings of comfort in his arm and to fill his arm completely with comfort until there was simply no room for any other feeling. He rapidly developed a strong transference to the therapist and began to share her confidence that he could conquer his phobia. His enjoyment of adolescent bravado further contributed to his motivation for success. After three hypnosis sessions, he tolerated restarting of his IV without requiring restraint. A few days later, with the therapist present, he tolerated a lumbar puncture with only moderate anxiety. By the end of his hospital stay, his anxiety was minimal and his cooperation excellent. He called the therapist some months later to report that he had had no difficulty when he required a tetanus shot after a minor injury. Other methodologies include hypnoanesthesia, such as revivification of a recalled local anesthetic numbness (such as a prior dental anesthesia or anesthetic for suturing), or metaphors to facilitate dissociation. A representative case history involving hypnoanesthesia for needle phobia follows.

Marty was 14 years old when he was referred by his pediatric endocrinologist to learn hypnosis for needle phobia associated with the need for daily growth hormone injections. Marty had long been afraid of needles but had managed to cope with intermittent blood tests or immunizations. The idea that he could self-administer injectable growth hormone seemed impossible not only to Marty but also, perhaps more significantly, to his mother. When the idea that he might someday do his own injections was presented, his doctor, nurse, and mother all agreed with him that he couldn't (but really wouldn't) be expected to do this to himself from the start. The missed opportunity to shift his expectation, belief, and behavior from the beginning served to perpetuate his phobic response to needles.

His mother administered the injections. With each subsequent injection, his behavioral-avoidant, phobic response was more pronounced. This usually took the form of delaying tactics, the demand that everything be "just so" before beginning, and increasing anxiety – for example, "Wait, wait, not yet, not yet ... I'll tell you when ... not yet," resulting in 60- to 90-minute ordeals at home for what should have taken less than 5 minutes. Increasingly, individual injection times were complicated by the mother's growing frustration expressed as complaints and denigrations of Marty, such as "you're taking up too much of my time" or "you're acting like a baby." She also used threats, such as "I'm not going to give them, and then you won't grow." Physicians counseled the mother to stop giving the injections in order to empower Marty to do so. For almost 6 months her fear that he would not grow if she didn't personally give the injections ("he'll never do it; I know he won't – he's too afraid") served as a major barrier to Marty's slowly developing skill and confidence that he could give himself the injections.

A timid and relatively socially isolated young adolescent, Marty lacked self-confidence in most areas of his life. His favorite activities, watching movies alone all day in the theater or at home, were also isolating. During his first visits to learn hypnosis skills, rapport was established slowly, and hypnosis was presented in a naturalistic, Ericksonian fashion: "This is not magic, I wish it was ... but you might be surprised to discover when you're ready that it might seem like magic, because I'm sure that when you're ready you'll be really surprised how effective it will be ... you'll probably really surprise yourself the most of all, don't you think?" It is essential that the clinician have a clearly and strongly held *personal belief and faith* in these suggestions so that the child or adolescent can and will apply suggestions to their own needs.

Marty was taught hypnosis with favorite place imagery of being at the movies or of riding his bike. Hypnotic suggestions emphasized themes of competence and autonomy for ego strengthening, as well as the importance of practicing self-hypnosis "just to get good at feeling relaxed and comfortable whenever you need to do so. And the more you do it, the better you'll get." After several practice sessions, therapeutic suggestions were offered in menu format, again with the focus being to facilitate personal choice and a sense of control and empowerment by letting Marty choose the (hypnotic) method by which he would indeed solve the dilemma of being able to give himself an injection. Ericksonian double-bind types of suggestions were given often – for example, "I don't know exactly how you're going to give the injection each time, whether it will be by letting your jaw be numb like it was at the dentist and then transferring that numb feeling with your mind and your hand down to the leg that will get the injection, or whether you'll just imagine that your leg isn't even there – although it is – and not notice it, or whether you'll just do it some other way." After about 6 months Marty came for an appointment. In the waiting room his mother smiled broadly and said, "You won't believe it; he'll tell you about it!" She was consciously unaware of the potential negative impact and power of her own words and tone, and of the confusing nature of her obvious pride mixed with her own struggle to allow her son to grow up, figuratively and literally.

Marty reported with awkward embarrassment and pride that he had given his own injection the night before and that "it took about 20 minutes, but I finally did it … and I could feel it, but it wasn't as bad as I thought it would be." Beyond purposely exuberant congratulations, we reviewed and reinforced success in and out of hypnosis by focusing on "how did you *do* it?" Marty proceeded to administer his own daily injections for the next 4–5 months without much difficulty or tension. The benefit to his maturation and self-esteem seemed to be dramatic, but then he relapsed for no apparent reason. His mother quickly became reinvolved in preparing and administering his growth hormone and thereafter he never gave himself another injection. To her credit, the mother was able to set specific limits. She and Marty agreed that she would give his injections only if he would not argue, fight, complain, or use delaying tactics. This accommodation was said to be mutually acceptable and continued until he discontinued the growth hormone at the end of his senior high school year.

Of note, and undoubtedly complicating this case of needle phobia, was the emergence in Marty of a full-blown panic disorder. After no contact for more than a year, Marty called the therapist because of anticipatory test anxiety that became manifest during examinations in his senior year. "Too anxious" to use his self-hypnosis, he requested and benefited from anxiolytic medication, which also allowed him to access his self-relaxation skills more easily. He had three clinic visits to develop comfort with these symptoms. Most recently, his continued struggle with autonomy was reflected in the desire to drive himself to college rather than to be "stressed" by his family taking him several hundreds of miles and then leaving him. Although this initial separation seemed to work, he soon became unhappy with his first college roommate, suffered great sadness at the long separation from his girlfriend, and dramatically quit college, returning home to live with his parents. At his most recent visit, he acknowledged his continuing anxiety and noted that he still turns to self-hypnosis to help himself relax, "sometimes."

In evidenced-based support of hypnosis training for Marty and many others in our clinical experience, numerous controlled studies have been performed. In 2008, Uman and colleagues (Uman, Chambers, McGrath, & Kisely, 2008) reported on an abbreviated Cochrane Review of randomized controlled trials for psychological interventions for needle-related procedural pain and distress in children and adolescents. Strict criteria were utilized for inclusion in their systematic review and meta-analysis of cognitive behavioral interventions for pain and distress. Though they did not specifically identify studies or participants as having needle phobia, they included both published and unpublished trials that had at least five children or adolescents (between 2 and 19 years) in each study arm. Needle procedures included venipunctures, immunizations, finger pricks, injections (subcutaneous or intramuscular), lumbar punctures, bone marrow aspirates or biopsies, peripheral or central IV or catheter insertions, laceration repairs, arterial punctures, portacath accesses, and thoracentesis or paracentesis. Exclusions included children undergoing surgery. Types of interventions reviewed included cognitive interventions (those which involved identifying and altering negative thinking styles related to anxiety about the medical procedure and replacing them with more positive beliefs and attitudes), behavioral interventions (based on principles of behavioral science and learning by targeting specific behaviors), or combined cognitive behavioral interventions.

Although their list of cognitive interventions included and distinguished between cognitive distraction, imagery, hypnosis, preparation and information, thought stopping, coping self-statements, suggestion, memory change, and parent training (Uman et al., 2008), we believe that each of these, except perhaps for parent training, represents a mind–body technique or strategy that is in fact hypnotic or includes elements that are hypnotic (Kohen, 2010a). Analogously, their list of behavioral interventions also includes many approaches that we would define as intrinsically reflecting hypnotic characteristics. These include behavioral distraction (tapes, games), muscle relaxation, breathing exercises, modeling, rehearsal, desensitization, and virtual reality (Uman et al., 2008), all of which have as significant ingredients the narrowing and focused, absorbed attention of the child and imaginal involvement – characteristics of the hypnotic experience.

This significant contribution to evidence-based medicine concluded that sufficient evidence was identified "to support the efficacy of (a) combined CBT for observer-reported distress and behavioral measures of distress; (b) distraction for self-reported pain; (c) distraction + suggestion for self-reported pain; *(d) hypnosis for self-reported pain, self-reported distress, and behavioral measures of distress* [emphasis added]; (e) providing information and preparation for observer-reported pain and improving pulse rates; (f) nurse coaching + distraction for behavioral measures of distress; and (g) parent positioning + distraction for observer-reported distress" (Uman et al., 2008). Among other conclusions, the authors noted – and we strongly agree – how important it is that health professionals and families be informed of and aware of the value of incorporating hypnosis training and related psychological strategies for procedural pain and distress into practice with children. In so doing, and particularly early in the course of a child's experience with needles, we will be able to not only effectively treat existing needle phobia but also likely prevent many more from developing. Berberich and Landman (2009) demonstrated the value of positive "waking hypnotic" suggestion with child friendly imaginative techniques in a randomized controlled trial to reduce the discomfort of immunizations in children 4–6 years old. Beyond the evidence provided from this study is the demonstration that effective randomized controlled studies of hypnosis can be conducted reasonably efficiently in a private practice setting.

## Animal Phobia

Crasilneck and Hall (1985) reported a case of animal phobia in which hypnosis was used to understand the dynamics and to help the child master the problem.

## Weather Phobia

Many children and adolescents develop weather phobia from experiencing an actual weather event such as a hurricane or watching weather events on television or observing adults who have weather phobia. There are books to help children prepare for and cope with weather disasters (Dean, 2020). Children with weather phobia benefit from learning self-hypnosis to use for relaxation when weather events are predicted.

## Obsessive–Compulsive Disorders

Obsessive–compulsive disorder (OCD) in children and adolescents can be very debilitating and interfere substantially with daily functioning. OCD is characterized by persistent intrusive thoughts, experience of inappropriate images or impulses that may cause marked anxiety, or by persistent repetitive behaviors such as ordering and checking or, in some, handwashing. As such, some of these repetitive, habituated behaviors may be responsive to hypnosis training in a manner similar to approaching other habit problems (see Chapter 9). For more debilitating or persistent forms of OCD, medication may be helpful, and our experience has been that the addition of self-hypnosis training to medication has been more effective than medication alone. Children with OCD with whom we have worked hypnotically report benefit from rehearsing split-screen imagery in hypnosis, in which they imagine the undesired compulsive behavior on one side of a split screen and the desired or alternative behavior on the opposite side. They then either watch the undesired image becomes smaller and smaller while the positive image becomes bigger or watch the undesired image get dimmer while the other becomes brighter. As with all self-hypnosis approaches, children are taught and encouraged that "the more you practice, the better you get, and the more you practice when you are *not* experiencing the problem, the better you will become at being able to quickly and easily apply the self-hypnosis when you *do* have the problem." Another useful strategy has been to offer the hypnotic suggestion that the very first sign of the intrusive thought or compulsive behavior is "your signal to yourself to do your self-hypnosis and picture either a huge *stop sign* or a *traffic light* in your imagination, and then just notice how the thought or behavior stops because you teach it to do that through your hypnotic utilization of the *stop sign* or of watching a *traffic light* go from green to red."

A Cochrane Review (O'Kearney et al., 2006) identified only four randomized control trials (involving 222 participants) evaluating the benefits of behavioral and CBT approaches. The results of two of the studies (Barrett, Healy-Farrell, & March, 2004; Franklin, Foa, & March, 2003) showed that BT/CBT is an effective treatment for reducing symptoms and for lowering the risk of OCD after treatment as compared to a wait-list or pill placebo control group. The overall review demonstrated that BT/CBT when combined with medication was superior to medication alone but not to BT/CBT alone. As noted earlier, these CBT programs all include relaxation and self-talk components that are hypnotic strategies.

## Posttraumatic Stress Disorders

Children, as adults, suffer complications of trauma, and these often extend for a lifetime. When one considers the number of children in the world who experience the early loss of their parents, the terror of war, dislocation from homes into refugee camps, earthquakes, tornadoes, mental and physical assaults, or traumatic medical and dental procedures, it is clear that the residual posttraumatic stress disorder (PTSD) will vary in severity, depending on the presence of a parent or other trusted adult, coping abilities of the family, early opportunities to express their perceptions and feelings about the event, whether the event was isolated or repetitive, and whether or not there was much associated deprivation of daily needs. Hypnosis training is increasingly being described as helpful for both adults and children who have suffered PTSD.

Friedrich (1991) described case histories of four children with PTSD. He speculated that a trance-like phenomenon occurred at the time of the trauma. A second trance, in the form of therapeutic hypnosis, was extremely helpful in integrating the trauma so that optimal, pretrauma functioning could be obtained. Rhue and Lynn (1991) described storytelling and hypnosis in the treatment of sexually abused children. They emphasized provision of a mental safe place as well as images of personal power and control via hypnosis.

Crasilneck and Hall (1985) described their work with an adolescent girl suffering psychogenic amnesia (in today's nomenclature, this would be understood as part of PTSD) after a severe trauma. In our hypnosis training with amnesic patients, we give an additional permissive suggestion for reinstatement of the amnesia: "When you come out of hypnosis, you can remember as much as you are now ready to cope with, now ready to face. Whatever you need to forget, you will be able to forget until a later time when you are ready to deal with it." This wording does not authoritatively impose reinstatement of amnesia, a maneuver that we think often has more to do with the anxiety of the therapist than with the needs of the patient. Instead, it communicates respect for the patient's defenses and ego strengthening by also implying that the patient may – either now or in the future – be strong enough to face and integrate the traumatic material. Sometimes a child has good recall of a traumatic event and wants to talk about it, but he or she is unwilling to do so for any of several reasons. Here again, the combination of hypnotic relaxation and heightened positive transference often provides a setting in which the child feels free enough to communicate.

In forensic cases it is sometimes suggested that hypnosis be used to assist children in recalling details of crimes in which they were victims and witnesses. Although hypnotic interrogation is sometimes valuable in criminal investigation, the process is fraught with pitfalls that sometimes lead to serious miscarriages of justice. Both the *International Journal of Clinical and Experimental Hypnosis* (Frankel & Perry, 1994; Orne, 1990) and the *American Journal of Clinical Hypnosis* (Mutter, 1990) have published monographs on the important subjects of the uses and misuses of forensic hypnosis and the relationship of hypnosis to memory. Therapists working with children must realize that techniques suitable for helping a child recall and master an emotional trauma differ in significant ways from appropriate techniques for working with the same child in the context of criminal investigation. The most competent child health professional should obtain additional special training before engaging in forensic hypnosis. We recommend that he or she take care to understand individual state or national laws regarding forensic hypnosis. We also recommend that he or she refuse to assist in obtaining evidence from children unless there is prior agreement that the information revealed will be used to guide investigators in their search for evidence but that neither the child nor therapist will be called to testify. It is also essential that there be a neutral observer present when he or she is doing hypnosis with the child and that each session be recorded.

Both before and since the tragedy of the 9/11 attack, with the occurrence of many natural disasters and with the prevalence of wars, sadly large numbers of children and adolescents have experienced PTSD (Olness, 2022). Fortunately, there have also been many efforts and increasingly thoughtful approaches to help these children, and not only have therapies been provided to those in need, but they have also been evaluated and reported so that more therapists may learn and more young people in need may benefit from timely, appropriate intervention (Adler-Nevo & Manassis, 2005; Catani et al., 2009; Cohen, Kelleher, & Mannarino, 2008; Ehntholt & Yule, 2006; Gordon et al, 2008; Lesmana, Suryani, Jensen, & Tiliopoulos, 2009; Nikulina et al., 2008; Salcioglu & Basoglu, 2008; Shooshtary et al., 2008; Smith et al., 2007; Stallard et al., 2006; Stein et al., 2003).

Lesmana and colleagues (2009) reported the effectiveness of a faith-based hypnosis program ("spiritual-hypnosis assisted therapy") provided to children between the ages of 6 and 12 years who experienced the 2002 terrorist bomb blasts in Bali, Indonesia. In a longitudinal, single blind randomized controlled study, 48 children comprising the experimental treatment group were compared to 178 in the control group who received no therapy. These 226 children were diagnosed with PTSD and were among 514 children who were initially screened 6 weeks after the bombings and exhibited symptoms directly attributable to the bomb experience. Most (87.5%) of the 3.5 million people on Bali are Hindu and thus believe that humans comprise mind, body, and spirit. The spirit is the source of energy, the source of personal awareness, a repository of knowledge, and a kind of subtle intelligence within the individual. The authors explain that a hypnotic approach was a natural for this population because Balinese Hindus tend to meditate from an early age, as part of their ritual of prayer, and a large number have experienced trance or mass hypnotic states in the context of annual religious ceremonies. The spiritual hypnosis was described as follows:

> It began with a meditation-trance induction. (They were) … instructed to meditate with their eyes closed, and after 5 minutes were instructed to breathe deeply through their nose and slowly exhale through their mouth. Instructions were repeated five times, and deep breaths lasted for one minute, … then the participants' breathing remained constant and deep without any further guidance, at approximately 5 breaths per minute. … The researcher monitored certain behavioral cues of the participants, such as arm rigidity and immobilization, eye catalepsy, and inability to communicate, all of which the authors accepted as indicators of a hypnotic state. When in trance participants were guided through suggestion to be sensitive of their own spirit and were advised to identify and reframe the meaning off traumatic memories that may have been at the root of a strong tendency to obscure their spirit. It was suggested that they express emotions and visualize the past and that their spirit would lead them to choose the particular traumatic memory related to the bomb … not to imagine or visualize the traumatic moment, but rather to let the process happen in a natural way. They were directed to express undesirable feelings with crying, shouting, or by inhaling deeply and exhaling slowly. The purpose was for them to release all emotional burdens that been stored in their memories. They were led to their *culturally familiar* [emphasis added] concept that the power of God would help them gain strength to cope with their emotions. As they re-experienced hidden emotions they were advised to see the problem from the perspective of the moment … guided to see the environment around them, their family, friends, and to visualize walking through the site where the bomb blast occurred … and guided to accept that the experience was in the past … and that what happened in it would enable them to face new challenges without the burdens of the past trauma. (pp. 26–27)

The group session lasted about 30 minutes. Statistically significant results showed a 77.1% improvement rate (compared to 24% improvement in the control group) and concomitantly significantly lower PTSD symptom scores in the treatment group compared to the control group. The authors note, appropriately, that their method is highly dependent on the skill of the therapist and, concurrently, the patient's trust of the therapist. As we have emphasized throughout this text, a highly positive rapport is essential to effective hypnosis work, and in the study by Lesmana et al. (2009), this is not only exemplified but amplified by the added ingredient of a shared faith system among patient participants, families, and therapists.

Gordon and colleagues (Gordon et al., 2008) reported an analogous successful group approach in helping adolescents in postwar Kosovo learn self-regulation strategies to help themselves cope with PTSD symptoms. Eighty-two adolescents were randomly assigned to a 12-session mind–body group program or a wait-list control group. Hypnosis and self-hypnosis strategies described included guided imagery; breathing techniques; meditation; self-expression through drawings, words, and movement; and autogenic training and biofeedback. Results showed statistically significant lower PTSD scores (Harvard Trauma Questionnaire) in the intervention group compared to the wait-list control group and later in the wait-list control group after they, too, received treatment, compared to their pretreatment PTSD scores. A 3-month follow-up showed maintenance of symptom reduction. Of particular note in this study is that the participants had significantly positive PTSD symptom scores 5 years after the war had ended. The authors emphasized that a variety of mind–body techniques were utilized, and they made no attempt to determine the effectiveness of any single modality. They emphasized that teaching a variety of techniques provided the opportunity for individual students to practice those techniques that they personally found most effective, and they speculated that the success of the program was related to a number of factors, including social support in the group setting, opportunities for a variety of self-expression, stress-reduction via mind–body techniques, and the students' use of imaginative techniques to solve problems. The significant role of hypnosis in this program seems clear, even though the words *hypnosis* and *hypnotherapy* do not appear in the text of the report.

In a similar report of group therapy, Ehntholt and colleagues (Ehntholt, Smith, & Yule, 2005) reported the effectiveness of a group CBT program in reducing PTSD symptoms and related emotional and behavioral problems in young refugees from different war-torn countries. This was a six-session, school-based program, which, as those described above, focused on normalizing reactions to the traumas and especially on developing self-hypnosis strategies, which they described as "visual imagery, relaxation exercises, coping self-statements." In a follow-up paper, Ehntholt and Yule (2006) provided an overview of treatments available to refugee children and adolescents and emphasized the importance of primary care clinicians being sensitive to and identifying symptoms of PTSD toward providing optimum intervention.

In a comprehensive review of studies to date, Nikulina and associates (Nikulina et al., 2008) summarized and defined the field of PTSD diagnosis and treatment, amplifying the value of group and school-based treatment programs and, again, emphasizing the value of hypnotic strategies, including relaxation training, imagery, and cognitive restructuring. Efficacy was described whether the groups were inner-city children 8 to 13 years old exposed to the 2001 World Trade Center attack (Brown, McQuaid, Farina, Ali, & Winnick-Gelles, 2006) or refugees from war in various countries. They concluded that taken together the studies suggest that 12-session manualized interventions have been feasible, acceptable, and efficacious with children and adolescents of multicultural backgrounds and that trauma-specific CBT has been found to decrease symptoms of anxiety, depression, and conduct problems as well as PTSD-specific symptoms (Nikulina et al., 2008).

Similar positive outcomes of the effectiveness of hypnosis for trauma (as part of a CBT program) have been reported recently regarding PTSD symptoms in adolescents following a 2004 earthquake in Iran (Shooshtary et al., 2008), PTSD in children following the tsunami in Sri Lanka in 2004 (Catani et al., 2009), and PTSD in children and adolescents following earthquakes worldwide (Salcioglu & Basoglu, 2008). Our colleague, Culbert developed "comfort care kits" for children and families with cancer and other severe and chronic illnesses. These kits, which include many activities for children, include a focus on "imagination exercises" and "progressive relaxation" and were very helpful to many children and families devastated by and coping with the recent tsunami in Thailand. Another colleague, Dr. Srivieng, translated Culbert's comfort kits into Thai and distributed 10,000 of them in Thailand after the tsunami. Clinical observation reports that they were very helpful (Pairojkul, 2010).

## Everyday PTSD and Acute Stress Disorder

It is clear that children and adolescents are vulnerable to the development of PTSD when they have been exposed to or experienced war and terrorism, physical and sexual abuse, and natural disasters such as floods and earthquakes. Additionally, however, PTSD symptoms may develop in the context of witnessing domestic violence, experiencing and navigating catastrophic illness (in themselves or family members), and in accidents and injuries such as motor vehicle accidents. The consequences of these experiences are myriad and may include developmental delay, increased propensity to anger, suicidal ideation, substance use, aggressive behavior, increased anxiety and depressive symptoms, and regressive behaviors.

Childhood traumatic grief – or what could also be called PTSD by proxy – represents the complex relationship between traumatic experiences and bereavement (Brown, Pearlman, & Goodman, 2004), and young children experiencing this are vulnerable to PTSD, anxiety, depression, anger, and associated behavioral problems. In the treatment of traumatic grief, hypnotic elements (progressive relaxation, cognitive restructuring to change thoughts and feelings, visualization) are key ingredients described in traumatic grief CBT programs, illustrated in one report of a 5-year-old boy whose firefighter father died in the line of duty on September 11, 2001 (Brown et al., 2004). Among the hypnotic suggestions utilized, but not identified at all as hypnosis, were suggestions offered as a metaphor for the child to change the channel of an imagined TV screen when or if the images seen internally were too bothersome, and by so doing he could change the physiology, behaviors, and negative thoughts associated with the previous channel's images and feelings.

Finally, we note that, despite the foregoing reports, PTSD remains a relatively young, or new, diagnosis in pediatrics, and much has yet to be defined in terms of diagnostic criteria or best methods of treatment. Adler-Nevo and Manassis (2005) reviewed 742 articles dealing with the treatment of pediatric trauma and identified only 10 as relevant to the treatment of pediatric PTSD following single-incident trauma, or Type I traumas (the result of one sudden blow, such as a motor vehicle accident or terrorist attack), as opposed to Type II traumas (resulting from long-standing repeated ordeals, such as war or repeated or ongoing child sexual abuse). As in the preceding discussion, most of those ten reports employed CBT treatment programs, all were school based, and all included elements we would consider hypnotic, especially progressive relaxation and visualization procedures for reduction of anxiety. Linden (2007) provided a comprehensive overview of an understanding and application of hypnosis in various forms of childhood trauma. Readers interested in further research directions are also encouraged to examine this review in detail.

## Performance Anxiety

We are often asked to help children who experience stress in school in the form of test anxiety as well as those who experience other performance anxiety, such as the anticipatory anxiety of musical recitals, stage fright regarding a school play or community orchestra, or hockey, football, track or related sports competition. Nath and Warren (1995) described a program of stress reduction for adolescents preparing for major examinations. This successful program incorporated relaxation and hypnosis within a cognitive behavioral framework (see also chapter on Medical Problems).

## Sleep Disorders

### *Fear of Going to Sleep*

Jacobs (1962, 1964) described three children, ages 6, 8, and 9 years, who suffered anxiety with going to sleep. He emphasized the importance of understanding the dynamics that, in these cases, included equating sleep with death, associating sleep with anesthesia and postoperative pain, and psychic trauma resulting in generalized feelings of insecurity. Jacobs directed his treatment to the underlying anxiety, reminding the children in hypnosis of their parents' love for them and assuring them that they could feel increasingly safe and confident. In all three cases, normal sleep patterns returned within several weeks.

Our experience with many such cases of so-called sleep onset anxiety or insomnia confirms Jacobs' report that these usually do not represent a sleep disorder but rather are a manifestation of anxiety expressed at bedtime. Most often the child's fears have not previously been expressed except through the symptom of insomnia. Accordingly, attention to rapport and elucidation of unexpressed worries with or without hypnosis will allow the clinician to then utilize a variety of hypnotic strategies to promote an easy and comfortable transition to sleep. Although most such sleep-onset anxiety cases are simple and straightforward, some are quite complex but potentially amenable to relatively easy symptom management. A representative case history follows.

Kohen (1995a) described an 11-year-old boy who was referred with a discrete 3-month history of what his family called "panic attacks," which occurred before he went to sleep at night, resulting in taking 2 hours to fall asleep, and later awakened him during the night for 1–2 hours. He described feelings of great fear at the time of the episodes and also when he worried that the events would happen again during the night or on the following night. He reported that the first episode occurred the night after the first day of school. They had occurred nightly since then.

The history also revealed that the family had moved recently from their home of many years and that the patient missed his friends. Further, the father had returned to the home part-time while remaining in a day-treatment, sexual-offender program for the molestation of the patient's sister, who had been removed from the home. The boy also missed his maternal grandmother, who had died 3 years earlier. He had never spoken about these events before and did so in a detached, spontaneously hypnotic fashion. In response, the therapist spoke to him in hypnotic fashion, offering positive, ego-strengthening, reframing, reassuring suggestions in the absence of any formal hypnotic induction. The patient was told that the therapist was certain he could be of help and that he was quite confident that the boy would soon find it easy to go to sleep. In what may have been a pivotal and valued hypnotic suggestion, the therapist ended the first visit by assuring the boy that his mother had a picture of the grandmother that she would give to the patient as his very own so he could keep it with him at bedtime. He agreed to do so.

To investigate the possibility of partial complex seizures, an electroencephalogram (EEG) was obtained the following day; it was normal. Six days later, the patient returned and reported happily that he had not had any trouble going to sleep and, for the first time in 3 months, he had not experienced any "panic attacks." He and his mother nonetheless requested medication, and a prescription for a low dose of imipramine (a medication of choice for panic attacks) was given. He returned a week later having remained free of panic attacks or sleep difficulties. The prescription had not been filled because of insurance problems. The boy spoke openly of sadness about his grandmother's death, anger with his father, and missing his friends from his hometown. At the fourth visit, he remained free of further panic attacks.

Although no formal hypnotic invitation was offered, in this case, elements of hypnotic behavior and hypnotic suggestion were clearly operative in beginning therapy with this youngster. Early in the clinical relationship, his diagnoses included sleep-onset anxiety and panic attacks. Separation anxiety regarding the family move, prolonged grief, bereavement regarding the death of his grandmother, and perhaps PTSD by proxy of delayed onset regarding the sexual abuse in the family may each have contributed to his symptoms.

Anbar and Slothower (2006) identified 75 children and teens who experienced sleep-onset insomnia or night-waking. In their retrospective review, 90% of those who had a sleep-onset delay more than 30 minutes reported a reduction in time to fall asleep. In addition, for those with night-waking more than once a week, over half (52%) completely resolved this symptom after learning self-hypnosis and an additional 38% reported improvement. The authors proposed that substantial benefit can and does occur with hypnosis for sleep problems, as most (2/3) of the reported successes occurred after only one or two hypnosis training sessions.

In single case reports, Howsam (1999) described the effective use of hypnosis in the treatment of individual children with insomnia, nightmares, and night terrors, and Merritt (1991) and Contos (1999) described its use for nightmares and fears of going to sleep. In each case, treatment was relatively short (four or five therapeutic hypnosis/relaxation and imagery sessions), and follow-up showed no recurrences at 3- and 7-month follow-ups.

## *Nightmares*

Although all children occasionally have nightmares, some children have them so frequently that they become truly disruptive, making the child afraid to go to sleep and causing the parents to be aroused at night. In contrast to night terrors (sleep terror disorder), the child usually is able to recall some details of the nightmare. If there is a known precipitating event, the child can be encouraged to recall that event in hypnosis and then be reminded that he or she is now older or safer or in some way able to deal with the problem. Whether or not there is a known precipitant, the child can be asked to experience hypnotic safety and then to re-dream the nightmare in hypnosis but this time changing the ending so as to emerge the master rather than the victim of the situation. The child is then told that it is possible to do the same thing when actually sleeping, if the nightmare should recur. Children enjoy this challenge, and their nightmares usually cease after one or two sessions of clinical therapeutic hypnosis (Gardner, 1978b).

King, Cranstoun, and Josephs (1989) described three children (ages 6, 8, and 11 years) with whom "emotive imagery" was utilized to allay anxiety associated with nighttime fears and nightmares. In addition to self-monitoring and behavioral assessment of "darkness toleration," each child was presented with therapeutic imagery suggestions based on favorite fantasies and interests. Although the authors did not identify this work as therapeutic hypnosis, a perusal of their scripts clearly reflects elements of positive imagery, posthypnotic suggestions, future-oriented suggestions, and ego-strengthening suggestions for safety and comfort (e.g., "What a brave boy you are; you slept in your bed by yourself all night"). Two of the three children showed fewer behavioral disturbances over the intervention period. In their multiple-baseline design study, the authors concluded that a combination of treatment procedures can be utilized to help children with these problems, including emotive imagery and hypnotherapeutic-like strategies, along with systematic desensitization, relaxation, and parent counseling.

St-Onge and colleagues (St-Onge, Mercier, & De Koninck, 2009) reported a randomized controlled study of imagery rehearsal therapy (IRT) in children 9–11 years of age with a history of moderate to severe nightmares (i.e., one or more nightmares a week for 6 months) and no history of PTSD. Results indicated that following a baseline period (for data collection), IRT training reduced the frequency of nightmares ($p < .04$) in the treated group (9 children) compared to the wait-list group (11 children), and nightmare reduction was maintained over a 9-month follow-up period. IRT is described as the most successfully used and frequently studied treatment for adults with nightmares (Halliday, 1987). St-Onge and associates described the ingredients of the IRT the children learned, and in our opinion this clearly represents a hypnotic and self-hypnosis methodology, although it is not described or characterized as such. The treatment protocol was taught to be applied the night following a nightmare. If a nightmare was remembered in the morning, children were asked to record their memory of it on a tape. The next evening before bed they were instructed to modify the nightmare any way they wanted to so that it would no longer be a nightmare for them and to record this new version on tape. A suggestion was given that there were thousands of ways of changing the nightmare but they only had to pick one, try it, and change it in another way if it didn't work. The second step was to lie in bed with their eyes closed in a relaxed state, and they were asked to rehearse mentally (and verbally if desired) the modified version (new dream) for 10 minutes, making sure to view the images in their head. Integral to the research was a third step in which they were asked to complete a daily intervention journal asking how long they had rehearsed the new version of their dream and how they felt afterward. We believe this study clearly describes the effectiveness of training in a method of self-hypnosis for nightmare modulation and management.

Parent counseling is a reasonable and appropriate concomitant to therapeutic hypnosis strategies with children. This is important for some parents who, in their efforts to help their child, have been unwittingly reinforcing a behavior; for example, some well-intentioned parents may overdo the recommendations for a comforting nighttime ritual by developing a series of measures such as a snack, a back rub, a story or favorite song, getting up to watch television, or sleeping in bed with the parents (or *vice versa*). Parents can be reassured that attention to underlying anxiety and the teaching of simple self-hypnotic exercises are often and usually quickly successful in eliminating the troublesome behavior. For preschool children, it may be helpful to ask parents to facilitate the hypnotic strategy through the technique of favorite stories or other strategies outlined earlier (Chapter 5). Linda Thomson's metaphorical tales for children in *Harry the Hypnopotamus* (Thomson, 2005; Thomson, 2009) have been very successful adjuncts for parents and children in facilitating the falling asleep process. Similarly, the series on meditation for children by Garth (1997) provides many relaxation and imagery ("meditative") techniques that parents can utilize to help children or that older children may read for themselves to help "calm themselves to sleep." It is our belief that by any name these meditations are in fact hypnotic and self-hypnotic in substance and function (Kohen, 2010a, p. 292).

## *Night Terrors (Sleep Terrors) Disorder*

Partial arousals from sleep include nocturnal behaviors ranging from quietly sitting up in bed to so-called bloodcurdling screaming associated with heightened autonomic arousal. These partial arousals typically occur in the first third of the sleep cycle, usually 60–90 minutes after sleep onset and during completion of the first period of slow-wave sleep. During these arousals, children are caught between deep (slow-wave) sleep and full arousal. Characteristics of this state include (1) high arousal threshold, (2) lack of response to the environment, and (3) mental confusion. Although clinical symptoms vary, they include three basic categories: quiet sleepwalking, confusional arousals, and night terrors, or sleep terrors. Although symptoms vary, all of these disorders of partial arousal are similar in pathophysiology, timing in the sleep cycle, duration, clinical features, and genetics (family history is positive in up to 60%). The feature that clearly distinguishes night terrors from nightmares is that children (or adults) are amnesic for night terrors.

Because children do not recall night terrors, one cannot use the hypnotic dream alteration method employed for nightmares. As with all problems, clinicians should, however, seek to clarify the history and any information known regarding possible precipitating events. Acute life-event changes or stressors are often identified as apparent triggers, as are acute, febrile illnesses; however, methods for establishing a cause-and-effect relationship have not been defined. In taking a careful history, one can clarify the precipitating event and then employ hypnotic imagery to increase the child's sense of confidence and safety. Taboada (1975) used this method with a 7-year-old boy who had had night terrors for 15 consecutive nights after a frightening incident at camp. The night terrors ceased after one hypnosis session, with no recurrence at a follow-up 18 months later.

Kramer (1989) described hypnotic intervention for a 10-year-old boy with a 6-year history of night terrors that had themes of changing into a werewolf or of being physically mutilated or hurt. He was amnesic for the events, but his mother reported the content he expressed during the night terrors. Induction of hypnosis was accomplished with a "finger-lowering technique" in which the middle two fingers were raised, and he was given a metaphoric suggestion to watch his fingers go to sleep. Therapeutic suggestions consisted of repetitive and methodical explanation of sleep physiology, emphasizing the regularity and continual movement of the cycles of sleep. After two hypnosis sessions, he became free of night terrors and remained free of recurrence for 2 years of known follow-up. He was reported as happier and able to watch scary movies, which had, in the past, seemed to trigger the night terror behavior. The author appropriately identified the need for further research to understand how hypnosis affected the night terrors.

Koe (1989) described a 16-year-old male adolescent with sleep terror disorder that had occurred nightly for 7 years and had been resistant to interventions including benzodiazepine medication, behavior modification, and psychotherapy. A typical episode began with repetitive screaming, leaping out of bed, running around his room, and often becoming violent, including breaking his mother's nose during one episode and smashing a window and furniture. Embarrassed and motivated to change, he explained the night terror as a fear of dying in his sleep but could not explain how or why the fear had begun. Koe utilized hypnosis to identify that the patient utilized external stimuli (i.e., noises) to (unconsciously) cue himself to the night terror/ partial arousal. While he was in a hypnotic state, suggestions were given that he was in a deep sleep, the stage in which he usually had night terrors. In response to the hypnotic suggestion, autonomic arousal (increased respiratory rate, agitation) occurred, and the noise of a pencil tapping on the desk evoked a full-blown night terror with screaming and running about and associated confusion. Subsequent hypnotic sessions focused repeatedly and only upon the post-hypnotic suggestion that, while asleep, he would gradually become less and less aware of outside sounds and sensations. The night terrors decreased from several per night to a total of three during the following week. Three months later he experienced no further night terrors.

Kohen, Mahowald, and Rosen (1992) described the use of self-hypnosis for four children, ages 8–12 years, who had frequent, prolonged, or dangerous disorders of arousal documented by a polysomnogram (in a regional sleep disorders center) that showed sudden arousals out of slow-wave sleep associated with the complex behaviors of sleep terrors. After demystification of their symptoms through methodical education about sleep physiology (unlike Kramer noted above, education was provided before, not during, trance), and because of the dangerous or prolonged nature of their sleep terror behaviors, these children were treated pharmacologically first. Each responded to a short course of imipramine while also being taught relaxation and mental imagery (self-hypnosis). In each case, the medication was discontinued while self-hypnosis was reinforced, and in each case the children remained free of further arousals over 2–3 years of follow-up. Invitations to learn hypnosis and deepening were individualized with favorite place imagery, and then each child was offered the opportunity to "let me know, with a finger signal, when you are ready to learn how to use this very nice feeling and imagination to reprogram that computer we call the brain to sleep very well." Superimposed on the waking-state information they received about sleep cycles and "accidentally getting stuck" between a state of deep sleep and wakefulness, each child was given the simple therapeutic suggestion that "as you practice this each night, and before you go to sleep, remind yourself to have a peaceful, restful, quiet night's sleep in your own bed and wake up in the morning happy and proud." Audiotapes of the office hypnotic suggestions were provided for reinforcement.

As success with these four children became evident, we then offered hypnosis to children without prior pharmacological treatment. Successful reduction and elimination of night terrors occurred in six of seven children (21 months to 16 years old) who were treated only with the described hypnotic approach. Later data analysis (G.R. Rosen, pers. comm.) revealed that polysomnograms previously believed to be diagnostic for night terrors in these children are, in fact, not distinguishable from matched siblings. Polysomnograms also showing partial arousals from slow-wave sleep occur in the siblings of night terror patients but with no clinical night terror behaviors.

We concluded, as did Kramer (1989), that hypnosis was successful in eliminating the troubling night terror behaviors but that we do not yet understand the mechanism by which change was effected. Research continues in this fascinating area.

## Psychophysiological Disorders

The problems discussed here have in common a presenting complaint of a physical problem for which the basis is primarily psychogenic. We include conversion disorders, psychogenic seizures, pain where there is no identifiable organic origin, and anorexia nervosa. In some cases, the psychological disorder is precipitated by a *bona fide* physical problem; in other cases, the origins are psychogenic. In all cases, however, psychological factors play a major role in maintaining or aggravating a somatic complaint, as noted by M.S. Smith (1983). Stressors triggering these symptoms may be environmental or physical stressors and psychological (emotional) stressors.

In their evaluation of such symptoms, Rickert and Jay (1994) recommended the severity, affect, family, and environment (SAFE) interview strategy. The severity of symptoms should be assessed in the beginning of the interview. The affects of both the patient and the parent or guardian should be evaluated. Efforts should be made to understand ongoing family concerns and conflicts as well as the patient's environment, including peers, school, and community. We have found that a helpful approach in meeting with the family together is to ask each parent, "What does your body do when you are nervous or anxious?" or "When I am anxious, my hands feel cold – what does your body do when you are nervous or anxious?" This question is always answered, and family members are often surprised to learn that other family members sometimes feel anxious. Children with somatoform disorders, however, often do not know immediately how their bodies react to distress.

## Conversion Reactions

Conversion reactions have been conceptualized as expressions of neurotic conflict that may center around issues of hostility or independence or sexual wishes. Conversion reactions may occur in children and in borderline or psychotic individuals as well as in neurotic individuals. Williams and Singh (1976) reported a case of conversion reaction manifested by hysterical amblyopia in an 8-year-old girl. We encourage the reader to consult the original report or to read it in its entirety in the third edition of our text (Olness & Kohen, 1996), as it is an excellent example of careful diagnostic assessment, detailed description of hypnosis treatment, and appropriate follow-up. Williams and Singh briefly reported other cases of childhood conversion reaction:

1. A 12-year-old boy presented with a 9-month history of abdominal pain with flexion of the trunk and inability to walk. After two sessions of hypnosis over 1 week, the patient began walking during the following week.
2. A 12-year-old girl with a seizure disorder presented with inability to walk and blindness of 1 day's duration. Her ability to see and walk was restored after one hypnosis session.
3. A 13-year-old girl complained of a 6-month history of polyarthralgia of hips, knees, and ankles with gait impairment. Her joint pains resolved completely after three weekly hypnosis sessions.

In all of these cases, continued individual and family therapy were recommended. Follow-up ranged from 7 to 16 months. There were no cases of symptom substitution, although some symptoms transiently recurred, usually associated with situational stress or premature termination of outpatient psychotherapy.

Williams (1979) reported the therapeutic hypnosis treatment of a 13-year-old boy with lower-back pain, eventually diagnosed as a conversion disorder. His method was essentially the same as that used by Williams and Singh (1976). The pain disappeared after one hypnosis session. At the time of Williams' report, the boy had remained symptom-free for 2 years.

Sarles (1975) briefly described a 16-year-old girl who was hospitalized after sudden onset of total paralysis from her neck down. Physical examination revealed no organic disease. Psychiatric evaluation disclosed hysterical features and a precipitating event in which the girl had been berated for kissing a boyfriend and warned that her parents would "watch every step she took." During an 8-week course of family counseling and hypnosis that used regressive techniques to explore the dynamics of the paralysis, the girl made a complete recovery. No follow-up data were given in this report.

In a paper on pediatric hypnosis, Olness and Gardner (1978) included a short case report of a conversion reaction. We present the case here in more detail, with special emphasis on the use of hypnosis and its role in the larger treatment context:

> Kit was a bright, active 8-year-old boy, the youngest of eight children in a middle-class, intact, Catholic family. He developed documented streptococcal pharyngitis and, soon thereafter, experienced pain and weakness in his extremities, progressing over 2 weeks to the point that he could not walk or use his arms and required total care. He was admitted to the neurological service of a large hospital, where diagnostic work-up revealed no organic basis for his complaints. Psychological evaluation pointed to conflict in the area of independence–dependence of which the boy was partially aware. He said he enjoyed the role of baby in the family, including special attention from mother; at the same time, he wished he was old enough to have more of the privileges enjoyed by his older siblings. Kit's mother acknowledged that she had always loved babies and derived gratification from continuing to think of Kit as her baby. Kit was aware of his mother's feelings, and his wish to please her contributed to his conflict. It seemed that the strep throat had tipped the balance, providing Kit with even more maternal attention. He unconsciously attempted to resolve the conflict by becoming a baby, thereby gratifying both himself and his mother. At the same time, the conversion reaction allowed unconscious expression of hostility toward the mother who seemed to interfere with his developmental needs. The therapist explained the dynamics to the boy and his mother, assuring them that Kit was not malingering. The mother was shocked that her feelings could have such a profound effect on her son, and she immediately asked for help with her problems. Both Kit and his mother were relieved that there was no permanent physical disability, and they readily accepted the recommendation of brief hypnosis training for Kit to alleviate his symptoms, followed by individual and family therapy to work through the underlying conflicts.
>
> That afternoon, in the first of two hypnosis sessions, the therapist talked further with Kit about mind–body relationships, the dynamics of his conversion reaction, and the way hypnosis could help him get conscious and unconscious wishes in better alignment. He was fascinated with the idea that, while consciously he could not move his arms, he probably could do so in the altered state of hypnosis. As an initial demonstration, the therapist used an arm levitation hypnotic induction with eyes open, to which Kit readily responded.

> Then the therapist employed the method of combined age regression and age progression to facilitate the recovery of a lost skill. First Kit was asked in hypnosis to recall a specific time when he walked or ran with confidence and enjoyment and to relive that past experience. Having accomplished this, he was then asked to let go of the situational details of the memory but to hold on to the good, strong feelings in his legs, now experiencing them in the present. He said, "My legs feel very strong; I don't think they could feel any stronger." It was then suggested that he could imagine using his strong legs in the future. He did so. Then he was told that, if he was ready, he could remain in hypnosis and walk across the room. Having followed this suggestion with obvious pleasure, he was given a posthypnotic suggestion that he could, if he wished, choose to retain the use of his legs when he came out of hypnosis. He did so, generally happy, but disappointed that we had not yet "cured his arms." The therapist said he could work on that the next day, planning to use the interim to observe his response to the partial recovery.
>
> By the following morning, Kit had maintained his gains with no evidence of new problems. The second hypnosis session proceeded along the lines of the first, now focusing on his arms. He achieved hypnotic arm rigidity and experienced normal strength and sensation first in hypnosis and then in the waking state. He was discharged from the hospital later that day. The symptoms briefly recurred the next day but then disappeared totally.
> Kit and his family were followed in outpatient therapy over several months, and the basic conflicts were satisfactorily resolved. Annual cards from Kit's mother have indicated that he has been symptom-free for more than three years and once more leads an active, happy life.

Sometimes cultural factors suggest that nontraditional methods in the general domain of hypnosis will be most useful. Carla was a 10-year-old Mexican–American girl with nonorganic total body paralysis and a diagnosis of conversion reaction. The child was hesitant to relate to Anglo–American doctors and responded only minimally to one session of traditional hypnosis. Although adequate history was difficult to obtain, it eventually came out that the child had been hexed. We then contacted a *curandera* (faith healer) who saw the child for three sessions. She produced a necklace and suggested that the power of the necklace could be transferred to the child. By touching the necklace, Carla regained movement of her arms and upper torso in two sessions. She also regained her ability to walk, although at a slower rate because she had been confined to a wheelchair for 4 months. She was given the necklace to wear as a continuing reminder of her own power and as a symbol to the community that she could no longer be hexed.

One must not conclude from these reports that hypnosis is always the treatment of choice to achieve rapid symptom relief in conversion reactions. Conversion reaction may occur in the context of a borderline psychotic state, serving a major defensive purpose. In such cases, hypnosis should be employed – if it is used at all – first for ego strengthening and only later and very gradually to aid in symptom removal or amelioration. In a recent report, Bloom (2001) presented a detailed discussion of his hypnotherapeutic work with a 12-year-old girl and a couple of years later with a 15-year-old boy with near total body paralysis conversion disorders. Although the elements of the cases are interesting in their own right, we believe that the author's conclusions about the process are indeed most instructive, not only for our uses of hypnosis with conversion disorders but also, indeed, for any of our clinical work with hypnosis.

Even in the abstract, Bloom characterized his clinical work with these two patients as a "journey," emphasizing throughout what and how much he had learned from the process, particularly in attending to the issues of transference and countertransference, which were operative and instrumental in the therapy. He emphasized that, "The use of hypnosis in the treatment of conversion disorder creates a unique opportunity to create an alternative solution to life problems in an acceptable context for change" (Bloom, 2001, p. 245), explaining that, because patients and families may not consider hypnosis as either a medical or a purely psychological treatment process, that hypnosis affords the patients a way to get well without necessarily deciding whether the origin of the problem was physical or emotional. After highly positive and fairly rapidly successful hypnosis results with the 12-year-old girl with (conversion) paralysis from the neck down, Bloom described his much more arduous and personally frustrating course of treatment with the 15-year-old boy with functional paralysis from the neck down who 2 years later was a patient in the same psychiatric inpatient unit as the 12-year-old girl. He approached the young man with confidence, utilizing similar strategies that had been so effective with the 12-year-old girl earlier. Little positive response ensued, but after many weeks he was surprised when the patient angrily announced his frustration and declined any further hypnosis. A couple of months later other members of the clinical inpatient team invited the author to resume therapy and the patient was surprisingly receptive.

A distinctively different approach was taken. Bloom (2001) explained pointedly the need for clinicians to be aware of their own countertransference and described the subsequent, very different, and ultimately successful therapeutic hypnosis approach. When the patient was asked by the clinician for advice about their relationship, the young man said, "It is the differences in people, not their similarities of diagnoses, that make for true therapy." He went on to say that "it was only after I got to know him as a different and unique individual that we could begin to work together so that he could change … of course he was right" (Bloom, 2001). The patient had heard about the 12-year-old girl who had been treated on the same unit 2 years earlier and had the impression, correctly, that the therapist had assumed that because his diagnosis was the same as the girl's that the treatment would be the same. As Bloom concluded, and as a reinforcement for Erickson's dictum to "go with the child" (Erickson, 1958b), "recognizing [unique] differences openly and using them to form a deep personalized contact unique to each patient creates a valid context for healing."

## Psychogenic Seizures

In cases of psychogenic seizures, psychological problems play a major role in precipitating seizure activity. The patient may or may not also have an organically based seizure disorder. Although not conscious during a true seizure, the patient often has heard descriptions of the details of the seizure activity. Sometimes the child has witnessed true seizures in relatives or close friends. Although it is difficult for casual observers to differentiate between true and psychogenic seizures, there are distinguishing characteristics; for example, if the patient exhibits dramatic movements that look like a grand mal seizure but does not lose consciousness, has no incontinence, and experiences no stupor or lethargy immediately afterwards, one should suspect that the seizure has a psychogenic origin (Glenn & Simonds, 1977).

Gardner (1973) described her treatment of Tracy, an 8-year-old girl with familial seizures, whose first generalized convulsion occurred at age 9 months. From age 3 years, her EEG showed a petit mal variant disturbance, with seizure activity manifested chiefly by eye-fluttering spells. Seizure frequency increased markedly when the child was in kindergarten, and the problem worsened over the next 2 years despite several medication changes and a trial ketogenic diet. At age 8 years, Tracy was diagnosed as having both true and psychogenic seizures. No longer able to function either at home or at school, she was highly motivated to improve seizure control. Treatment lasted for 18 sessions, consisting of a combination of hypnosis, play therapy, and parent counseling.

The therapist avoided suggesting any sensations associated with the seizures such as eye closure, drowsiness, amnesia, or time distortion. The hypnotic induction consisted of relaxation with eyes open, followed by hand levitation as a metaphorical demonstration that the child could learn new ways to control her body. In hypnosis, she was given repeated suggestions that it could be fun to keep her eyes open and see what was going on. Ego-strengthening suggestions were also utilized that praised her for cooperation and improvement and reminded her of the happy consequences of positive changes. She learned self-hypnosis and enjoyed home practice sessions focused on "being able to keep her eyes open more and more."

By the fifth session, Tracy showed clear improvement. She then developed a new problem: difficulty getting to sleep at night. This problem quickly resolved when the therapist reminded her that there were times when it was appropriate to close her eyes. Play therapy emphasized carryover of the hypnotic behavior to the waking state and modification of low self-esteem. The parents were counseled to reinforce behavioral improvement and to ignore periods of eye fluttering. We did not deal with other complex family issues that would have required long-term therapy. At the time of termination, the seizure frequency was markedly reduced, and the child was enjoying success both at home and at school. Ten months after initiation of hypnosis training, she continued to make good progress in all areas. About 8 months later, Tracy's symptoms returned. In the second course of hypnosis, she made marked gains initially but then deteriorated again. Therapy was terminated after about 6 months. The parents sought help for the child elsewhere, and no further follow-up was available.

Glenn and Simonds (1977) treated a 13-year-old girl who had been having psychogenic seizures for about 2 weeks. There was no identifiable underlying organic seizure disorder. The child did have a 4-year history of emotional problems, apparently precipitated by the death of her father. Early in hypnoanalytic treatment she experienced a seizure concurrent with describing a vivid rape fantasy, probably related to conflicts over emerging sexual desires. The treatment included hypnotically induced seizures and training the patient to prevent the seizures by pressing her right thumb and forefinger together. She was also taught to verbalize her fantasies. She participated in an inpatient behavior modification program with emphasis on improving self-esteem. Her mother and stepfather were seen twice monthly for counseling. There were no seizures after the first week of a 4-month hospitalization, and follow-up revealed that the patient remained seizure-free for 2 years after discharge. It is not clear in this report whether hypnosis continued during the 2 years after discharge or was limited to the period of inpatient treatment.

Williams and Singh (1976) briefly described two cases of psychogenic seizures. In the first case, a 15-year-old girl presented with a 4-year history of both true and psychogenic psychomotor seizures, markedly exacerbated in the last month. She was seizure free after a 10-day hospitalization that included both hypnosis and family therapy. During 14 months of continued outpatient therapy, both individual and family, she had only occasional seizures, associated with situational stress. In the second case, a 12-year-old girl presented with a 4-year history of mixed-type seizures, both organic and psychogenic, unresponsive to medications. After initial improvement in a hospital program including hypnosis, behavior modification, and family therapy, the girl's condition worsened after discharge. She improved again after readmission and maintained her gains over the next 12 months at home where she continued in supportive psychotherapy.

Elkins and Perfect (2007) described hypnosis training of a 10-year-old with uncontrolled seizures. Connecting with the patient through the child's science fiction fascination, Elkins invited the child to imagine he was in a spaceship with the mission to "shoot down enemy rockets." The hypnotic suggestion was that each rocket represented part of a seizure and as the parts disappeared (by being shot down) the seizures would reduce, and he would relax more and more.

## Psychogenic Pain

The diagnosis of psychogenic pain must be made with great care. We have had numerous experiences of evaluating children who were referred to us with the diagnosis of psychogenic pain and who later proved to have a biological basis for the pain symptom. Many of these children presented with headaches or abdominal pain or leg pain. It is also possible for children to have pain with both biological and psychological components. Williams and Singh (1976) described an 11-year-old boy with a long history of recurring abdominal pain, complicated by many factors including serious organic illness that had been misdiagnosed as psychogenic. The child was seen for brief hypnosis aimed at understanding sources of tension and using relaxation to reduce and eliminate pain. He was symptom-free in 48 hours. He was followed in outpatient psychotherapy for 20 months during which there was only one transient recurrence of abdominal pain, possibly attributable to gastroenteritis.

Sarles (1975) treated a 14-year-old girl with a 12-week history of severe hip pain determined to be of psychogenic origin, probably related to family discord. Her pain was relieved after one session of hypnosis, and she walked 3 days later. She successfully used self-hypnosis whenever the pain recurred. Follow-up revealed that she had returned to school and that the family was involved in family therapy. When psychogenic pain serves major defensive functions or provides significant secondary gain, it is much less likely to respond to hypnosis. Kelly was a 14-year-old girl referred because of knee pain that began when she dislocated her knee 12 months earlier. Corrective surgery had been deemed successful, but the pain continued. Nerve blocks and various medications had been of little help. In the first session, Kelly was constricted and markedly depressed, expressing doubt that hypnosis would be of any value. Despite the fact that she responded well to hypnotic invitation, she derived no benefit from several hypnotic approaches designed to alleviate her pain. Diagnostic interviews and psychological testing suggested that the pain might be binding severe anxiety and might also be providing significant secondary gain, including passively expressing hostility and dependency needs, neither of which she could admit into consciousness. The girl vigorously denied any sort of emotional distress and responded negatively to the suggestion of extended psychotherapy. She terminated hypnosis after four sessions, her condition unchanged. Although her parents were hesitant to accept the idea of a psychological basis for her pain, 1 month later they did take her to a psychotherapist nearer their home.

Anbar (2001a) reviewed the efficacy of self-hypnosis in helping five children help themselves with recurrent abdominal pain, or so-called functional abdominal pain (see also Chapter 12). Elkins and Perfect (2007) reported their comprehensive assessment and therapeutic approach to childhood somatoform disorders and described in detail an example of a hypnotic approach effective for a 14-year-old boy with severe, persistent headache requiring hospitalization. A hypnotic strategy that included creative imagery and relaxation was provided and proved to be very effective.

## Anorexia Nervosa

The syndrome of anorexia nervosa may result from a number of causes, including biological ones; however, regardless of the cause, the life-threatening aspects of continued voluntary starvation mandate whatever interventions ensure food retention. Crasilneck and Hall (1985) reported that they begin hypnotic treatment with direct suggestions for increased food intake. When the patient begins to gain weight and the medical situation is stabilized, they then begin psychodynamic exploration, both with and without hypnoanalytic techniques. Their technique is illustrated in detail in case reports.

Gross (1984) reported the successful use of hypnosis in treating 50 patients with anorexia nervosa. Torem (1987, 1991) reported similar success in using hypnosis as an adjunct. Most of the patients with anorexia we see in a tertiary-care setting are dangerously ill, often having lost 50% of their normal body weight. The threat of death demands immediate increase in food intake. We therefore begin with a strictly controlled behavior modification program in which the patient either eats and retains frequent small meals or is tube fed an equivalent amount. Hypnosis and conventional psychotherapy are used for anxiety reduction, to facilitate coping, to improve self-esteem, and for dynamic exploration and conflict resolution. Malnourished individuals often have cognitive processing problems and irritability as a result of the malnutrition. We have found that it is difficult to work with severely ill anorexic adolescents until nutritional rehabilitation has begun and there is some improvement in nutritional status

## Depression

Depression as a diagnosis in children was not even acknowledged until the late 1950s and early 1960s (Gabriel, 1989). Even then it was said to be unusual, and pediatric residency training in the 1960s and 1970s hardly included mention of depression as a diagnosable condition in children. Despite the virtual explosion of pharmacologic therapy for children and adolescents with a variety of depression-related diagnoses, and relatively few controlled studies thereof, therapy for depression in children has remained largely in the realm of psychotherapies, typically psychodynamic-oriented CBT and, more recently, brief solution-oriented therapies. With an awareness of the growing prevalence of depression in children and adolescents, and with the recognition that depression in young people is a major risk factor for adult depression, it is incumbent upon child health clinicians to not only make accurate diagnoses of depression and depression-related conditions in children but also to provide interventions that allow children to help themselves and reduce the likelihood of depression and related comorbid conditions (e.g., anxiety) into adulthood (Garber, Kriss, Koch, & Lindholm, 1988; Harrington, Fudge, Rutter, Pickles, & Hill, 1990; Kohen & Murray, 2006).

In recent database literature reviews (Medline, PubMed, PsychInfo), we found no controlled studies of hypnosis for depression or for related disorders with depressed mood (such as dysthymia or adjustment disorder with depressed mood), although a few studies were identified in which depressed mood or depression was identified secondarily as being improved in response to hypnosis provided for a primary medical disorder. Kohen and Murray (2006) offer a framework of considerations for the application of hypnosis principles to individual patients. These include emphasis on the evolution of a careful history in the context of a focused rapport and the essential ingredient of finding the hypnosis in the encounter. They emphasize the universality of ego-strengthening as an almost pivotal tool in hypnotic work with children struggling with depression, amplify the importance of future orientation in the hypnotic work, and offer two cases illustrative of the significance of sensitivity to both behavioral and developmental differences in the uniqueness of each patient.

Clinicians have provided rich examples of applications of hypnosis for depression in its various forms. These case descriptions are wonderful resources for child healthcare professionals and include Gabriel's (1989) description and discussion of an 11-year-old child with depression, Mills' (Mills, 1989; Mills & Crowley, 1986) creative storytelling metaphors for helping children with fears and depression, the storytelling and imagery approaches of Doris Brett in her *Annie Stories* (1986, 1992), and Kohen's (2007) description of the treatment of "B" for almost 4 years from age 5 years to almost 9 years. As in so many cases, B's improvement was attributed to "a blend of effective parent counseling, … skill development in self-hypnosis, intermittent … adjunctive use of medication, and, in the context of his history, his family and his maturation" (p. 194). Thomson's metaphorical tales with *Harry the Hypnopotamus* (2005, 2009) provide clinicians and parents alike with wonderful resources for helping children help themselves. Like the *Annie* stories, the *Harry* stories are readily accessible and malleable for parents to change and fine-tune to the needs of their child; they can utilize the story templates to fashion their own creative, positive imagery and associated relaxation toward improved affect and self-esteem, confidence, and problem modulation. In his book, Yapko (2009, pp. 178–298) offers an entire chapter devoted to guidance for depressed parents ("Learn to Reduce Your Child's Depression Inheritance"). Replete with ideas and guidance of how to "be hypnotic" in the service of reducing the possibilities of depression in your children, this section should be reviewed by child health clinicians who can then decide which of their families might benefit from the parent training this provides.

## Conclusions

Hypnosis can be useful in helping children with a great variety of emotional problems, both recent and of long duration, with children of all ages. Poor results are usually associated with lack of motivation, unrecognized learning disabilities, deep-seated conflicts that the patient refuses or is unable to acknowledge, severe underlying pathology for which the symptom serves as a major defense, significant secondary gain from the symptom, missed biological causes, and premature termination of treatment. Parental attitudes also play an important role, especially in cases where parents deny that physical symptoms are chiefly the result of psychological problems. When the child's problems are the most obvious manifestation of complex family pathology, hypnosis is likely to fail unless family therapy is also accepted as a treatment modality.

## References


Achenbach, T. (1991). *Manual for Child Behavior Checklist 4–18, 1991 Profile*. Burlington VT: University Associates in Psychiatry.

Adler-Nevo, G. & Manassis, K. (2005). Psychosocial treatment of pediatric posttraumatic stress disorder: the neglected field of single-incident trauma. *Depression and Anxiety*, *22*, 177–189.

Ambrose, G. (1968). Hypnosis in the treatment of children. *American Journal of Clinical Hypnosis*, *11*, 1–5.

American Psychiatric Association. (2013). *Diagnostic and Statistical Manual of Mental Disorders, Fifth Edition (DSM-5)*. Arlington: American Psychiatric Association.

Anbar, R.D. & Slothower, M.P. (2006). Hypnosis for treatment of insomnia in school-age children: a retrospective chart review. *BMC Pediatrics*, *6*(*23*), 10.1186/1471-2431-6-23.

Anbar, R.D. (2001a). Self-hypnosis for the treatment of functional abdominal pain in childhood. *Clinical Pediatrics*, *40*, 447–451.

Aviv, A. (2006). Tele-hypnosis in the treatment of adolescent school refusal. *American Journal of Clinical Hypnosis*, *49*(1), 31–40.

Barrett, P., Healy-Farrell, L., & March, J.S. (2004). Cognitive–behavioral family treatment of childhood obsessive–compulsive disorder: a controlled trial. *Journal of the American Academy of Child and Adolescent Psychiatry*, *43*(*1*), 46–62.

Berberich, F.R. & Landman, Z. (2009). Reducing immunization discomfort in 4- to 6-year-old children: a randomized clinical trial. *Pediatrics*, *124*(*2*), e203–e209.

Bloom, P.B. (2001). Treating adolescent conversion disorders: are hypnotic techniques reusable? *The International Journal of Clinical and Experimental Hypnosis*, *49*(*3*), 243–256.

Brown, E.J., McQuaid, J., Farina, L., Ali, R., & Winnick-Gelles, A. (2006). Matching interventions to children's mental health needs: feasibility and acceptability of a pilot school-based trauma intervention program. *Education and Treatment of Children*, *29*, 257–286.

Brown, E.J., Pearlman, M.Y., & Goodman, R.F. (2004). Facing fears and sadness: cognitive–behavioral therapy for childhood traumatic grief. *Harvard Review of Psychiatry*, *12*, 187–198.

Brett, D. (1986). *Annie Stories*. Victoria, Australia: McPhee Gribble Publishers.

Brett, D. (1992). *More Annie Stories: Therapeutic Storytelling Techniques*. New York: Imagination Press.

Catani, C., Kohiladevy, M., Ruf, M., Schauer, E., Elbert, T., & Neuner, F. (2009). Treating children

traumatized by war and tsunami: a comparison between exposure therapy and meditation-relaxation in North-East Sri Lanka. *BMC Psychiatry*, *9*(22), 10.1186/1471-244X-9-22.
Cohen, J., Kelleher, K.J., & Mannarino, A.P. (2008). Identifying, treating, and referring traumatized children: the role of pediatric providers. *Archives of Pediatrics and Adolescent Medicine*, *162*(*5*), 447–452.
Contos, A. (1999). The case of how the boogie man disappeared. *Australian Journal of Clinical and Experimental Hypnosis*, *27*, 125–135.
Costello, E.J., Egger, H.L., & Angold, A. (2004). Developmental epidemiology of anxiety disorders. In T.H. Ollendick & J.S. March, Eds., *Phobic and Anxiety Disorders in Children and Adolescents* (pp. 61–91). New York: Oxford University Press.
Crasilneck, H.B. & Hall, J.A. (1985). *Clinical Hypnosis: Principles and Applications*, 2nd ed. New York: Grune & Stratton.
Dean, J. (2020). *Freddy the Frogcaster and the Huge Hurricane*. Washington DC: Regnery Publishing.
Deckro, G.R., Ballinger, K.M., Hoyt, M., Wilcher, M., Dusek, J., Myers, P., Greenberg, B., Rosenthal, D.S., & Benson, H. (2002). The evaluation of a mind/body intervention to reduce psychological distress and perceived stress in college students. *Journal of American College Health*, *50*, 281–287.
Ehntholt, K.A. & Yule, W. (2006). Practitioner review: assessment and treatment of refugee children and adolescents who have experienced war trauma. *Journal of Child Psychology and Psychiatry*, *47*(12), 1197–1210.
Ehntholt, K.A., Smith, P.A., & Yule, W. (2005). School-based cognitive–behavioural therapy group intervention for refugee children who have experienced war-related trauma. *Clinical Child Psychology and Psychiatry*, *10*, 235–250.
Elkins, G.R. & Perfect, M.M. (2007). Hypnotherapy for the treatment of childhood somatoform disorders. In W.C. Wester II & L.I. Sugarman, Eds., *Therapeutic Hypnosis With Children and Adolescents* (pp. 227–239). Bethel, CT: Crown House Publishing.
Emslie, G. (2008). Pediatric anxiety: underrecognized and undertreated. *New England Journal of Medicine*, *359*(26), 2835–2836.
Erickson, M.H. (1962). The identification of a secure reality. *Family Process*, *1*, 294–303.
Erickson, M.H. (1958b). Pediatric hypnotherapy. *American Journal of Clinical Hypnosis*, *1*, 25–29.
Esch, T., Fricchione, G.L., & Stefano, G.B. (2003). The therapeutic use of the relaxation response in stress-related diseases. *Medical Science Monitor*, *9*, RA23–RA34.
Faigel, H.C. (1983). Learning disabilities in adolescents with high IQ scores. *Journal of Developmental and Behavioral Pediatrics*, *4*, 11–15.
Frankel, F.H. & Perry, C.W., Eds. (1994). Hypnosis and delayed recall, Part 1. *International Journal of Clinical and Experimental Hypnosis*, *42*(4), 259–446.
Franklin, M.E., Foa, E., & March, J.S. (2003). The pediatric obsessive–compulsive disorder treatment study: rationale, design, and methods. *Journal of Child and Adolescent Psychopharmacology*, *13*(Suppl. 1), S39–S51.
Friedrich, W.N. (1991). Hypnotherapy with traumatized children. *International Journal of Clinical and Experimental Hypnosis*, *39*(*2*), 67–81.
Fromm, E. & Gardner, G.G. (1979). Ego psychology and hypnoanalysis: an integration of theory and technique. *Bulletin of the Menninger Clinic*, *43*, 413–423.
Gabriel, R.M. (1989). Therapeutic diagnosing in cases of childhood depression. In M.D. Yapko, Ed., *Brief Therapy Approaches to Treating Anxiety and Depression* (pp. 171–183). New York: Brunner/Mazel.
Garber, J., Kriss, M., Koch, M., & Lindholm, L. (1988). Recurrent depression in adolescents: a follow-up study. *Journal of the American Academy of Child Psychiatry*, *27*, 49–54.
Gardner, G.G. (1973). Use of hypnosis for psychogenic epilepsy in a child. *American Journal of Clinical Hypnosis*, *15*, 166–169.
Gardner, G.G. (1976a). Attitudes of child health professionals toward hypnosis: implications for training. *International Journal of Clinical and Experimental Hypnosis*, *24*, 63–73.
Gardner, G.G. (1978b). The use of hypnotherapy in a pediatric setting. In E. Gellert, Ed., *Psychosocial Aspects of Pediatric Care*. New York: Grune & Stratton.
Garth, M. (1991). *Starbright: Meditations for Children*. New York: HarperCollins.
Garth, M. (1992). *Moonbeam: A Book of Meditations for Children*. San Francisco, CA: HarperOne.
Garth, M. (1997). *Earthlight: New Meditations for Children*. San Francisco, CA: HarperOne.
Glenn, T.J. & Simonds, J.F. (1977). Hypnotherapy of a psychogenic seizure disorder in an adolescent. *American Journal of Clinical Hypnosis*, *19*, 245–250.

Goldbeck, L. & Schmid, D. (2003). Effectiveness of autogenic relaxation training on children and adolescents with behavioral and emotional problems. *Journal of the American Academy of Child and Adolescent Psychiatry, 42(9)*, 1046–1054.

Gordon, J.S., Staples, J.K., Blyta, A., Bytyqi, M., & Wilson, A.T. (2008). Treatment of posttraumatic stress disorder in postwar Kosovar adolescents using mind–body skills groups: a randomized controlled trial. *Journal of Clinical Psychiatry, 69(9)*, 1469–1476.

Gray, J.A. (1987). *The Psychology of Fear and Stress*. Cambridge, U.K.: Cambridge University Press.

Gross, M. (1984). Hypnosis in the therapy of anorexia hysteria. *American Journal of Clinical Hypnosis, 26*, 175–181.

Grynkewich, M.A. (1994). *The Use of Mental Imagery Strategies to Improve School Performance*, unpublished manuscript. University of Arizona.

Gualtieri, C.T., Koriath, U., Van Bourgondien, M., & Saleeby, N. (1983). Language disorders in children referred for psychiatric services. *Journal of the American Academy of Child Psychiatry, 22*, 165–171.

Halliday, G. (1987). Direct psychological therapies for nightmares: a review. *Clinical Psychology Review*, 7, 501–523.

Harrington, R. Fudge, H., Rutter, M., Pickles, A., & Hill, J. (1990). Adult Outcomes of Childhood and Adolescent Depression. *Archives of General Psychiatry*, 47, 465–473. 10.1001/archpsyc.1990.01810170065010.

Hatzenbuehler, L.C. & Schroeder, H.E. (1978). Desensitization procedures in the treatment of childhood disorders. *Psychological Bulletin, 85*, 831–844.

Hendricks, C.G. & Wills, R. (1975). *The Centering Book*. New York: Transpersonal Books.

Howsam, D.G. (1999). Hypnosis in the treatment of insomnia, nightmares and night terrors. *Australian Journal of Clinical and Experimental Hypnosis, 27*, 32-39.

Huynh, M.E., Vandvik, I.H., & Diseth, T.H. (2008). Hypnotherapy in child psychiatry: the state of the art. *Clinical Child Psychology and Psychiatry, 13*, 377–393.

James, A., Soler, A., & Weatherall, R. (2006). Cognitive behavioural therapy for anxiety disorders in children and adolescents. *The Cochrane Database of Systematic Reviews* (4).

Jacobs, L. (1962). Hypnosis in clinical pediatrics. *New York State Journal of Medicine, 62*, 3781–3787.

Jacobs, L. (1964). Sleep problems of children: treatment by hypnosis. *New York State Journal of Medicine, 64*, 629–634.

Kaffman, M. (1968). Hypnosis as an adjunct to psychotherapy in child psychiatry. *Archives of General Psychiatry, 18*, 725–738.

Kagan, J. (1994). *Galen's Prophecy*. New York: Basic Books.

Kaiser, P. (2014). Childhood anxiety and psychophysiological reactivity: hypnosis to build discrimination and self-regulation skills. *American Journal of Clinical Hypnosis*, 56, 343–367.

Kellerman, J. (1981). Hypnosis as an adjunct to thought-stopping and covert reinforcement in the treatment of homicidal obsessions in a twelve-year-old boy. *International Journal of Clinical and Experimental Hypnosis, 29*, 128–135.

Kendall, P.C. (1994). Treating anxiety disorders in children, results of a randomized clinical trial. *Journal of Consulting Clinical Psychology, 62*, 100–110.

Kendall, P.C., Flannery-Schroeder, E., Panichelli-Mindel, S.M. et al. (1997). Therapy for youths with anxiety disorders: a second randomized clinical trial. *Journal of Consulting Clinical Psychology, 65*, 366–380.

King, N.J., Cranstoun, F., & Josephs, A. (1989). Emotive imagery and children's nighttime fears: a multiple baseline design evaluation. *Journal of Behavior Therapy and Experimental Psychiatry, 20*(2), 125–135.

Koe, G.G. (1989). Hypnotic treatment of sleep terror disorder: a case report. *American Journal of Clinical Hypnosis, 32*(1), 36–40.

Kohen, D.P. (2010a). A pediatric perspective on mind–body medicine. In T.P. Culbert and K. Olness, Eds., *Integrative Pediatrics* (pp. 267–301). New York: Oxford University Press.

Kohen, D.P. (2007). Depression. In W.C. Wester and L.I. Sugarman, Eds., *Therapeutic Hypnosis With Children and Adolescents* (pp. 179–198). Bethel, CT: Crown House Publishing.

Kohen, D.P. & Murray, K.M. (2006). Depression in children and youth: applications of hypnosis to help young people help themselves. In M.D. Yapko, Ed., *Hypnosis and Treating Depression: Applications in Clinical Practice* (pp. 189–216). New York: Routledge.

Kohen, D.P., Mahowald, M.W., & Rosen, J.R. (1992). Sleep terror disorder in children: the role of self-hypnosis in management. *American Journal of Clinical Hypnosis, 34(4)*, 233–244.

Kohen, D.P. (1995a). Childhood grief and mourning: applications of hypnotherapy, paper presented at the Minnesota Society of Clinical Hypnosis, Minneapolis, MN.

Kovacs, M. (1992). *Children's Depression Inventory Manual.* North Tonawanda, NY: Multi-Health Systems.
Kramer, R.L. (1989). The treatment of childhood night terrors through the use of hypnosis: a case study – a brief communication. *International Journal of Clinical and Experimental Hypnosis, 37*, 283–284.
Lawlor, E.D. (1976). Hypnotic intervention with "school phobic" children. *International Journal of Clinical and Experimental Hypnosis, 24*, 74–86.
Lazar, B.S. & Jedliczka, Z.T. (1979). Utilization of manipulative behavior in a retarded asthmatic child. *American Journal of Clinical Hypnosis, 21*, 287–292.
Lembke A. (2021). *Dopamine Nation: Finding Balance in the Age of Indulgence.* Dutton: Boston MS.
Lesmana, C.B.J., Suryani, L.K., Jensen, G.D., & Tiliopoulos, N. (2009). A spiritual-hypnosis assisted treatment of children with PTSD after the 2002 Bali terrorist attack. *American Journal of Clinical Hypnosis, 52(1)*, 23–34.
Linden, J. (2007). Hypnosis in Childhood Trauma. In W.C. Wester II & L.I. Sugarman, Eds., *Therapeutic Hypnosis With Children and Adolescents* (pp. 135–160). Bethel, CT: Crown House Publishing.
Masia, C.L., Klein, R.G., Storch, E.A., & Corda, B. (2001). School-based behavioral treatment for social anxiety disorder in adolescents: results of a pilot study. *Journal of the American Academy of Child and Adolescent Psychiatry, 40*, 780–786.
Mellor, N.H. (1960). Hypnosis in juvenile delinquency. *General Practitioner, 22*, 83–87.
Merritt, J.E. (1991). Reducing a child's nighttime fears. *Elementary School Guidance and Counseling, 25*, 291–295.
Mills, J. (1989). No more monsters and meanies: multisensory metaphors for helping children with fears and depression. In Yapko, M.D., Ed., *Brief Therapy Approaches to Treating Anxiety and Depression* (pp. 150–170). New York: Brunner/Mazel.
Mills, J. & Crowley, R.J. (1986). *Therapeutic Metaphors for Children and the Child Within.* New York: Brunner/Mazel.
Mutter, C.B. (1990). Hypnosis with defendants: does it really work? *American Journal of Clinical Hypnosis, 32*(4), 257–262.
Nath, S. & Warren, J. (1995). Hypnosis and examination stress in adolescence. *Contemporary Hypnosis, 12*(2), 119–124.
Nikulina, V., Hergenrother, J.M., Brown, E.J., Doyle, M.E., Filton, B.J., & Carson, G.S. (2008). From efficacy to effectiveness: the trajectory of the treatment literature for children with PTSD. *Expert Review in Neurotherapy, 8*(8), 1233–1246.
O'Kearney, R.T., Anstey, K.J., & von Sanden, C. (2006). Behavioural and cognitive behavioural therapy for obsessive compulsive disorder in children and adolescents. *The Cochrane Database of Systematic Reviews* (4). Article No. CD004856.
Ollendick, T.H. & King, N.J. (1998). Empirically supported treatments for children with phobia and anxiety disorders; current status. *Journal of Clinical Child Psychology, 27*(2), 156–167.
Olness, K. & Gardner, G.G. (1978). Some guidelines for uses of hypnotherapy in pediatrics. *Pediatrics, 62*, 228–233.
Olness, K. & Libbey, P. (1987). Unrecognized biologic bases of behavioral symptoms in patients referred for hypnotherapy. *American Journal of Clinical Hypnosis, 30*, 1–8.
Olness, K. (2022). Children's mental health at times of disasters: a narrative review. *Pediatric Medicine, 5*, 171. http://dx.doi.org/10.21037/pm-20-85
Orne, M.T., Ed. (1990). Forensic hypnosis (special issue). *International Journal of Clinical and Experimental Hypnosis, 38*(4), 219–319.
Pairojkul, S., Siripul, P., Prateepchaikul, L., Kusol, K., & Puytrakul,T. (2010). Psychosocial first aid: support for the child survivors of the Asian Tsunami. *Journal of Developmental and Behavioral Pediatrics*, 31, 723–727.
Petty, G.L. (1976). Desensitization of parents to tantrum behavior. *American Journal of Hypnosis, 19*, 95–97.
Reynolds, C.P. & Kamphaus, R.W. (2002). *The Clinician's Guide to the Behavior Assessment System for Children (BASC).* New York: Guilford.
Rhue, J.W. & Lynn, S.J. (1991). Storytelling, hypnosis and the treatment of sexually abused children. *International Journal of Clinical and Experimental Hypnosis, 39*(4), 198–214.
Rhue, J.W., Lynn, S.J., & Kirsch, I., Eds. (1993). *Handbook of Clinical Hypnosis.* Washington, D.C.: American Psychological Association.
Rickert, V.I. & Jay, S.M. (1994). Psychosomatic disorders: the approach. *Pediatrics in Review, 15*, 448–454.
Roberts, D. (1998). The use of hypnosis and brief strategic therapy with a case of separation anxiety and school refusal. *Contemporary Hypnosis, 15*(4), 219–222.

Rogeness, G.A., Javors, M.S., & Pliszka, S. (1992). Neurochemistry and child and adolescent psychiatry. *Journal of the American Academy of Child and Adolescent Psychiatry, 31*, 765–781.

Salcioglu, E. & Basoglu, M. (2008). Psychological effects of earthquakes in children: prospects for brief behavioral treatment. *World Journal of Pediatrics, 4*(3), 165–172.

Sarles, R.M. (1975). The use of hypnosis with hospitalized children. *Journal of Clinical Child Psychology, 4*, 36–38.

Scaini, S., Belotti R., Ogliani A., Battaglia. M.A. (2016) Comprehensive meta-analysis of cognitive-behavioral interventions for social anxiety disorder in children and adolescents. *Journal of Anxiety Disorders, 42*,105–112.

Schowalter, J.E. (1994). Fears and phobias. *Pediatrics in Review, 15*, 384–388.

Shooshtary, M.H., Panaghi, L., & Moghadam, J.A. (2008). Outcome of cognitive behavioral therapy in adolescents after natural disaster. *Journal of Adolescent Health, 42*, 466–472.

Smith, M.S. (1983). Acute psychogenic stridor in an adolescent athlete treated with hypnosis. *Pediatrics, 72*, 247–248.

Smith, P., Yule, W., Perrin, S., Tranah, T., Dalgleish, T., & Clark, T.M. (2007). Cognitive–behavioral therapy for PTSD in children and adolescents: a preliminary randomized controlled trial. *Journal of the American Academy of Child & Adolescent Psychiatry, 46*(8), 1051–1061.

Solovey, G. & Milechnin, A. (1955). Conduct problems in children and hypnosis. *Diseases of the Nervous System, 16*, 249–253.

Stallard, P., Vellerman, R., Salter, E., Howse, I., Yule, W., & Taylor, G. (2006). A randomized controlled trial to determine the effectiveness of an early psychological intervention with children involved in road traffic accidents. *Journal of Child Psychology and Psychiatry, 47*(2), 127–134.

Stein, B.D., Jacycox, L.H., Kataoka, S.H. et al. (2003). A mental health intervention for school children exposed to violence: a randomized controlled trial. *Journal of the American Medical Association, 290*(5), 603–611.

Steinberg, A.M., Brymer, M.J., Decker K.B., Pynoos R.S. (2004). The University of California at Los Angeles post-traumatic stress disorder reaction index. *Psychiatry Reports*, 6, 96–100.

St-Onge, M., Mercier, P., & De Koninck, J. (2009). Imagery rehearsal therapy for frequent nightmares in children. *Behavioral Sleep Medicine*, 7(2), 81–98.

Taboada, E.L. (1975). Night terrors in a child treated with hypnosis. *The American Journal of Clinical Hypnosis, 17*, 270–271.

Thomas, J. (2019 ). VIDEOS. Videos developed by Dr. Thomas are accessed on The Meg Foundation website at www.megfoundationforpain.org

Thomson, L. (2005). *Harry the Hypno-potamus: Metaphorical Tales for the Treatment of Children*. Bethel, CT: Crown House Publishing.

Thomson, L. (2009). *Harry the Hypno-potamus: More Metaphorical Tales for Pediatric Problems*. Bethel, CT: Crown House Publishing.

Torem, M.S. (1987). Ego-state therapy for eating disorders. *American Journal of Clinical Hypnosis, 20*, 94–103.

Torem, M.S. (1991). Eating disorders. In W.C. Wester II & D. O'Grady, Eds., *Clinical Hypnosis with Children* (pp. 230–257). New York: Brunner/Mazel.

Uman, L.S., Chambers, C.T., McGrath, P.J., & Kisely, S. (2008). A systematic review of randomized controlled trials examining psychological interventions for needle-related procedural pain and distress in children and adolescents: an abbreviated Cochrane Review. *Journal of Pediatric Psychology, 33*(8), 842–854.

Walkup, J.T., Albano, A.M., Piacentini, J.C., Birmhaer, B., Compton, S.N., Sherrill, J.T., Ginsburg, G.S., Rynn, M.A., McCracken, J., Waslick, B., Iyengar, S., March, J.S., & Kendall, P.C. (2008). Cognitive behavioral therapy, sertraline, or a combination in childhood anxiety. *New England Journal of Medicine, 359*(26), 2753–2766.

Williams, D.T. (1979). Hypnosis as a therapeutic adjunct. In J.D. Noshpitz, Ed., *Basic Handbook of Child Psychiatry*, Vol. *3*. New York: Basic Books.

Williams, D.T. & Singh, M. (1976). Hypnosis as a facilitating therapeutic adjunct in child psychiatry. *Journal of the American Academy of Child Psychiatry, 15*, 326–342.

Yapko, M.D. (2009). *Depression Is Contagious*. New York: Free Press.

Zaider, T.I. & Heimberg, R.G. (2003). Non-pharmacologic treatments for social anxiety disorder. *Acta Psychiatrica Scandinavica, 108*(Suppl. 417), 72–84. www.pedstest.com/AboutOurTools/LearnAboutPEDS/Introduction to PEDS.html (accessed January 11, 2022). https://www.sdqinfo.org/aO.html (accessed January 11, 2022).

# 9

# THERAPEUTIC HYPNOSIS FOR YOUTH WITH AUTISM SPECTRUM DISORDERS

## Introduction

Numerous studies have suggested that the prevalence of diagnosed autism spectrum disorders (ASDs) has increased dramatically in decades. A report based on a 2007 national survey of parents of children ages 3–17 years suggested that the prevalence of diagnosed ASD is higher than previous US estimates. The prevalence was 110 per 10,000 children (1.1%), representing an estimated 673,000 US children 3–17 years with a current diagnosis of ASD. Interestingly, for nearly 40% of all the children reported to have ever had an ASD diagnosis, a parent or caregiver reported a past but not current ASD diagnosis (Kogan et al., 2009). In 2021 the CDC's Autism and Developmental Disabilities Monitoring Network reported a 2018 survey in which 1 in 44 children had ASD (CDC, 2021). Between this prevalence and the substantial increased social awareness of ASD through advocacy groups, our schools, and the media, it is predictable that providers of child health care will have ongoing contact with more than just a few children who are "on the spectrum" and who present and reflect unique challenges and problems in addition to the usual diversity of issues encountered during child and adolescent development and acclimation to their society. Here we ask how children with ASD can benefit from clinical and therapeutic hypnosis and how hypnosis for this group of children is the same or different from their more typically developing peers.

The *DSM-5* (American Psychiatric Association, 2013) characterizes ASD by "persistent deficits in social communication and social interaction across multiple contexts, including deficits in social reciprocity, nonverbal communicative behaviors used for social interaction, and skills in developing, maintaining, and understanding relationships … The diagnosis of ASD requires the presence of restricted, repetitive patterns of behavior, interest or activities …. Many individuals previously diagnosed with Asperger's disorder would now receive a diagnosis of autism spectrum disorder without language or intellectual impairment. This latest edition of DSM" (pp. 31–2, 51) goes on to say that "Individuals with a well-established DSM-IV (American Psychiatric Association, 2000) diagnosis of autistic disorder, Asperger's disorder or pervasive developmental disorder not otherwise specified should [now] be given the diagnosis of autism spectrum disorder. Individuals who have marked deficits in social communication, but whose symptoms do not meet criteria for autism spectrum disorder (*DSM-5*, 2013), should be evaluated for social (pragmatic) communication disorder."

DOI: 10.4324/9781003243687-11

Although there is no single specific diagnostic test for ASD, screening tools and follow-up diagnostic questionnaires and rating scales are available that allow for early identification and referral/treatment as indicated. These include the Modified Checklist for Autism in Toddlers (M-CHAT) (Kleinman et al., 2008; Mawle & Griffiths, 2006; Pinto-Martin et al., 2008; Robins, 2008; Robins, Fein, Barton, & Green, 2001), and the M-CHAT Follow-up Interview (Robins, 2008).

All are clear in emphasizing specific aspects of the three areas traditionally understood to be affected in individuals diagnosed with ASD (i.e., communication, social interaction, and behavior). Although a detailed discussion of the diagnosis of ASD is beyond the scope of this volume, clinicians should be clear that, as we have emphasized throughout, one should not consider focusing upon utilizing therapeutic clinical hypnosis with a child with ASD or problems incident to their ASD unless one is familiar with and works with youth with ASD without therapeutic hypnosis.

Because history and rapport are essential ingredients that precede and guide ongoing clinical hypnotic communication, it becomes a special and unique challenge to identify and decide whether the communication differences in an individual child with ASD preclude effective therapeutic hypnosis or, more likely, serve to guide that therapy. What do we know?

## Pervasive Developmental Disorder

Gardner and Tarnow (1980) published a case report describing the use of therapeutic hypnosis with Tom, a 16-year-old boy diagnosed as mildly autistic at age three and one-half years or 42 months. The child had made gains in traditional psychotherapy and in special education programs, although he remained socially isolated and unable to integrate new experiences. He had a longstanding habit of biting his finger in response to frustrating situations, and he had developed a large callus on his finger, with intermittent bleeding and infection. At age 16, it seemed that Tom might be able to transfer to a regular high school, but his continued finger-biting behavior – refractory to previous treatment – seemed certain to elicit peer rejection and interfere with school adjustment. He was referred for clinical hypnosis in an attempt to eliminate this problem.

Unresponsive to traditional hypnotic invitation methods, Tom mentioned that Aria No. 47 from Bach's "Saint Matthew Passion" helped him feel calm; thereafter, when the therapist played him a recording of this aria, he easily entered hypnotic trance. Skilled in music, he wrote two short musical compositions for use in therapeutic hypnosis treatment. He listened to the first, entitled "Frustration in C Minor," after recalling a frustrating experience, with the suggestion that recall of the music could replace the finger-biting behavior. Then he listened to the second composition, "Happiness in C Major," with the suggestion that recall could strengthen feelings of confidence and increased self-control. The therapist also discussed the construction of the Bach aria, focusing on the way it implied different possible responses to particular events. The finger biting, which had occurred two to three times weekly prior to therapeutic hypnosis, extinguished entirely after 4 weeks, with the exception of an episode when both Tom's parents and his primary therapist were out of town. He maintained his gains over a follow-up period of 18 months.

Interestingly, Tom was able to describe frustrating events with greater detail and understanding when he was in hypnosis. At first, there was a marked difference between hypnotic and waking-state verbalizations. Later, the hypnotic communication skills generalized to the waking state. Improvement also generalized to other areas of behavior at home and at school where he continued a satisfactory adjustment in regular classes and became a member of the school jazz band. Throughout the treatment, the therapists emphasized competence and mastery in several ways (Gardner & Tarnow, 1980, p. 178):

Involving the patient in treatment planning from the very beginning of the process
Communicating to the patient that he was acceptable, while agreeing that aspects of his behavior were unacceptable

Focusing immediately on developing a solution rather than getting bogged down in discussing the problem

Praising the patient for cooperation and responding quickly to his efforts (e.g., using his compositions before he had achieved a hypnotic trance)

Utilizing the patient's obsession with music as a strength on which to base therapeutic strategy rather than perceiving it negatively as resistance or as an obstacle in the way of progress

Helping the patient observe his own progress, thus further enhancing his confidence in his ability to master problems in living

The authors concluded that therapeutic hypnosis may be a suitable technique for youngsters with severe ego deficits, provided invitation techniques are modified to suit special needs and interests and therapeutic suggestions focus on patient skills and ego strengthening rather than on stressful uncovering of repressed material.

More recent clinical reports, research, and our own experience support and reinforce the clinical impressions and recommendations of Gardner and Tarnow (1980). Sofronoff and colleagues (Sofronoff, Attwood, & Hinton, 2005) reported a randomized controlled study in Australia of a cognitive behavioral therapy (CBT) intervention for anxiety in children with Asperger syndrome (AS). Seventy-one children ages 10–12 years with AS participated, and all were diagnosed with anxiety symptoms by brief parental report. Children were randomly assigned to an intervention for the child only, intervention for child and parent, or a wait-list control. Both intervention groups demonstrated significant decreases in parent-reported anxiety symptoms after intervention and at follow-up, as compared to controls.

As with other references to, and discussions of, CBT in this volume, this study made no specific mention of hypnosis or hypnotherapy; however, as in prior studies and discussions, it seems quite clear to us that substantial elements of hypnosis are integral to the CBT program described in this study, in which each child received a workbook for the six 2-hour sessions. Each session ended with a project assignment that was the focus of discussion for subsequent sessions. Thus, homework, or home practice and review of the strategies, was integral to this intervention, much as self-hypnosis practice is essential to effective development of self-regulation. The authors observed that "a metaphor was created of the child as scientist or astronaut exploring a new planet," adding that children with AS in this age group had been noted to have a special and often highly focused interest in science and science fiction. This approach is thoughtful and creative and resonant with the theme throughout this text of careful history taking and the evolution of matching hypnotic approaches to the communication and learning style and interests of the child. The authors noted that the first session focused on happiness and relaxation. The second focused on recognition of the changes that occur in physiology, behavior, thinking, and speech in association with anxious feelings and the creation of a toolbox to fix the feelings. Emphasis was placed both on physical tools, such as running or playing on a trampoline, and relaxation tools, including listening to music or reading a book. Subsequent sessions focused on ways to measure one's anxiety (e.g., a thermometer, or scale) and social stories (Gray, 1998). Results of the study demonstrated that the program was effective in reducing parent-reported anxiety symptoms.

There are no definitive research studies related to hypnosis or biofeedback for treatment of ASDs. Two articles from Canada (Thompson, Thompson, & Reid, 2010a, b) describes a review of neurofeedback training with 150 clients with AS and nine clients with ASDs, of whom 117 were children and 30 were adolescents. These clients were seen over a consecutive 15-year period. The authors reported an average gain for the Full Scale IQ score of 9 points and other positive outcomes of decreased difficulties with attention, anxiety, aprosodies, and social functioning. The described protocols included training in diaphragmatic breathing and progressive relaxation. The authors noted that clients needed to remind themselves on a daily basis to relax their shoulders and breathe diaphragmatically. They stated that children with a diagnosis of autism might require over 100 sessions of training; children who did so demonstrated clear improvement in socialization skills.

Coben and colleagues (Coben, Linden, & Myers, 2010) published a review of the literature on treatment for ASDs, including several case studies of neurofeedback for children. Coben and colleagues noted that all studies reported significant clinical improvements but they must be viewed cautiously because they were uncontrolled studies. One of these studies involved 180 Thai children with autism (Limsila et al., 2004). Coben and colleagues also reviewed five controlled group studies with a total of 180 subjects; however, these studies largely included non-randomized samples, and neither participants nor therapists were blind to the treatment condition. The authors noted that a randomized, double-blinded, placebo-controlled study is necessary to evaluate the efficacy of neurofeedback for persons with ASDs (Coben et al., 2010).

A recent systematic literature review describes the treatment of anxiety in ASD using cognitive behavioral therapy (Lang, Regester, Lauderdale, Ashbaugh, & Haring, 2010), and another provides an overall review of approaches to anxiety in children and adolescents with ASD (White, Oswald, Ollendick, & Scahill, 2009). Both reports mention the use of relaxation and imagery or storytelling as integral tools in CBT in some of the studies but not others.

In a compelling, detailed case report in an *Anthropology* journal, Park (2008) described the imaginative practices of a child with autism in interaction with his therapist during a sensory integration-based therapy session. In describing and examining the intimate interactive details of imaginary play between the child and his occupational therapist, Park observed how the method of an *enacted narrative* (which we believe equals imaginative play equals the hypnotic work of children with the therapist) reveals how imaginative practices reflect the ways in which desire and hope are integral to the healing process. Park stated that "making scenes is integral to a healing of belonging. … Narrative as an imaginative practice may be integral to the healing and transformation of belonging for individuals facing the contingencies of chronic illness or lifelong disability. Enacted narratives … foreground the intimate ties between action and the realization of imagined possibilities" (Park, 2008, p. 248).

A number of recent reports have described the effectiveness of neurofeedback training (electroencephalography alone or combined with other forms of biofeedback) for patients with ASD and, more specifically, AS (Coben & Padolsky, 2007; Coben et al., 2010; Thompson et al., 2010a, b). These reports describe outcome details following, in most cases, many neurofeedback sessions (as many as twice weekly training). We were unable to identify in these reports efforts to discern any potential differential effects on outcome of therapist suggestion, concurrent relaxation or imagery suggestions, or expectations of the therapist, patient, and parent. As discussed in Chapter 15, we remain curious about and await further controlled prospective research in this important arena.

As many as 45–83% of children with ASD have a sleep problem as defined by either parent report or actigraphy (Honomichl, Goodlin-Jones, Burnham, Gaylor, & Anders, 2002; Moore, Meltzer, & Mindell, 2008; Wiggs & Stores, 2004; Yapko, 2003). We have had consistent success in helping children and teens with ASD modify and resolve sleep difficulties with the use of hypnosis and biofeedback-assisted hypnosis.

Robert had just turned 10 years old when I (DPK) met him early in 2009. As his mother explained, he had been known since toddlerhood to have "intense sensory sensitivity and tactile defensiveness" and had the diagnosis of ASD. Although they had worked with a variety of clinicians, Robert's difficulties had evolved into a highly dysfunctional set of behaviors for him and his family. His difficulties were described as including explosive behaviors in response to the smallest change, refusal to bathe aside from his weekly swims at the YMCA, being a picky eater, refusal to wear a seatbelt in the car because of "how bad it feels," ritualistic difficulties getting dressed every day and refusal to wear all but one specific pair of pants, difficulty falling asleep and staying asleep, and "restless leg syndrome."

As we have noted throughout, rapport is an essential first step with all of our young patients and their families, and nowhere is that more important than with a child with ASD whose communication skills and style and memory may be problematic both for child and interviewer (Bruck, London, Landa, & Goodman, 2007; Yapko, 2006). Accordingly, my intent from the beginning was to be patient, slow, and focused with Robert, to both the surprise and delight of his parents. An obviously bright boy, Robert at first responded non-verbally or with monosyllabic or two- or three-word crisp replies at best. By the end of the first visit, however, he had agreed that certain things (such as new clothes, getting dressed, the seatbelt in the car, or taking a bath) made him nervous and that they felt bad.

Learning of his interest in numbers and measuring things, I retrieved from my desk drawer a plain, wooden 12-inch ruler (one of my favorite visual aids for almost any patient). I asked him to tell me what it was for, and he appropriately identified it as being "for measuring stuff." He understood when I asked, "So, what could we measure with it?" (Note the purposeful use of "we" to continue to engage him in developing our early rapport and to solving a nonthreatening problem together.) Predictably concrete, he suggested that we could measure my pencil, or his finger, or, surprising me with what I think was a joke, "your beard!" I then asked him, "What if we could measure your nervous feelings?" He was perplexed, but I persisted: "If the *worst* nervous feeling is a 12 – this end of the ruler – and the *no* nervous feeling at all is a 0 – this end of the ruler – where is your *usual* nervous feeling?" He identified it as 6 or 7 and proceeded gradually to note where it was for the different situations (e.g., getting dressed, thinking about a bath, wearing the seatbelt). I asked him what number it would have to be for him to wear different clothes, fall asleep easily, or wear a seatbelt, for example, and he concretely identified a number for each, thereby setting a goal. I asked him if would be okay to find a way to get to those numbers, and although he was hesitant and anxious, he said it was. This conversational hypnosis and contextualization represented the beginning of his success. As Yapko (2006) observed, "The goal is to associate the desired response with the appropriate context." Robert agreed to keep track of his numbers on a calendar that he brought to each visit.

With the addition of the emWave Personal Stress Reliever®, a home biofeedback device that utilizes heart-rate variability, paced breathing, and positive imagery (www.heartmath.com), he agreed to practice relaxation and imagination every morning and every evening to help lower the ruler before going to school and before going to bed. Within five visits over 4 months, Robert was falling asleep easily and sleeping through the night, bathing weekly, and getting dressed without any of the previous hassles. His mother wrote in an e-mail: "He's been taking a weekly bath perfectly well ever since you saw him!!! It's been awesome. He has had little or no trouble putting clothes on the next day … and he is willing to see what it's like to wear the seatbelt!" As we have emphasized throughout this volume, Robert's success was a function, first and foremost, of our rapport, followed by an identification of his patterns and ways of thinking and talking, followed by utilization of his own patterns and style to teach him discrimination strategies to develop complementary patterns and new skills (Yapko, 2006). Of course, success breeds success, so, in addition to feeling good about being able to do something he had not perceived himself as able to do before, Robert was reinforced in his new successes by the joy, approval, and compliments (and relief) reflected by his very loving and supportive parents.

Kaslovsky and Gottsegen (2015) reported how learning hypnosis helped a 12-year-old boy with ASD and Vocal Cord Dysfunction. He had an intense interest in electronics and automobiles and wanted to buy his mother a van. The pediatrician asked him to imagine that he was in the driver's seat of his van, driving wherever he wanted. He was asked to imagine the cool air flowing easily through his airways and to imagine ice cream cooling his esophagus. He was given the post-hypnotic suggestion to gently pinch his ear if he had any symptoms of wheezing or shortness of breath and that this would bring him right back to his comfortable place, in his imaginary van. At the next visit his mother said he was practicing self-hypnosis whenever he felt stressed. During the visit, he was reading the Berenstein Bears book, *Trip to the Moon*. The pediatrician used this to reinforce the previous hypnosis, saying that he thought the Berenstein Bears could leave their worries on the moon and that the boy could leave his worries behind while driving his van. After these two visits, the boy had no further episodes of wheezing requiring urgent care visits and far fewer absences from school.

In a research study, Bruck and colleagues (Bruck et al., 2007) developed two paradigms to examine autobiographical memory and suggestibility in children with ASD. Thirty children with ASD were matched with 38 typically developing age-matched children from 5 to 10 years of age. They were asked about details of current and past personally experienced events (based on information gathered from their parents) and later participated in a staged event in which they were later provided with true and false reminders about the event. Finally, they were later interviewed about the staged event. Results showed that children with ASD had significantly poorer autobiographical memory compared to controls, with their memory being particularly poor for early-life events. They were, however, as suggestible as the typically developing children. In the evolution of the study's development, the authors proposed two different hypotheses about the suggestibility of children with ASD. One posits that children with ASD may be less suggestible than typically developing children because their social and pragmatic deficits may make them insensitive to the social cues of misleading questions (i.e., answering to go along with or to please the interviewer); consequently, children with ASD would be less likely to acquiesce to an interviewer's suggestion. They also wondered, however, if children with ASD might, on the other hand, be more suggestible because of cognitive deficits; thus, they may parrot an interviewer's words that contain misleading information and this might become incorporated into memory. As noted, the children with ASD were not found to be any more or less suggestible; however, they did show substantially poorer memory. In applying the results of their study, the authors emphasized that interviewing children with developmental disabilities (such as ASD) presents unique challenges for families and professionals who care for them. High-functioning children can and do provide basic details that are mainly accurate, but their accounts of both recent events and events experienced long ago are sparse compared to typically developing children. The data support the importance of developing interviewing and questioning strategies for children with ASD whose recall may be limited because of inability to recall details of their lives (Bruck et al., 2007, p. 92).

This experimental report provides value-added support to our continued emphasis of matching or joining with the patient, pacing and leading, finding the hypnosis in the encounter. More and more, and perhaps particularly with this group of young people, we are interested in and aware of conversational hypnosis (inductions and our use of therapeutic language, embedded metaphors, expectancy, post-hypnotic suggestions, and their utilization in context). As Yapko (2006) observed, these will include but not be limited to:

> Metaphors containing embedded suggestions (e.g., the child as scientist, gardener, or whatever hero with whom he or she identifies)

Relaxed scenario experiences that are content or process oriented (i.e., in what situations is the child most comfortable, content, or happy?)

Accessing previous hypnotic experiences (e.g., "Remember when you …? Just do that now, as if you were there now, because you can be in your mind's imagination. That's right!")
Varying the ratio of internal to external foci

Much as Haley (1985) showed us through his description of Erickson's use of carefully crafted storytelling and as Mills and Crowley (1986) and Thomson (2005, 2007) related the value of the integral use of stories in the care of a wide variety of childhood problems, so have Gray (1987) and others demonstrated the effectiveness of stories in helping children with ASD to help themselves. This is, as we have seen repeatedly, entirely consistent with Erickson's insistence that we "go with the child" (Haley, 1985) and Sugarman's (2007) more recent interpretation and urging that we find (and cultivate) the hypnosis in the encounter.

## References

American Psychiatric Association. (2000). *Diagnostic and Statistical Manual of Mental Disorders*, 4th ed. (Text Revision). Washington, D.C.: American Psychiatric Association.

American Psychiatric Association (2013). *Diagnostic and Statistical Manual of Mental Disorders – Fifth Edition – DSM-5.* Washington, DC: American Psychiatric Publishing

Bruck, M., London, K., Landa, R., & Goodman, J. (2007). Autobiographical memory and suggestibility in children with autism spectrum disorder. *Development and Psychopathology*, *19*, 73–95.

Centers for Disease Control (CDC). (2021). www.cdc.gov

Coben, R., Linden, M., & Myers, T.E. (2010). Neurofeedback for autistic spectrum disorder: a review of the literature. *Applied Psychophysiology and Biofeedback*, *35*, 83–105.

Coben, R. & Padolsky, I. (2007). Assessment-guided neurofeedback for autistic spectrum disorder. *Journal of Neurotherapy*, *11*, 5–23.

Gardner, G.G. & Tarnow, J.D. (1980). Adjunctive hypnotherapy with an autistic boy. *American Journal of Clinical Hypnosis*, *22*, 173–179.

Gray, C. (1998). Social stories and comic strip conversations with students with Asperger syndrome and high functioning autism. In E. Schopler, G.B. Mesibov, & L.J. Kunce, Eds., *Asperger Syndrome or High Functioning Autism*. New York: Plenum Press.

Gray, J.A. (1987). *The Psychology of Fear and Stress*. Cambridge, U.K.: Cambridge University Press.

Haley, J., Ed. (1985). *Conversations with Milton H. Erickson, Vol. 1.* Rockville, MD: Triangle Press.

Honomichl, R.D., Goodlin-Jones, B.L., Burnham, M., Gaylor, E., & Anders, T.F. (2002). Sleep patterns of children with pervasive developmental disorders. *Journal of Autism and Developmental Disorders*, *32*, 553–561.

Kaslovsky, R. & Gottsegen, D. (2015). Hypnosis for Asthma and Vocal Cord Dysfunction in a patient with autism. *American Journal of Clinical Hypnosis*, *58*, 195–203.

Kleinman, J.M., Robins, D.L., Ventola, P.E., Pandey, J., Boorstein, H.C., Esser, E.L., Wilson, L.B., Rosenthal, M.A., Sutera, S. et al. (2008). The modified checklist for autism in toddlers: a follow-up study investigating the early detection of autism spectrum disorders. *Journal of Autism and Developmental Disorders*, *38*, 827–839.

Kogan, M.D., Blumberg, S.J., Schieve, L.A., Boyle, C.A., Perrin, J.M., Ghandour, R.M., Singh, G.K., Strickland, B.B., Trevathan, E., & van Dyck, P.C. (2009). Prevalence of parent-reported diagnosis of autism spectrum disorder among children in the U.S., 2007. *Pediatrics*, *124*, 1395–1403.

Lang, R., Regester, A., Lauderdale, S., Ashbaugh, K., & Haring, A. (2010). Treatment of anxiety in autism spectrum disorders using cognitive behaviour therapy: a systematic review. *Developmental Neurorehabilitation*, *13*, 53–63.

Limsila, P., Toomim, H., Kijvithee, J., Bunthong, W., Pookjinda, J., & Utairatanakit, D. (2004). Hemoencephalography (HEG): an additional treatment for autism, http://www.biocompresearch.org/Thai_autism_study.htm.

Mawle, E. & Griffiths, P. (2006). Screening for autism in pre-school children in primary care: systematic review of English language tools. *International Journal of Nursing Studies, 43*, 623–636.
Mills, J. & Crowley, R.J. (1986). *Therapeutic Metaphors for Children and the Child Within*. New York: Brunner/Mazel.
Moore, M., Meltzer, L.J., & Mindell, J.A. (2008). Bedtime problems and night wakings in children. *Primary Care: Clinics in Office Practice, 35*, 569–581.
Park, M. (2008). Making scenes: imaginative practices of a child with autism in a sensory integration-based therapy session. *Medical Anthropology Quarterly, 22*, 234–256.
Pinto-Martin, J.A., Young, L.M., Mandell, D.S., Poghosyan, L., Giarelli, E., & Levy, S.E. (2008). Screening strategies for autism spectrum disorders in pediatric primary care. *Journal of Developmental and Behavioral Pediatrics, 29*, 345–350.
Robins, D.L. (2008). Screening for autism spectrum disorders in primary care settings. *Autism, 12*, 537–556.
Robins, D.L., Fein, D., Barton, M.L., & Green, J.A. (2001). The modified checklist for autism in toddlers: an initial study investigating the early detection of autism and pervasive developmental disorders. *Journal of Autism and Developmental Disorders, 31*, 131–144.
Sofronoff, K., Attwood, T., & Hinton, S. (2005). A randomized controlled trial of a CBT intervention for anxiety in children with Asperger syndrome. *Journal of Child Psychology and Psychiatry, 46*, 1152–1160.
Sugarman, L.I. (1997/2007). *Hypnosis in Pediatric Practice: Imaginative Medicine in Action* [video and instructional manual]. Bethel, CT: Crown House Publishing.
Thomson, L. (2005). *Harry the Hypno-potamus: Metaphorical Tales for the Treatment of Children*. Bethel, CT: Crown House Publishing.
Thomson, L. (2007). Hypnosis for children with elimination disorders. In W.C. Wester II & L.I. Sugarman, Eds., *Therapeutic Hypnosis with Children and Adolescents* (pp. 387–416). Bethel, CT: Crown House Publishing.
Thompson, L., Thompson, M., & Reid, A. (2010a). Functional neuroanatomy and the rationale for using EEG biofeedback for clients with Asperger's syndrome. *Applied Psychophysiology and Biofeedback*, 35, 39–61.
Thompson, L., Thompson, M., & Reid, A. (2010b). Neurofeedback outcomes in clients with Asperger's syndrome. *Applied Psychophysiology and Biofeedback, 35*, 63–81.
White, S.W., Oswald, D., Ollendick, T.H., & Scahill, L. (2009). Anxiety in children and adolescents with autism spectrum disorders. *Clinical Psychology Review, 29*, 216–229.
Wiggs, L. & Stores, G. (2004). Sleep patterns and sleep disorders in children with autistic spectrum disorders: insights using parent report and actigraphy. *Developmental Medicine and Child Neurology, 46*, 372–380.
Yapko, D. (2003). *Understanding Autism Spectrum Disorders: Frequently Asked Questions*. Philadelphia, PA: Jessica Kingsley Publishers.
Yapko, D. (2006). Utilizing Hypnosis with Children on the Autistic Spectrum, paper presented at the XVII International Congress of Hypnosis, Acapulco, Mexico.

# 10

# THERAPEUTIC HYPNOSIS FOR HABIT DISORDERS

## Introduction

Childhood habit problems potentially responsive to hypnosis include habitual coughs (or so-called cough tics), enuresis, thumb-sucking, fecal-soiling, nail-biting, hairpulling, verbal dysfluencies, sleepwalking and related parasomnias, certain eating disorders, and drug abuse. Although many habits may at one time have had emotional significance for the child, often the habit has long lost its original meaning and become functionally autonomous by the time the child is referred for treatment. Sometimes habits seem to develop without any identifiable underlying emotional significance or antecedent trigger and are perpetuated simply by repetition in association with certain situations. In this way they behave for all intents and purposes like conditioned responses. As discussed further in this chapter, these understandings are not only important but also may well be critical to discuss and explain as such to patients and families as part of the therapeutic education and communication process before moving into applying therapeutic hypnosis strategies. As in many situations, often such education provides comfort in context and may in itself alleviate negative parental (and child) expectations and fears that may have been inadvertently perpetuating the habituated behavior.

As with any other clinical problem, before beginning hypnosis clinically for a habit problem, it is important to determine if and whether the habit (still) serves any important psychological function – that is, whether there is any continuing so-called secondary gain from maintenance of the problem behavior. For example, does the child unconsciously achieve a position of control in his or her family through the prominence of their habit in family life? By reason of the habit behavior does the child have the power, for example, to delay leaving the house in a timely fashion to go certain places? Or, does the child take pleasure in making the parents angry in a passive way that avoids punishment? In the event that such significant secondary gain seems to be present, it may be preferable to postpone a symptom-oriented clinical hypnosis approach, at least until such time as one or another form of insight-oriented individual or family-oriented psychotherapy can help the family identify, acknowledge, and work through underlying problems. Not uncommonly children are able to resolve dynamic issues concurrently with a symptom-oriented, solution-focused approach.

Even in the absence of apparent or important secondary gain, the clinician/therapist must of course carefully assess the child's motivation for overcoming the habit. This is often easily

DOI: 10.4324/9781003243687-12

accomplished in the context of a comprehensive history obtained matter-of-factly and preferably from the child, who, of course, knows the most about and is the "expert" regarding their problem. Such assessments can be made directly through verbal questioning, indirectly through naturalistic inquiries as part of history taking, or indirectly by ideomotor signaling in hypnosis. Beyond the standard and traditional obtaining of a clinical history, we have had consistent success with naturalistic, Ericksonian utilization approaches that tend to allow for bypassing critical judgment and the elicitation of spontaneous "true" responses from the unconscious. In response to direct verbal inquiry, children's responses may or may not reflect active defenses; however, in response to an inquiry that is direct, humor based, and perhaps an abrupt shift of context, defenses are more likely to be equally abruptly bypassed, thus allowing more honest and definitive answers to questions. As an example, consider the following conversation between a child and a therapist regarding a thumb-sucking problem:

Therapist: So, how come you came over to see me?
Child: Well, see, uhhhh, well, it's'cause they [parents] said I had to.
Therapist: Because ...?
Child: Well,'cause I suck my thumb sometimes.
Therapist: Oh ... when?
Child: Sometimes.
Therapist: Oh. Well, mostly where are you when it *happens*?

Note that this is a purposeful shift in language to the problem "happening" rather than the child "doing" it. As an implication, it is designed to let the child begin to shift and to hear that the therapist understands that he does not feel like he is in charge of it, at least some of the time.

Child: You mean like at home or school or ...?
Therapist: Yeah.
Child: Well, usually at home.
Parents: You can tell him. It's when you're going to bed or when you're watching TV, and Ms. Smith told me that at kindergarten sometimes you suck your thumb during story hour.
Child [anguished]: MOM!!!!
Therapist: Say, are you going to *miss that* thumb-sucking *when* it's gone?

This represents a double or triple kind of shift and example of naturalistic suggestions and inquiry. The child has just been embarrassed through the mother's revealing that he sucks his thumb at school sometimes. Rather than take direct acknowledgment or mention of that, the therapist instead seemingly changes the subject, thus at one level helping to defuse the embarrassment. At another level, the future-oriented suggestion is offered or planted like a seed that the problem will be gone by inquiring about when (not "if") it is gone. Finally, the critical inquiry about whether the habit will be missed is embedded in the middle of the sentence in the abruptly offered query, thus easing it into the unconscious, making it a question more likely (though of course not guaranteed!) to be answered spontaneously from the unconscious.

Although children, of course, answer these questions in different ways, the answers, like those from ideomotor signals, seem to be more consistently reliable. Thus, in the example, if there is ambivalence, it is *commonly obviously* there. Usually this will be revealed quite clearly by the nature or content of the response, or both. So, in answer to "Say, are you going to miss *that* thumb-sucking when it's gone?" many say, "No, of course not, are you kidding?" and look at the clinician incredulously for asking such a foolish question. Others, such as those who are ambivalent, are more likely to hesitate, hem and haw, or perhaps even to say openly, "Yeah, I need to suck my thumb to get to sleep at night"; they then want to change the subject. Note also the use of "that" thumb-sucking as a dissociative suggestion instead of "your" thumb-sucking. The theoretical advantage of these conversational questions and suggestions over ideomotor signaling responses in hypnosis is that the latter are not usually able to be introduced, of course, until hypnosis has been formally introduced, discussed, and taught. With ideomotor signaling, unconscious conflict is more likely to be easily revealed, as, for example, when the child's "yes" and "no" fingers lift simultaneously in response to questions asked "to the fingers" during hypnosis.

For any habituated or chronic problem, it is valuable to determine how the child thinks life will be different when the problem is resolved. If, for example, a child still obtains much pleasure from a given habit, has little desire to give it up, and has come for therapy chiefly as a result of parental pressure, there is likely to be little benefit from a therapeutic approach with hypnosis. In such a case, the clinician might suggest that the parents postpone treatment for the child and spend some time instead perhaps discussing realistic parental expectations. Sometimes parents expect too much of a young child who is not developmentally ready to change a certain behavior. Accordingly, treatment for the habit with the child may be postponed while perhaps the clinician helps the family with issues related to unrealistic expectations.

In therapeutic clinical hypnosis for habit disorders, we have not found symptom substitution to be a problem, although we sometimes hear dire warnings in this regard. Our experience suggests that children either gladly give up habits or indicate a continuing need for them, sometimes despite an earnest spoken or unspoken desire to the contrary. In general, a trial of four to six sessions of therapeutic clinical hypnosis, if that many, suffices to learn whether the child is really ready for habit change. In the case of some habits, successful treatment depends on removal of misconceptions about the problem. Sometimes such misconceptions can be resolved by verbal explanations; at other times, the clinician may choose to use diagrams to explain anatomical or physiological relationships that may in turn enable a child to develop suitable images for success consciously or during hypnosis. Many parents have also benefited from such explanations. In order to detect persisting confusion, it is helpful to request that the child bring his or her own drawing or diagram to the clinician on the next visit. Alternatively, it is often useful to invite the child to create their own drawing as part of the next session. Children and parents (and clinicians) alike not only enjoy this opportunity but also are often pleasantly surprised to see how very much the child has learned from but a single guided explanation (even 1–2 weeks before) about how the body works (with respect to the child's particular problem).

Whenever a habit may be a symptom of an underlying physical disorder, it is crucial that the child be appropriately evaluated from a medical perspective prior to initiation of any clinical hypnosis. Because this possibility is most likely in cases of enuresis (bedwetting) and encopresis (fecal soiling), we always include issues of differential diagnosis in our discussion of these problems. These habits may have both psychological and medical components, and too often the former are emphasized while the latter are ignored. A psychotherapist, for example, must not yield to parental pressure for hypnosis to "fix it" without proper diagnostic evaluation of the problem as indicated.

Finally, clinical hypnosis approaches to habit problems should focus on the patient's competence and ability for mastery, emphasizing that it is ultimately the child, not the clinician or therapist, who makes the change. Hypnotic suggestions should include images of future recognition that the problem is solved/resolved. For someone working on a thumb-sucking habit, one might say, for example: "Just picture yourself on that video in your mind, and notice the date is some time later this year, I don't know which month, but you'll notice it … good … then notice what a nice evening you have, first finishing your homework, then playing a game with your sister. Then notice yourself getting ready for bed and listening to a story and notice your hand and thumb comfortably down by your side under the covers." For their part and their role, parents should be asked to focus on family life without the problem, thus affirming their confidence and trust in their child's ability (and commitment) to overcome it.

## Enuresis

Through the ages, nocturnal enuresis has been the most common chronic behavioral problem faced by the pediatrician (Olness, 1977b). Glicklich (1951) reported that this problem was discussed in a 16th-century pediatrics text in a section entitled, "Of Pyssying in the Bedde." One study has estimated that enuresis has occurred in approximately 20 million Americans over the age of 5 years (Cohen, 1975). It is generally agreed that the symptom does not warrant extensive investigation or treatment under age 5–6 years unless information from history and physical examination suggests organic causes. The majority of bedwetting beyond age 5 years is associated with no discernible organic or psychological causes and thus may be understood as equivalent to a habituated response, or habit problem. In his *Lectures on Diseases of Children* (1882/1994), the famous pediatrician Dr. Edward Henoch noted that so little was known of the causation of nocturnal enuresis that "there is a certain justification for the doubt whether this is a diseased condition or an acquired habit" (pp. 257–258). A very recent review of the role of sleep monitoring in children with nocturnal enuresis (Zhu et al., 2021) proposes that subtle changes in polysomnography (PSG) may be significant in distinguishing Nocturnal Enuresis from its comorbidities. While they suggest that continued research is essential, they are very definitive in not recommending that PSG be included as routine or "first-line" evaluation of nocturnal enuresis.

In view of the foregoing nocturnal enuresis may be not only best understood but also perhaps best explained to children and families as a developmental or maturational variant, or as an "accidental habit," that has become stuck and inadvertently perpetuated. Using this kind of language in particular defuses blame.

## Evaluation

The approach to evaluation of enuresis varies depending on whether or not the symptom is primary (i.e., the child has never had a prolonged period of consecutive dry beds) or is secondary (e.g., the child had 6 months of dry beds followed by a relapse) (Culbert & Banez, 2008; Olness, 1977b; Schmitt, 1990). It is also important to ascertain whether the enuresis is at night only or is a combination of diurnal (daytime) and nighttime wetting. The presence of concurrent day and night enuresis indicates that more intensive investigation is needed to rule out organic causes that might include diabetes mellitus, occult spinal dysraphism, urinary tract infections, congenital anomalies of the urinary tract, or seizures (Anderson, 1975; Kolvin, 1973; Neveus et al., 2006; Olness, 1977b). Chronic constipation is a common, yet often unrecognized, cause of both daytime and nighttime wetting and should be carefully searched for in any patient with enuresis. Rarely, the presence of nocturnal enuresis is caused by hyperthyroidism, diuretic medications, or a child's habit of consuming large amounts of caffeine drinks such as coffee or colas. There is also a likely association between documented allergies and the presence of nocturnal enuresis; the mechanism is unknown (Gerrard, Jones, Shokier, & Zaleski, 1971; Olness & Immershein, 1977).

Initial evaluation of enuresis must include questions regarding the meaning of the symptom for the family. Although there may have been no original emotional trigger, emotional problems often develop as bedwetting persists. It is important to ascertain in particular the expectations of the parents regarding the ultimate achievement of dry beds. If, for example, the parents believe that "all children should be dry by age 3," it is possible that unreasonable parent pressure has contributed to the child losing confidence even when neurophysiological maturity has developed somewhat later than 3 years. In the case of secondary bedwetting, it is essential to know about stresses that may have triggered the abrupt onset of the symptom (Doleys, 1977; Lawless & McElderry, 2001; Robison, 2009). These may be events that we all would agree are or could be stressful, such as an emergency appendectomy for the child, emergency surgery for a parent, death of a pet, death of a grandparent, or a move to a new home resulting in increased distance from bed to bathroom. Or, the stress might be something the adults in the child's life may not have perceived as a major stressor but may well have been very stressful for the child and contributed to or triggered the symptom. These may include having been somehow embarrassed in school in front of the class, not getting their desired role in the school play, a friend moving away, getting an unexpected lower grade on a homework assignment or examination, or any of a myriad of similar childhood life experiences. A model questionnaire for assessment of enuresis can be found in the Appendix of the fourth edition of this text.

Physical examination should endeavor to rule out the rare neurological etiologies of enuresis. Therefore, it is important to undertake a careful neurological assessment with emphasis on lower extremity muscle tone and strength, sensation, gait, and deep tendon reflexes. Examination of the spine and back (for dimples, tufts of hair as suggestive of spinal dysraphism), abdomen, external genitalia, and perineum is important (Robison, 2009). If concomitant soiling is present, it is crucial that a rectal examination be performed. Impacted stool present in the rectal ampulla might suggest constipation that is causally associated with enuresis. Poor anal sphincter tone or an abnormal anal wink response might suggest a neurological impairment. The physician should also observe the urine stream of the child.

Each child presenting with the complaint of enuresis should have a urinalysis done. If there are symptoms or physical findings suggestive of a urinary tract infection, a urine culture, of course, should also be done. Radiologic studies are not indicated unless physical findings suggest physical abnormalities.

## General Management

Given the high incidence of enuresis and of its spontaneous remission or resolution, it seems logical that, in general, bedwetting should not be regarded as a major problem. Unfortunately, the perceptions of physicians, parents, and children often differ in defining when it is a problem, and sociocultural norms and expectations also play a strong role in whether this common and usually maturational phenomenon is experienced as a problem. If the youngster is less than 5 years old and has no historical or physical findings that suggest an underlying medical problem, then the possibility of maturational delay regarding nighttime urinary continence should be explained to the parents who may then accept patience as the most desirable approach. For children, bedwetting is usually regarded as a problem when the possibility of camping or sleepovers develops. At this time, the symptom may engender a sense of social incompetence and a feeling of being different from (or even teased by) siblings and peers. If the parents and child wish treatment, it is important to agree on a plan that is acceptable to all parties involved, especially the child. Studies indicate that the most successful treatment methods are those reinforcing the child's own responsibility for success (Marshall, Marshall, & Richards, 1973; Schmitt, 1990). One such method is therapeutic clinical hypnosis.

## A Therapeutic Hypnosis Approach

Initially, we meet with the child and parents together. Statistics about the incidence of enuresis are presented along with a brief review of ideas concerning current understanding of cause. We routinely ask for the child's perception about the cause of the problem, as well as the parents' perceptions, in that order. Asking the child before the parents usually facilitates the elicitation of a more spontaneous and authentic response reflecting what the child really thinks. We tend to frame this specifically by asking what they wondered might be the reason for the problem or what went through their mind, rather than asking them specifically what they think was the "cause." Occasionally a child, particularly in the case of secondary enuresis, will recall some trigger event that the parents did not know about, have not considered significant, or did not even remember.

It is our custom to focus an initial interview on obtaining a history of the presenting problem in the context of developing rapport with the child and family. Beyond knowing about the presenting problem, goals to be accomplished include that the child leaves the first visit with (1) a feeling that he or she can trust us; (2) a belief that we are quite certain that we can be of help; (3) curiosity about what was said and in what ways we will be able to be of help; (4) a sense of having been believed, respected, and liked; and (5) a beginning idea that they can have fun and get help at the same time. In an eclectic, often humor-based approach, an effort is made first and foremost to do what Milton Erickson said was critical in helping children; that is, "go with the child" (Haley, 1985). In trusting that the child knows best about their own problem and, in this case, their habit, questions regarding secondary gain can be asked directly and abruptly, often catching the child slightly off guard, and as such having the quality of going directly to the unconscious and in turn evoking a response likely to be quite honest. An example would be to ask a child with enuresis if he or she is going to miss the problem when it's gone. Perhaps predictably, most find this either confusing or amusing or both, and they say, "No, of course not!" Those who understand it and hesitate may in fact have more secondary gain than we realized, and that factor may require attention before focusing on further work on the enuresis.

We determine the child's words for urination and defecation. Anatomy is discussed with the aid of diagrams. Some therapists like to use printed diagrams (e.g., from texts), but we tend to draw a new picture each time, like the one shown in Figure 10.1. We believe that this personalized approach then becomes part of the therapeutic process, anchoring the rapport, increasing the focused attention, and as such facilitating understanding, interest, and commitment to creating change. We ask the child to review the diagram and our discussion about it before going to bed, and we may ask the child to bring a similar drawing for us at the time of the next visit or to reproduce his or her own rendition of the drawing in the office as part of the next session. We explain that success will depend upon the child's involvement and commitment to practice self-hypnosis. We ask parents specifically to NOT remind the child to practice, again emphasizing the child's responsibility in the treatment process. We give the parents a printed summary concerning enuresis and their part in the self-hypnosis treatment program and ask them to leave or prepare them for the fact that subsequent visits with their child will be in private.

In therapeutic clinical hypnosis sessions with children with enuresis, we discuss in detail the best time to practice suggested exercises. It is usually not a good idea to practice just before bedtime if the child is very tired. We recommend practice just after dinner or an hour before bedtime. We review the path from bed to bathroom and sometimes have the child draw us a map of this path. We encourage the child to decide on a specific reminder to themselves to practice self-hypnosis (e.g., a string around the toothbrush handle, ribbon around the neck of a favorite stuffed toy, sign on the bedroom door or the wall). We emphasize that the bladder is a muscle and that the patient has previously learned control of many muscles, such as in the many muscles

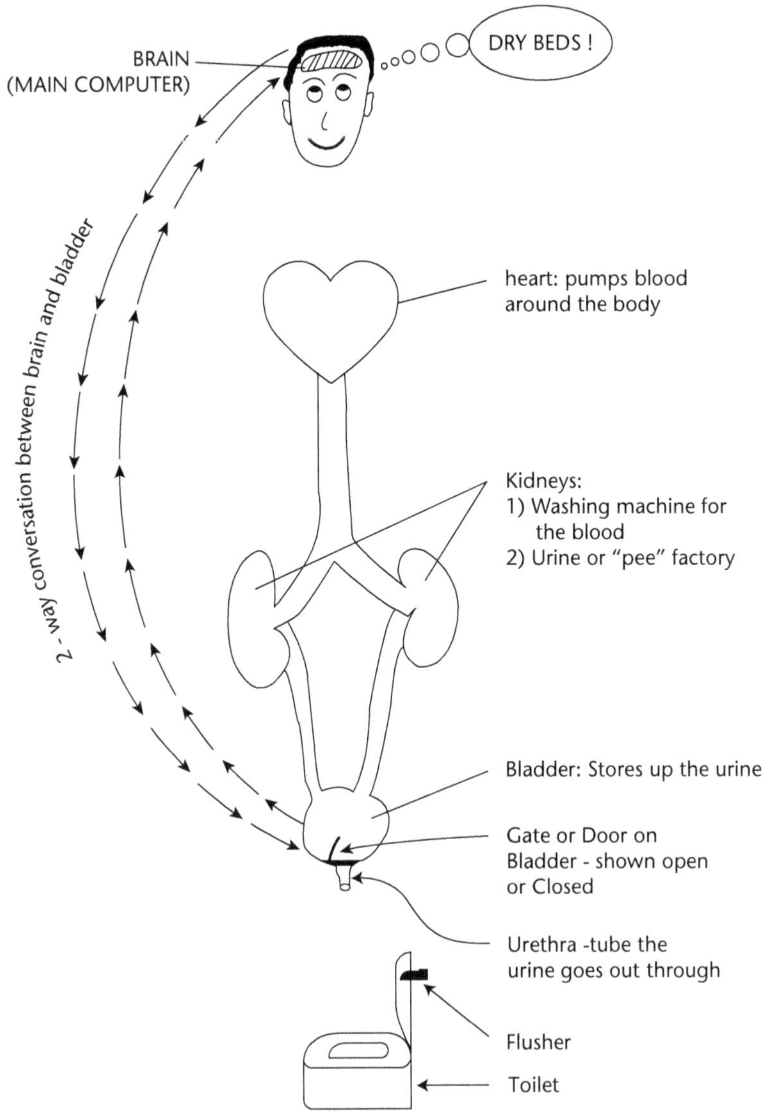


**FIGURE 10.1** "Brain-Bladder Communication"

*Source: Simplified diagram of physiology and anatomy of urine for use with children with enuresis (See text).*

required to ride a two-wheeler bicycle (Kohen, 1990), or to walk, play soccer, etc. We also use the analogy of the clinician being the coach asking the patient to practice muscle control, thereby further placing ultimate responsibility on the child.

We proceed to ask the child to explain likes and dislikes such as hobbies, interests, favorite colors, videos or computer games, or favorite dreams. We then choose an invitation method that seems appropriate. Following the invitation, we often ask the child to show us a "yes" finger and a "no" finger and then ask a series of questions, most irrelevant such as "Do you like the color purple?" or "Do you like to eat chocolate ice cream?" Without changing pace, we insert the question "Would you like to have all dry beds?" or "Are you ready to work on solving the problem of wet beds today?" If the answer is "no," as it is occasionally, this suggests that the child may be receiving significant secondary gain from the problem (e.g., being allowed to get into bed with parents when own bed is wet), or simply that there is not sufficient motivation to work on the problem at this time.

Following a "yes" response, we ask the child to imagine being in a favorite place and to signal a "yes" when ready to give instructions to his or her bladder. At this point, we might say something similar to the following:

> Tell yourself that you will sleep well tonight. Tell your bladder to send a message to your brain to awaken you when it is full of urine [or pee]. When you awaken, tell yourself to get out of your dry bed, walk across the room, through the door, and down the hall to the bathroom. Turn on the light and open the bladder gate to let the urine out in the toilet where it belongs. When it is empty, close the gate, flush the toilet, wash and dry your hands, turn the light off, and return to your nice, warm, cozy, dry bed. Then think of yourself awakening in a nice, warm, cozy, dry bed, knowing you will have a good day, and go back to sleep. Enjoy knowing that your bed is dry because of your efforts, because you're the boss of your bladder muscle gate. Enjoy the good feeling of waking up in a dry bed as long as you like. Then, before you finish this nice imagination practice which you are doing so well, remind yourself that every time you practice this it gets easier and easier to do, and you get better and better at teaching yourself to wake up every day in a nice, warm, cozy, dry bed. Then when you're ready, you can open your eyes and enjoy the rest of the day.

Both during the last portion of the hypnotic trance and after return to the usual state of alertness, the child is encouraged and engaged in a commitment to practice this self-hypnosis exercise daily. We have described similar approaches with the addition of multiple Ericksonian strategies including double-bind suggestions, metaphors for control, dissociative suggestions (e.g., for the bladder and the brain talking to each other), positive expectancy, and reframing (Kohen, 1990).

In general, the initial visit takes from 45 to 60 minutes. Depending on the individual child and his or her history, a hypnosis exercise may or may not be taught at the first visit. If the complexity of the history or child and family circumstances suggest to the clinician's judgment or intuition that hypnotic rapport may take a bit longer, then formal hypnosis training as described may be deferred to the next or a subsequent visit when the child in his or her relationship with the therapist is determined to be ready to learn. At a minimum, however, our first visit always includes teaching about how the body works, a commitment to keeping track of the number of dry beds at home, and a commitment to just think about the communication between the brain and bladder prior to the next visit. Subsequent visits are tailored to the particular child. Many older children do very well after a couple of visits and are followed by letter and/or phone. Younger children sometimes seem to require more professional reinforcement and may have return visits every 2 weeks for several months. We ask most children, and particularly younger ones, to keep calendars or cumulative graphs of their successes. After termination of in-person office visits, we ask the children to mail (or e-mail) their calendars on a monthly basis for several months. This process of continued communication appears to be of multipurpose value in that it: (1) provides the continuing anchor through a connection with the clinician coach; (2) eases the termination process of a usually very positive, intimate therapeutic relationship; and (3) facilitates ongoing ego strengthening through reinforcement of the self-monitoring, practice, and self-regulation process.

## Observations about Special Cases

Occasionally, children do better with a personal audio reminder that can be prepared on a digital recorder or recorded on the clinician's and/or patient's smartphone and placed on a CD or added to their other portable media players for personal listening. These reminders can be prepared by recording a therapeutic hypnosis practice session during a regular office visit. Ordinarily, we wish to wait until the children have demonstrated understanding of, and facility with, self-hypnosis practice before making a recording for their home use. In theory, this is to avoid or reduce the possibility of developing (complete) dependency on the clinician and to reinforce the concept that what happens with clinical hypnosis is both because of and inside of the child, and not due to the clinician/therapist alone or to the recording. Children are asked to listen to the recording each evening or to alternate practicing on their own and with the recording. We do not know any way to predict in advance which children can benefit most from such personal recordings.

Occasionally, children as young as 4 years old will do very well in spite of our belief and concern that many this age are not physiologically capable of nighttime bladder control. In one case, a clinician refused to work with a 4-year-old, saying he was too young, but she did work with his 6-year-old brother. A week later they returned, and in the interim the 6-year-old had taught the 4-year-old and both were dry! We have seen similar unexpected and unpredictable outcomes among other sibling pairs.

We have occasionally worked with siblings concurrently up to a maximum of five in a single family. The siblings seem to reinforce each other in these situations, although most siblings prefer to be seen privately. From time to time even being seen separately by the same therapist can be problematic, and the clinician must be mindful of, and creative about, managing potential differential success and the risk of negative consequences of competition between and among siblings.

A mother who is also a nurse adapted what she called the "quarter trick" (coin induction) from an article on treatment of enuresis with self-hypnosis. Her 6-year-old son had never had a dry bed. After 5 days of practice, he had no further wet beds. Generally, however, the process goes less well if parents teach, reinforce, or are otherwise involved in a process that we believe should be largely the child to practice and master. Several physician-parents have reported total failures in working with their own children who then were able to do well when referred to a non-relative for therapeutic hypnosis.

Children may relapse after more than a year of dry beds; however, when they review self-hypnosis, they usually recapture control quickly and easily, often after only one or two such reviews. Occasionally, children who fail with self-hypnosis exercises will move on to use one of the several available alarm systems with rapid success. When children ask for our assistance in maximizing the effectiveness of these alarm systems, we offer suggestions for integrating the alarm into a hypnotic approach (or the therapeutic hypnosis into the alarm approach). One such simple suggestion is to ask the child to give themselves a challenging message during self-hypnosis such as:

> Tonight while I'm sleeping, bladder, when you fill up with urine be sure to send the message to the brain that you're full. And, brain, be sure to keep the gate on the bladder shut until you wake me up so I can get out of my dry bed, walk to the bathroom, open the bladder gate, and let the pee out in the toilet where it belongs. Brain, be sure to do that right so you can *beat the buzzer.* Wake me up before the buzzer does.
>
> In general, we believe that self-hypnosis emphasizes more self-control than does the alarm. At present, we have no way to predict which children will benefit most from therapeutic hypnosis and which from some other form of treatment.

Although the various alarms have been the most widely studied and recommended methods for control of nocturnal enuresis (Robison, 2009), none of the randomized controlled studies explains the precise mechanism by which alarms work. It is our impression that positive suggestion plays a significant role in the efficacy of alarms, whereas the attribution of success is typically made about the device itself. Moreover, we believe that all of the alarms seem to "work" in a way that is counter-productive because they all buzz/ring/vibrate ONLY when urination has begun, and the moisture triggers the signal to activate the alarm and awaken the child. While all of that seems to be "fine," we think it is counterproductive as even with this alarm the child has already become wet before it "works" to awaken them.

## Results of Therapeutic Hypnosis for Nocturnal Enuresis

Several published accounts report the successful use of clinical therapeutic hypnosis with children with enuresis. Some are single case reports (Jacobs, 1962; Olness & Gardner, 1978; Tilton, 1980). Solovey and Milechnin (1959) described their hypnotherapeutic approach to the problem but presented no data concerning results. Collison (1970) employed clinical hypnosis with nine children, ages 9–16 years, with onset (secondary) enuresis. Treatment lasted 6–20 weeks and included direct suggestion, ego-strengthening methods, and insight therapy. All nine children achieved dry beds and remained dry during follow-up lasting 1–5 years.

Baumann and Hinman (1974) reported improvement in 64 of 73 boys ages 7–13 years with enuresis who were treated with hypnotherapy in combination with imipramine and other medical management, parental instruction, and monetary rewards for dry beds. Duration of treatment and duration of follow-up were not reported. Gottsegen (2003) reported complete resolution of nocturnal enuresis in four children ages 9–12 years each after only one visit. He was very thoughtful to note that not only did complete resolution of enuresis occur in one visit and was maintained over time, but also that in three of the four cases hypnotic suggestions, education, and positive expectations were provided without benefit or apparent need for a formal clinical hypnosis induction experience.

In writing about nocturnal enuresis, Thomson (2005, 2007, 2009) reported several individual case vignettes and discussed metaphorical storytelling as an example of successful hypnotherapy for enuresis. While at George Washington University, Olness (1975) taught self-hypnosis to 40 children with enuresis, ages 4–16 years. Treatment focused on direct suggestions that the children were asked to review daily. Parental involvement was minimal. Of the 40 children, 31 resolved their bedwetting, most within the first month of treatment. Six others improved. Of three children who did not improve, one said he did not want dry beds and was experiencing significant secondary gain from his symptom. A second child refused to practice self-hypnosis at home. The third child had significant urological anomalies that had required surgery. The successful children required no more than two visits before improvement was apparent. Follow-up lasted 6 to 28 months. No concurrent medications were employed.

Stanton (1979) included background music along with a variety of hypnotic techniques in his treatment of 28 children with enuresis, ages 7–18 years. After one to three sessions, 20 children stopped wetting. Of these, 15 remained dry after 1-year follow-up. The five who relapsed were among the younger children. Characteristics of the eight who did not improve were not described.

Edwards and van der Spuy (1985) reported a study of 48 boys with enuresis, ages 8–13 years. They were randomly assigned to four treatment conditions: no intervention, trance plus suggestions, suggestions without trance, and trance alone without suggestions. One difficulty in interpreting this study relates to the high frequency of secondary or onset enuresis (50%) in this group. This raises the possibility, for example, that stool retention was a cause of enuresis in the secondary group. Groups were not matched for this variable. In this study, suggestions for trance with or without suggestions were given through headphones, and suggestions were tape-recorded. These were aimed at general tension reduction and enhancement of self-confidence and contained suggestions for: (1) increased bladder capacity, (2) reduction of fluids before bedtime, (3) visiting the toilet before bedtime, and (4) awakening at night to go to the toilet if the bladder was full. The authors found that subjects responded equally well whether they received trance plus suggestions or suggestions alone. Those who received trance alone or no treatment showed no changes over the initial 6-week treatment period. Those who received trance induction, however, improved only to the level of the other intervention groups by the second 6-week follow-up interval. At 6 months, the non-treatment group averaged three dry nights per week, and the treatment groups averaged between four and five dry nights per week. The authors noted a greater relapse among those with secondary enuresis. The results of this study are consistent with other studies related to self-regulation of autonomic responses in children; that is, formal trance induction is not essential for suggestions to be effective. It is possible that poorer response in those with onset enuresis is related to unrecognized stool retention or, perhaps, to some other as yet unrecognized biological problem.

Kohen and associates (Kohen, Colwell, Heimel, & Olness, 1984) reviewed data for 257 children with enuresis treated with hypnosis at the Behavioral Pediatrics Program at the Minneapolis Children's Medical Center. In all, 44% achieved complete dryness, defined as 30 consecutive dry beds and requiring a 12-month follow-up without relapse. Another 31% showed significant improvement. Most children referred had already tried two or three other treatment methods, including an alarm system, imipramine, and other drugs. Failures related primarily to lack of motivation on the part of the child and excessive involvement by parents; for example, if parents said, "We had two dry beds last week," pre-empting the child's own personalized report, failure was likely. If parents reminded children to practice their self-hypnosis exercises, progress was much slower. Many parents would say, "I know I shouldn't, but I can't help it." In these cases, further exploration of the parent–child relationship or family counselling was sometimes useful.

Banerjee and colleagues (Banerjee, Srivastav, & Palan, 1993) compared treatment with hypnotherapy to treatment with imipramine in two groups (25 children each) of children with enuresis, ages 5–16 years. Comparable results were found between groups after 3 months of treatment, with 76% of the imipramine group and 72% of the hypnosis group achieving positive responses (as defined by all dry beds or decreased frequency of wetting). After 3 months of treatment and reinforcement, imipramine was discontinued, and active follow-up visits were discontinued for both groups; however, the hypnosis group was encouraged to continue self-hypnosis practice. At subsequent follow-up 6 months later, only 24% of the imipramine group had maintained a positive response, whereas in the hypnosis group 68% had maintained a positive response, without clinical reinforcement. In an interesting finding, the authors noted that, in children under age 7 years of age, hypnosis was less effective than imipramine after 3 months of treatment. Six of seven children treated with imipramine had a positive response, whereas only two of eight in this age group treated with hypnosis had a positive response. It is unclear from the authors' report whether any of the children in this age group either ultimately became dry (in the hypnosis group) or were in the smaller group (24%) who sustained dryness (in the imipramine group) at the 9-month follow-up. As the authors noted, methodological considerations limit the generalizability of these results and are important for future studies. In addition to random selection and group assignment, such comparative studies should consider designs that include a group or groups receiving time and attention equal to that of the groups receiving hypnotherapy or other treatment approaches, or they should include a group learning hypnosis (e.g., mental imagery and relaxation) without receiving specific hypnotic suggestions for enuresis control. Measuring hypnotizability with the Stanford Hypnotic Clinical Scale for Children (SHCS-C), the authors found no difference in responsivity between the imipramine treatment and the hypnosis-treated groups.

A report by Minosh, Schwartz, and Badalyan (2013) noted the use of hypnosis with 53 children with anxiety disorders, nocturnal Enuresis, or Insomnia. They described that of the 17 children with enuresis 59% experienced good or excellent ratings of long-term success. They emphasized that "rapport is arguably the most important factor" that the enduring positive benefit is tied to patient (and parent) expectations and consistent self-hypnosis practice.

A review of "Controlled outcome studies of child clinical hypnosis" (Adinolfi & Gava, 2013) concluded that "hypnosis can be used effectively for habitual disorders such as nocturnal enuresis" and may have the added benefit of improvement in quality of life and self-esteem.

Two studies (Kohen et al., 1984; Stanton, 1979) concluded that clinical hypnosis is not likely to help children with enuresis if there is no marked improvement over the first three or four sessions. Prolonging treatment rarely produces gains commensurate with the investment of time and money involved, unless the focus has shifted to dealing with family dilemmas and associated parent or family counselling.

## Soiling

### *Evaluation and Medical Management*

A recent review noted that constipation is classified as a functional gastrointestinal disorder (FGID) in the Rome Foundation IV standardized diagnostic criteria but the term, encopresis, is omitted from Rome IV. Encopresis, however, is defined by the American Psychiatric Association in the Fifth Edition of the Diagnostic and Statistical Manual of Mental Disorders (Leleiko, Mayer Brown, Cerezo & Plante, 2020).

The symptom of soiling or encopresis in a child past usual toilet training age represents constipation until proved otherwise. Pure encopresis (soiling without stool retention) is rare, although parents will often insist that their child's symptoms do not represent constipation (Fleisher, 1976; Levine, 1982). The presence of primary fecal incontinence in association with urine incontinence should lead the examiner to suspect a neurological problem. Occasionally, a congenital defect (e.g., spinal dysraphism) will not manifest itself by symptoms of fecal or urinary incontinence until the child is 5 or 6 years of age (Anderson, 1975).

Much emphasis has been placed on the psychological concomitants of fecal incontinence (Clayden & Lawson, 1976; Halpern, 1977). There is no doubt that many secondary emotional problems develop in a child with this symptom, but the original cause is more often physical than psychological. It is important to note that psychotherapy, while often indicated for the ego damage caused by soiling, cannot unblock a stuffed colon! Practitioners may reflexively send a child with fecal incontinence to a mental health professional before undertaking a complete evaluation. Inasmuch as secondary emotional effects are common and may be profound and inasmuch as the ongoing stress of chronicity and relapses are trying for the patient and the family, we emphasize, as do others (Buchanan & Clayden, 1992), that the initial evaluation should be carefully focused and comprehensive to prevent misconceptions about causation and treatment from contributing inadvertently to chronicity. Thus, the following information is essential before undertaking treatment:

- *How often and when does the child soil?* Children with underlying constipation are likely to soil several times a day, whereas the child with pure encopresis may have a normal bowel movement once a day into a place other than the toilet.
- *Does anyone else in the family have bowel problems?* This question is important with respect to the vaguely defined entity of familial constipation, which may reflect family eating habits or

intrinsic slow motility. The question may aid in assessment of the family focus on bowel function and expectancies with respect to outcome.

- *What was the child's stool pattern in early infancy?* Constipation in early infancy may be present in the case of congenital aganglionosis (Nixon, 1964) or in the irritable colon syndrome described by Davidson and Wasserman (1966).
- *How was the child fed in early infancy?* Feeding habits established in infancy may potentiate later constipation; for example, continuation of large amounts of cow's milk into the second year of life may contribute to constipation.
- *Was there any change in diet, family constellation, caretaker, or bathroom options around the onset of constipation?* Frequently, one finds that, just prior to onset of bowel problems, the family moved and the bathroom changed; the family went camping and the child didn't like outdoor toilets; the child had a febrile illness and was dehydrated, following which he or she had a hard, painful stool; or the child suddenly began drinking an extra quart of milk a day.
- *Ask the parents to describe the child's accidents.* Information concerning size and appearance of stool aids in determining whether or not there is constipation with overflow soiling or pure encopresis. Overflow stools tend to be runny and small in amount. Occasionally, particularly after an enema or suppository, the stool of a chronically constipated child will plug the toilet.
- *Is the child taking any medicines?* Certain medications such as imipramine, codeine, and Ritalin® are constipating, and their use must be considered in any management plan (Fleisher, 1976). Occasionally, parents or physicians misinterpret the problems as diarrhea and inadvertently prescribe kaopectate, which will exacerbate the problem.
- *Has the child complained of tingling, numbness, or funny feelings in his or her legs or is there poor coordination?* It is important to look into the possibility of lower extremity paresthesias that might suggest the presence of spinal dysraphism.

With respect to planning management, it is important to know how the child currently handles the problem, how siblings and schoolmates respond, what interventions have been tried and how they work, and what the family believes to be the cause of the soiling.

A thorough evaluation requires a physical examination that includes a careful neurological examination as well as abdominal palpation. A rectal examination is reasonable in the context of a positive rapport between the clinician and patient and after careful preparation of the child for this portion of the examination. If the examination does not confirm constipation, it may be necessary to obtain x-rays of the abdomen to determine whether or not stool is present or is in excess. A diagnostic anal manometry may be indicated if there is a question of rectal aganglionoses. Thyroid function tests should be done if there are any signs of hypothyroidism. If history and physical examination uncover occult spinal dysraphism, aganglionoses, hypothyroidism, or other conditions requiring specific treatment, these conditions must be treated.

If a diagnosis of constipation with overflow soiling is made, as it commonly is (Buchanan & Clayden, 1992), then appropriate intervention is as follows:

1. Anatomy should be explained carefully, with the aid of drawings.
2. Mechanical problems associated with prolonged retention should be carefully explained.
3. If the patient currently has significant retention, a series of enemas or oral polyethylene glycol solution for thorough evacuation should be prescribed.
4. Concurrently, the diet should be regulated. Dietary changes should be explained in detail to the child with emphasis on graduated re-introduction of proscribed foods (e.g., milk, apples, bananas, rice, gelatin, carrots) after a period of 4–6 weeks.

5. Unprocessed bran or another high-fiber supplement should be added twice daily to the child's diet.
6. The child should make a commitment to choose to sit on the toilet either after breakfast for 10 minutes or after supper for 10 minutes (or one minute for each year of age). This decision should be communicated to the parents.
7. In the initial period some enemas may have to be given. It is recommended that an enema be given every 48 hours if the child has not voluntarily defecated. If this rule is broken, the ultimate curative process is only delayed by the continued excessive stretching of the lower colon.

Parents may find children-friendly YouTube videos helpful in engaging and teaching their children about constipation (and soiling). Also, a variety of books geared to children may be helpful not only for children with delayed toilet training but also for constipation.

### *Therapeutic Hypnosis*

Fleisher (1976) and Buchanan and Clayden (1992) stressed the need for children to be given responsibility in the treatment of soiling. Conventional medical and surgical management do not do this. Clinical hypnosis alone, in patients who have had the problem for many years, is unlikely to affect the mechanical components. It does, however, give the child personal responsibility and the opportunity to remain in control of his or her bowels while eliminating an undesirable habit. Parents as well as children can benefit from greater understanding of the problems connected with soiling. We ask parents to refrain from reminding the child to practice self-hypnosis exercises, however, and to indicate in their praise of the child's successes that they know that their child was responsible for the happy and proud outcome.

Some children with longstanding soiling may continue to have some residual soiling, although they learn to defecate regularly. This problem may be due to long-term stretching of the anorectal sphincters.

In some clinical reports, hypnosis has been directed at dynamic issues with little or no attention paid to the need for medical management. While in such cases there may be improvement, the problem is rarely fully resolved. Goldsmith (1962) described therapeutic hypnosis with a 9-year-old girl with constipation who soiled herself several times each day. The poor bowel control was interpreted as an unconscious expression of aggression toward the mother, and the therapeutic hypnosis was directed at understanding these underlying issues, as well as including direct suggestions for symptom relief. The child was told in hypnosis that she would not be able to eliminate until she was actually sitting on the toilet. Over the next week the child had no major accidents but experienced continuous seepage. Medical aspects of the problem were still not addressed, and the seepage was again interpreted as an expression of hostility toward the mother. Further dynamic psychotherapy and therapeutic clinical hypnosis resulted in some improvement, but the child continued to have an occasional lapse, again thought to represent hostility.

Silber (1968) did distinguish between soiling based on mechanical problems and encopresis, which he defined as psychologically motivated soiling. He employed clinical hypnosis in combination with enemas for nine children with encopresis ages 5–9 years. Treatment, which lasted approximately three sessions, helped the child focus on anthropomorphic images related to defecation such as the anal sphincter as an intelligent watchman. Dynamic issues were then dealt with only through these images, and all nine children were reported as cured.

Olness (1976) reported successful clinical hypnosis treatment of four children with functional megacolon, of whom three were in the 3–5-year-old range. All were taught self-hypnosis and gave themselves daily suggestions regarding their ability to control their bowels in appropriate ways. Olness concluded that success was chiefly the result of the children being given responsibility for their own solutions. Parents were involved only to the extent that they praised the child for improvement and reinforced emerging feelings of mastery.

Others (e.g., Thomson, 2007, 2009) have described creative uses of hypnotherapy and storytelling to help children help themselves in the context of a comprehensive plan as we have outlined. In the context of an integrated, comprehensive medical approach as described, these approaches have the potential to be especially effective as they emphasize the value of the positive relationship with the clinician and an abiding faith in the child's ability to work on and solve the problem.

An Italian group described a study of 52 children who had encopresis without constipation. Twenty-six children enrolled in a program of play therapy plus toilet training for six months. The other 26 children were enrolled in a toilet training program only. After six months the first group had an average frequency per month of 6.46 soiling episodes per month and the group that experienced toilet training only had 12.04 soiling episodes per month (Esposito et al., 2013).

## Speech and Voice Problems

### *Stuttering*

The problem of stuttering has been described from many perspectives, with treatment approaches derived from presumed neurological, educational, and psychological causes. Hypnosis has been found to be a helpful therapeutic adjunct in the context of differing treatment approaches. A key factor in success may be the children's feelings of mastery and confidence in the therapeutic clinical hypnosis relationship. Published accounts consist of technical considerations, with isolated case reports (Falck, 1964; Moore, 1946; Silber, 1973). Silber (1973) utilized fairy tales, folklore, and symbols to help children who stutter to get in touch with potential verbal fluency and self-esteem and to strengthen their ability to cope effectively with environmental stress. He used his own imaginative skills to engage the child's creative abilities in working toward a solution to the problem. Lockhart and Robertson (1977) described the effectiveness of therapeutic hypnosis when combined with speech therapy in completely eliminating symptoms in those with mild stammering and reported substantial improvement in the majority of 30 patients ages 15–33 with more severe stammering. In the latter group, an extensive speech therapy program was supplemented with weekly hypnotherapy sessions for at least 8 weeks. The authors emphasized the role of ego strengthening and self-confidence/self-esteem as essential ingredients in the therapeutic hypnotic suggestions and relationships.

We have worked with several latency-aged children (8–12 years old) with stuttering who continued to have daily stuttering difficulties, despite years of appropriate speech therapy. As with so many people with these difficulties, their stuttering was worse during times of stress. Hypnotic approaches were geared both to creating increased internal awareness of fluency and to modulation, control, and coping with stress. In each of the children we have seen with stuttering, their stuttering definitively and dramatically decreased or disappeared during hypnosis. Though this was a source of joy and pride and was accordingly able to be utilized as a positive affect bridge to "bring the fluent, smooth speech back with you to your usual state of mind and alertness," none made this ultimate transition with any consistency, and each gave up on the hypnotic strategy much as they had on other treatments that had helped them "a little" or "for a while."

We note for completeness that a recent systematic review of research regarding treatments for stuttering included no studies involving hypnosis, imagery, imagination, visualization, or relaxation. Although the studies reviewed included ones examining therapeutic approaches of response contingencies and regulated breathing, and two studies incorporated EMG biofeedback of mouth/lip musculature, none appeared to include or incorporate hypnotic-like work (Bothe, Davidow, Bramlett, & Ingham, 2006).

### Defects of Articulation

Silber's (1973) therapeutic hypnosis approach to children with significant articulation problems again focused on imaginative use of fairy tales, folklore, and symbols. He described his successful work with a 10-year-old boy, seen for 26 sessions over a period of 18 weeks. The child continued to speak clearly 2 years later. Silber concluded that success was related to the fact that the "patient is committed by cooperation and participation in a creative endeavor of the imagination" (p. 281).

### Voice Problems

Laguaite (1976) reported her therapeutic hypnosis treatment of 18 children, ages 4–10 years, with deviant voices, usually associated with excessive shouting. In some cases, the problem was related to vocal nodules or hypertrophy of the vocal bands. Five children had normal larynges, and two could not be visualized adequately. Three children did not complete the course of treatment. For the remaining 15, hypnosis treatment focused on encouraging the patients not to yell so much, ego strengthening, and insight-oriented techniques. Thirteen of these 15 children showed improvement in the appearance of the larynx or complete disappearance of the nodules. Laguaite noted that another group of children who were treated for nodules without hypnosis also showed improvement but required an average of 14 sessions of treatment as opposed to only 10 sessions for the hypnosis group.

Gildston and Gildston (1992) reported their clinical hypnosis treatment of two children, an 8-year-old girl and a 12-year-old boy, with voice disorders secondary to recurring juvenile laryngeal papillomatosis, caused by the human papillomavirus. In both cases, the use of hypnotic strategies had multiple foci: retard, regress, or prevent recurrence of the papillomas; facilitate vocal techniques; and improve vocal function. In the 8-year-old girl, the papillomas diminished considerably after seven sessions and were almost gone by the 16th session; they diminished spontaneously, as these are known to do 50% of the time, or in response to hypnotic suggestion. The 12-year-old boy had had multiple surgical procedures for juvenile laryngeal papillomas between the ages of 3 and 9 years; his voice was sharply reduced in pitch and loudness and thought of as annoyingly hoarse and breathy with speech that was very difficult to understand. Hypnosis was used in an intermittent and integrated fashion with voice rehabilitation therapy. After 2 months of treatment, he was described as having achieved significant improvement in the office setting, although carryover into conversational speech was sporadic. The authors concluded that, for these two children, therapeutic hypnosis was an excellent approach for increasing motivation and speeding up the acquisition of vocal skills.

One of our patients was an 11-year-old boy who had swallowed lye at age 21 months and subsequently underwent numerous surgical procedures. He had not spoken normally since esophageal surgery at age 9 years. When asked questions in the therapist's office, the patient whispered answers. In the preliminary conversation, he said that fishing was one of his favorite pastimes and that he looked forward to being able to sing when he recaptured his voice. He was told that there may have been a temporary organic cause of his loss of voice, such as swelling around the vocal cords associated with surgery, and perhaps he had continued to whisper as a habit. His mother said that she believed this because she had heard him speak aloud in his sleep. At the first visit, the boy learned progressive relaxation, synchronized with breathing. He then imagined himself in a favorite place.

He later reported that while imagining himself in a favorite place he went fishing and caught three walleye pike. Following the therapist's request, he then recalled a time in the past when he was enjoying singing a particular favorite song, and he carried this forward to a time in the future when he could imagine himself singing the same song aloud. He appeared very relaxed throughout the 15-minute exercise. He was asked to review it at home twice daily.

The patient returned a week later. After review of progressive relaxation and favorite place imagery, he visualized a calendar going backward week by week. He used previously arranged ideomotor signals to indicate that the problem leading to his loss of voice occurred in September 1977. As the therapist described moving from week 3 to 2 in September, he coughed, had a choking expression, and tensed his left hand. Asked to return to his favorite place, he reviewed the suggestions of the first visit. In checking records of his outpatient visits to the surgeon's office, it was noted that he was seen by the surgeon on September 15, 1977, with a chart notation of "surgery to follow."

The third visit occurred 2 weeks later. The parents reported that they now heard the boy speak in a normal voice interspersed with whispering. At this visit, he reviewed the progressive relaxation and favorite place imagery. He was taught the clenched fist self-hypnosis technique (Stein, 1963) as a device for letting go of something that might be bothering him and might be related to the vocal loss. Following this he was asked to describe his favorite place, and he said "fishing" in a normal voice. He was encouraged to speak immediately following relaxation exercises at home and was asked to call the therapist when his voice returned.

He called 2 weeks later to say that he could speak again, but he would like to come for an additional visit. He explained that he heard himself singing loudly as he completed one of his relaxation exercises. His mother confirmed, "He's talking and doesn't need to come back, but he wants to come back once more." His mother said he was very happy after school on the day following the return of his voice. He said, "School is more fun when you can talk." On the second day, though, he returned home saying, "Talking can get you into trouble." At follow-up 4 months later, he continued to speak normally.

A more recent study from the Netherlands reported a retrospective study of 116 patients with nonorganic voice disorders and the efficacy of mental imagery in treatment (Voerman, Langeveld, & van Rossum, 2009). Of those who lost their voice, 92% were female; the median age was 39 years, but the range was from 10 to 77 years, and 15 subjects were less than 21 years old. Over half of the patients (61%) presented with aphonia and the rest with dysphonia. All were treated with mental imagery as the strategy of choice. The authors report restoration of normal voice typically at the conclusion of the first session, ranging from 10 minutes to up to 2 hours. Of the 116 patients, 86% were reported as cured, and 81% (94 patients) retrieved their normal voice within one session; 67 of these 94 were cured through mental imagery or mental imagery in combination with "laryngeal shaking." The multisensory mental imagery treatment process was described as including instructions: (1) to recall and visualize in their mind's eye a past, emotionally neutral situation in which the voice sounded normal; (2) to mentally listen carefully to their voice, noting its pitch, loudness, and quality; and (3) to mentally simulate (imagine) the action of speaking, counting from 1 to 10 (motor imagery), and to concentrate on the mental sensation of speaking (what the authors call *kinesthetic motor imagery*) (Voerman et al., 2009). Once patients indicated an ability to mentally hear and experience how their voice sounded, they were asked to audibly reproduce their voice, and most were able to do so.

## Vocal Cord Dysfunction

Vocal cord dysfunction (VCD) is a disorder in which the vocal cords close paradoxically during inspiration (instead of during expiration), resulting in a wheezing-like sound due to the narrowing of the glottis allowing only a small amount of air to pass. This involuntary adduction of the vocal cords on inhalation is often associated with shortness of breath and appears to be contributed to by high levels of sympathetic nervous system arousal and increased or exaggerated muscle tension in the muscles of the throat, face, neck, and shoulders. Competitive athlete adolescents, the most commonly affected group, typically experience wheezing, tightening sensation of the throat and chest, dyspnea, voice changes, and dry cough. Though not the same as asthma – and typically not responsive to the commonly used rescue albuterol inhalers effective in asthma – VCD may be misdiagnosed as asthma and may occur with or without concurrent asthma. Although the pathophysiologic symptoms are quite real, they are often triggered by psychological stressors and may become worse before better when treatments offered (such as those offered for acute episodes of asthma) are not effective. Not improving as desired and expected commonly drives the sense of worry and fear and, in turn, symptomatic distress. The most commonly effective treatment described has been diaphragmatic breathing, which results in throat muscle relaxation and improves airflow (Newsham, Klaben, Miller, & Saunders, 2002).

Banez and Culbert (2005) described their success with an integrative approach utilizing clinical hypnosis strategies, including diaphragmatic breathing with relaxation, imagery, and biofeedback, emphasizing, as we have throughout this volume, the importance of teaching adolescents about how their body works to empower them in informed fashion to develop the control that they desire. Anbar and Hehir (2000) described the use of hypnosis to facilitate the diagnosis of VCD in an 11-year-old who had been diagnosed with asthma since he was 4 years old. Hypnosis was used to reproduce his episodic symptoms and in turn to teach him to alleviate his symptoms. Using the case study of a 16-year-old elite male swimmer with VCD as an example, Rhodes (2008) reviewed the diagnostic and therapeutic considerations for VCD, amplifying the hypnotherapeutic strategies of hypnosis and biofeedback.

Anbar and Fernandes (2016) recently published a thorough review of an understanding of the pathophysiology of VCD (also called Paradoxical Vocal Fold Motion), including a description of research to date, and discussion of the variety of clinical presentations that may at first impression often seem to be due to asthma. However, it is noted that whether asthma is present or not, the recommended and customary oral and aerosolized/inhaled treatments for asthma do not resolve the symptoms of VCD. A case example describes the all too common situation of a 15-year-old who had a 2-year history of developing shortness of breath during cross-country competitions. She was seen initially by her primary care physician, and was treated with inhaled medications usually used for asthma, but without improvement. Subsequent referrals included next to an Allergist, followed by a consultation with an otolaryngologist without improvement of her shortness of breath. A tonsillectomy and adenoidectomy were performed which resolved mild snoring but provided no relief of the shortness of breath. Only after referral to a pulmonologist was the history elicited and identified that her shortness of breath was associated with inspiratory stridor and difficulty with inhalation, characteristic of and diagnostic for VCD (Anbar and Fernandes, 2016). After the pulmonologist taught the young woman how to do self-hypnosis to calm herself and she practiced self-hypnosis regularly, within a month she reported no further shortness of breath with exercise, no further fear of it occurring, and no further VCD as result of anxiety about it.

Various clinical hypnosis strategies for VCD are described in detail, and the authors also provide a list of psychological stressors that can trigger VCD in children.

Kaslovsky and Gottsegen (2015) reported a complex case of a patient with multiple psychiatric problems including autism who had severe recurrent wheezing and stridor as a result respectively of asthma and VCD. Hypnotic strategies were considered major factors in successful symptom control.

## Intractable Cough aka Cough Tic or Habit Cough

Many children develop cough habits that are annoying to parents, teachers, and peers and may become the focus of frustration, eventuating sometimes in blame, reprimand, punishment, and ongoing conflict. Although such cough habits often represent prolongation of a response to an infectious or allergic disease, results of thorough (or even over exhaustive) evaluations typically show no evidence of underlying reactive airways disease or other physical causes. As contrasted with asthma patients who may have nighttime cough variant asthma, children with this problem typically stop coughing during their sleep. Although many children may obtain so-called secondary gain by having to miss certain classes at school or stay home, no particular psychological profile characterizes such youngsters. As with most habits, it is likely that the preceding illness or problem (e.g., an allergy or a respiratory infection) provided the children and adolescents with an (unconscious) model for the symptom, which then became self-perpetuating. A review of the literature (Gay et al., 1987) reported follow-up information on 24 pediatrics patients with habit cough who were treated successfully with some type of suggestion therapy; 23 of these patients were cough free 1 year later. In most, successful treatment was evident even within a few days of beginning treatment.

Several authors have described the successful application of therapeutic hypnosis strategies for the treatment of habit cough (Anbar & Hall, 2004; Bauer, Magers, McCubbin, & Black, 2001; Labbé, 2006). Bauer and colleagues (2001) described the efficacy of voice therapy and discussed successful applications in nine children between the ages of 8 and 15 years. The treatment protocol applied seems to us to be clearly hypnosis/hypnotic in its ingredients: training in diaphragmatic breathing; learning to relax the throat; reducing muscle tension in neck, chest, and shoulders; teaching the child to interrupt early cough sensation with swallowing and relaxed breathing; substituting a mild cough for a racking cough; interrupting a cough sequence with diaphragmatic breathing; and increasing awareness of initial sensations that trigger cough.

Anbar and Hall (2004) provided a retrospective review of 56 children and adolescents (mean age, 10.7 years) with habit cough, 51 of whom utilized hypnosis. The cough resolved during or immediately following the initial hypnosis session in 78% and within a month in an additional 12%. Ingredients of the hypnotherapeutic work emphasized: (1) learning and practicing self-hypnosis with self-induction (various methods), (2) progressive relaxation and relaxation, (3) favorite place imagery, (4) cough-related imagery (e.g., what might a cartoon character causing the cough do instead, find a switch to turn off the cough), (5) teaching an anchoring gesture to cue (posthypnotic suggestion) the relaxation response, (6) noticing how the cough diminishes with self-hypnosis (ratification and reinforcement), and (7) reinforcing the value of home practice of self-hypnosis. The authors very appropriately and wisely emphasized the importance of careful diagnosis and searching for antecedent causes, as well as appropriate evaluation for psychosocial stressors and necessary treatment for identified comorbid disorders.

Labbé (2006) described the value of biofeedback training (peripheral skin temperature) to teach relaxation during coughing episodes in an 11-year-old girl with habit cough. She became cough free after six visits and remained free of cough 2 years later. Anbar (2007) published a case report describing the not very quick resolution of habit cough in a 12-year-old boy despite his very rapid learning and successful application of self-hypnosis skills. In the discussion of ensuing follow-up visits and reinforcement of self-hypnosis, Anbar described and thoughtfully emphasized the necessary integration of rapport-based therapy and family therapy with self-hypnosis training in order to achieve the desired successful outcome and permanent resolution of the habit cough. This message, a significant and recurrent theme throughout this volume, is essential to the appropriate understanding and application of clinical hypnosis with children.

We have observed that hypnotic strategies are very effective in helping young people with cough habits to help themselves (Kohen & Olness, 1987). The following demonstrates one approach to this problem. A 13-year-old patient was referred to us by a pediatrician for a trial of self-hypnosis in treatment of a cough that had been present for 6 months. Three months after onset of the cough, the patient was hospitalized for a bronchoscopy, the results of which were normal. He also had normal pediatric and psychological evaluations and negative allergy tests. The patient and his mother associated the onset of the cough with the time when he helped his father with a soybean harvest. He and the therapist discussed the possibility that the cough may have begun as a response to inhaled irritants from the harvest dust and had later become an annoying habit. The therapist drew diagrams of anatomy, the bronchial tree, and the cough reflex. She also explored at length the patient's interests, hobbies, likes, and dislikes, noting that he especially enjoyed bicycle riding.

The patient was approached from the perspective of symptom relief to be achieved through daily practice of a self-hypnosis exercise. Self-induction used backward counting followed by imagining a favorite place and then increasing relaxation by imagining a long bicycle ride. When he felt relaxed, he was asked to focus on the image of his bronchial tree and cough reflex and to suggest cessation of the cough to himself. He also focused on future anticipated happy events that he could enjoy without the cough. During the exercise he did not cough. The patient practiced the exercise twice daily for a week and returned for a follow-up visit. He reported having no severe coughing episodes since the last visit and said he was sleeping without coughing interruptions. He continued practice for an additional month. Subsequently, the mother sent a letter which said that the patient was doing fine, and she thought his symptoms had been "like those of a virus."

## Giggle Micturition

Although rare, this entity is seen occasionally by physicians and may represent a conditioned reflex as demonstrated in the following case histories. A 14-year-old boy was referred for the problem of giggle micturition. Although he was popular among his peers and a good student, he was embarrassed by the problem of urinating whenever he laughed. His mother believed the problem had its origins in toilet training when she discovered that he would urinate if she tickled him. The patient had been evaluated by several urologists and pediatricians without improvement.

During the first visit, the boy was given diagrams to help him understand urinary tract anatomy and bladder reflexes. After he had agreed to practice twice daily, he was taught a relaxation–imagery exercise. He relaxed by focusing on a favorite place of his choosing and used imagery of stair descent to increase the depth of relaxation. He was asked to give himself suggestions for bladder control and to imagine himself in a laugh-provoking situation in which he could laugh freely without concurrent urination.

At the second visit a week later, he stated he was much improved and very pleased with his progress. He stated that he had "lost a few drops of urine" only three times while laughing. At the third visit, 2 weeks after the second, he reported only one accident. Subsequent follow-up was by phone over the next 4 months. He was completely dry. Five months after his last call, his mother called saying he had no accidents in school but occasionally wet during group outings. He was no longer practicing the relaxation–imagery exercise. The mother was told that because he had solved the primary problem of control during school, perhaps he did not regard the residual problem as serious enough to warrant further practice. The mother was asked not to encourage him to return for therapy unless he made the request. He returned for an additional visit 3 months later with the report that he had laughed frequently and had had no accidents of any kind during the preceding 4 weeks. He spoke of his plans to become a lawyer or psychiatrist, his plans to go to summer camp, and of his recent honor grades in geometry. Follow-up over the subsequent year indicated no recurrence of giggle micturition.

A 14-year-old girl with mild intellectual disability and moderately severe speech and hearing problems was referred to Behavioral Pediatrics for help with daytime and nighttime wetting. At the time of referral, she and her mother reported (and later recorded) a starting dryness rate of approximately 40–50% at night and 20% in the daytime. Thus, about 5–6 days a week she would have some daytime urinary accidents, and about 3 days a week she would wet the bed at night. A detailed history revealed that daytime wetting occurred most commonly when she would become involved in prolonged laughing jags with friends during school recess or when roughhousing with her teenage brother at home. Her mother repeatedly reassured us that the brother and sister were very close and the wrestling was all in good fun. The patient was very embarrassed, especially by the daytime wetting. Her mother reported that pediatricians and urologists had found no physical reason for the problem, and psychologists who had followed her development suggested that the ongoing problem was related to her neuro-maturational problems and a function of inattentiveness and not being aware of social cues.

The focus of the first visit was to develop a relationship with, and to assess the communication abilities of, this young girl. To assess understanding, motivation, and the potential role of secondary gain, she was asked directly, "Would it be okay to have dry pants every day and a dry bed every night?" and she became very excited and said "Yes!" with a broad smile. Toward the end of the first visit, a simple diagram of urinary tract anatomy and communication between the bladder and the brain was drawn. In the midst of education about the manner in which the bladder lets the brain know when it is full, she jumped up, much as a 5- or 6-year-old might, and said, "I have to go to the bathroom!" and ran out of the room, making it to the bathroom without an accident. Her mother was astonished and said that that was the first time she had ever seen her react and respond so abruptly to the need to urinate. The child agreed to the simple request to "take this picture home, put it on your wall, and every night before bed just think in your inside thinking about how the bladder sends messages to the brain and the brain tells the bladder what to do, when you're awake and laughing, and when you're asleep," as well as to keep track of dry days and nights. By the second visit, 2 weeks later, nighttime dryness was improved to 70%, and by the third visit 2 weeks after that daytime dryness had improved to about 30% of days. A matter-of-fact, Ericksonian approach was utilized for reinforcement with emphasis on "being so grown up" compliments and adding a more formal imagery exercise of "doing your thinking with your eyes closed sometimes." Nocturnal enuresis resolved completely over the next several months. Daytime accidents seemingly related to not paying attention to the need to urinate decreased steadily, and after a year of monthly visits these had decreased to no more than one to two per month. Although the giggle micturition component had been the slowest to respond, at the 18-month follow-up, she and her mother reported only one occasion of giggle micturition during a major laughing episode at summer camp. She is proud of now being able to be tickled by her brother without urinating and enjoys "faking him out" this way.

## Hairpulling, Nail-biting, and Thumb-sucking

These habits may have their origins in anxiety, emulation of a peer or an adult role model, or unsatisfied oral needs. They are certainly nonlethal and of little physical medical significance, unless a child should ingest parasites, bacteria, or viruses in the course of biting or sucking or unless excessive hairpulling includes eating the hair and the formation of a gastric trichobezoar or hairball that may require surgical removal. They may be exceedingly annoying to observers, however, and often to the patients themselves as they develop increasing feelings of helplessness around their sense of their *apparent* inability to resolve the habit. Frequent reminders from parents and resistance in the child may lead to significant family problems. The use of therapeutic hypnosis for these problems may provide an acceptable way out.

As is true in the management of all habit problems, it is useful to structure intervention in such a way that the child's confidence, sense of personal responsibility, and mastery are reinforced. The initial interview should be structured in similar fashion to those related to problems such as enuresis and soiling. We emphasize that the original cause for the problem may no longer be important because the child is older and sees things in a different perspective. At the same time, however, we recognize that for some children the original circumstances may still be important to discuss and resolve. Of course, each situation must be individually assessed.

One 8-year-old girl was brought in for help for repeated scratching of her scalp with resultant bleeding, scabbing, and picking of scabs. Fortunately, no fungal or bacterial infection was identified; and some hair was missing from vigorous scratching but not from being pulled out.

She was asked what she thought this is and she said "It's a HABIT!" and when asked what a HABIT is she said "It's like something you do and you do it a lot and it just gets stuck in your head to do it over and over …" to which the waking suggestion response offered was a conclusion that "UNTIL it STOPS and the STOP gets stuck instead!" She liked that a lot and this was the beginning of 3-weekly visits that completely eliminated the habit without any formal hypnosis but with the utilization of her own language (and understanding) to re-frame the understanding and create change.

After discussion about the child's interests, likes, and dislikes, we plan an appropriate self-hypnosis exercise. Given the importance of comfort and rapport for the evolution of a successful hypnotherapeutic relationship, hypnosis would not ordinarily be taught until a second or subsequent visit, though occasionally rapport will develop rapidly, and therapist and child alike will be ready to do hypnosis at a first visit, as reflected in the case of scratching just described.

Following rapport, history, and discussion about hypnosis, initiation of hypnosis may begin and the child may be taught the use of ideomotor signals and asked questions related to the desire to be rid of the habit, desired rate of progress, and other details. If it is evident that the child wishes to proceed, we ask the child to devise an appropriate suggestion. These may be variations of the following:

> "Whenever your hand begins to lift toward your hair or your mouth, move it instead to the other hand and give yourself a little pat for not pulling, sucking, or biting."
>
> "Whenever your hand begins to lift, tell yourself that you can feel as comfortable as you do in your favorite place – as you do now – without any need to bite or suck or pull."
>
> "Whenever that hand [dissociative suggestion] begins to lift, let that be the signal to the other hand to lift up, come over to help, and say, 'I'll be your friend and I'll help you' as it gently pushes downward to help that hand stop lifting and return to the lap."
>
> "At the close of your exercise, tell yourself to sit down with a clock and suck each finger for 5 minutes to treat them all fairly." [This often results in rapid extinguishing of the symptom of finger- or thumb-sucking.]
>
> "You will bite all of your fingernails except your thumbnails. You will then let your pointer finger nails grow out" [and so forth in sequence until all are grown].
>
> "See yourself without the symptom, buying nail polish and putting it on your lovely nails, and hearing your friends admire your nails and the color of nail polish … seeing a baby sucking his thumb and wishing you could help him the way you helped yourself … going on a trip and thinking 'I don't suck my thumb anymore' … looking in the mirror of your

> mind and seeing yourself a little older (maybe a week or a month or 4 months or a year from now) with your hair and eyelashes full and beautiful and just the way you want them, buying barrettes for your lovely hair, and going for a haircut and styling."

In general, it is not a good idea to reinforce these suggestions with the image of parental praise, for that may encourage the child in the midst of striving for autonomy to resist.

Mohlman (1973) recommended that, after the patient is in trance, suggestions to eliminate thumb-sucking should be as follows: "Instead of putting your thumb in your mouth, would it be all right to put your thumb in your fist?" After receiving a "yes" reply, the therapist says, "This will be even more pleasant to you than putting it in your mouth, and it will be easier because your fist is nearer your thumb."

Erickson (1958a) recommended prescribing the symptom of thumb-sucking to a rebellious 16-year-old girl who rapidly lost interest in the habit after ten evenings of deliberately irritating her parents with loud thumb-sucking. Staples (1973) reported successful use of hypnotherapy in the case of a 4-year-old girl who sucked her thumb. Hypnosis was induced by having her imagine she was holding her sleeping teddy bear. Following initiation of hypnosis, suggestions were made that the patient was growing bigger every day, that soon she would get so big that she would not suck her thumb anymore, that she might be big enough next week or next month. Secter (1973) recommended a similar approach to those who suck their thumbs.

Although these approaches, stressing maturation and elimination of the symptom, are often successful, they may embarrass older children who are clearly beyond the age of thumb-sucking, bedwetting, and other preschool behaviors. In the case of older children, it seems more appropriate to provide a substitute comfortable feeling for the symptom and to enhance mastery by focusing on the patient's previous successes and future anticipated events without the symptom.

Gardner (1978a) reported successful use of therapeutic hypnosis with an 8-year-old girl who twisted and pulled out her hair, leaving obvious bald patches. As is true of many children with habit problems, she claimed to be unaware of the behavior and was highly motivated to change it. The symptom and resulting attention were interpreted as a manifestation of the child's need for power and control in her family. In hypnosis, she was told that she could find a way truly to be in control of her hair. She was given suggestions for awareness of the hairpulling behavior as soon as she lifted her hand for this purpose, and she was told that she could recall the phrase "Stop, please do not hurt" from the part of her that wanted pretty hair. In the first of three hypnotic sessions, the child added her own creative details to these ideas. When she lifted her hand to begin hairpulling, it trembled as it got near her head, then returned to her lap. She reported the sensation of a "force field," an impenetrable barrier similar to the one on the TV program *Star Trek*. When not thinking of hairpulling, she could touch her head easily and enjoy new habits of good hair grooming. Although this child refused to practice self-hypnosis, she responded well to posthypnotic suggestions. After 2 weeks, the scalp lesions were healed, and there was new hair growth. After another 2 weeks, there was further hair growth, and the child was no longer wearing a bandana. Follow-up 2 months later revealed no further hairpulling and improvement in other behavior patterns.

Kohen (1992) described a successful therapeutic hypnosis approach with a 10-year-old boy who had several habit problems, including hairpulling and tongue sucking. His hairpulling had begun at age 3 years. It stopped briefly with home daycare rather than at a large daycare center and having toys to occupy his hands, but it recurred. When his mother married, a psychologist helping with adjustment to a newly constituted family instructed the parents to use a trigger word to remind him when he was pulling his hair. This worked only sometimes, and he was referred for help with hypnosis.

Like most, he professed a lack of awareness of the habit ("I don't always know when I do it") but would speculate that it happened more when he was nervous or bored. As he loved baseball, imagery of playing baseball was utilized for initiation and intensification of hypnosis. A metaphor for personal control was introduced by discussing how he had learned to ride a bicycle, emphasizing "how you did it without purposely giving out-loud instructions to each muscle about what to do to ride" and noting that he could now ride a bike without really thinking about it. Playing baseball successfully was used as another metaphor for control of muscles and movement. Progressive relaxation reinforced the analogy that the brain could be the boss of the body. Dissociative suggestions for control and comfort were then introduced: "Those hands can help each other, because they are friends. And, because your brain is the boss of your body, you can reprogram that computer we call the brain to teach those hands to help each other. Let one hand go up toward the head, then use the other hand to gently push it down. They can be friends and help each other."

At the second visit, he and his mother reported improvement, and he said, "I imagine baseball, relax from my head to my toes, have one hand go up to my head and the other help it down." At the fourth visit 3 weeks later, he was proud, and his mother confirmed a dramatic disappearance of hairpulling. He reported again that, "I close my eyes, I relax, I think of baseball or something, then I teach my hands." At the fifth visit, 6 weeks later, hairpulling was reported to be 90% gone, and new hair growth was evident. The hypnosis practice session was video-recorded "to help other doctors and other kids learn this." He experienced a relapse 3 months later, however, perhaps related to the mother's continued overinvolvement. In spite of his progress, she had told him, "Since you have had it so long, since you were 3 years old, it might take a real long time to get rid of and be real hard to change." Although intended to be supportive, her statement served as a strong negative suggestion, and in hypnosis efforts were made to reframe her statement: "Some kids are surprised by how easy it turns out to be when they let their inside mind do it by practicing the way you already know you can and did." For reinforcement, he was given an article describing how self-hypnosis had helped a famous baseball player to improve his batting average. Four weeks later no bald spots were evident. He was proud, his mother had stopped bugging him, and he had a full head of hair by the time school began for the fall term. Three months later, he had his first haircut in a year and a 2-year follow-up showed no recurrence.

Grayson (2012) provided an excellent review of the habit of thumb-sucking and the variety of still unfortunately commonly used physical and aversive conditioning methods used to treat it. By contrast he described his preference for a "positive and comfortable method of treatment," and he described his detailed therapeutic hypnosis approach to helping a nearly 7-year-old girl eliminate the habit with one clinical hypnosis session. The key ingredients described the use of simple relaxation and mental imagery, inviting the young child to imagine a favorite Disney character such as Hannah Montana as portrayed by the actress, Miley Cyrus. The patient reported enjoying this image. A hypnotic suggestion followed that she might picture the character sucking *her* thumb and the patient surprised the clinician by beginning to laugh. The clinician acknowledged that perhaps the character Hannah Montana as a "big girl" looked pretty silly sucking her thumb, and that she – the patient – might also look silly doing so. The patient nodded her agreement with this. The clinician provided several reinforcements of this imagery and the concept of "big girl" before re-alerting. A follow-up call from the parents a week later reported no thumb-sucking in the interim since that initial visit. Telephone contact 6 months later and in-person visits at 13 and 20 months later all affirmed the continued absence and presumed elimination of the habit (Grayson, 2012).

Trichotillomania merits special mention beyond the foregoing case examples. In DSM-IV-TR (American Psychiatric Association, 2000), trichotillomania (312.39, TTM, "Trich") is described as a chronic impulse control disorder characterized by repetitive pulling out of one's own hair. Diagnostic criteria include (1) recurrent hairpulling with noticeable hair loss; (2) an increasing sense of tension before pulling or upon attempting to resist the urge to pull; (3) pleasure, gratification, or relief when pulling; (4) not being due to a general medical condition or some other mental disorder; and (5) the disturbance causes clinically significant distress or impairment in social, occupational, or other areas of functioning. Some have challenged these diagnostic criteria in view of the fact that at least younger children (i.e., younger than adolescents) may deny either the increasing tension before pulling or the sense of gratification thereafter, saying that the pulling takes place outside of their conscious awareness. Whether the absence of these characteristics represents a difference in the disorder between younger children and adolescents and adults or whether they reflect a difference in cognition more typical of younger children is unclear. We have speculated that perhaps TTM in younger, preadolescent children represents a different kind of problem or an earlier form of the problem, behaving more like a habit problem (e.g., like thumb-sucking) than like an impulsive or OCD-like disorder with the likelihood of multiple mental health comorbidities such as anxiety or depression (Kohen, 1996b).

A recent study (Tolin, Franklin, Diefenbach, Anderson, & Meunier, 2007) appropriately noted that no studies had examined the efficacy of cognitive behavioral therapy (CBT) or pharmacologic interventions for childhood TTM. They amplified the importance of early, effective, and efficient treatment for children and adolescents with TTM in order to minimize the likely adverse effects of pulling and alopecia on socialization and social identity. In their two-part study, Tolin and colleagues described 46 children and adolescents who had sought treatment for TTM. Most reported pulling from various sites, had visible alopecia, reportedly spent 30–60 minutes a day pulling or thinking about pulling, and experienced substantial distress regarding the pulling. There were high rates of comorbid psychopathology in the children and their families. Of these 46, 2 enrolled in an open trial of individual CBT with particular attention to relapse prevention. TTM severity was reportedly decreased significantly to 77% immediately after treatment and to 64% at 6-month follow-up. As in many other applications of CBT, the CBT described for TTM was based on manual describing weekly training sessions. These included eight weekly sessions with an "emphasis on increasing awareness of pulling, teaching new strategies for preventing pulling (not described), and assigning homework for practicing strategies."

The first session focused on establishment of rapport, history taking, and psycho-education; the second through fourth sessions involved training and rehearsal in competing response prevention (i.e., learning a behavior incompatible with pulling) and stimulus control (changing the environment to reduce pulling); the fifth session focused on progressive muscle relaxation; the sixth and seventh sessions focused on cognitive restructuring, including "guided self-dialogue"; and the eighth session involved training in relapse prevention, including "children imagining and describing themselves responding well to stressful situations without resorting to pulling" (Tolin et al., 2007, p. 138). In the second phase of treatment, relapse prevention, four biweekly sessions were interspersed with 15- to 20-minute telephone contacts, emphasizing in both the in-person and phone contacts the value of enhanced awareness and practice of learned strategies. Although the authors did not, and we cannot, discern which of the several elements of this overall approach were more or less operative or contributed significantly to the positive outcomes described, it seems clear to us that the significant therapeutic hypnosis elements of relaxation and mental imagery were integral to this CBT approach described by Tolin and colleagues.

In addition to our clinical report (Kohen, 1996b), several other clinical case reports demonstrate effective therapeutic hypnosis approaches to trichotillomania. Cohen and colleagues (Cohen, Barzilai, & Lahat, 1999) described their experience with three children between 8 and 11 years old who were seen for 8 consecutive weekly visits and treated with relaxation/mental imagery strategies modeled after Kohen (1996b). Two of the three were symptom-free after 7 to 8 weeks and the other after 16 weeks. Follow-up at 12–18 months revealed no recurrence. Working in Israel, Zalsman and associates (Zalsman, Hermesh, & Sever, 2001) described the successful application of Ericksonian strategies in response to adolescents who characterized their hair as "weak and in need of protection." Therapeutic suggestions included assigning the patient the role of "patron of the hair" which was expanded and reinforced in ongoing therapy. Hairpulling was described as significantly reduced in response to this intervention, and improvement was sustained at 6-month follow-up.

In a different therapeutic approach with hypnosis, Iglesias (2003) focused on offering direct hypnotic suggestion to emphasize sensitization to and increasing awareness of impending hairpulling behaviors. This approach was prompted by histories in the three described children of no awareness of hairpulling until after hair had been twisted and pulled out. Beyond increasing awareness, hypnotic suggestions were given to be able to first clearly notice the urge to pull and then to be free to choose to pull or not to pull. No explicit suggestion or directive was offered to stop pulling the hair. A likely powerful and agreed-upon condition of treatment was parental agreement that the children were the sole owners of their hair and that the children therefore had sole responsibility for care and maintenance of their property. Hairpulling disappeared after seven visits in all three children, and no evidence of relapse was noted up to 6 months later.

A recent review of the management of Trichotillomania discusses various pharmacologic and non-pharmacologic therapies, highlighting CBT and notably Habit Reversal Training (HRT) as the most well-studied approaches (Henkel, Jaquez, & Diaz, 2019). Although there is an emphasis on the paucity of controlled studies and recommendation for further studies, particularly of hypnosis, they noted the recent 2017 randomized controlled study of HRT in which there was a 76% response rate with encouraging maintenance of success at 1 and 3-month follow-ups compared to placebo control (Rahman, McGuire, Storch, & Lewin, 2017). Henke at al. (2019) specifically mention hypnotherapy as an "alternative behavioral intervention" and reference our clinical report (Kohen, 1996) as one case series with complete or near complete resolution with low relapse rate. It is interesting to note that in the discussion of HRT Henke et al. (2019) specifically mention that one of the key elements of HRT focuses upon "*Relaxation* techniques such as diaphragmatic breathing, progressive muscle relaxation (*PMR(), or guided imagery are another component to HRT and involve teaching the patient how to actively enter a relaxed state" (p. 805). As we have noted elsewhere in this text, it is clear that HRT and other forms of CBT often (usually? always?) include a focus upon self-regulation training. Here emphasis is placed upon "relaxation and guided imagery … and how to actively enter a relaxed state." Clinician practitioners of hypnosis readily recognize and understand these to be essential ingredients of effective clinical hypnosis even though these authors do not identify them as such. Many CBT studies for various psychological problems include relaxation and imagery as one of several components of a therapeutic program, but while research reports the success of the program and its combination of ingredients, rarely do they study or report upon the relative value or significant effect of one or another of the individual components.

We of course concur that randomized controlled studies of therapeutic hypnosis for trichotillomania would add appropriate credence to its utilization.

## Nail-biting

Nail-biting is a very common oral habit in children, teenagers, and young adults (Ghanizadeh & Shekoohi, 2011; Leung & Robson, 1990). It is also commonly understood to be the most common habit in the general population being found in 10% of the adult population (Infante, 1976). Some estimate that as many as one-third of children 7–10 years and 45% of adolescents experience nail-biting (Leung & Robson, 1990). In a survey of primary school children in Iran, Ghanizadeh and Shekoohi (2011) noted that 24.4% of boys and 209% of girls reported nail-biting. This presence of nail-biting in 10% of adults and of up to 33% in children and 45% in adolescents surely raise the question of whether these behaviors in youth should even be considered "abnormal" or "disorders" given their prevalence.

In a recent extensive literature review Kohen (2017) noted the variety of clinical reports describing effective utilization of therapeutic hypnosis for nail-biting dating from 1980 and beyond. No comprehensive or controlled study was identified. Our clinical experience and that of others as described teach that training in self-hypnosis when provided appropriately by experienced, skilled clinicians is a safe, easy, and very effective treatment to eliminate the habit of nail-biting. A detailed description of an effective "waking hypnosis" strategy is described in detail by Kohen (2017). A 16-year-old young man was brought in primarily for "test anxiety." As they were leaving the office and were assured that the clinician was "100% certain" that he could help the young man with the test anxiety beginning at the second visit, only then did his mother say "Oh and by the way he is a "nail-biter." In the very few minutes that were left the clinician explained his belief that there are no such people as "nail-bit**ers** or thumb-suck**ers** or hairpull**ers** or epilep**tics** or diabe**tics"**; amplifying that "people are not [defined by] their problem or disorder/disease," and noting that though he (the clinician) happens to have Diabetes type II, he does not ever think of or call himself a diabe**tic.** This re-framing from "nail-biter" to one who bites fingernails *sometimes* turned out to be very important and was referred to in the second visit when a somewhat more formalized therapeutic hypnosis strategy was undertaken. Storytelling was key and was the beginning purposely about an 18-year-old guy who had previously been brought to see the clinician by his mother because he *used to have (past tense on purpose)* a thumb-sucking habit problem. After telling the story the 16-year-old patient was asked to do an "experiment" and "please show me" HOW he *used to* bite his fingernails, but to do so in slow motion much as I had described asking the 18-year-old who had sucked his thumb to do in the story.

He complied with the "experiment" and even with my STOPPING him several times, noting that he was "going too fast." After several of these "pattern interruptions" he was asked to STOP when his hand was near to mouth, close his eyes, and picture a STOP SIGN. Though no formal hypnotic "technique" or "strategy" was employed, he was nonetheless in a spontaneous hypnotic state with eyes closed, arm and hand suspended in a levitated state, stillness in his chair, and relaxed. He was told that the clinician would touch his *other* hand and in so doing lifted it gently, placing it on top of the hand suspended in air and gently pushing it toward his lap, noting "those hands have known each other all their lives and know how to help each other create a new pattern of behavior to replace that old pattern (not 'habit') that is of no value anyway." He was asked to do this on his own again, and then to repeat it while doing the "opposite" (he knew intuitively that this meant "switching hands" so that each hand knew how and had experience to help the other). Further details of the verbalizations utilized and the success of this approach can be found in the detailed description (Kohen, 2017).

## Sleepwalking

The problem of sleepwalking has not been adequately studied to determine precise etiological factors. Although the symptom may reflect anxiety, it also seems to be associated with certain developmental periods and to be more frequent in certain families. Although it usually is a benign symptom, those who sleepwalk may occasionally fall downstairs and injure themselves or may even leave their homes clad unsafely and inappropriately for the nighttime weather. This is frightening to other family members, who are likely to request investigation and treatment, while the person doing the sleepwalking is likely to at least initially remain unconcerned, largely because he or she is usually amnesic for the event of sleepwalking. Amnesia notwithstanding, children may become frightened simply from hearing their parents' repeated expressions of concern and stories about themselves about which they have no personal memory. The following case history describes our use of therapeutic hypnosis in one such instance of parasomnia or disorder of arousal.

The patient was an 11-year-old boy who had been having sleepwalking episodes since he was approximately 4 years of age and had increased to walking around the multilevel house at least once every night. His parents were concerned about possible injury, and having heard about his activities he, too, had become afraid to stay at the homes of friends or relatives. He was taught the coin induction (invitation) method of relaxation, with the addition of favorite place imagery and a nice, long walk down a hill during which time he became more and more comfortable. Prior to this, sleep levels had been discussed with him, and because sleepwalking is thought to occur in the transition between REM and non-REM sleep, he was asked to program himself to remain in bed during this transition period. He practiced this every night prior to sleeping. There was an immediate decrease in sleepwalking incidents to two or three a week, and within 2 months the sleepwalking had ceased. His mother stated that she felt he was using his newly found abilities for self-control in other areas such as school and personal relationships (see also the discussion on parasomnias in Chapter 8).

## Chronic Overeating

In the past decade there has been a serious and very disturbing increase in the prevalence of obesity in childhood. It is estimated that 16.3 % of US children and adolescents are obese, as defined by a body mass index that is ≥95th percentile for age and for gender (Ogden, Carroll, & Flegal, 2008). Although researchers agree that multidisciplinary approaches with family intervention are essential to treatment as well as prevention of obesity (Barlow, 2007; Epstein et al., 2007), no agreed-upon methodology has yet been defined, and no defined role for therapeutic hypnosis has been studied in a controlled trial. Haber, Nitkin, and Shenker (1979) reported uniformly unsuccessful results for therapeutic clinical hypnosis in eight obese adolescents. Suggestions included maintenance of an appropriate diet, aversive response to fattening foods, increased exercise, and positive self-esteem. Four patients were not responsive to the hypnotic induction(s) utilized. Of the other four, three experienced negative sequelae of hypnosis, including feelings of depersonalization, increased anxiety, and dissociative behavior. We have not found such a large incidence of untoward effects of hypnosis. The problems might have been due to peculiar patient characteristics.

In a previously unpublished study at George Washington University, therapeutic group hypnosis was offered to 60 obese post-menarche female adolescents (Olness, Fallon, Coit, Fry, & Bassford, 1974). Pre-study evaluations included many laboratory studies, psychological testing, and physical examinations. Criteria for inclusion in the study included weight greater than 140 pounds, weight 20% above the weight norm for the subject's age and height, and obesity by skinfold measurements.

Patients were divided into three groups. Group A patients were taught self-hypnosis, Group B patients spent equal time with a control physician who gave them support and counseling, and Group C patients had no treatment. All patients were seen regularly by a nutritionist and nurse clinician. After undergoing the pre-study evaluations, patients were weighed on a monthly basis for 1 year. At the end of 1 year, the subjects in Groups A and B had lost an average of 5.8 pounds. Non-intervention Group C had gained an average of 5.0 pounds per person; however, within the group there were some significant differences that correlated with the ability of the girls to visualize themselves as thinner in the future – for example, buying clothing of a smaller size. Those girls had an average weight loss of 9.7 pounds. Those subjects who described clear images of changes in their life with the desired weight loss were those who lost weight and were able to maintain the loss. Although this study officially ended after 1 year of follow-up, the girls in Groups A and B were weighed again after a second year. Those in Group A had maintained their weight loss or continued to lose weight, even those who had not lost appreciably during the first year. Those in Group B had gained weight in similar fashion to the control group.

A report of 505 children with behavior problems treated with therapeutic hypnosis mentions five children with obesity who lost weight during periods when they practiced self-hypnosis (Kohen, Colwell, Heimel, & Olness, 1984); however, only one child maintained significant weight reduction. Treatment approaches followed those of other habit problems. Specific suggestions included the following: enjoying eating the appropriate amount of food for health and correct weight, feeling comfortable between meals without eating snacks, and visualizing looking thinner, buying smaller sizes, being complimented for one's appearance, and seeing one's height and weight as compatible on a growth chart. Our clinical impression is that it is important that obese children review the self-hypnosis exercises several times daily for several weeks and that frequent visits in the first months of treatment are essential and much more necessary than in management of other habit disorders.

## Tics and Tremors

We find that children with tics and tremors are frequently referred for a trial of clinical hypnosis and that these referrals not only come from pediatricians or neurologists but also from psychologists and other counselors and therapists. Increasingly, referrals also come from school personnel, including school nurses, social workers, or psychologists. These symptoms, perhaps more than many habit problems, sometimes seem to be the symbolic expression of unresolved conflicts. For this reason, we recommend psychological evaluation with an emphasis on family interaction. This may be accomplished by the primary treating clinician skilled in family assessment and treatment (pediatrician, family physician, psychologist) or by consultation and collaboration with an appropriate therapist. Although it may not be necessary or appropriate to mention the hypothesis of psychogenic determinants of the child, it is essential to have a reasonable working hypothesis before beginning a clinical approach with therapeutic hypnosis.

Approaches are similar to those for all habit problems with the addition of the jettison technique in which the child is taught to release both tension and the problem from his or her clenched fist. Suggested imagery should emphasize mastery and the child's own control and should include a focus on future happy events in which the patient no longer has a tic or tremor. The following case demonstrates the utilization of a jettison technique.

A. was a well-developed, attractive 14-year-old girl who was referred by her pediatrician for "hypnosis to control a hand tremor." She described a series of psychophysiological complaints, including headaches, epigastric pain, and lower abdominal pain for each of which she had prior extensive (and normal) medical evaluations. She was a good student who mentioned a desire to finish school and study medicine. As she described her previous symptoms and evaluations through grade school, she said, "I always knew there wouldn't be anything really wrong. I was just nervous." When asked why she thought she was nervous, A. hesitated and said, "Well, I'm nervous about my mother's boyfriend who attacked me when I was around 8 or 9." She stated that she had never discussed these episodes of sexual abuse with her mother and that her mother continued to see the boyfriend, whom A. said she couldn't stand to be around. She said she was angry at her mother, who "knew what was going on and did nothing." She stated that she had been asked out by a boy for the first time a few weeks before, and that the hand tremor had begun at the same time. She did not wish to discuss the problem with her mother or the boyfriend. A. was taught progressive relaxation and favorite place imagery, and she was then taught the clenched fist technique for releasing what bothered her. During the first session she opened and closed her fist several times. On a return visit, 2 weeks later, she said she had no recurrence of the tremor and was coping much better. The therapist hypothesized that the hand tremor represented aggressive or sexual impulses but did not share this idea with A., as such insight might produce unnecessary conflict about discussing the problem with her family.

Heimel (1978) reported a case of tic disorder that required a longer course of therapeutic hypnosis. E.P., a 10-year-old boy, had a tic consisting of shaking movements of the head and shoulders that occurred repeatedly each day for a 9-month period prior to presentation in the pediatrician's office. He was seen on 15 occasions over 16 months. Because E.P. found it very difficult to discuss his problems with the therapist, the dynamic meaning of the tic remained unclear for quite some time. Eventually, some information became available through the use of ideomotor signaling in hypnosis. The patient had a very poor self-image and feelings of non-acceptance by his parents, grandparents, and peers. He believed that his sister was much more accepted by family members. His father seemed to be very passive and played no active role in the patient's life. As these feelings were shared with his parents, they made efforts to improve the family relationships. The dynamics of E.P.'s tic were never entirely clear; the head shaking might have served as unconscious expressions of hostility while at the same time ensuring increased attention and concern from the family. The relatively long duration of the symptom, together with the ongoing emotional difficulties, made rapid resolution unlikely.

Initially during hypnosis, E.P. was taught progressive relaxation and given ego-strengthening suggestions. When there seemed to be no response after a few weeks, the clinician offered him the jettison technique: "wrapping or packing up what was bugging him and sending it far away on a freight train or plane." During these sessions, the patient was noted to smile several times as he clenched his fist in the process of eliminating troublesome thoughts or ideas.

After addition of this technique, E.P.'s parents and teachers noted a 90% reduction in frequency of the tic; however, when the tics disappeared, the patient developed a chronic cough. Consultation with an otolaryngologist was obtained, and no pathology was found. E.P. was again offered therapeutic hypnosis, which he accepted. He was gently confronted with the possibility that he had used the cough as a substitute for the tic. The coughing disappeared within a few weeks after two sessions with clinical hypnosis. In follow-up 3 years later, the family stated that E.P. was adjusting well as a sophomore in high school. He had no tics, coughs, or other habit symptoms, and he seemed happy and relaxed.

A boy was referred to us just before his tenth birthday with a history of a lip-licking tic that had begun 2 years before as a sniffing and coughing habit and disappeared until 5 months prior to referral when this began. At the time of the first visit, the tic had been gone for 3 weeks. There was no other history of tics. During further history taking at the second visit, the patient and his mother were asked to think back to September when the tic had begun and if anything important or worrisome or bad had happened or was going on around the same time. The clinician had all but decided that this was probably due to stress from returning to school after summer vacation, but in fact he loved school and they said nothing bad had occurred. They were asked to consider the preceding month, August, and they also said no. When they were asked to think back to July they both seemed about to say no when the mother abruptly gasped, "Oh …," and put her hand to her mouth as a look of recognition and remembrance came across her face. She and her son looked at one another. She said, "Remember?" They both began to weep. The mother then told the story of how the patient and his sister were with their grandparents while the parents were visiting close friends on their farm. They were out for a horse and buggy ride when a car traveling at high speed ran into them broadside, killing both close friends and the horse and seriously injuring and hospitalizing the parents in two different hospitals. When he visited his father in the hospital, the patient was terrified at his father's confused state of mind. Tics began 2 months later.

Visits to the pediatrician and allergist eventuated in referral to Behavioral Pediatrics. Seventeen months after the accident, the father continued to be out of work, and the mother, though back to work, continued to have problems with memory. The patient had tics, became withdrawn, was tearful, and "kept everything inside." Supportive counseling was provided for the patient and his parents. An Ericksonian approach was taken in helping the child to develop mastery over his tic behaviors. He was told methodically and matter-of-factly that "back then," when he was younger, he was appropriately so scared and saddened by the scary and sad things that happened that he didn't know even how to talk about it, so he kept it inside because he was so young *back then*. Now that he was older and could talk about and understand how strong those feelings were to a younger child, the feelings didn't have to come out in different ways (such as tics). During therapeutic hypnosis, additional metaphors were provided for the manner in which the brain controls the movements of muscles of the body – for example, "You don't have to think about walking, do you? Your brain sends messages to all of the right muscles to move in the right way at the right time, without even thinking about it." His tics disappeared, and though there was a brief recurrence for a few weeks 9 months later, a subsequent 2-year follow-up showed no recurrence. (See also discussion on applications with hypnosis for Tourette syndrome in Chapter 13 and with posttraumatic stress disorder in Chapter 8.)

## Habitual Drug Abuse

Baumann (1970) reviewed his experience with students from grades 6 to 12 who abused a variety of drugs. With most of these patients, the hypnotic approach focused on asking the youngsters to develop a "hypnotic high" in which they used their own imaginative abilities to experience feelings even better than the similar feelings they had had following actual drug ingestion. Other forms of psychotherapy were also employed with many patients. Initially pleased with the finding that 50% of 80 marijuana users were no longer using the drug 1 year after learning and utilizing self-hypnosis, Baumann reviewed data for 80 more marijuana users who had not been treated for this problem. Again, about half had stopped drug use after 1 year. Neither group considered the drug physically harmful, and those who stopped did so from boredom, lack of satisfaction, or fear of the law. Baumann concluded that clinical hypnosis could not be considered an effective approach or therapeutic modality for this group.

Among adolescents who used drugs that they thought to be physically dangerous, Baumann (1970) found that his methods were more successful. Of 30 teenagers who had only "good trips" with LSD, 26 stopped taking the drug completely, and 4 reduced the frequency of usage. There was little change, however, for 12 other patients who had experienced "bad trips" with LSD; it was difficult to adapt the technique in these cases. Of 17 adolescents who were "shooting speed" (amphetamines), all of them stopped injecting the drug, although 4 turned to oral amphetamines. Of 28 users of oral amphetamines, 6 stopped altogether, 20 decreased usage, and 2 remained unchanged. Of 10 patients who frequently used overdoses of barbiturates, 9 showed significant improvement following therapeutic clinical hypnosis. Because this group had no "high" experiences, imagery was directed more toward helping the youngsters satisfy other needs more appropriately. The treatment was not considered effective for two patients who used heroin or for two others who used multiple drugs.

Baumann (1970) concluded that therapeutic hypnosis can be a useful adjunct in the management of adolescent drug abusers, provided that they are well motivated for habit change. The greatest motivating factor seemed to be fear of physical damage to the patients themselves or to their children. We have had little ongoing or clinical hypnosis experience with adolescents who abuse drugs; however, we have sometimes adapted Baumann's imagery technique to help patients get rapid and maximal effect from prescribed sedatives and analgesics. Some of our patients have used hypnotic sedation and comfort to obviate the need for preoperative sedation or postoperative chemical analgesia. The technique might also be adapted in the therapeutic hypnosis treatment of other habit disorders, providing the child with emotional gratifications and obviating the need to engage in the habit. Gardner's (1978a) emphasis on giving the child with hairpulling a sense of controlling her hair is one example in which the basic need (i.e., control) was not changed but rather was re-channeled in more appropriate directions.

## Misophonia

Misophonia is a relatively newly described condition/disorder which has yet to be classified in DSM-V (American Psychiatric Association, 2013). There is no known prevalence data regarding this condition through publications of large surveys (Brout et al., 2018; Claiborn et al., 2020; Danesh & Aazh, 2020; Schroder, Vulink, & Denys, 2013; and Wu et al., 2014) consistently note over 80% of adolescent and adult patient reports indicate both onset of misophonia symptoms in early childhood (as young as 5 year old) and either absence of any treatment or absence of success/benefit from any therapeutic intervention. No randomized controlled studies have been conducted/reported (Brout et al., 2018) but all recent reports reviewed (Brout et al., 2018; Claiborn et al., 2020; Danesh & Aazh, 2020; Schroder et al., 2013; and Wu et al., 2014) indicate consistent psychiatric co-morbidities including anxiety, depression, tics and Tourette syndrome, and others.

History: Misophonia has been described as a "complex neurophysiological and behavioral syndrome characterized by heightened physiological responsivity and a high magnitude of emotional reactivity resulting from intolerance to specific auditory stimuli" (Brout et al., 2018; Jastreboff & Jastreboff, 2014; and Wu, Lewin, Murphy, & Storch, 2014). Misophonia was first described as a specific syndrome initially by Jastreboff's (Jastreboff & Jastreboff, 2001). Readers interested in details of the evolution of the "Jastreboff model" are referred to Brout et al., (2018), and Jastreboff & Jastreboff (2001, 2014). As described in detail by Brout et al. (2018) most literature published has reported on case descriptions or a series of case reports, focusing upon adult self-reports.

So-called trigger sounds, or the stimuli that evoke patients' often dramatic "misophonic" responses have typically been [complaints of] other people (e.g., family members) chewing, swallowing, smacking lips, coughing, throat-clearing, sniffing. Others have described aversions [less often] to mechanical noises from air conditioners, refrigerators, pet "sounds."

Proposed neurophysiology: Utilizing fMRI (functional magnetic resonance imagery) along with psychophysiological heart rate and galvanic skin response, Kumar, Hancock, Sedley, Winston, Callaghan, and Allen (2017) studied a group of participants with misophonia and age-matched controls. Each group was presented with three sets of sounds: so-called trigger sounds, unpleasant sounds (i.e., aversive but non-misophonic sounds) and neutral sounds. In the participants with misophonia an expected strong reaction occurred in response to the "trigger" sounds but not to unpleasant/annoying sounds or to neutral sounds. In the fMRI, those with misophonia showed definitive increased activation in the bilateral anterior insular cortex (AIC) compared to controls while no differences were found between the groups in response to the other two sounds presented. The conclusion was appropriately made that the AIC as a neural structure may play a significant role in the processing of misophonic triggers. Brout et al. (2018) discuss some of the limitations of the Kumar et al. (2017) study, but nonetheless conclude that "… this research validates the experience of sufferers of misophonia by demonstrating that … misophonic cues do elicit automatic sympathetic arousal and negative affect states." Though not mentioned per se by Brout the implications for the value of hypnosis intervention are clear, i.e., if hypnosis can be helpful in reducing and/or eliminating misophonic reactions and behaviors and associate negative affect, this would seem to us to be prima facie evidence for yet additional proof that hypnosis can be effective in altering physiologic responses to negative stimuli. Case descriptions below are provided as examples of these outcomes.

## Cases Described

Several case studies have been reported utilizing variation of cognitive behavioral approaches. (Bernstein, Angell, & Dehle, 2013; McGuire, Wu, & Storch, 2015, Schneider & Arch, 2017; Webber, Johnson, & Storch, 2014). Self-report surveys of adults with misophonia emphasized almost universal onset of symptoms in childhood with none indicating any successful intervention during their childhood, and most reporting no intervention at all (Brout et al., 2018).

In their thorough review "Investigating Misophonia …." Brout et al. (2018) strongly recommended a multidisciplinary approach to provide patients with coping skills to learn to both prevent and respond effectively and efficiently to their symptoms. They went on to suggest that "contemporary cognitive behavioral therapies offer empirically supported principles of change that could be considered as reasonable strategies as part of a coping skills strategic based approach even though CBT has not been tested for misophonia in controlled trials." Though they specifically note CBT, mindfulness, change-based behavioral interventions, self-regulation strategies such biofeedback and [self] hypnosis are notably absent from their recommendation. They conclude that "clinical guidelines for the management of misophonia should emphasize the use of coping skills grounded in empirically supported principles of change, as there is no evidence-based behavioral or pharmacological treatment shown to be efficacious for misophonia" (Brout et al., 2018).

By contrast, Pearson's recent review (2017) seems to be the only one which describes not only a description of many (over 200) prior cases, but also presents details of a "sequent repatterning model" for treatment. He describes sequent repatterning as "… often referred to as sequent repatterning hypnotherapy for misophonia," adding that "Hypnosis does … provide an ideal platform from which a neuropsychotherapeutic change can be achieved. It allows individuals to enter a nurturing, comfortable, and safe state of mind in an enriched environment, receptive and ideal for learning" (Pearson, 2017, p. 4). We very much appreciate reading Pearson's detailed description of his approach as it is reminiscent of, and entirely consistent with, our recurring emphasis on the essential features of rapport, history, and noticing as not only integral, but also in a true sense, *mandatory* ingredients for, and antecedents to, doing hypnosis, formally, informally, or conversationally. (See Chapter 5 on Initiation/Induction and Chapter 7 on Therapeutic Language for Clinicians and Families.) Pearson describes sequent repatterning as a bottom-up approach to therapy, intended and planned over 8 weekly sessions. A first stage – the "bottom" or Foundation begins a clear structure for the therapeutic process beginning with introduction history-taking and explanations = the "pre-therapy sequence" followed by the foundation that is "all about safety, comfort, and the moment of now." Pearson notes that "Hypnosis does provide an ideal platform from which neuropsychotherapeutic change can be achieved; and allows individuals to enter a nurturing, comfortable, and safe state of mind in an enriched environment, receptive and ideal for learning." A summary of 204 patients treated between 2013 and 2017 showed that 197 completed a programme of sequent repatterning, with seven having dropped out early in the process. The results after intervention were a greater than 50% reduction in symptoms, and in 101 of the 197 completing the program, a follow-up 6 months later showed the improvement to be sustained.

Within this group there were some who experienced a complete transformational change of 100% symptom remission. The author is clear that this was not a research study and that his preference would be to have had a year to 2 years follow-up. There was no description in this report of what percentage of his patients were male/female or adults/teens/or children (Pearson, 2017).

## Case Examples

**BK was 11 and 1/3 years old** when she was referred by her pediatrician for help with Misophonia first noted 18 months earlier. The family had recently moved from another state where a psychiatric nurse practitioner was treating mother's anxiety and older sister's "mood disorder" for several years with psychotropic medications. Due to this family history the nurse clinician prescribed Imipramine and Abilify for BK's misophonia even though according to BK's mother the clinician had "never heard of Misophonia before." These medications provided no benefit and were discontinued.

At the beginning of the second visit BK said she had not discussed the visit with her Dad. She was invited to pretend that the clinician (DK) was her Dad and tell him what she would say that she learned. She thought momentarily before saying:

> "I'd tell him that I learned to change and train my brain to change the habit (of Misophonia)!"
>
> Asked what she had done or been "noticing" in the intervening 2 weeks since visit #1, she said "Well, one time I was sitting sort of near X, (14 yo older sister) and she was chewing and the TV was on so I [told myself to] was
>
> *focusing on the TV and kind of turning UP the volume on that (TV) and turning it down on her … but then after a little while it didn't*
>
> *'work' any more so I got up and left the room."*

Her characterization of this was "it didn't work," to which the clinician (DK) replied simply but pointedly "YET!" Intended to sound like "ordinary conversation" the clinician then explained that all people have lots of regular behaviors that are habits but we don't call them that because they are "regular," and good and these days most people call something a habit when it's a "bad habit" or in some way undesirable; and one never hears people having "good habits." But of course we do have good "habit behaviors"; and walking was described as a habit *because we don't tell our feet out loud "left foot go here, right foot go there" and we really don't even* ***think*** *it, we just DO IT, kind of "automatically" or "sub-consciously." And that's the way most habits "work" or "happen," kind of subconscious as though we aren't aware of it, but of course we really ARE aware of what we're doing."* She agreed. Seeming to shift, the clinician re-affirmed that she had this misophonia pattern for 1–1/2 years, that "in that computer we call the brain, there is a small file called 'Misophonia' which has 1–1/2 years of Memory – she agreed. BUT also in that computer there is another, BIGGER file called BEFORE, or 'NO MISOPHONIA', which has been there for more than 9–1/2, nearly 10 years!! WHICH ONE IS BIGGER?" As the clinician used his hands to depict "higher" or "lower" amount of "MEMORY" required for each of these "files," BK quickly said that the left hand, representing the NO MISOPHONIA file, was MUCH HIGHER than the MISOPHONIA, much smaller, much lower (closer to the floor) memory file. She uses a Google Chrome Computer in school and on it one gets rid of a file by clicking on it and then hitting DELETE.

I asked her which one she thought would be easier, faster to delete. She quickly and matter-of-factly said "The Misophonia one."

Closing my eyes as a model for what I was about to describe and invite her to do, I suggested that each night for 5 minutes before bed she *could* "close your eyes, picture yourself sitting at that computer we call the brain, and see the desktop and see the Misophonia file, click on it, and then push delete. Then do it again 3 or 4 or 5 times which should take a few minutes and then turn off your light and go to bed and tell your brain; just keep working on and repeating that while I'm sleeping in your own words." I amplified this by reminding her that the brain is awake all the time and at night has more "free time" to take care of working on stuff since it doesn't have to go to school, pay attention there, etc. etc. I reminded her that she could ALSO do this during the day when she has time, but NOT to close her eyes during class! I also suggested she continue to rehearse doing what she had told me did when sister X was chewing, "because the more you do it, the better you'll get, that's what all actors, musicians, dancers, singers, athletes know … that's why they practice, rehearse." She agreed. This was the conversational hypnosis invitation, therapeutic suggestion and teaching and modelling of self-hypnosis to be practiced daily and at bedtime.

At the initial visit it was established readily that she was motivated to make these changes: BK was asked a few simple questions:

1. What do you think about this Misophonia? >> "I wish I didn't have it."
2. Do you need it for anything? >> "NO!"
3. Will you MISS it WHEN it's GONE? >> "NO!"

In response to these the clinician said "Well, since you wish you didn't have it, don't need it and won't miss it WHEN it's GONE, then I'm 100% certain that I can help you help yourself with it."

At the third visit BK said "I've been doing the practice at night like you said and at first I didn't think it was going to work but then it started helping and it's getting a little better."

She was asked to "rehearse" and "just go ahead and start and then I'll talk with you." She closed her eyes, moved into a spontaneous state of self-hypnosis evident by slowing of respirations, relaxation, and stillness on the couch. Suggestions were then provided:

- "Imagine that computer [desktop] in your mind (nods) and over in the corner somewhere see that LITTLE misophonia file … and THIS TIME notice what color and shape it is (later she reported 'rectangular, cream colored'."
- "Now imagine putting it inside a bag (She later told me it was pink.) and tie the bag closed tightly. THEN, put the bag inside of a box (later reported the box was a regular cardboard box, brown color) and tape it shut with that really good sealing tape …" (she nodded, ideomotorically).
- "NOW, take it outside and maybe there's a pick-up truck there, and put it on the back of the truck; and then NOTICE the driver gets in and starts to drive away slowly at first, and as you watch him drive away, you'll notice that the box (with the bag inside and the misophonia file inside of the bag) gets smaller … … and smaller… … and smaller … until you can barely see it at all … except maybe as a TINY DOT way off in the distance (and, implied, 'until it's gone …')."

"And every time you do it, it gets easier and everyone knows that the more you practice, the better you get."

BK's final visit was almost 7 weeks later. Her Mom reported that in the interim BK seemed much less bothered by noises and if she is bothered she is coping with it very well and hasn't mentioned anything to parents at all. BK beamed and said "I'm a LOT BETTER! It (noises) just doesn't bother me any more. No further follow-up was requested or needed."

**JP was 10 and 1/2 years old when she was referred to** me in our developmental-behavioral pediatrics clinic a few years ago for help with "Issues with sounds." In the telephone intake her Mom said JP "has issues with sounds like chewing, sniffles to the point where we don't eat together at all! It's pretty all consuming and becoming debilitating (for Mom)." After rapport development and about 15 minutes into the visit JP was asked:

> "How come you came over here?" Later she would say she didn't know what would happen here, but hoped she would "get some help" and agreed (see below) that she did. She said "because chewing and human noises (coughing, sniffling, sneezing) bother me." >> "How do you KNOW? where do you notice bother?" >> "It makes me feel ANGRY, in my brain. I feel sad, and sometimes have tears, and frustrated … I ONLY get angry with my family because that's the only place where I feel safe." She said that in the cafeteria at school there are a lot of chewing noises but it's not as bad or problem "… because there's so much (conversation) noise that I don't notice … [the chewing sounds] …" de facto acknowledging but not being consciously aware that she selectively is NOT bothered by din of the conversation and hearing IT allows her to selectively in-attend to chewing sounds.

In the context of at once developing rapport, providing empathy, learning the history, and attending to the specificity of responses, the clinician said in a spontaneous conversational hypnotic fashion "please help me understand – kind of in slow motion – what I might see if I had a video of a usual/typical kind of 'event' of your frustration at home …" and pointed to the only blank wall in the office, noting "There's the video screen … where are we looking?" In a spontaneous eyes-open and dissociated trance, she proceeded to describe: "… we're in the living room – me and Mom. Mom is eating …" "Mom is sitting on the chair and eating a nutrition bar and I'm on the couch …" JP was invited to describe "kind of in slow motion what *happens* …" >> "Well … I hear her chewing and it triggers my brain to get sad and frustrated … I make a sound (of irritation), I might almost yell, like 'STOP!!' and I might storm away or hide my face so I can't see her chewing … and/or plug my ears … even looking at her chewing makes it worse …"

> When Mom was asked about HER response in such a situation, and the clinician offered some speculation about options – such as being angry, sending JP to her room, telling JP in turn that it hurts her (Mom), etc. Mom said "It varies, sometimes we (her and Dad) take it personally, other times I get sad. Other times we are understanding."
>
> JP was asked what her first memory was of being sensitive to sound. She said she remembered she had this in her "old house" but they just moved in the past year, and the previous move was less than a year before that. She remembers her fifth birthday party and says she thinks she remembers chewing bothering her then, but not the singing of Happy Birthday. She doesn't recall what she "did" or how she "reacted" at the time but she is quite sure she didn't run away, hide under the table, yell "STOP!", etc.
>
> As we were talking JP said "Dad has Misophonia too" though neither she nor Mom had mentioned this or the name misophonia before. Mom said she had to be "careful how loud I was swallowing when we were dating …!" JP said that her Dad "had gotten used to it … he says it still triggers him but he doesn't react." I asked her if someone has something and they don't react, then "does it MATTER?" She hesitated only briefly before saying "not really!"

When a nurse friend told Mom that this (misophonia) is a "real thing" (diagnosis) they took her to a psychologist. The psychologist reportedly told her "you seem pretty normal to me, what's the problem?" When JP explained her sound sensitivity the psychologist reportedly said "Well, that's pretty weird!" and suggested they see an occupational therapist. On the way home JP told Mom "I don't think that lady is going to be able to help me!" Mom agreed and they didn't return. A year before the referral to DBP they saw an audiologist who recommended white noise machines which "helped some."

Nearing the end of the first visit JP and her Mom were invited to do an "experiment" and they agreed:

> "There is no work for you to do. All you have to do is close your eyes and listen. You sit there and I'll sit here."

- They closed their eyes and within moments both were very still, RR had slowed, and muscle relaxation was evident though none of that was either suggested or mentioned or acknowledged.
- Suggestion was offered to pay complete attention to the sound of air flowing in the room; and to 'let your head nod' (request for an ideomotoric signal) when you can hear it. >> They each nodded typical ideomotoric affirmative nods, almost in unison.
- Suggestion was given to "notice a volume knob or lever somewhere in the side of your mind … and turn it up to about a 7 on a 0–10 scale. I don't know what the knob or button will look like, maybe like on a TV or CD player or whatever, maybe it turns and clicks, or maybe it's smooth, or maybe it's like a dimmer light switch. Let me know when you notice it at 7" and they both nodded.
- "Now, turn it up to 8 … let me know >>> nods."
- "After it's at 8 for a while, BLAST IT! all the way up to 10!"

PAUSE

- "After you can't stand it any longer, turn it ALL THE WAY DOWN TO 1 or zero."
- Before I could say anything further, they alerted – nearly simultaneously – and Mom said WOW!! and JP smiled, agreed, and said it really turned OFF … I added "And NOW can you hear it sort of there a little? and they both agreed."

JP said her "button" was an "old remote from a TV and she pushed an UP and a DOWN button AND pictured the numbers on a screen (of an imagined TV). Mom said *her* imagined volume control was a 'slider on speakers' and reiterated her sense of 'WOW!'"

Asked if they knew or figured out the PURPOSE/REASON for the experiment, neither had a reply and they were told simply: "IT'S all about PERCEPTION … we can DECIDE." (Earlier we had talked about the five senses: Visual, Hearing, Smell, Taste, and Touch/movement/feeling.)

When JP was asked what she had **learned,** she said:

> "Maybe I could find another noise that is happening when there is chewing and I could turn that one UP …." to which I replied "OR …." and she added "OR, I could turn [my perception of] the chewing DOWN."

At the end of our time I asked JP expectantly "What will be different WHEN the problem is GONE?" She replied, "I will do it (we spoke earlier about DO or DO NOT, there is NO TRY ...) and I will be able to CONTROL IT and I will be able to eat with my family."

At the second visit JP announced "I *did* it, and it didn't work." After thanking her for reporting this, there was a purposeful shift to asking HOW she got GOOD at DANCE and at SOFTBALL, and she said "by doing it over and over, practicing!"

At the third visit JP was asked to describe her SH as though she was telling a friend, she said "I focus on one sound and I picture the remote in my mind with the volume control button or slider and I turn it down. *And the more you do it, the easier it becomes.*"

A week later JP's Mother began by saying that she wanted help in "how to respond when JP is having trouble and when she reacts." She went on to explain with the example that occurred the day before while they were watching a movie. Dad was eating popcorn and "the noise" was too much for JP and, as she said,

> before I could do anything I screamed "STOP!" and then Mom "sniffled" (she later impersonated this rather than describing it, sniffing-in loudly) and JP said "I just got up and stormed out before Mom could scream at me."

Mom noted it is very frustrating to hear JP scream and in helplessness she (Mom) *screams*. In response JP is upset and storms out to her room. Waking suggestions were offered to "slow down time in a blink of an eye and lower the volume of the chewing and your own volume." Mom was offered waking suggestions to "Whisper" her responses and a brief formal hypnosis session followed, reinforcing the earlier waking suggestions by imagining slowing down time while also lowering volume.

Two weeks later – JP reported practicing self-hypnosis/RMI and the specific three and six technique with a new focus on the breath, breathing in slowly to a count to three through the nose and breathing out more slowly through pursed lips to a slow count to 6, noticing relaxation of shoulders during exhalation.

At a follow-up 2 months later JP asked "are there any other strategies?" The idea of practicing self-hypnosis when it was NOT needed was reviewed in order to habituate and condition the NEW pattern of responding in order to replace the old and undesirable habit behavior, Analogies were made to how she "tuned out" the newly arrives "sound machine" in our office.

A week later – JP brought was introduced to the Biofeedback program, Heartmath and the "games" available on "Emwave"; and most notably the way that alteration of Heart Rate Variability through SH/RMI could be manifest (and reinforcing) by increased progress. success, "winning" on the video game. She quickly and spontaneously moved into a state of hypnosis even as the electrode for HRV was placed and before the imagery on the screen had even begun! Information was given to review the website for Heartmath (www.heartmath.com).

No further appointments were scheduled; and she was "lost to follow-up."

**AB was 15-year-old at the time of referral**. His pediatrician had been treating him with anti-depressants for depressed mood when AB brought up a concern that he is "very disturbed by various noises," so much so that he told his parents that he has a pretty dramatic sense of a "Fight or Flight" response when he becomes aware of sounds. At the time of this "reveal" he had been experiencing this x 5 years and never mentioned it before. It "came up" as he was anticipating a ski trip with a friend and his family and he was afraid he'd have a dramatic response to his friend's gum-chewing

First visit: Rapport, history, notice, re-framing:

> *"I'm here because I don't like sounds of eating – chewing (he agreed that this is 'BOTHER' and later called it an 'issue, not a problem.'*
>
> *He explained that ONSET was about 10 yo, that he didn't know or remember a reason, and over time it had become 'more irritating' saying it had been 'escalating since then.'*
>
> *When I asked what he DID to help it, he said 'Well, I tried ....'*
>
> *In response to which the clinician said with clear intent but jocularity 'try' was not*
>
> *allowed in his office and directed AB's attention to the green sign on the wall of YODA 'Do or Do NOT, there is NO TRY!' A Star Wars fan, AB was able to explain the details of the scene in which YODA says that during the Episode V film that this 'The Empire Strikes Back,'*
>
> *Between 10–11 yo 'It was not as bad (as now) so I ignored it back then.'* >> 'HOW did you DO that?' >> '*I don't know.*' Do you think PART OF YOU knows? You don't have to answer that now, just think about it and we can talk some more about it next time."
>
> *Between 12–13 yo "I tried to ... uh, I avoided the situation, some situations ... like at restaurants or lunchrooms it's not an issue because the ambient noise is so loud that I can't hear and so it doesn't bother me there."*
>
> At home at dinner "*My Dad is not very proficient at chewing with his mouth closed ... so what do I DO? I try to get out of there (= sitting at the dinner table) as fast as I can ... I either finish fast or go to another room?"* When asked if anyone "quarrels" with this, he said that one time he left the table and took his homework to go down to the basement. His Dad followed shortly and "yelled at me" that "other people have imperfections too, like having your arms on the dinner table all the time." When asked "HOW do you accept/cope/manage? He said COPE is the right word and *"I cope by focusing on my own chewing ..."*

AB said his pediatrician was seeing him "more for ANXIETY than for depression" and had increased his dose of Sertraline (Zoloft) from 50 through 75 to 100 mg /day.

When AB first nodded his head in response to a question he was purposely interrupted with "Did you notice what you just DID? >> No, what did I do? >> What DID you do? I asked a question and you did what? >> 'I guess I nodded'." This led to a discussion of how long he had known that nodding meant YES and shaking head side to side mean NO. He estimated he was around 1 or 2 yo, and correctly "guessed" that he had learned NO before he had learned YES as do most toddlers. Returning to "now" he was asked "But HOW did you DO your head nod just now?" I did not hear you say "I don't feel like talking right now to answer YES so I'll just nod my head." He agreed he had NOT said that; nor had he *thought it*. He said he guessed it "just *happened*" and agreed when I said *"automatically?"* And then we enjoyed a laugh when I wondered aloud rhetorically "OR, does your Mom have a remote and SHE caused the head to nod??"

I asked both AB and his Mom to "do another experiment" and asked them to close their eyes and turn all of their attention to the sound of the (2) sound machine(s) in the room; and to "let your head nod when you notice it." Both nodded in this spontaneous hypnotic state with ideomotoric nodding (coming from the unconscious mind in response to the hypnotic suggestion to "LET your head nod," rather than the qualitatively *different* and conscious "nod your head").

- They were invited to [each] notice a dial or lever which controls the volume, as might be found on a CD player. A nod confirmed they could see it … then the suggestion continued "Perhaps it goes like from 1 to 7 … Notice what it's on now… (nods) … now turn it up a notch or 2 (nods) … pause… … NOW turn it ALL THE WAY UP… pause … and WHEN you can't stand it that loud any more, turn it all the way down… off … click."
- Moments later they opened their eyes and alerted. Mom was asked first to describe what she had "noticed." She said it was a horizontal line – slide like control and the number it was on was RED … Hers started at 4 and went up to 5 and "I tried to make it softer but only got it back to 4 and it was hard to turn it off."
- Ben said his dial was "like a round one on an OVEN" and it started at 3 and then went up to 4 and then to 10 and "then I turned it off." He said he thought I'd done a "good job" in this first visit, gave me a "thumbs up" and agreed to schedule additional visits.

At the second visit the "experiment" from the first visit was reviewed. He was asked if the metaphor should be explained and he said "No, I got it." He was told that perhaps he could learn some biofeedback at the next visit.

At the third visit AB was introduced to and experienced Heart Rate Variability biofeedback with the Emwave system from Heartmath (www.heartmath.com). Though just his initial visit, he quickly became aware that the state of mind with biofeedback was/could easily be understood as identical to or at least very similar to a hypnotic state. He achieved a very high Coherence level (Heartmath.com) and was given the Heartmath website and encouraged to read there about Emwave and the Innerbalance app which would allow use/rehearsal on his smartphone.

During the next visit the focus was upon introducing the concept that "What you think about, and focus on, your mind amplifies," AB remained annoyed by his Dad's chewing noises at dinner time but at no other time, and in no other venue. He reported that they had obtained a "personal stress reliever home biofeedback unit from Heartmath" (www.heartmath.com). During a subsequent parents-only visit – and first-time visit including Dad – Dad reported AB had definitely improved responses to Dad's chewing; resulting in the family having dinner together now four times a week Mom noted "He (AB) is very intuitive and when he learns something he believes in/likes, he puts his mind to it and does it."

At the fifth visit "self-rating" was introduced suggesting a 0–10 scale on which 10 = worst. AB said he is a "9.5" while saying he is a "little better." He was encouraged to think about "How will I get from 9.5 to 7, or 9.5 to 6, or to 4, or to '1' or '0'" where there is "no bother." He was asked HOW he does it in other settings. He said "I SUFFER!" and noted that in cafeteria with "all the chewing! I clench my fists, grind my teeth for 2 minutes up to an hour!"

During visit #10 AB reported feeling very stressed due to Final Exams and said "It's almost as if the Misophonia is worse." The focus reinforced "What we focus on we amplify" and lead to an emphasis on the value of practicing turning down sound when we DON'T need it in order to habituate and create a new pattern that would ultimately "kick in almost automatically (like a head nod) when needed."

A few visits later his mood was improved and AB said he had been practicing SH/RMI daily. He was offered recording of the clinician guiding a hypnosis practice session, OR ideas about making a recording for self. Emphasis was placed on explaining how a recording could help when one part of his mind KNOWS it would be important to practice and another part "doesn't feel like it." This was left up to AB to decide and let me know if he wanted me to prepare a recording. He never asked.

In 2020 follow-up visits were switched to TeleHealth visits due to the Pandemic. The Telehealth platform did not seem to be problematic for AB or for our interaction, likely because by this time the rapport and relationship were long established. In response to his stated need the focus of several subsequent visits was upon the STRESSES of Pandemic, the murder of

George Floyd and the associated racial tensions, protests, et al. AB said he would have participated in protests if there was no Pandemic. Despite all of this he said he was less depressed but "… the sound issues are worse I guess because we have more meals together each day with the Schools on hybrid or all Online." AB agreed with the clinician's suggestion that he chats with his Dad about what Dad might DO he helped with AB's stress response to Dad's chewing. He said he would. He decided that monthly visits were preferrable to every 2 weeks.

In November 2020 – the 20th visit – AB said he was not sure if he was better re: Misophonia and he was encouraged to empower himself by answering the question "What will I DO to improve it?" This turned out to be the last visit. Four months later his Mother sent an email noting that AB's anxiety was now "severe" and depression worse, and that his pediatrician changed his medication to a new antidepressant Desvenlafaxine 25 mg/d. She said that the hardest for her is that AB was spending a lot of time on video gaming to "numb" the "pain, sadness, anxiety" that he is suffering because of all the stress of COVID-19. Nonetheless, he is happy to be back in school in person 4 days a week whereas most of early 2020 were virtual or hybrid at best. Though he is very worried that he'll get COVID and has been dismayed and upset that his *parents did NOT do THEIR thing by responsibly being masked or socially distancing and AB found that to be very disturbing*. Despite his "high scores" for Anxiety and moderate for Depression, he was described as

> *functioning pretty well i.e. has a job at 'the Mall' in a Game shop, is in an E-sports League and functioning well in the family:* He does chores when asked, albeit reluctantly but without too much grousing. He eats dinner with his parents – his older brother is now away at College this 2020–21 year for Freshman year – and while there is still occasional hanging out in the bathroom privately before coming to dinner, and an occasional abrupt leaving the table in response to "chewing sounds," parents believe his misophonia is much better and expressed her gratitude. No other follow-up is available.

## Conclusion

Therapeutic hypnosis appears to be valuable in the treatment and ultimate resolution of a wide variety of habit disorders, provided: (1) there is no underlying/untreated organic medical problem, (2) the child is well motivated, (3) the child is willing to assume primary responsibility for change, and (4) treatment for any co-morbidities is facilitated. As compared with many other approaches, clinical hypnosis is less expensive, less time-consuming, and less dangerous. Therefore, it would be advantageous to consider a therapeutic hypnosis approach early on rather than as a last resort as has often been the case in the past. On the other hand, some of the better controlled studies have found that patients who resolve a habit problem after clinical hypnosis may not do it because of hypnosis but for different reasons. Accordingly, better controlled prospective studies are essential to determine which children with which habit problems are most likely to benefit the most from which therapeutic hypnosis strategies. As a reminder, while many – though not all – habit problems may have concurrent associated mental health challenges (e.g., anxiety, depression, sadness due to or in association with their habit problem) clinicians must be attuned to assuring assessment and management for these or other co-morbidities either concurrently or following successful treatment for the habit problem, if co-morbidities persist.

## References

Adinolfi, B. & Gava, N. (2013). Controlled outcome studies of child clinical hypnosis. *Acta Bio-Medica de/ Ateneo Parmense*, *84*(2): 94–97.

American Psychiatric Association. (2013). *Diagnostic and Statistical Manual of Mental Disorders – Fifth Edition – DSM – 5* American Psychiatric Publishing, Washington, D.C.: American Psychiatric Association.
American Psychiatric Association. (2000). *Diagnostic and Statistical Manual of Mental Disorders*. 4th edition (Text Revision). Washington, D.C.: American Psychiatric Association.
Anbar, R.D. (2007). User friendly hypnosis as an adjunct for treatment of habit cough: a case report. *American Journal of Clinical Hypnosis*, *50*(2), 171–175.
Anbar, R.D. & Hall, H.R. (2004). Childhood habit cough treated with self-hypnosis. *Journal of Pediatrics*, *144*, 213–217.
Anbar, R.D. & Hehir, D. (2000). Hypnosis as a diagnostic modality for vocal cord dysfunction. *Pediatrics*, *107*(2), e21.1–e21.4.
Anbar, R. & Fernandes, B.A. (2016). Vocal Cord Dysfunction Chapt 47. In Elkins, G.R. (Ed.) *Handbook of Medical and Psychological Hypnosis: Foundations, Applications, and Professional Issues* (pp. 429–434). Springer Publishing Company. (English language)
Anderson, F.M. (1975). Occult spinal dysraphism: a series of 73 cases. *Pediatrics*, *55*, 826–835.
Banerjee, S., Srivastav, A., & Palan, B.M. (1993). Hypnosis and self-hypnosis in the management of nocturnal enuresis: a comparative study with imipramine therapy. *American Journal of Clinical Hypnosis*, *36*(2), 113–119.
Banez, G.A. & Culbert, T.P. (2005). An integrative approach to vocal cord dysfunction in young athletes. *Biofeedback*, *33*(2), 54–57.
Barlow, S.E. (2007). Expert committee recommendations regarding the prevention, assessment, and treatment of child and adolescent overweight and obesity: summary report. *Pediatrics*, *120*(Suppl. 4), S164–S192.
Bauer, M.L., Magers, C.A., McCubbin, M.M., & Black, P.G. (2001). How to recognize and treat habit cough in children. *The Journal of Respiratory Diseases for Pediatricians*, *3*(3), 141–145.
Baumann, F.W. (1970). Hypnosis and the adolescent drug abuser. *American Journal of Clinical Hypnosis*, *13*, 17–21.
Baumann, F.W. & Hinman, F. (1974). Treatment of incontinent boys with non-obstructive disease. *Journal of Urology*, *111*, 114–116.
Bernstein, R.E., Angell, K.L., & Dehle C.M. (2013). A brief course of cognitive behavioural therapy for the treatment of misophonia: a case example. *The Cognitive Behaviour Therapist*, 6:e10, 1–13.
Bothe, A., Davidow, J.H., Bramlett, R.E., & Ingham, R.J. (2006). Stuttering treatment research 1970–2005. I. Systematic review incorporating trial quality assessment of behavioral, cognitive, and related approaches. *American Journal of Speech-Language Pathology*, *15*, 321–341.
Brout, J.J., Edelstein, M., Erfanian, M., Mannino, M., Miller, L.J., Rouw, R., Kumar, S., & Rosenthal, M.Z. (2018). Investigating misophonia: a review of the empirical literature, clinical implications, and a research agenda. *Frontiers in Neuroscience*. 10.3389/fnins.2018,.00036
Buchanan, A. & Clayden, G.S. (1992). *Children Who Soil: Assessment and Treatment*. Chichester, U.K.: Wiley.
Claiborn, J.M., Dozier, T.H., Hart, S.L., & Lee, J. (2020). Self-identified misophonia phenomenology, impact, and clinical correlates. *Psychological Thought*, *13*(2), 349–375. 10.37708/psyct.v13i2.454
Clayden, G.S. & Lawson, J. (1976). Investigation and management of longstanding chronic constipation in childhood. *Archives of Diseases of Childhood*, *51*, 918–923.
Cohen, H.A., Barzilai, A., & Lahat, E. (1999). Hypnotherapy; an effective treatment modality for trichotillomania. *Acta Paediatrica*, *88*, 407–410.
Cohen, M.W. (1975). Enuresis. *Pediatric Clinics of North America*, *22*, 545–560.
Collison, D.R. (1970). Hypnotherapy in the management of nocturnal enuresis. *Medical Journal of Australia*, *1*, 52–54.
Culbert, T.P. & Banez, G.A. (2008). Wetting the bed: integrative approaches to nocturnal enuresis. *Explore: The Journal of Science and Healing*, *4*(3), 215–220.
Danesh, A. & Aazh, H. (2020). Misophonia; a neurologic, psychologic, and audiologic complex. *The Hearing Journal*, *73*(3), 20, 22, 23 10.1097/01.HJ.0000657984.74790d5
Davidson, M. & Wasserman, R. (1966). The irritable colon of childhood. *Journal of Pediatrics*, *69*, 1027–1038.
Doleys, D.M. (1977). Behavioral treatments for nocturnal enuresis in children: a review of the literature. *Psychological Bulletin*, *84*, 30–54.
Edwards, S.D. & van der Spuy, H.I. (1985). Hypnotherapy as a treatment for enuresis. *Journal of Child Psychology and Psychiatry*, *26*, 161–170.
Epstein, L.H., Paluch, R.A., Roemmich, J.N. et al. (2007). Family-based obesity treatment, then and now: twenty-five years of pediatric obesity treatment. *Health Psychology*, *26*, 381–391.
Erickson, M.H. (1958a). Naturalistic techniques of hypnosis. *American Journal of Clinical Hypnosis*, *1*, 3–8.

Esposito, M., Gimigliano, F., Ruberto, M. et al (2013). Psychomotor approach in children affected by non-retentive fecal soiling (FNRFS): a new rehabilitative purpose. *Neuropsychiatr Dis Treatment, 9*, 1433–1441.

Falck, F.J. (1964). Stuttering and hypnosis. *International Journal of Clinical and Experimental Hypnosis, 12*, 67–74.

Fleisher, D.R. (1976). The diagnosis and treatment of disorders of defecation in children. *Pediatric Annals, 5*, 700–722.

Gardner, G.G. (1978a). Hypnotherapy in the management of childhood habit disorders. *Journal of Pediatrics, 92*, 838–840.

Gay, M., Blager, F., Bartsch, K., Emergy, C.F., Rosenstiel-Gross, A.K., & Spears, J. (1987). Psychogenic habit cough: review and case reports. *Journal of Clinical Psychiatry, 48*(12), 483–486.

Gerrard, J.W., Jones, B., Shokier, M.K., & Zaleski, A. (1971). Allergy and urinary infections: is there an association? *Pediatrics, 48*, 994–995.

Ghanizadeh, A. & Shekoohi, H. (2011). Prevalence of nail-biting and its association with mental health in a community sample of children. *BMC Res Notes, 4*, 116. 10.1186/1756-0500-4-116.

Gildston, P. & Gildston, H. (1992). Hypnotherapeutic intervention for voice disorders related to recurring juvenile laryngeal papillomatosis. *International Journal of Clinical and Experimental Hypnosis, 40*(2), 74–87.

Glicklich, L.B. (1951). An historical account of enuresis. *Pediatrics, 8*, 859–876.

Goldsmith, H. (1962). Chronic loss of bowel control in a nine-year-old child. *American Journal of Clinical Hypnosis, 4*, 191–193.

Gottsegen, D.N. (2003). Curing bedwetting on the spot: a review of one-session cures. *Clinical Pediatrics, 42*, 273–275.

Grayson, D.N. (2012). Hypnotic intervention in a 7-year-old thumbsucker: a case study. *American Journal of Clinical Hypnosis, 54*(3), 195–201.

Haber, C.H., Nitkin, R., & Shenker, L.R. (1979). Adverse reactions to hypnotherapy in obese adolescents: a developmental viewpoint. *Psychiatric Quarterly, 51*, 55–63.

Haley, J., Ed. (1985). Conversations with Milton H. *Erickson, Vol. 1*. Rockville, MD: Triangle Press.

Halpern, W.I. (1977). The treatment of encopretic children. *Journal of the American Academy of Child Psychiatry, 16*, 478–499. Heartmath – www.heartmath.org

Heimel, A. (1978). Use of hypnosis in pediatric clinical practice: a report of 68 patients [abstract]. *Proceedings of the Northwestern Pediatric Society*, Minneapolis, MN.

Henkel, E.D., Jaquez, S.D., & Diaz, L.Z. (2019). Pediatric trichotillomania: review of management. *Pediatric Dermatology, 36*(6), 803–807.

Henoch, E. (1994). *Lectures on Diseases of Children: A Handbook for Physicians and Students, special ed.* New York: Gryphon Editions (original work published 1882).

Iglesias, A. (2003). Hypnosis as a vehicle for choice and self-agency in the treatment of children with trichotillomania. *American Journal of Clinical Hypnosis, 46*(2), 129–137.

Infante, P.E. (1976). An epidemiologic study of finger habits in preschool children, as related to malocclusion, socioeconomic status, race, sex, and size of community. *ASDC Journal of Dentistry*, 43, 33–38.

Jacobs, L. (1962). Hypnosis in clinical pediatrics. *New York State Journal of Medicine, 62*, 3781–3787.

Jastreboff, P.J. & Jastreboff, M.M. (2001). Components of decreased sound tolerance: hyperacusis, misophonia, phonophobia. *ITHS Newsletter, 2*, 5–7.

Jastreboff, P.J. & Jastreboff, M.M. (2014). Treatments for decreased sound tolerance (hyperacusis and misophonia). *Seminars in Hearing, 35*, 105–120.

Kaslovsky, R. & Gottsegen, D. (2015). Hypnosis for asthma and vocal cord dysfunction in a patient with autism. *American Journal of Clinical Hypnosis, 58(2)*, 195–203.

Kohen, D.P. (1990). A hypnotherapeutic approach to enuresis. In D.C. Hammond, Ed., *Handbook of Hypnotic Suggestions and Metaphors* (pp. 489–493). New York: W.W. Norton.

Kohen, D.P. (1991). Applications of relaxation/mental imagery (self-hypnosis) for habit problems. *Pediatric Annals, 20*(3), 136–144.

Kohen, D.P. (1992). Hypnotherapeutic management of pediatric trichotillomania: experience with five Children, paper presented to the *12th International Congress of Hypnosis, International Society of Hypnosis*, Jerusalem, Israel.

Kohen, D.P. (1996b). Management of trichotillomania with relaxation/mental imagery (self-hypnosis): experience with five children. *Journal of Developmental and Behavioral Pediatrics, 17*, 328–334.

Kohen, D.P. (2010). A pediatric perspective on mind-body medicine. *Ch 14, 267-301.* In T.C. Culbert &

K. Olness (Eds.), *Integrative Pediatrics. a volume in Integrative Medicine Library Series – Senior Editor:* Andrew Weil Oxford University Press, New York.

Kohen, D.P. (2017). Nail Biting. In G.R. Elkins (Ed.) *Handbook of Medical and Psychological Hypnosis: Foundations, Applications, and Professional Issues. Chap 34* (pp. 321–325). Springer Publishing Company.

Kohen, D.P. & Olness, K.N. (1987). Child hypnotherapy: uses of therapeutic communication and self-regulation for common pediatric situations. *Pediatric Basics, 46*, 4–10.

Kohen, D.P., Colwell, S.O., Heimel, A., & Olness, K.N. (1984). The use of relaxation/mental imagery (self-hypnosis) in the management of 505 pediatric behavioral encounters. *Journal of Developmental and Behavioral Pediatrics, 5*(1), 21–25.

Kolvin, I., Ed. (1973). *Bladder Control and Enuresis*. Philadelphia, PA: Lippincott.

Kumar, S., Hancock, O.T., Sedley, W., Winston, J.S., Callaghan, M.F., Allen, M. et al (2017). The brain basis for misophonia. *Current Biology, 27*, 527–533.

Labbé, E.E. (2006). Biofeedback and cognitive coping in the treatment of pediatric habit cough. *Applied Psychophysiology and Biofeedback, 31*(2), 167–172.

Laguaite, J.K. (1976). The use of hypnosis with children with deviant voices. *International Journal of Clinical and Experimental Hypnosis, 24*, 98–104.

Lawless, M.R. & McElderry, D.H. (2001). Nocturnal enuresis: current concepts. *Pediatrics in Review, 22*, 399–406.

Leleiko, N.S., Mayer-Brown, S., Cerezo, C., & Plante, W. (2020). Constipation. *Pediatrics in Review, 41*(8), 379–392. 10.1542/pir.2018-0334

Leung, A.K.C. & Robson, L.M. (1990a). Nailbiting. *Journals.sage.pub.med* 10.1177/000992289002901201

Leung, A.K.C. and Robson, L.M. (1990b). Childhood obesity. *Postgraduate Medicine, 87*(4), 123–133. 10.1080/00325481.1990.11704600

Leung, A. K. & Robson, L. M. (1990). Nailbiting. *Clinical Pediatrics*, 12(120), 690–692.

Levine, M.D. (1982). Encopresis: its potentiation, evaluation, and alleviation. *Pediatric Clinics of North America, 29*(2), 315–330.

Lockhart, M.S. & Robertson, A.W. (1977). Hypnosis and speech therapy as a combined therapeutic approach to the problem of stammering: a study of thirty patients. *British Journal of Disorders of Communication, 12*(2), 97–108.

Marshall, S., Marshall, H.H., & Richards, P.L. (1973). Enuresis: an analysis of various therapeutic approaches. *Pediatrics, 52*, 813–817.

McGuire, J.F., Wu, M.S., & Storch, E.A. (2015). Cognitive behavioral therapy for 2 youths with misophonia. *Journal of Clinical Psychiatry, 76*(5), 573–574. 10.4088/JCP.14cr09343

Minosh, C., Schwartz, R.H., & Badalyan, V. (2013). Hypnosis in 53 children with anxiety disorders, nocturnal enuresis, or insomnia. *International Journal of Clinical Pediatrics, 2*(2), 61–67 *(open access).*

Mohlman, H.J. (1973). Thumbsucking. In *A Syllabus on Hypnosis and a Handbook of Therapeutic Suggestions.* Des Plaines, IL: American Society of Clinical Hypnosis Education and Research Foundation.

Moore, W.E. (1946). Hypnosis in a system of therapy for stutterers. *Journal of Speech Disorders, 11*, 117–122.

Neveus, T., von Gontard, A., Hoebeke, P. et al. (2006). The standardization of terminology of lower urinary tract function in children and adolescents: report from the Standardization Committee of the International Children's Continence Society. *Journal of Urology, 176*, 314–324.

Newsham, K.R., Klaben, B.L., Miller, V.J., & Saunders, J.E. (2002). Paradoxical vocal cord dysfunction: management in athletes. *Journal of Athletic Training, 37*(3), 325–328.

Nixon, H.H. (1964). Review: Hirschprung's disease. *Archives of Diseases in Childhood, 39*, 109–115.

Ogden, C.L., Carroll, M.D., & Flegal, K.M. (2008). High body mass index for age among U.S. children and adolescents, 2003–2006. *Journal of the American Medical Association, 299*, 2401–2405.

Olness, K. (1975). The use of self-hypnosis in the treatment of childhood nocturnal enuresis: a report on forty patients. *Clinical Pediatrics, 14*, 273–279.

Olness, K. (1976). Autohypnosis in functional megacolon in children. *American Journal of Clinical Hypnosis, 19*, 28–32.

Olness, K. (1977b). How to help the wet child and the frustrated parents. *Modern Medicine, 45*, 42–46.

Olness, K. & Gardner, G.G. (1978). Some guidelines for uses of hypnotherapy in pediatrics. *Pediatrics, 62*, 228–233.

Olness, K. & Immershein, R. (1977). Association of nocturnal enuresis and allergy [abstract], paper presented to the *Ambulatory Pediatric Association*, Washington, D.C.

Olness, K., Fallon, J., Coit, A., Fry, G., & Bassford, M. (1974). Group hypnotherapy in management of obesity in teenage girls, paper presented at the *annual meeting of the American Society of Clinical Hypnosis*, New Orleans, LA.

Pearson, C. (2017). Reviewing misophonia and its treatment. *International Journal of Neuropsychiatry, 5*(1), 2–10.

Rahman, O., McGuire, J., Storch, E.A., & Lewin, A.B. (2017). Preliminary randomized controlled trial of habit reversal training for treatment of hair pulling in youth. *Journal of Child Adolescent Psychopharmacol, 27*, 132–139.

Rhodes, R.K. (2008). Diagnosing vocal cord dysfunction in young athletes. *Journal of the American Academy of Nurse Practitioners, 20*, 608–613.

Robinson, S., Hedderly, T., Conte, G., Malik, O., Cardona, F. (2018). Misophonia in children with tic disorders: a case series. *Journal of Developmental & Behavioral Pediatrics, 39*(6), 516–521.

Robison, W.L.M. (2009). Evaluation and management of enuresis. *New England Journal of Medicine, 360*(14), 1429–1436.

Schmitt, B.D. (1990). Nocturnal enuresis: finding the treatment that fits the child. *Contemporary Pediatrics, 2*, 70–97.

Schneider, R.L. & Arch, J.J. (2017). Case study: a novel application of mindfulness – and acceptance – based components to treat misophonia. *Journal of Contextual Behavioral Science, 6*, 221–225.

Schroder, A., Vulink, N., & Denys, D. (2013). Misophonia: diagnostic criteria for a new psychiatric disorder. *PLoS One, 8*(1), e54706, 10.1371.journal.pone,0054706

Secter, I.I. (1973). Thumbsucking. In *A Syllabus on Hypnosis and a Handbook of Therapeutic Suggestions*. Des Plaines, IL: American Society of Clinical Hypnosis Education and Research Foundation.

Silber, S. (1968). Encopresis: rectal rebellion and anal anarchy? *Journal of the American Society of Psychosomatic Dentistry and Medicine, 15*, 97–106.

Silber, S. (1973). Fairy tales and symbols in hypnotherapy of children with certain speech disorders. *International Journal of Clinical and Experimental Hypnosis, 21*, 272–283.

Solovey, G. & Milechnin, A. (1959). Concerning the treatment of enuresis. *American Journal of Clinical Hypnosis, 3*, 22–30.

Stanton, H.E. (1979). Short-term treatment of enuresis. *American Journal of Clinical Hypnosis, 22*, 103–107.

Staples, L.M. (1973). Thumbsucking. In *A Syllabus on Hypnosis and a Handbook of Therapeutic Suggestions*. Des Plaines, IL: American Society of Clinical Hypnosis Education and Research Foundation.

Stein, C. (1963). The clenched fist technique as a hypnotic procedure in clinical psychotherapy. *American Journal of Clinical Hypnosis*, 6, 113–119.

Thomson, L. (2005). *Harry the Hypno-potamus: Metaphorical Tales for the Treatment of Children*. Bethel, CT: Crown House Publishing.

Thomson, L. (2007). Hypnosis for children with elimination disorders. In W.C. Wester II & L.I. Sugarman, Eds., *Therapeutic Hypnosis with Children and Adolescents* (pp. 387–416). Bethel, CT: Crown House Publishing.

Thomson, L. (2009). *Harry the Hypno-potamus: More Metaphorical Tales for Pediatric Problems*. Bethel, CT: Crown House Publishing.

Tilton, P. (1980). Hypnotic treatment of a child with thumbsucking, enuresis and encopresis. *American Journal of Clinical Hypnosis, 22*, 238–240.

Tolin, D.F., Franklin, M.E., Diefenbach, G.J., Anderson, E., & Meunier, S.A. (2007). Pediatric trichotillomania: descriptive psychopathology and an open trial of cognitive behavioral therapy. *Cognitive Behavioral Therapy, 36*(3), 129–144.

Voerman, M.S., Langeveld, A.P.M., & van Rossum, M.A. (2009). Retrospective study of 116 patients with non-organic voice disorders: efficacy of mental imagery and laryngeal shaking. *The Journal of Laryngology & Otology, 123*, 528–534.

Webber, T., Johnson, P.L., & Storch, E.A. (2014). Pediatric misophonia with comorbid obsessive-compulsive spectrum disorders. *General Hospital Psychiatry, 36*, 231–e1.

Wu, M.S., Lewin, A.B., Murphy, T.K., & Storch, E.A. (2014). Misophonia: incidence, phenomenology, and clinical correlates in an undergraduate student sample. *Journal of Clinical Psychology, 70*, 994–1007. D01:1002/jclp.22098

Zalsman, G., Hermesh, H., & Sever, J. (2001). Hypnotherapy in adolescents with trichotillomania: three cases. *American Journal of Clinical Hypnosis, 44*(1), 63–68.

Zhu, B., Zou, K., He, J., Huang, X., Zhu, W., Harb, A.H.A., Wang, J., & Luo, A. (2021) Sleep monitoring of children with nocturnal enuresis: A narrative review. *Frontier. Pediatrics, 9*, 1–6. https://doi.org/103389/fped2021.701251

# 11

# HYPNOSIS FOR PROBLEMS IN LEARNING, PERFORMANCE, AND ATTENTIONAL DISORDERS

## Introduction

Many children experience problems both in learning certain materials and skills and in performing or demonstrating that they have mastered the material or skills. Increasingly, children, adolescents, and their teachers, coaches, and parents are turning to hypnosis for help, spurred on by encouraging reports in the press and in professional journals. Some reports of hypnosis for learning problems contain a measure of optimism that is not really warranted by the data. Hypnosis can often be beneficial as either a primary or an adjunct therapy in treating emotional problems such as low self-esteem or anxiety that may impede learning; however, a clinician utilizing hypnosis must take care to distinguish these emotional problems from true learning disabilities. Diagnostic evaluation should include psychological, neuropsychological, and psychoeducational evaluation (of child and family); in some cases, a child will also require and benefit from evaluation by a speech pathologist, a neurologist, and an ophthalmologist.

When clinical evaluation suggests that hypnosis might be helpful for patients with learning difficulties, we think it is of critical importance that they understand that the process is under their own control and that they are, in large part, accordingly responsible for the outcome to the extent that their learning abilities allow this. Integral to this emphasis is our recommendation for the daily practice of self-hypnosis with appropriate suggestions. This approach serves to help identify children who are not (yet) really motivated for change or who derive so much secondary gain from their problem that other counseling or psychotherapy is indicated before self-hypnosis could be expected to be of particular value.

Prior to teaching hypnosis, the clinician should discuss specific goals with the child – for example, to pass third-grade requirements, to increase reading level by 6 months, to complete math homework, to increase classroom participation, to pass a particular test, or to achieve some particular benchmark or milestone of performance. Generally, the emphasis should first be on small goals, and there should be clear feedback to the child. Often the clinician conducting hypnosis training will need frequent consultation with the child's teachers to facilitate understanding and agreed upon, consistent reinforcement in the classroom. When it seems clear the hypnosis will not be or has not been helpful, the patient and parents should be counseled as to more appropriate avenues of help. Parental pressure may make this referral process very difficult, particularly if the parents feel they are at the end of their rope or if they were inappropriately led

DOI: 10.4324/9781003243687-13

to believe that hypnosis could or would provide some sort of quick, magical, or miraculous solution to their child's ongoing learning or performance dilemmas.

The Behavioral Pediatrics Program at Minneapolis Children's Medical Center (now Children's Hospital and Clinics of Minnesota) conducted two pilot stress-reduction programs in local elementary schools. Both of these programs were successful. They included ten sessions a week apart and a review of stress-reduction strategies by teachers on a daily basis (Rusin & Wynne, 1987). A prospective study compared two groups of sixth-grade children who participated in the stress-reduction program. One group of children was in a regular classroom; the second group was in a special classroom because of their disruptive behaviors. The Piers–Harris Children's Self-Concept Scale and the Nowicki–Strickland Internal/External Locus of Control were administered to each child prior to the initial session and following the tenth session. In beginning sessions, Dr. Rusin talked with children about definitions of stress, how to recognize stressors in daily life, and how to strengthen inner controls. All of the children learned self-hypnosis exercises and played computer games that were linked to their autonomic responses. They all had the opportunity to learn and practice peripheral skin temperature biofeedback and galvanic skin resistance feedback. There was no difference between the Locus of Control test results before and after testing. Both groups showed similar and significant changes in reduction of anxiety (Piers–Harris Children's Self-Concept Scale) from week 1 to week 10. The special classroom group demonstrated a peripheral temperature increase of 9.5°F compared with an increase of 4.5°F in the regular classroom group. This significant difference may reflect a greater degree of chronic arousal present in children in the special classroom. Training in self-regulation via self-hypnosis and providing feedback from autonomic functions by using computer games may be very helpful to children who frequently demonstrate out-of-control behaviors (Culbert, Reaney, & Kohen, 1994).

## Applications of Hypnosis in the Classroom

It is clear that classroom experiences may be very stressful for children and may result in the development of undesirable autonomic responses and fear that may continue to affect them as adults. Many adults recall conscious memories of unhappy experiences related to elementary school such as reading aloud, taking a timed math test, participating in a spelling bee, or being teased by peers. Perhaps even more adults have repressed such memories, yet they manifest behaviors that have evolved from these or similar stressful grade school experiences.

There are many popular books, relaxation apps, and teacher's manuals that provide methods aimed at classroom stress. Many of these use verbal instructions similar, if not identical, to those used in hypnosis invitations and verbalizations. These may be very helpful to some children. The difficulty is that – like most teaching aids – they do not allow for flexibility and individual differences. Although most do, not all children have the ability to use visual images; some have auditory-processing disabilities that make it difficult for them to follow or recall verbal instructions.

Rusin and Wynne (1987) developed a model system for teaching stress reduction in the classroom which has been used successfully in entire classrooms. Its objectives are to help children recognize that their bodies respond to thoughts, that such body changes are measurable, and that the children can learn to control undesirable body changes and feelings by changing their thoughts. It might be very helpful to children if, during their early elementary school years, they could have the opportunity to experience and recognize the effects of thinking on body processes. Computer game biofeedback units are readily available, and they can be connected to computers or to smartphones. We believe that they should become standard equipment in children's museums and in hands-on science museums around the world (see Chapter 16).

Grynkewich (1994) developed a system of incorporating mental imagery strategies into cognitive behavioral strategies that are used in classroom education. She defines five components of mental imagery strategy instruction:

1. Student motivation, goal setting, and commitment to learn.
2. Student determination of effective mental images through interview with the counselor.
3. Student learning of effective relaxation techniques.
4. Incorporation and practice of relaxation techniques with effective mental images.
5. Self-management and regulation.

Grynkewich recommended determining effective mental images by asking students to identify favorite activities, places, vacations, books, movies, and people. In addition, it is helpful to know what thoughts, images, feelings, or sensations are perceived when the student experiences personal successes and problems. She notes that it is a mistake to recommend specific imagery based on general knowledge of students of the same age. Grynkewich recommends similar individualization in choice of relaxation methods.

Bothe and colleagues (2014) conducted a study of a stress-management intervention in a third-grade classroom. In this controlled prospective longitudinal study, teachers led daily practice of 1 minute of diaphragmatic breathing, 4 minutes of simple stretching, another 1 minute of diaphragmatic breathing, and 4 minutes of guided imagery (self-hypnosis). This practice continued for 4 months during which time the teacher of the control class read to the children for 10 minutes each day. A standardized anxiety scale and heart rate variability was measured in each child before the 4-month intervention, immediately after 4 months, and 1 year later. The children who participated in the experimental group showed significant reductions in total anxiety at 4 months and also at the 1-year follow-up. The control group showed no improvements. Qualitatively, children reported that they continued to do the breathing and guided imagery during stressful times at home and at school after the study ended.

## Hypnosis with Children Who Have Intellectual Disabilities

Parents of children with intellectual disabilities sometimes turn in helplessness or desperation to unusual or even bizarre treatment methods that have no known efficacy and may actually do more harm than good. Probably because of its magical appeal and reports of dramatic cures in other areas, hypnosis similarly has been sought out with the hope it could help children with intellectual disabilities. Clinical hypnosis researchers have also investigated this area, focusing on two issues: whether these children can learn self-hypnosis and whether it is possible to increase their performance in intelligence tests and related learning tasks. All researchers do not agree on the definition of intellectual disability.

Many cognitively impaired students have long histories of failure and low expectancies of success. These factors combine to produce passive behavior; the student approaches tasks reluctantly, and this may reinforce the feeling of helplessness. Mildly impaired and nonimpaired children (Shuck & Ludlow, 1984) between 10 and 16 years old, classified by groups according to suggestibility, were exposed to positive, neutral, or negative suggestions regarding their performance of a learning task. Highly suggestible cognitively impaired students showed greater improvement from the first task to the second; this finding permits the inference that suggestibility may enhance the learning of these learners. Group mean scores showed a trend toward better performance by subjects receiving positive suggestions than by those receiving neutral or negative suggestions. The fact that no difference was found between neutral and negative suggestions implies that students in general have low expectancies for success in tasks and that predicting that a task may be difficult does not affect performance any more than saying nothing at all about it. Prior reinforcement history may be the key determinant in conceptualizing success or failure.

## Hypnotic Responsiveness

The normative studies of hypnotic responsiveness cited in Chapter 3 did not include cognitively impaired children and therefore contribute nothing to the question of whether such children can experience hypnosis. Jacobs and Jacobs (1966) concluded that children with very low intelligence were generally not hypnotizable; however, that study did not utilize any standardized measure of hypnotizability. Sternlicht and Wanderer (1963) addressed themselves specifically to the question of whether cognitively impaired children are hypnotizable. Unfortunately, however, their study also had significant methodological limitations. The subjects were 20 "certified mentally defective" children who were institutionalized at the Willowbrook State School near New York City. The children's chronological ages ranged from 7 to 15 years (mean age, 11 years). All children had been tested with the Revised Stanford–Binet Intelligence Scale, Form L; they had IQs ranging from 37 to 68 (mean IQ, 52) and mental ages from 3 to 9 years.

The authors argued that the use of a standardized hypnotizability scale, such as the Children's Hypnotic Susceptibility Scale (CHSS) (London, 1963), would be inappropriate because the emphasis on verbal instructions would put cognitively impaired children, with their typically poor verbal skills, at a disadvantage as compared to subjects of normal intelligence. In place of a standardized scale, the authors used a "progressive anesthesia" induction technique (Watkins, 1962). The children were told that parts of their bodies would become more still and rigid and would be without any feeling. When this effect was achieved in the entire body, the children would then be "in a deep state of sleep" (p. 106). These verbal suggestions were enhanced with tactile stimulation on the children's fingers and hands. The children were first asked to move a finger in which they felt altered sensation. They were then asked to report how deep a state of sleep had been achieved by giving a number on a scale in which 0 meant none at all and 10 meant deeper asleep than ever before. Of the 20 children, eight did not pass the initial finger-moving test and were declared "non-hypnotizable." For the remaining 12 children, the scores were negatively skewed, with 10 reporting scores in the 7–10 range and the other 2 reporting a score of 1.

The authors concluded that 60% of their samples were hypnotizable. We cannot agree. The authors acknowledged the problem of using subjective reports of hypnotizability but defended their choice as the best available. We note the U-shaped curve of scores and come to a different conclusion. Institutionalized children who are cognitively impaired tend to fall into two groups, those who demonstrate minimal cooperation and those who exert tremendous effort to cooperate and to please adults, apparently thriving on bits of social reinforcement so often lacking in larger institutions. All 20 children in this study counted from 1 to 12 for the examiners, as part of the process of establishing rapport and to demonstrate ability to use the scoring system. We wonder whether they received verbal or nonverbal reinforcement for each higher number or for completing the task. If so, they may have concluded "the higher, the better" as do young children. If they were given this sort of reinforcement, they might have simply been seeking further praise by giving a high number when later asked to estimate their depth of "sleep." We become even more suspicious of the high scores when we notice the emphasis on "sleep," in light of the repeated findings that children often respond negatively to hypnotic induction methods that suggest sleep. In short, we think these data have more to do with social reinforcement and demand characteristics than with hypnosis, and we cannot conclude from the data that cognitively impaired children are hypnotizable. Obviously, the study suffers from other concerns, including the lack of a control group of institutionalized children with normal IQ and the lack of any evidence that the children really understood the anesthesia instructions. It may be notable that none of the 12 "hypnotizable" children responded to suggested age regression.

Before leaving the question of hypnotic responsiveness in cognitively impaired children, we should mention the issue of pseudo-retardation; that is, a child may test and function at a low level but may actually have normal intelligence. Gardner (1973) reported IQ data on an 8-year-old girl with psychogenic epilepsy. At the beginning of treatment, when she was virtually in petit mal status, her Stanford–Binet IQ was 72, in the borderline range. Eighteen months earlier, before exacerbation of her symptoms, her IQ on the Binet had been 93 (average); 3 months after initiation of psychotherapy, her Binet IQ was 103 (average). The fact that she was hypnotizable when her measured IQ was 72 obviously says nothing about the relationship between hypnotizability and intelligence, as the IQ score was not a true measure of her intellectual ability. In future research on hypnotic responsiveness of children with low intelligence, one must be careful not to include such cases of pseudo-retardation.

## Studies of Hypnosis Effects on IQ

We know of no long-term studies that utilize hypnosis as an adjunct in the educational programs of cognitively impaired children. The results were disappointing in one study (Woody & Billy, 1970) that included a single session of "clinical suggestion." Because the study was published in a hypnosis journal, we assume that the authors believed that they employed hypnosis but avoided that term – as did many authors cited in this chapter – perhaps because they feared it might not be acceptable in the school setting where the study was conducted.

Woody and Billy (1970) located 28 cognitively impaired boys, ages 9–13 years, in special-education classrooms. All had been given an individual intelligence test on which their IQs ranged from 50 to 75. The authors selected 32 boys from regular classes in the same schools. Each of these groups was then divided into an experimental and a control group, equated for age and IQ. The cognitively impaired and the normal cognition control groups were given the Peabody Picture Vocabulary Test (PPVT) on two occasions, 2 weeks apart. Apparently these groups received no intervening treatment or special attention. The two experimental groups received a "clinical suggestion session" immediately prior to the second PPVT administration. The suggestions focused on enhancing physical relaxation, minimizing anxiety over past test performance, and heightening motivation for and expectation of good performance. Neither of the groups showed any change in PPVT scores. The mean IQ increase for the cognitively impaired "clinical suggestion" group was 4.79 points, whereas the mean gain for the controls was 3.21 points. Although the authors indicated that the difference is statistically significant, neither difference is greater than the standard error of measurement for individual IQ tests. The authors concluded that differences of such small magnitude are hardly likely to have any practical significance. Further statistical analysis led the authors to state that "it does not appear that clinical suggestions are any more effective for cognitively impaired boys than they are for normal boys" (Woody & Billy, 1970, p. 270). They wondered whether several clinical suggestion sessions might have yielded different results. Based on the data from this study, we find no evidence that hypnotic suggestions can increase IQ in children who have cognitive impairment.

## The Utility of Hypnosis in Counseling Children with Cognitive Impairment

Although we do not think it has been demonstrated that cognitively impaired persons are hypnotizable, neither has it been shown clearly that they are not hypnotizable. Even if they do not seem to respond to hypnotherapeutic suggestions for enhanced intellectual performance, perhaps they can utilize hypnosis as an adjunct to counseling and psychotherapy. Woody and Herr (1967) surveyed 102 psychologists in clinical and academic settings, all trained in the use of hypnosis, concerning their opinions on the possible utility of hypnosis in counseling the mentally retarded. The 84 who responded tended to be uncertain rather than having clear positive or negative opinions; most had no experience using clinical hypnosis with this population.

Lazar (1977) reported successful hypnosis with a moderately intellectually impaired boy with behavior problems (see Chapter 8). Of course, in this and other single case reports, it is impossible to be certain whether the positive results should be attributed to hypnosis or to some other aspects of the therapeutic intervention. Lazar (1977) did not measure her patient's hypnotic responsiveness by any standardized scale, and one could conceptualize her techniques for extinguishing undesirable behavior as belonging more in the realm of behavior modification than hypnosis.

Based on available research and our own clinical experience with cognitively impaired children, we conclude that their capacity to respond to hypnotic induction is, at best, quite limited. In cases of true intellectual disability, we doubt that hypnosis can significantly enhance intellectual functioning. In treating such children for emotional and behavioral problems, we think behavior modification and parent counseling are probably the most effective approaches, although it certainly makes sense to consider the addition of strategies of relaxation and mental imagery (hypnosis) to counseling and behavior modification in given individual situations. It should be possible to design methodologically sound research studies that would further clarify these issues.

## Hypnosis for Children with Learning Disabilities

### *Attentional Disorders*

Among educators, psychologists, and others who work with children with learning difficulties, opinions vary as to the cause, frequency, and diagnosis of attentional disorders – most recently, frequently, and consistently referred to as attention-deficit/hyperactivity disorder (ADHD). Though the prevalence of this group of attentional disorders is estimated at 3–5% of the school-aged population, they remain among the most frequently renamed and redefined problems presenting to child health-care providers. A Mayo Clinic report placed the highest estimate of the cumulative incidence of ADHD at age 19 years at 16.0% and the lowest estimate at 7.4% (Barbaresi, Katusic, Colligan et al., 2002). Although their precise nature and best treatment approach remain a matter of ongoing debate and study, there is general agreement on diagnostic criteria. Reiff, Banez, and Culbert (1993) noted that children with attentional disorders share core symptoms that interfere with optimal functioning: (1) inattention, (2) impulsivity, and (3) overactivity inappropriate for their developmental level. Some investigators believe additional primary deficits include difficulty adhering to rules and instructions, impaired executive function, and excessive day-to-day variability in performing tasks or following directions. In this context, most clinicians agree that: (1) these children have normal intelligence with specific learning deficits (if any), (2) they experience repeated failure in school because of their academic and behavior problems, and (3) these difficulties result in low self-esteem, anxiety, depression, and poor attitudes toward learning. These children then may reduce their own efforts to succeed in school, thus lowering academic performance even more and creating a vicious cycle of ever-increasing problems.

An awareness that ADHD and related variants are now understood to represent biological disorders allows the further understanding that the attendant learning difficulties may be primary or secondary and associated emotional problems are most often secondary. A wide variety of special group and individualized educational strategies have been developed to remediate the variety of learning difficulties (general and specific) associated with attentional disorders. Also, evaluation, special education, and individualized educational plans (IEPs) are now widely available and mandated by law (Public Laws 94–142 and 101–476). Sometimes, however, the children's low self-esteem, negative attitudes toward learning, and related emotional problems may combine to make it almost impossible for them to benefit from remedial training. We agree with Crasilneck and Hall (1975) that hypnosis is not a primary treatment for attentional disorders, then known as minimal brain dysfunction (MBD). We believe, however, that hypnosis can often help the child with ADHD or related difficulties to manage common comorbidities such as reducing anxiety and improving the capacity to recognize emotional lability. It can be a useful tool in strategies designed to control emotional outbursts, manage associated problems such as sleep or interactional difficulties, and modify attitudes toward learning in general and school in particular.

Increasing numbers of studies of biofeedback in the treatment of ADHD are being conducted. The potential value of biofeedback and its relationship to hypnosis are discussed in detail in Chapter 16. In a critical review of the literature, Lee (1991) reviewed 36 studies in which biofeedback was used as a treatment for hyperactivity. He concluded that biofeedback treatments alone have not been effectively evaluated and that methodological difficulties with existing studies limit any generalizations that may be made from individual studies or patients to so-called hyperactive populations. He also concluded that, in conjunction with other self-regulation strategies such as hypnosis, biofeedback is promising in its potential for modulation of some of the behavioral concomitants of attentional disorders.

Blanton and Johnson (1991) described their use of computer-assisted biofeedback to help three children with ADHD to develop self-control. Two sixth-grade boys (11 years old) and one fourth-grade boy (10 years old) were selected by teacher and principal interviews as showing the most off-task behaviors in terms of being out of their seats and touching others, failing to pay attention, and failure to complete work assignments. They each were treated with biofeedback sessions lasting 20 minutes, including a baseline of 2 minutes, verbal instruction of 2 minutes, relaxation tape of 8–12 minutes, and relaxation period of 2 minutes. Electromyographic (EMG) readings were monitored during the baseline. Results indicated that all students were able to relax through the use of computer-assisted biofeedback, and one student demonstrated an increase in on-task behavior after implementation of the biofeedback. As described in detail in Chapter 16, biofeedback clinical studies and descriptions include and involve descriptions of relaxation and some form of imagery – analogous if not identical to what we know and define as hypnosis. In the report by Blanton and Johnson, they referred to "psychophysiologic relaxation training and biofeedback techniques," described the "biofeedback sessions" in which key features (of the longest duration) are an 8–12-minute relaxation tape with imagery suggestions and concluded that the results are a function of "implementation of the biofeedback." Whereas this is a reflection of the methodological dilemmas Lee (1991) noted in many studies, Blanton and Johnson's work is of interest for its demonstration of the value of creativity in combination with self-regulation strategies (biofeedback, imagery/relaxation) to promote improvement of behavior and learning in children with ADHD.

Tansey (1993) reported the stability of EEG biofeedback results for a hyperactive boy who failed fourth grade in a perceptually impaired class. The 10-year-old subject presented with a "developmental reading disorder" along with hyperactivity and an educational classification as being "perceptually impaired" since the second grade. He was trained in EMG biofeedback, and with an EEG 14-Hz biofeedback training regimen he became symptom-free within three sessions. He was reported to have remained free of motoric overactivity, high distractibility, low frustration tolerance, and poor self-control for over 10 years following. The author explained that the EMG session can be understood to introduce the child to a state of motoric calm, thought by the author to be a reflection of 14-Hz dominant posture from which 14-Hz brainwave training proceeded to functionally rectify the brain state activation abnormality reflected by the hyperactivity. Following the biofeedback training, this youngster was described as having shifted to a normal classroom when his learning difficulties, hyperactivity, and related (negative) behaviors had disappeared. The author described the biofeedback apparatus and procedure clearly, methodically, and in precise detail, and the results are impressive. The author also described his use of instructions for the boy to close his eyes; to become quiet, hollow, and heavy; and to "let the music come out," accompanied by much positive verbal reinforcement (Tansey, 1993).

To the clinician familiar with hypnosis, these instructions clearly include and reflect elements of a hypnosis intervention: hypnotic invitation (close your eyes), positive and permissive deepening imagery with a kinesthetic focus ("Just let yourself be a hollow, heavy rock"), ego-strengthening suggestions ("That's very good"), and posthypnotic suggestions ("The better your brain works, the better your ability to be calm and learn"). The author does not identify this as hypnosis but concludes, we believe mistakenly, that the described biofeedback process is responsible for the outcome described. Although we do not doubt the efficacy or potential value of biofeedback, we wish to emphasize the at least potential role and value of the hypnotic-like language described.

A study from Germany found distinct EEG effects related to neurofeedback training in children with ADHD. This randomized, controlled trial required children to use mental imagery strategies to control the neurofeedback animations such as a boy walking on a rope or directing a ball upward or downward (Gevensleben et al., 2009). Forty-six children were randomized to neurofeedback training, and 26 children were controls. In contrast to the control children, the children who did 36 units of 50 minutes of neurofeedback demonstrated a reduction of theta activity. Groeneveld and colleagues (2019) reported a retrospective study of Z-score neurofeedback and heart rate variability treatment for both adults and children with ADHD. One hundred children received 30 sessions of neurofeedback and heart rate variability training. The reward provided for improved EEG responses was playing a movie. Although specific instructions were not provided with respect to the training, children also received psychoeducation that included exercise, diet, deep breathing training, and "other coping skills." Eighty percent of children demonstrated clinical improvement.

A review of neurofeedback for autism spectrum disorders concluded that neurofeedback is possibly efficacious (Coben, Linden, & Myers, 2010) and that much more research is needed in this area. Another review of 159 children with autism (Thompson, Thompson, & Reid, 2010b) concluded that the use of neurofeedback was associated with a decrease in symptoms and improvements in social, intellectual, and academic performance; however, these studies were not controlled.

Illovsky and Fredman (1976) utilized hypnosis with 48 children, ages 6–8 years, who were selected from among 180 children referred to a clinic because of behavior and learning problems in school. Excluding children with major psychiatric disorders or perceptual difficulties, the authors selected children manifesting short attention span, acting-out behavior, and distractibility. All of these children had a history of good school attendance, an IQ above 85, and parental consent. Concurrently with hypnosis, the students received remedial academic instruction, as they had before the hypnotic sessions were begun, albeit with little success. On 55 occasions (no child was present for all sessions) the children listened to tape-recorded hypnotic suggestions under the supervision of one of their reading teachers. The taped hypnotic induction included eye fixation, eye closure, general relaxation, counting from 1 to 10, and imagining a pleasant outdoor scene. Suggestions for improved learning and increased ability to cope with emotional problems were then given. At each session, the teacher rated every child for the presence or absence of "relaxation," manifested by eye closure and motionless behavior, with the appearance of sleep. There was no measure of hypnotic responsiveness, and the authors themselves questioned whether relaxation and hypnosis should be equated. Teacher ratings of improved self-confidence correlated positively with the number of sessions attended by each pupil but correlated negatively with the percentage of sessions in which each pupil was judged to be relaxed. Ratings of relaxation were positively correlated with improved attention in class but were not related to five other academic and behavioral variables. The authors urged caution in interpreting the data because of teacher bias, lack of a control group, and lack of any real indication of hypnotic responsiveness. Noting the emphasis on eye closure in the induction, the young age of the children, and the fact that the sessions were supervised by teachers with whom the children may have had a relationship marked by failure and negative attitudes, we too doubt the validity of equating relaxation with hypnosis and are really not surprised at the paucity of positive results.

Young, Montano, and Goldberg (1991) described a hypnobehavioral procedure that integrated self-monitoring, self-hypnosis and progressive relaxation, and response prevention training. The combination of these self-regulation strategies was applied to helping a 10-year-old boy manage and overcome an adjustment disorder manifested by anxiety secondary to learning disabilities which was affecting his written language output. Evaluation in a multidisciplinary clinic revealed the boy to have an anxiety-induced tremor in one arm with no other abnormalities on examination. On the Wechsler Intelligence Scale for Children–Revised (WISC-R), he demonstrated an IQ of 111, but significant inter-scale scatter was noted, and reading was at grade level. Reversals were noted in cursive writing. In addition to educational recommendations that included guidance in task completion and study skills, as well as the use of recorded texts to improve comprehension, the evaluating team recommended training in self-management to reduce the negative effects of anxiety on school performance. Self-monitoring consisted of requesting that he keep track of the thoughts he had before anxiety-related experiences at home and school. This resulted in identification of three cues preceding anxiety-related thoughts and behaviors: fine tremors in the left hand, thoughts of failure, and feelings of anger.

Self-hypnosis training began with practice of imagery and progressive muscle relaxation, and initial follow-up sessions focused on reinforcing favorite place/activity imagery and on training in rapid induction of self-hypnosis. Response prevention was integrated into his hypnosis through instructions to imagine himself getting ready to write, becoming aware of the sensations associated with tremors and anticipatory anxiety, and then imagining himself doing the rapid induction of self-hypnosis to relax his arms and eliminate the anxiety response. By the fourth treatment session, the patient's anxiety level was significantly decreased; he reported no anxiety on 6 of 14 days, and on 6 other days he reported the easy conversion of anxiety to comfort through the techniques he had learned. His parents corroborated his improvement and reported dramatic improvement in handwriting productivity. Although his learning disability *per se* remained the same at follow-up 18 months later, he had maintained the effective application of his self-management skills, found school and writing much easier, was on the honor roll at school, and was engaged in many positive social activities. We agree that the description given by the authors (Young, Montano, & Goldberg, 1991) supports their conclusion that such hypnobehavioral, integrative approaches offer the clinician the opportunity to target specific behaviors, to identify the approach to altering that behaviors, and to easily assess both overall and individual strategy effectiveness. As they suggest, such combined approaches have promise as procedures to be evaluated within larger, systematic research studies.

Margolis (1990) described a variety of self-regulation strategies in a literature review from which he concluded that what he overall referred to as "relaxation training" has promising results in reducing symptoms of anxiety, impulsivity, hyperactivity, distractibility, and emotional lability of exceptional learners, while also positively influencing their self-concept, academic achievement, and classroom behavior. Although hypnosis was not specifically mentioned, he briefly described so-called common forms of "relaxation training," including progressive muscle relaxation, visual imagery, autogenics, and meditation.

Portes, Best, Sandhu, and Cuentas (1992) described the effects of relaxation training on anxiety and academic performance. Their study examined relationships among state anxiety, trait anxiety, and performance; it also estimated the value of a brief session of relaxation with music as compared to a lecture treatment across two subject areas. No improvement in performance was found for either treatment. The lecture condition was found to lower trait anxiety. They concluded that both state and trait anxiety may be reduced by autogenic (experiential) and lecture "treatments" with no improvement in test performance.

## Reading Disability

Illovsky (1963) studied the effect of group hypnosis with five nonpsychotic adolescent boys confined to a state hospital because of delinquency and severe behavior disorders. Five similar adolescent patients served as no-treatment controls. All subjects were nonreaders, with reading skills at or below first-grade level at the beginning of the study. Every day, before class began, the experimental group listened to a hypnotic induction followed by several suggestions for increased motivation, concentration, and performance in reading. Although no standardized hypnotizability scale was administered, these boys all responded to several informal measures similar to items from the Stanford Scales. One boy in this group cooperated minimally and was not included in the data analysis. After 6 months, the four remaining boys in the hypnosis group had gained an average of 2 years and 3 months in reading skills; the no-treatment controls had gained an average of 9 months. The author concluded that "hypnosis through its well-known hypermnesia can maintain and even enhance the reading ability of the hypnotized subjects." Such a conclusion seems unwarranted, in view of uncontrolled factors such as attention. At follow-up 2 months later, two boys in the experimental group showed no further improvement.

Jampolsky (1975) reported his hypnotherapeutic work with a small group of third- and fourth-grade children who were having difficulty learning to read. In a unique effort to overcome the negative reinforcement to which such children are repeatedly subjected, Jampolsky also used imagery techniques with the teachers and parents, encouraging them to visualize the children as successful readers. The research included a control group of poor readers who apparently received no treatment but were tested at the beginning and end of the study. The experimental group participated in an eight-step program over a period of three 45-minute sessions:

1. Because the children had already demonstrated problems with traditional visual learning, the group hypnotic induction minimized suggestions for visualization and focused instead on kinesthetic techniques such as feeling a weight pull their arm down or feeling fur on their face.
2. The children then imagined being in a pleasant place of their own choosing and concentrated on rhythmic breathing.

3. They were encouraged to get rid of painful associations to learning by mentally washing such bad feelings, dirt, and grime out of their brains.
4. They imagined themselves writing a small book about their favorite subject.
5. They used suggested tactile, auditory, and visual imagery to picture themselves on a motion picture screen reading their books with fluency, success, confidence, and joy, thus creating an ego ideal.
6. They climbed into their images on the screen, merging with the ideal self.
7. They imagined the new self-permeating all body tissues.
8. They were asked to repeat this process daily for 5–10 minutes before going to school and before going to sleep.

Jampolsky emphasized that this was a holistic approach to learning rather than the bit-by-bit process usually employed. Over a 1-month period, the experimental group averaged an increase in reading skill of 1–1/2 years, whereas the control group gained only 1 month. Self-esteem was markedly increased in the experimental group, and the parents and teachers reported decreased tension and increased energy. When the experimental group was retested a year later, their progress continued to be excellent compared to the control group. Jampolsky's results are encouraging, although the study contains methodological problems similar to those of the Illovsky study. Jampolsky presented no evidence that the subjects were really in hypnosis and, if so, that hypnosis and not some other variable accounted for the results.

Johnson, Johnson, Olson, and Newman (1981) studied the impact of group hypnosis and self-hypnosis on the academic performance and self-esteem of learning-disabled children, using the Jampolsky study (1975) as a model but extending the type of data gathered and analyzing it for more explanatory power. The authors suspect that, in practical application, group treatment may be highly feasible, but the effectiveness of the procedure may be better evaluated by individual techniques such as multiple correlations.

Krippner (1966) studied 49 children, ages 8–17 years and generally of average intelligence, enrolled in a 5-week remedial reading program. Hypnosis was utilized adjunctively with nine children whose parents specifically requested it. The median amount of reading improvement for the entire group was 5 months, as measured by a standardized reading test. In the hypnosis group, 8 children scored above the median and 1 at or below the median; in the control group, 16 children scored above the median and 24 at or below. The difference between the two groups was statistically significant, although the difference in actual amount of improvement (6 months vs. 5 months) was too small to be of much practical value. For the hypnosis group, Krippner tailored the induction to the expectations and needs of each child. The suggestions pertaining to reading focused on three areas: reducing tension and anxiety, enhancing the motivation to read, and increasing concentration and attention span. In discussing his results, Krippner noted the need for cautious interpretation. It is possible that parents in the hypnosis group were especially cooperative and optimistic about the entire remedial program, with unknown effects on their children's progress. The effect of special attention from the hypnosis teacher in the experimental group is also unknown. Finally, it is possible that the suggestions might have been equally effective in the absence of any hypnotic induction.

Crasilneck and Hall (1985) reported moderate to marked improvement in three-fourths of their child patients who presented with dyslexia. They described one adolescent with severe dyslexia, previously diagnosed as retarded who appeared to them to have normal intelligence and no severe emotional problems. After hypnosis practice lasting a few years, she graduated from high school and passed her driver's license exam. Their suggestions included ease in recognizing words which would make an impression on the unconscious brain so that word recall would be much easier in the future.

Prichard and Taylor (1989) reported a study of 32 remedial reading students who participated in a SALT program modified to include a creative writing exercise as a substitute for one-half of the relaxation and visualization activities normally employed by their classroom teachers. (SALT, Strategic Alternative Learning Techniques, is a University of Arizona program that promotes achievement of individuals with learning and attention challenges.) Students were tested before and after with the California Achievement Test. The average gain per month of instruction was 2.375 months, indicating a considerable decrease from the 3.86 months gain per month average. The authors believed that the most likely reason for the drop in reading success was the reduction by one-half of the opportunities for students to employ their visual imagery modality. The substitution of a creative writing activity, while enjoyed by students and thought worthwhile by teachers, appeared not to have exerted as strong an accelerative learning effect as did the full complement of relaxation and visualization exercises employed in previous years. These data were felt to provide support for instructional programs that set out to create a strong positive-suggestive atmosphere and to employ relaxation and visualization activities on a daily basis. Again, we note that hypnosis is not mentioned in this report; nonetheless, the operative ingredients of the study are indeed those of hypnosis as we understand and describe it – that is, of imagery and relaxation and of the concomitant awareness of the importance and value of the positive-suggestive atmosphere.

A study in England offered mental imagery training to nine children with specific language impairment (Joffe, Cain, & Maric, 2007). They were trained to produce mental images for sentences and stories in five 30-minute practice sessions. They were compared with 16 same-age, typically developing control children. Although the children improved in their ability to answer literal questions about the stories, improvement for inferential questions was not significant.

## Number Reversals

Jampolsky (1970) studied 10 children in grades 1–3 who were 6–9 years old and manifested number reversals. All the children had abnormal EEGs and various signs of attentional difficulties, then called MBD. The five children in the experimental group had a single hypnotic induction focusing on kinesthetic and tactile imagery and including suggestions that they would learn to write numbers properly. There was no determination of whether these children were actually in hypnosis. The single hypnotic session was followed by 2 weeks of remedial training in writing numbers, using a variety of special techniques for learning-disabled children. The five control children received no hypnotic induction and no remedial training. After 2 weeks, number of reversals were entirely eliminated in the experimental group; the control group showed a slight increase in reversals. The design of the study makes it impossible to determine whether the difference was due to hypnosis, to remedial training, or to other factors.

## Combination of Learning Problems and Text Anxiety

Wachelka and Katz (1999) reported a study of 15 public high school and 12 junior college students who had significant difficulties in reading, writing, or math. All reported that test anxiety was also a problem. The study was a randomized pre-test/post-test control group experiment. Thirteen students were randomly assigned to the treatment group, and 16 were assigned to a wait-list control group. Eleven students completed the 8-week intervention, which included progressive relaxation, guided imagery, and training in more rational self-talk. Sessions in weeks 7 and 8 focused on strategies for exam preparation. Text anxiety reduced significantly and self-esteem increased significantly in the treatment group. Students perceived the relaxation training as most helpful to them.

A study from the Netherlands reported improvements in spelling after quantitative electroencephalographic (QEEG)-based neurofeedback (Breteler, Arns, Peters, Giepmans, & Verhoeven, 2010). This randomized controlled treatment study of 19 children found that the experimental group improved considerably in spelling but had no improvement in reading. The 10 children in the experimental group received 20 sessions of neurofeedback training over a 10-week period. The neurofeedback instructions included encouragement to change mental imagery in a way that achieves the desired QEEG changes. During the neurofeedback training period both the experimental and control groups received additional counseling regarding reading and spelling.

## Test Anxiety

We sometimes see children whose IQs are at least average, whose study skills are adequate, and whose teachers insist that they have mastered classroom material as evidenced by workbook assignments, learning games, and other classroom activities. Yet, when these children are confronted with a formal test of their knowledge, they become markedly anxious and perform at a level much lower than would be expected. When children with test anxiety come to our office, they usually are aware that their anxiety is unwarranted and are often highly motivated to seek help. Sometimes the test anxiety is a clue to a more pervasive problem requiring intensive psychotherapy and accordingly, as always, a careful diagnostic assessment is essential. Often, however, the problem can be treated quite directly, usually with gains then spreading to other areas of the children's (commonly adolescents') lives. Our approach includes the following steps:

1. Having established the children's understanding of the irrationality of their anxiety and their motivation for assistance, we teach them to go into hypnosis by whatever method seems most appropriate and the best match for them.
2. During hypnosis, we invite them to imagine themselves in some activity unrelated to school in which they know they are competent and perform with minimal or no anxiety.
3. Having achieved a feeling of competence, they are then taught to let go of the specific content of the imagery, retain the feeling, and imagine an idealized self with the same good feelings in a classroom. This can be accomplished in many ways. It is often easily done with a split-screen idea or letting a screen be full, then blank, then full again with the new image.
4. They then experience a series of images, in a manner similar to systematic desensitization, beginning with a very brief and simple performance task such as distributing homework sheets. They move through images of more difficult tasks, culminating in an image of taking a major test or final examination, always retaining the feeling of confidence and competence and merging with each positive image as it becomes clear. If at any point anxiety develops, they may drop back to an easier image before progressing or utilize the imagery equivalent of thought-stopping by equally abruptly imagining, for example, a stop sign to abruptly interrupt the feelings of anxiety.
5. They are informed that this kind of rehearsal in fantasy often carries over into the actual situation.
6. They are given the posthypnotic suggestion that when actually required to perform (for example, take an examination), they can recall and experience the same good feelings as in the therapeutic sessions; they can do the same when preparing for the examination.
7. They are taught self-hypnosis, with the specific suggestion to review the positive images at an appropriate time and place, preferably twice daily for 5–10 minutes. They are encouraged as a posthypnotic suggestion and also out of hypnosis that "the more you practice the better you

get." In a future projection suggestion, they are encouraged to picture themselves successful before, during, and after an examination and being proud of that accomplishment.
8. Finally, they are reminded that no one performs perfectly all the time, and they are encouraged to set realistic expectations and to perceive failures as opportunities for new learning.

We find that two to five sessions are usually sufficient to master the problem, provided there is no significant psychopathology in the patients, their families, or the school environment itself.

## Conclusions

We have reviewed clinical and research reports that include many methodological problems that prevent us from definite conclusions about the value of hypnosis for enhancing learning and performance. Some of the more detailed approaches contain therapeutic suggestions that are interesting and might indeed prove valuable. There is clinical research evidence that training in self-hypnosis can reduce children's stress in classroom situations. A number of clinical studies describe the benefit of neurofeedback in helping children who have either attention-deficit or autism spectrum disorders. The biofeedback protocols that we have reviewed include procedures that are equivalent to hypnotic inductions in children. There is a great need for more research in this important area.

## References

Barbaresi, W.J., Katusic, S.K., Colligan, R.C., Pankratz, V.S., Weaver, A.L., Weber, K.J., Mrazek, D.A., & Jacobsen, S.J. (2002). How common is attention-deficit/hyperactivity disorder? *Archives of Pediatrics & Adolescent Medicine, 156*, 217–224.

Blanton, J. & Johnson, L.J. (1991). Using computer assisted biofeedback to help children with attention-deficit hyperactivity disorder to gain self-control. *Journal of Special Education Technology, 11*(1), 49–56.

Bothe, D., Grignon, J., & Olness, K. (2014). The effects of a stress management intervention in elementary school children. *Journal of Developmental and Behavioral Pediatrics*, 35, 62–67.

Breteler, M.H., Arns, M., Peters, S., Giepmans, I., & Verhoeven, L. (2010). Improvements in spelling after QEEG-based neurofeedback in dyslexia: a randomized controlled treatment study. *Applied Psychophysiology and Biofeedback, 35*, 5–11.

Coben, R., Linden, M., & Myers, T.E. (2010). Neurofeedback for autistic spectrum disorder: A review of the literature. *Applied Psychophysiology and Biofeedback, 35*, 83–105.

Crasilneck, H.B. & Hall, J.A. (1975). *Clinical Hypnosis: Principles and Applications.* New York: Grune & Stratton.

Crasilneck, H.B. & Hall, J.A. (1985). *Clinical Hypnosis: Principles and Applications*, 2nd ed. New York: Grune & Stratton.

Culbert, T.P., Reaney, J., & Kohen, D.P. (1994). Cyberphysiologic strategies in children: the biofeedback–hypnosis interface. *International Journal of Clinical and Experimental Hypnosis, 42*(2), 97–117.

Gardner, G.G. (1973). Use of hypnosis for psychogenic epilepsy in a child. *American Journal of Clinical Hypnosis, 15*, 166–169.

Gevensleben, H., Holl, B., Albrecht, B., Schlamp, D., Kratz, O., Studer, P., Wrangler, S., Rothenberger, A., Moll, G.H., & Heinrich, H. (2009). Distinct EEG effects related to neurofeedback training in children with ADHD: a randomized controlled trial. *International Journal of Psychophysiology, 74*, 149–157.

Groeneveld, K.M., Mennenga, A.M., Heidelberg, R.C., Martin, R.E., Tittle, R.K., Meeuwsen, K.D., Walker, L.A., & White, E.K. (2019). Z-Score Neurofeedback and heart rate variability training for adults and children with symptoms of attention-deficit/hyperactivity disorder: a retrospective study. *Applied Psychophysiology and Biofeedback, 44*, 291–308.

Grynkewich, M.A. (1994). *The Use of Mental Imagery Strategies to Improve School Performance*, unpublished manuscript, University of Arizona.

Illovsky, J. (1963). An experience with group hypnosis in reading disability in primary behavior disorders. *Journal of Genetic Psychology, 102*, 61–67.

Illovsky, J. & Fredman, N. (1976). Group suggestion in learning disabilities of primary grade children: a feasibility study. *International Journal of Clinical and Experimental Hypnosis, 24*, 87–97.

Jacobs, L. & Jacobs, J. (1966). Hypnotizability of children as related to hemispheric reference and neurological organization. *American Journal of Clinical Hypnosis, 8*, 269–274.

Jampolsky, G.G. (1970). Use of hypnosis and sensory motor stimulation to aid children with learning problems. *Journal of Learning Disabilities, 3*, 570–575.

Jampolsky, G.G. (1975). Hypnosis in the treatment of learning problems, paper presented at the 27th annual meeting of the Society for Clinical and Experimental Hypnosis, Chicago, IL.

Joffe, V.L., Cain, K., & Maric, N. (2007). Comprehension problems in children with specific language impairment: does mental imagery training help?. *International Journal of Language and Communication Disorders, 42*, 648–664.

Johnson, L.S., Johnson, D.L., Olson, M.R., & Newman, J.P. (1981). The uses of hypnotherapy with learning disabled children. *Journal of Clinical Psychology, 37*, 291–299.

Krippner, S. (1966). The use of hypnosis with elementary and secondary school children in a summer reading clinic. *American Journal of Clinical Hypnosis, 8*, 261–266.

Lazar, B.S. (1977). Hypnotic imagery as a tool in working with a cerebral palsied child. *International Journal of Clinical and Experimental Hypnosis, 25*, 78–87.

Lee, S.W. (1991). Biofeedback as a treatment for childhood hyperactivity: a critical review of the literature. *Psychological Reports, 68*, 163–192.

London, P. (1963). *Children's Hypnotic Susceptibility Scale*. Palo Alto, CA: Consulting Psychologists Press.

Margolis, H. (1990). Relaxation training: a promising approach for helping exceptional learners. *International Journal of Disability, Development, and Education, 37(3)*, 215–234.

Portes, P.R., Best, S.M., Sandhu, D., & Cuentas, T. (1992). Relaxation training effects on anxiety and academic performance. *Journal of the Society for Accelerative Learning and Teaching, 17*, 117–148.

Prichard, A. & Taylor, J. (1989). Creative writing and visual imagery activities in an experimental reading program. *Journal of the Society for Accelerative Learning and Training, 14(4)*, 297–310.

Reiff, M.I., Banez, G.A., Culbert, T.P. (1993). Children who have attentional disorders: diagnosis and evaluation. *Pediatrics in Review*, 14(12), 455–465.

Rusin, W. & Wynne, E. (1987). Stress Reduction Intervention Program in Grade School Children Using Computer Game Feedback, paper presented to the Society for Behavioral Pediatrics, Washington, D.C.

Shuck, A.U. & Ludlow, B.L. (1984). Effects of suggestibility on learning by retarded and nonretarded students. *Psychological Reports, 54*, 663–666.

Sternlicht, M. & Wanderer, Z.W. (1963). Hypnotic susceptibility and mental deficiency. *International Journal of Clinical and Experimental Hypnosis, 11*, 104–111.

Tansey, M.A. (1993). Ten year stability of EEC biofeedback results for a hyperactive boy who failed fourth grade perceptually impaired class. *Biofeedback and Self-Regulation, 18(1)*, 33–44.

Thompson, L., Thompson, M., & Reid, A. (2010b). Neurofeedback outcomes in clients with Asperger's syndrome. *Applied Psychophysiology and Biofeedback, 35*, 63–81.

Wachelka, D. & Katz, R.C. (1999). Reducing test anxiety and improving academic self-esteem in high school and college students with learning disabilities. *Journal of Behavior Therapy and Experimental Psychiatry, 30*, 191–198.

Watkins, J.G. (1962). *Hypnotherapy Postdoctoral Course*. Brooklyn, NY:American Psychological Association.

Woody, R.H. & Billy, H.T. (1970). Influencing the intelligence scores of retarded and non-retarded boys with clinical suggestion. *American Journal of Clinical Hypnosis, 12*, 268–271.

Woody, R.H. & Herr, E.L. (1967). Mental retardation and clinical hypnosis. *Mental Retardation, 5*, 27–28.

Young, M.H., Montano, R.J., & Goldberg, R. (1991). Self-hypnosis, sensory cueing, and response prevention: decreasing anxiety and improving written output of a preadolescent with learning disabilities. *American Journal of Clinical Hypnosis, 34*, 129–136.

# 12

# HYPNOTIC APPROACHES AND STRATEGIES IN THE MANAGEMENT OF PAIN

## Introduction – History

Historical accounts of hypnotherapy (therapeutic hypnosis) include many reports of its use for pain control, including that of James Braid, an English surgeon, who, in the mid-19th century, applied hypnotic training techniques to alleviate the pain of major surgery (Braid, 1843/1960). Milling, Valentine, LaStimolo, Nett, and McCarley (2021) published a comprehensive meta-analysis on hypnosis and the alleviation of clinical pain. Forty-two studies met the inclusion criteria and included both adults and children. Effect sizes suggested that the average participant using hypnosis reduced pain more than 75% of control participants. Authors also stated that hypnosis appears to be about as effective in alleviating clinical pain as distraction, cognitive behavioral therapy (CBT), biofeedback, and mindfulness. This comment is interesting because our experience suggests that the focus and absorption involved in distraction, CBT, biofeedback, and mindfulness are hypnotic.

Given that children generally have more hypnotic talent than adults and that the ability to control pain with hypnotic suggestion is positively correlated with hypnotizability (Hilgard & Hilgard, 1975), it should come as no surprise that children have been found to be more adept than adults in using hypnosis for control of pain (Wakeman & Kaplan, 1978).

Although these findings are true in terms of group comparisons, individual differences, of course, exist. Advantages to children who learn these methods of self-regulating pain include enhancement of self-confidence, personal participation in the therapeutic process, reduction of side effects, and increased ability to participate in normal daily activities. Articles report successful use of self-hypnosis techniques by children with a variety of chronic illnesses or recurrent pain, including malignancies, hemophilia, diabetes, sickle cell disease, abdominal pain, cystic fibrosis, migraines, and juvenile rheumatoid arthritis (Anbar, 2001; Barnes & Kohen, 2006; Dahlquist, Gil, Armstrong, Ginsburg, & Jones, 1985; Delivet, Dugue, Ferrari, Postone, & Dahmani, 2018; Dinges et al., 1997; Erickson, 1991; Gerik, 2005; Jong et al., 2020; Kohen & Zajac, 2007; Nunns et al., 2018; Olness, 1985; Olness & MacDonald, 1987; Russo & Varni, 1982; Tome-Pires & Miro 2012; Varni & Gilbert, 1982; Varni, Katz, & Dash, 1982; Vlieger, Menko-Frankenhuis, Wolfkamp, Tromp, & Benninga, 2007; Zeltzer, Dash, & Holland, 1979).

Interventions to help children cope with pain may reduce some of the acute and long-term psychological complications associated with hospitalization or procedures in other venues.

DOI: 10.4324/9781003243687-14

Colville and colleagues have documented the delusional memories children have after pediatric intensive care unit (PICU) experiences as well as the high risk of posttraumatic stress disorder for both hospitalized children and their parents (Colville, 2008; Colville, Kerry, & Pierce, 2008; Colville et al., 2009).

Hypnosis interventions are helpful as adjunct therapy in the management of childhood pain (Kuttner, 2010). Liossi and colleagues (Liossi, White, & Hatira, 2006) conducted a prospective controlled trial to compare the use of an analgesic cream (EMLA®), EMLA plus training in hypnosis, and EMLA plus attention in 45 Greek pediatric cancer patients for relief of discomfort from lumbar punctures. All children had experienced several lumbar punctures before the experiments. Those children randomized to learn hypnosis received one training session about 5 days before the next lumbar puncture. Children rated their pain and anxiety and nurses in the treatment room also completed observational scales. Children in the EMLA plus hypnosis group reported significantly less anticipatory anxiety and less procedure related pain and anxiety than the other groups.

A study from Australia (Cyna, Tomkins, Maddock, & Barker, 2007) reported on brief hypnosis for a 5-year-old boy who had severe needle phobia. He had received inhalational general anesthesia for intravenous cannulation on 58 occasions because of his severe distress and agitation about intravenous placement. Oral premedication with midazolam or ketamine did not help him. He was referred to learn hypnosis. After a 10-minute conversational hypnotic induction he was able to use switch-wire imagery to dissociate sensation in both arms and legs. Two days later he used his new skill and experienced painless vena puncture without the use of topical local anesthetic cream.

Some children may prefer to use self-hypnosis at some times and not at others. The following case report illustrates these complexities; it also reveals the power of the spoken word in a hypnotic context. Frank L., age 13, suffered electrical burns over much of his body after trying to retrieve a kite that had landed on a high-voltage wire. In the course of his hospitalization, he was taken to the department of physical medicine for a special test to determine the extent of nerve damage to his hand. During the test, he reported to the hypnosis coach a pain level of 8, on a 0–10 scale, in his right arm and back. He responded very well to suggestions for reduction of the pain in his arm, lowering it to a 0 level in a minute or so. He could not, however, do anything about the pain in his back. When questioned about this, he said that he did not want to relax and lie down on his back because his back would then stick to the sheet, and he would have to go through the severe pain of getting unstuck in order to get back to his own room and back to his bed. This pain was so severe that Frank could not use hypnosis at all to modify it. The therapist agreed with his logic and casually remarked, "That's okay. I'll go back upstairs with you and you can get rid of the back pain after you are in your room and back in your own bed."

Because the therapist knew that Frank had had little success using self-hypnosis for severe pain, of course she intended to communicate that she would help him. She accompanied Frank back to his room. A few minutes after he was in bed, she told him that he could now begin work to get rid of the pain in his back. He smiled and said that as soon as he got into bed the back pain disappeared. He had indeed taken the therapist's casual remark as a posthypnotic suggestion. Interestingly, he then reported the return of pain in his arm, which disappeared after a brief session of about 5 minutes. He was possibly responding to the demand characteristics of the therapist's seeming expectation that he would still have pain when he got into bed.

Accardi and Milling (2009) conducted a comprehensive methodological review of hypnosis for reducing procedure-related pain in children and adolescents. They identified 13 studies meeting review criteria and found that hypnosis was consistently more effective than control conditions in alleviating discomfort associated with procedures such as lumbar punctures, bone marrow aspirations, voiding cystourethrograms, and postsurgical pain. Another review from England (Richardson, Smith, McCall, & Pilkington, 2006) found seven randomized controlled clinical trials and one controlled clinical trial involving children with cancer. Studies reported statistically significant reductions in pain and anxiety or distress. A number of methodological limitations were identified, and the authors recommended further research into the effectiveness and acceptability of hypnosis for children with cancer.

Child health professionals who teach hypnosis sometimes approach the problem of pain in children in a trial-and-error fashion, randomly offering hypnoanalgesic techniques with which they are most familiar with little thought as to why one method might be preferable to another in a particular instance. Research in school-age children (Ross & Ross, 1984) indicates that the perception of pain in children is dependent on past experiences, education about pain, and the psychological and social contexts in which pain occurs. The following material deals with aspects of a child's experience of pain that might influence choice of technique.

## Variations in the Experience of Pain

### *Age*

Neonates can perceive pain, as reflected by their crying and by autonomic changes; however, because of their incomplete cortical development, there may be no conscious memory of painful experiences in the neonatal period. Fortunately, much research was done in the 1980s on pain experienced by newborns, including premature infants (Anand, 1990; Fitzgerald, Millard, & McIntosh, 1988; Schecter, Bernstein, Beck, Hart, & Sherzer, 1991). This led to increased efforts to provide analgesia and anesthesia for infants. By the end of the first year of life, the child can identify and localize pain, and by the end of the second year there is clear evidence of memory. Young children quickly learn to avoid painful stimuli such as a hot bulb on a lamp or a roasted marshmallow just out of the fire, and they may begin to cry at the mere sight of a doctor who has previously given some painful treatment. Because most children as young as 2 years have developed skills in imagery and in receptive language and can perceive adults as sources of help, these factors together with motivation to avoid pain should make young children receptive to hypnosis techniques for pain control. The main problems involve a poorly developed sense of time and of cause and effect. Thus, a 2-year-old probably could not benefit from a statement such as, "If you will do this or think about that, then the pain might go away." More naturalistic techniques, such as storytelling, which capture the child's attention and therefore focus attention away from pain, can often be successful (Kuttner, 1991). Generally, a child of 4 or 5 years should be able to utilize hypnotic suggestions for pain control unless past or present experience has taught a contrary expectation. An online survey of 35 child health professionals indicated that clinicians vary their use of hypnotic strategies primarily as a function of a patient's age (Tome-Pires et al., 2016).

## Individual Differences in Tolerance

Children vary greatly in their ability to tolerate pain; they vary more than do adults. Given three children who have apparently equal amounts of pain, the first may continue playing, the second may ask someone to "kiss it and make it all better" and will then continue playing, and the third may experience complete disruption of play and behave as if a catastrophe had occurred. In Petrie's (1967) terms, these children are reducers, moderators, and augmenters, respectively, and they tend to distort their perceptions of pain. In a study of adolescents and adults, Petrie (1967) found that juvenile offenders and youngsters involved in contact sports tended to be reducers. Alcohol and aspirin, both of which are associated with increased tolerance of pain, significantly lessened pain for augmenters but had little or no effect with reducers. Likewise, we would speculate that hypnosis for pain control might be more effective for augmenters than for reducers; however, the moderators might prove to be the most responsive to hypnosis, especially if the augmenters have some emotional investment in experiencing or expressing the experience of pain. It is not clear whether the differences among Petrie's groups reflect biological or psychological differences or both. Schecter has reviewed neuroanatomical and neurochemical factors that may ultimately explain individual differences in pain perception (Schecter, Berde, & Yaster, 2003).

## Cultural Differences

Different cultures have varying beliefs about pain. These beliefs impact how persons express discomfort, how they interpret their own pain levels, and how they believe pain should be treated. The International Children's Palliative Care Network has designed an app that is useful in many different cultural or ethnic contexts (ICPCN, 2015). It is important that cultural difference be considered before offering self-hypnosis training to a child and his family.

## Emotional Significance

For some children, pain has little emotional significance and is perceived mainly as a nuisance or a bad experience to be terminated as soon as possible. For other children, pain may have a variety of meanings and may serve a variety of psychological functions: (1) punishment for real or imagined sins; (2) getting attention and love, especially for children who tend to be ignored when "everything is okay"; (3) identification or merging with a loved one who has had similar pain, especially if there has been real or threatened abandonment by that person; (4) avoiding feared or unwanted situations that would be inevitable if the child were not in pain; (5) remaining close to a loved one whom the child feels a need to protect or in whose absence the child does not feel secure (most school-phobic pains fall into this category); (6) gaining status in certain families or cultural contexts where expressions of pain are socially acceptable and highly valued; (7) unconscious expression of hostility toward parents or siblings ("I'll make you feel bad to see me in pain"); (8) controlling others, especially for children with passive–aggressive tendencies ("I'll make you stay home with me, I'll ruin your day, and you can't get mad at me because you have to feel sorry for me because I'm in pain"); or (9) ensuring continuation of life, especially in sick children who have been taught that God uses death to take away pain. These are only a few of the ways in which pain can have emotional meaning; one must always be on the alert for other idiosyncratic kinds of significance. Hypnoanalgesic suggestions are likely to have no effect if the therapist has not dealt with the emotional significance of pain, either directly or indirectly.

## Context of Pain

Many aspects of the child's reality affect the extent to which pain will be tolerated. Previous pain experiences may have shaped the child's expectations that the present experience will be dreadful. For many children, the repeated invasive procedures associated with chronic diseases such as cancer or sickle cell disease are more distressing than any other aspect of illness or treatment (Fowler-Kerry, 1990; Kuttner, 1989; Savedra, Tesler, Holzemer, & Ward, 1989). Certain coexisting bodily states such as fatigue or physical discomfort will probably reduce pain tolerance. Coexisting psychological states are also important. Anxiety and depression usually reduce pain tolerance. Excitement and anticipatory joy, such as the time of a birthday, will often enhance pain tolerance.

A child's response to pain may depend partly on understanding its purpose, including: (1) no understanding in a very small child; (2) no purpose for the pain (e.g., an accident); (3) an unjust purpose (e.g., a wound resulting from a fight to defend oneself); or (4) a logical purpose (e.g., a dressing change for burns). When a child understands the purpose or source of pain, his or her reaction may also be influenced by the response of others. A parent who responds with anxiety and confusion will elicit a more negative reaction in a child than will a parent who responds with acceptance and with clarity about what needs to be done (Eland & Anderson, 1977).

Children's reactions to pain are often influenced by the context of their expectations concerning adults' response as much as by the response itself. Helen H., age 9 years, sustained a small laceration of her hand after a fight on the school playground. Frequently ridiculed and punished by her parents, the child was terrified that she would be punished for her misbehavior. She made no effort to report the accident and hoped to conceal it entirely by wiping the blood on her red dress. Although blood loss was minimal, she fainted a few minutes later. The fainting probably was an unconscious expression of her need to avoid "facing the consequences." The child was frankly disappointed when the pediatrician, after some deliberation, decided that sutures (painful punishment) would not be necessary. We would expect that this child would not have responded to hypnoanalgesic suggestions, had they been offered, despite her good imaginative skills.

In general, we would expect children to benefit less from hypnosis for pain that occurs in a negative context than from pain that occurs in a more neutral context; therefore, we recommend that pediatricians and other child health specialists counsel parents regarding optimal ways of responding to pain in their children. Of course, doctors and other medical staff also play an important role in creating or modifying the reality context of pain in children. The doctor who communicates that pain is inevitable and may become even more severe will tend to have patients who experience a great deal of pain. On the other hand, if all members of the medical team approach the child with a calm and positive manner, then the child may well be able to fulfill the expectation that the situation is manageable and may even be enjoyable. Because children lack the preconceptions of adults, because they may be influenced positively or negatively, and because their future perceptions concerning pain may be permanently affected, it is incumbent on all adults to choose words related to pain very carefully when speaking to children.

The following is an example of a therapeutic approach to a child who had been negatively conditioned to needles and to people and places associated with needles. Six-year-old David had become conditioned to manifest fear, tantrums, and physical resistance whenever he saw a nurse, a physician, or even the hospital doctors. David had leukemia and had been in remission since shortly after his diagnosis 14 months earlier. With respect to the disease, he was doing well; emotionally, however, he was not.

What factors could have led to his pathological fear of needles? We cannot be sure, of course, but several influences may have affected David. His father had a dental phobia, which required him to take tranquilizers before going to the dentist even for a routine cleaning. David's first nurse in the hospital had an unresolved memory of an unpleasant experience, dating from when she had first received ether anesthesia at age 6 years. The lab technician who drew blood from David the first time explained nothing to him about the procedure. We do not know what other children may have said to frighten David or if he had seen something on television that had also contributed to his fear. Whatever the causes, a finger stick became an unpleasant and dreaded experience, not only for David but also for his family, the nursing staff, and the laboratory staff.

David was sedated for intravenous injections and was given general anesthesia for bone marrow exams and spinal taps. After he had an allergic reaction to sedation, his physician sought alternative approaches. David was referred to us to learn self-hypnosis for control of his needle phobia. At the time of his initial visit, we chatted with David and his parents about his interests, likes and dislikes, fears, and learning styles. We learned about games he liked, stories he liked, and music he preferred. Then we tailored a simple relaxation exercise for David and asked him to practice his exercise twice a day until the next visit a week later.

David was a quick learner and demonstrated good retention at the time of the second visit. We reviewed the exercise with him, this time giving him the opportunity to play computer games that reflected his state of relaxation (by monitoring peripheral temperature and galvanic skin resistance). As he succeeded, we explained that he was showing that he was the boss of these body processes and that his brain was directing the changes he saw on the computer screen. We also made drawings of his nervous system and explained how nerves carried messages to his brain, which his brain then figured out. We asked him to make a similar drawing at home. He was reminded to practice the relaxation exercise once a day. We saw David a third time a week later, and he brought the drawing with him. He was eager to play the computer game again. After one practice session with the computer, we gave David a small needle and began to rehearse procedures, using stuffed animals as models. David participated, and we asked him to review these procedures at home under his parents' direction. We also told him that he should continue to practice the relaxation exercise at home once a day. During the fourth visit, David reviewed his relaxation exercise and then began to program himself to turn on and off the switches in the brain that controlled his nerves. We allowed David to let us know when he was ready, and he turned off the switch to his left hand. With his permission, we touched his hand with the needle. He was elated when this did not bother him. Again he practiced at home, and a week later he tolerated a venipuncture with no difficulty. Subsequently, after watching a videotape of another child undergoing a lumbar puncture and bone marrow puncture while doing the relaxation exercises, David underwent his next bone marrow and lumbar puncture procedures with comfort and competence.

Ross and Ross (1984), in a study of 994 school children, found no clearly defined age trends in the children's pain concept; however, they did find much evidence for early maladaptive behavior in coping with pain. These authors expressed concern that, if unchecked, such behavior might persist into adulthood. Ross and Ross also noted that the children were generally ignorant about how to cope with pain, and they suggested that pain be a topic in school science curricula.

We believe that healthcare professionals working with children who have pain should analyze themselves with respect to their own childhood experiences with pain, the persistence of their own fears of painful procedures, and their own strategies for coping with pain. Such analysis may not only help the therapist to understand the perceptions of the child patient but may also keep him from projecting his own negative expectations onto the child.

## Toward Understanding Hypnoanalgesia

Most researchers and clinicians who work with therapeutic hypnosis agree that the phenomenon of hypnoanalgesia is real and that patients and subjects are not faking in order to please the experimenter or therapist. Whereas it is possible to deny the limited pain involved in a laboratory experiment, the idea of faking becomes farfetched in severe clinical pain such as one sees in surgical procedures or in advanced cancer. Some skeptical researchers have deemphasized the role of hypnotic suggestion in favor of such constructs as role playing or expectation (e.g., Barber & Hahn, 1962; Stam & Spanos, 1980). We agree that role playing and expectation can enhance one's ability to modify pain, but we also believe that these factors are neither necessary nor sufficient for hypnoanalgesia. Crasilneck and Hall (1973), for example, demonstrated hypnotic pain reduction with naïve children and with culturally unsophisticated subjects not acquainted with the expectations of the person who was teaching hypnosis. We have had similar clinical experiences. It is one thing to accept the phenomenon of hypnoanalgesia as real; it is another to explain the mechanism by which it occurs. Two lines of research, one psychological and the other physiological, have been pursued.

## A Psychological Lead: Alternative Cognitive Controls

It is often the case in science that new ideas occur almost by chance, beginning in unrelated areas and finding new direction by virtue of the creative ability of the scientist. Thus, the contribution of Hilgard and Hilgard (1975) toward explaining hypnoanalgesia began with a demonstration of hypnotic deafness that had nothing at all to do with pain. In a classroom demonstration, a subject who had been given suggestions for hypnotic deafness failed to respond to loud noises or to questions from classmates. Another student, noting that nothing was wrong with the subject's ears, asked if there might be some part of him that actually did hear. When the subject was asked to lift one finger if some part of him other than the part in hypnosis could hear, he lifted one finger. The subject then asked Hilgard to restore his hearing so he could tell him what he did to make him raise his finger. The part of him not in hypnosis was able to give a full account of what had occurred after Hilgard gave him the signal (touching the arm).

It occurred to the Hilgards that a similar mechanism might be operating in the case of hypnotic pain control, and a series of subsequent experiments demonstrated this to be true. Subjects who were capable of hypnotic pain control were asked if some other part of them knew more of what was going on than the part in hypnosis. In about half of the cases, the part in hypnosis reported low levels of pain, but the other part reported pain at higher levels. The Hilgards described this other part as a "hidden observer," emphasizing that it is a metaphor for something occurring at an intellectual level but not available to the consciousness of the person in hypnosis. In attempting to explain their findings, the Hilgards postulated alternative cognitive controls, which may or may not be in ascendance at any given time. These ideas also offer an explanation for the fact that subjects who are hypnotically analgesic demonstrate physiological signs of pain (e.g., increased heart rate) while reporting no felt pain. The theory of alternative cognitive controls, also called *neodissociation theory*, is further described in E.R. Hilgard's *Divided Consciousness* (1977).

One of us (KO) successfully underwent orthopedic surgery on a finger for 50 minutes with hypnosis as sole anesthesia. Preparation consisted of listening to an audiotape of a meditation exercise for 1 hour. The coach, or teacher, was Dr. Kohen, who reinforced my self-hypnosis. I felt comfortable throughout the procedure, which was videotaped. Physiological measures, including cardiac rate, respiratory rate, and blood pressure, remained steady throughout the procedure. Electroencephalographic (EEG) monitoring recorded primarily theta activity, although there was a period of 15 minutes near the end of the procedure when there was no measurable alpha, beta, or theta activity. When the operation ended, the EEG recorded primarily alpha and beta activity. I used both dissociation and direct pain-control strategies and concluded that both were important to the successful anesthesia. Postoperative pain did occur, and I also controlled that with self-hypnosis. During the surgery, I felt no pain, nor did my autonomic measures suggest that some other part of me was perceiving pain.

## Functional Magnetic Resonance Imaging Studies Clarifying Cortical Dimensions of Pain

Rainville and colleagues have conducted research on the cortical representations of sensory and affective aspects of pain for many years, using functional magnetic resonance imaging (fMRI) to determine where these representations are located (Albunese, Duerden, Rainville, & Duncan, 2007;

Rainville, Duncan, Price, Carrier, & Bushnell, 1997). They have demonstrated clearly that emotions modulate both cortical and spinal pain processes (Roy, Piche, Chen, Peretz, & Rainville, 2009). They have also documented that sensory and affective dimensions of pain are impacted by hypnotic modulation (Rainville, Carrier, Hoffbauer, Bushnell, & Duncan, 2001). Their exciting work has demonstrated shared brain mechanisms whether the intervention is hypnosis or meditation (Grant & Rainville, 2005). Furthermore their work has demonstrated that the length of meditative practice is associated with increased cortical thickness in the pain-related brain regions and is associated with decreased pain sensitivity (Grant, Courtemanche, Duerden, Duncan, & Rainville, 2010). Studies from France have also demonstrated neuroimaging changes when children use self-hypnosis for pain control (Wood & Bioy, 2008).

## Neuropeptides and Pain

Endorphins, endogenous morphine-like peptides, were discovered in 1975. Concurrently, another neuropeptide, substance P, was recognized to be a transmitter of pain impulses. With respect to pharmacological management of postoperative pain, opioid analgesics have the cornerstone. Opioids produce analgesia by binding to opioid receptors both within and outside the central nervous system. They are classified as full agonists, partial agonists, or mixed agonist–antagonists, depending on how they interact with opioid receptors. Many different receptors exist, and they accept various opioid agonists such as morphine and codeine. Unfortunately, most opioid agonists cause side effects, including major problems such as respiratory depression and sedation and lesser problems such as constipation, nausea, urinary retention and addiction. These side effects limit the dose that may be safely given (US Department of Health and Human Services, 1992). This is why nonpharmacological treatments such as hypnosis may be valuable as adjuncts to opioid treatment. It is important to keep in mind that a child who has had opioids recently cannot learn self-regulation methods such as self-hypnosis as well as a child who is fully alert.

Studies to determine whether or not hypnotic strategies trigger release of endogenous endorphins have had conflicting results. It has been demonstrated that naloxone does not negate hypnotically achieved analgesia in adults (Goldstein & Hilgard, 1975). A study by Katz and colleagues (Katz et al., 1982) measured beta-endorphin reactivity in the cerebrospinal fluid of 75 children with leukemia who were undergoing lumbar punctures. This study analyzed beta-endorphin levels with respect to the children's reports of their pain and their fear, as well as measures of distress noted by observers. Levels of beta-endorphin generally decline with increasing age of the children. Nurse ratings of the children's anxiety positively correlated with beta-endorphin levels; this suggests that beta-endorphin elevations reflected stress and might have represented the body's attempts to modulate unpleasant perceptions. This study also found that girls had higher levels of distress during lumbar puncture procedures than did boys.

Varni et al. (1982) summarized research strategies used to elucidate the physiological, neurochemical, and behavioral implications of endorphin peptides for humans. These include administration of narcotic antagonists to displace opiates from opiate receptors, direct administration of synthetic endorphins while behavioral alterations are observed, direct assays of various endorphins in biological fluids such as blood, and direct measurement of endorphins before and after the introduction of interventions believed to affect pain. Thus far, none of these strategies in adults or in children has led to conclusive evidence with respect to whether or not endorphin release is affected by hypnosis. This area of inquiry remains an important one. Hypnotic responsiveness in children is associated with physiological changes that reflect neurotransmitter changes. It remains conceivable that the self-regulatory processes associated with voluntary pain control are mediated by release of endogenous endorphins or some other neurotransmitters.

The effectiveness of either hypnosis or pharmacological treatments for pain may be dependent on dietary factors, fatigue, medication interactions, or geomagnetic effects on neurotransmitters. We recognize that the following section may be much too general and that eventually we will have specific, practical methods to assess individual differences and guide the choice of pain treatment more precisely for both children and adults.

## Pain-Rating Scales and Assessments

Patient self-report is the gold standard for assessment of pain intensity. Whatever the method used, it is important to use the same system at each visit with the child and to compare pain intensity between visits and from one visit to the next. Many studies in recent years have attempted to develop pain-rating scales that could be replicated and validated. Some have been observational; others require some type of subjective assessment from the child (Eland & Anderson, 1977; Haslam, 1969; Jay, Ozolins, Elliott, & Caldwell, 1983; LeBaron & Zeltzer, 1984; Ross & Ross, 1984; Schecter et al., 2003). These methods have included color selections to represent pain intensity, visual analog scales (such as rulers), scales made up of happy or sad faces, and the selection of pain descriptors from a list of words or audiotaped sounds.

A study (West, Oakes, & Hinds, 1994) compared the Faces Pain Scale (FPS) and Poker Chip Tool (PCT) in 30 children, ages 5 to 13 years, who were hospitalized in a pediatric oncology intensive care unit. Parents and patients completed these scales, and each patient's nurse completed the Objective Pain Scale (OPS). Patients' ratings on the FPS correlated significantly with parents' ratings but not on the PCT. Nurses' ratings on the OPS correlated moderately with patients' FPS ratings. The majority of children, parents, and nurses expressed a preference for the FPS. In the final analysis, child health professionals should accept the pain rating of the child rather than that of parents or other caretakers.

Varni and colleagues (Varni, Thompson, & Hanson, 1987) developed the Pediatric Pain Questionnaire (PPQ), which attempts to assess empirically the complexities of chronic pain in children. The PPQ includes a combination of several types of pain assessments including a visual analog scale as well as questions about the location of pain, pain history, and socioenvironmental situations that may influence pain perception. In a study of 25 children with juvenile rheumatoid arthritis, they found that correlations were highly significant for the PPQ results with respect to present pain and worst pain. This instrument may provide a step toward achieving reliable methodology for understanding the experience of and for measuring the level of pain experience in children with chronic pain. We developed a pain questionnaire for use with children who have chronic or recurrent pain such as Migraine which includes not only descriptors of pain but also information about the child's interests, likes, and preference for different types of imagery. The latter helps guide our choice of strategies for teaching the child a self-management method.

Birnie, Noel, Chamers, Uman, and Parker (2018) did a review of self-report pain intensity measures for children and adolescents. They strongly recommended use of the 11-point numeric rating scale (NRS-11), FPS-Revised and the Color Analogue Scale(CAS) for self-report of acute pain. They could make only weak recommendations for self-report of postoperative and chronic pain and no recommendations for any measures for children younger than six years.

Young children may manifest pain by crying, fussing, or being irritable; withdrawal from social interaction; sleep disturbances; facial grimacing; guarding; inconsolability; poor appetite; or disinterest in play. These behavioral indicators should be assessed for any young child who may have pain and should be recorded. Additional assessment of pain includes a careful medical and psychosocial history, physical examination, and review of prior investigations and treatment. It is helpful, when possible, to include an assessment of autonomic responsivity. Some children may not verbalize significant pain but may demonstrate changes in autonomic measures such as increased heart rates or electrodermal activity, and these may reflect pain. It seems likely that the most reliable pain rating scales will include both physiological and subjective measures. Hypnotic interventions to reduce pain may be applied more reliably after careful assessments; however, this may be impractical in acute, emergency situations.

## General Principles and Guidelines for Teaching Hypnoanalgesia

In working with more than 1500 children who have learned hypnotic pain control for various conditions, we have found the following principles and guidelines to be useful:

- *Assess one's personal experience about pain.* The clinician needs to analyze his or her own attitude toward discomfort. Most of us, by the time we reach adulthood, because of our childhood experiences and our training, have certain negative notions about pain that we may project onto our patients. A therapist who lacks faith in a child's ability to overcome pain is unlikely to succeed in helping the child.
- *Assess parental perceptions and expectations about pain.* Expectations of parents regarding discomfort are important variables, and parents may also benefit from self-hypnosis exercises. In fact, in certain situations, it may be preferable for the parent to learn concurrently with the child. Children are less conditioned to the necessity for pain, suffering, and mental anguish if not overwhelmed by the negative expectations of their parents and other caretakers regarding how one manages pain.
- *Consider the impact of the pediatric treatment team.* Whether interventions for pain relief are to be pharmacological, nonpharmacological, or a combination of the two, the attitudes and perceptions of adults on the treatment team may have significant effects on the outcome. Caregivers may have unresolved anxieties stemming from their own perceptions of pain suffered in hospitals or in dentists' offices as children. These can be reflected in subtle changes in voice, demeanor, or behavior when they are confronted with a child in pain or one about to undergo a painful procedure. Such anxiety may be perceived by the child and increase his or her own distress.
- *Consider the age and development of the child.* One must decide whether or not the child is able to learn a formal technique. For the very young, music, massage, or rocking are natural adjuncts to pharmacological pain management. For the toddler, a distraction technique such as blowing may be most appropriate. Some bright, verbal 2-year-olds can learn self-hypnosis. All children think concretely; abstract reasoning skills do not develop until mid to late adolescence. Failure to recognize this is a major impediment to successful adult–child communication. Adults tend to assume children have more abstract reasoning capacity than they actually have. Children often misinterpret expressions such as "she was fired" (interpreting it as "she was set on fire"), "patching the eye" (interpreting it as "sewing a piece of cloth on my eye"), or "frog in the throat" (interpreting it as a Kermit, the *Sesame Street* frog, in the throat). When fear seems out of proportion to the situation, the child may have misinterpreted an adult's statement as somehow threatening. The practice of hypnosis tends to help child health professionals become more aware of the importance of word choice; this benefits all of their interactions with children.
- *Consider learning styles, strengths, and learning handicaps.* Parents often can provide information about how their children learn best – by observing, listening, or reading. Many children enjoy learning via computers. Parents may also be aware of learning handicaps. Research has

documented that children may develop learning handicaps after receiving cancer therapy. In a long-term follow-up of children with cancer (Olness & Singher, 1989), some of the children who learned quickly during the initial training period had developed learning disabilities after a few years and had difficulty in remembering their self-regulation methods. Information about learning also helps in choice of an appropriate pain assessment tool. If a child does not grasp a sequence of numbers, then use of a ruler scale is not a good idea.

- *Consider a child's interests, likes, and dislikes.* It is helpful to know what the child enjoys and does not enjoy in terms of play, environment, social media, games (including video games) music, and sports. Does he or she like books? Which television programs does he or she enjoy? What are family interests and hobbies? The task of teaching self-hypnosis is much easier if the therapist asks the child to focus on something that he or she enjoys.
- *Emphasize the child's control and mastery.* Learning self-regulation strategies provides an opportunity for children with chronic diseases, such as cancer, to develop a sense of coping ability and personal mastery. Many children with chronic illnesses have little or no control over most aspects of treatment, but they can be in complete control over self-hypnosis. We emphasize this to children from the first visit, explaining that we are like a coach or teacher, but that the child is in control just as he or she is when learning to play soccer or the piano. We provide choices such as what imagery a child will use and what reminders to use for practice. We also acknowledge the child's personal mastery when he or she succeeds. Children may not always want to use their pain-control skills depending on fatigue or secondary gain issues or other unknown factors. When this is the case, they must be allowed to have the choice of not using hypnosis, and the adults around them must understand and accept this as well.
- *Explain what you plan to do and what the child may do in appropriate language.* The initial discussion of hypnotic pain control should be tailored to the child's interests and developmental level, the parents' wishes, and the therapist's strengths. For some adolescents, explanations may be lengthy and involve descriptions of the nervous system and pain pathways. For most young children, brief explanations are preferable. Some preschoolers benefit from watching a videotape of children of similar ages who are demonstrating hypnotic pain control. Children of grade school age understand the concept of similar sound signals being interpreted differently by the brain. For example, the sound of "b" may be interpreted by the brain as "bee," "be," or "B"; "c" may be interpreted as "see," "sea," or "C." Similarly, the signal from the entrance of a needle into the skin may be interpreted in multiple ways, and the child can decide how to control this. School children can understand that one cannot focus on more than two or three stimuli at one time. This can be demonstrated easily by asking the child to pay attention to the feeling of his or her right foot inside the sock, at the same time to pay attention to the feeling of the shirt on the back of his or her neck, and at the same time to pay attention to the feeling of the watch on his or her wrist. The child cannot focus on all three stimuli at the same time. We explain that each of us is constantly choosing which stimuli we pay attention to and that we do this unconsciously; however, we can also learn to do this with our own controls such as when we learn to shut off pain signals to our brain. We then ask the child to consider what sort of a control system is in his or her brain, possibly some sort of computer system or a switch system, that allows him or her to turn signals on or off. We also explain to the child and parents that practice is important but that parents should not remind the child to practice. They may help him or her to select a practice reminder system.
- *Avoid prescribing the child's images, or pain perceptions.* Although it is incorrect to say that something will not hurt, it is also incorrect to say that something will hurt. It is helpful to give the child options in his or her descriptions. The therapist can say, "Some children say this feels like cold ice, and some say it feels like a thorn from a rose bush, and some say it feels like

a hairbrush. I wonder what it will feel like for you?" This gives the message that the child can decide how it feels and describe the feeling for himself or herself. The child's description may then be incorporated into a therapeutic suggestion – for example, "If you like, you can let that pecking bird fly away." The therapist should also avoid being too specific about when and how the pain will go away. One can rapidly back oneself into a corner by such statements as "The pain will be gone in 10 minutes" or "The hurting will go away when I count to five." If the prophecy is not fulfilled, the therapist loses credibility, and thereafter even appropriate suggestions may have no effect.

## Positive Side Effects

Hypnosis for pain control may have a variety of side benefits, especially in the case of children with chronic or life-threatening illness. These include reduction of anxiety, enhancement of mastery and hope, increased cooperation, and increased comfort among family members and among other members of the health-care team.

## Techniques of Hypnoanalgesia

The following techniques represent methods we have used with our patients. We often use several in combination. Every technique involves suggested dissociation, either directly or indirectly; for example, notice how the phrase "that arm" rather than "your arm" facilitates dissociation. As with invitation/induction techniques, our list is by no means complete. Others who teach hypnosis to children will prefer variations of our methods or will develop other methods.

## Direct Suggestions for Hypnoanesthesia

- *Request for numbness.* "You know what a numb feeling is. How does numbness feel to you?" Child responds. "Good, just let that part of your body get numb now. Numb like a block of ice [or whatever image the child has used]."
- *Topical anesthesia.* "Just imagine painting numbing medicine onto that part of your body. Tell me when you're finished doing that."
- *Local anesthesia.* "Imagine putting an anesthetic into that part of your body. Feel its flow into your body and notice the change in feeling as the area becomes numb."
- *Glove anesthesia.* "First, pay attention to your hand. Notice how you can feel tingling feelings in that hand. Then let it become numb. When it is very numb, touch that hand to your jaw [or other body part] and let the numb feeling transfer from the hand to the jaw."
- *Switchbox.* The therapist explains the idea that pain is transmitted by nerves from various parts of the body to the brain, which then sends a pain message back to the body. The therapist can describe nerves and their pathways or can ask the child to provide a color for nerves. The importance of accuracy varies with the age and needs of the child. The child is then asked to choose some sort of switch that can turn off incoming nerve signals. The therapist can describe various kinds of switches, such as flip, dimmer, pull, or even a television computer push-button panel or control panel of lights. Having chosen a switch, the child is asked to begin practicing turning off the switches or the lights that connect the brain and certain areas of the body. It is useful to ask the child to turn off the incoming nerve signals for defined periods of time (e.g., 10 minutes, 15 minutes, 90 minutes). The success of the exercise is judged by touching the child with a small-gauge needle or some other sharp object and asking for a comparison with feelings on the other side where the nerve signals are unchanged.

## Distancing Suggestions

- *Moving pain away from the self.* "Imagine [or pretend] for a while that that arm [or other body part] doesn't belong to you, isn't part of you. Think of it as part of a sculpture or a toy or picture just floating out there by itself." Some patients comfortably imagine having only one arm; others imagine three arms, one of which is dissociated.
- *Transferring pain to another body part.* "Imagine putting all the discomfort of the spinal tap into the little finger of your right hand. Tell me how much discomfort is in that little finger. Give it a number rating and let me know if it changes. Good. Now let it float away."
- *Moving self away from the pain.* "You said you like to go to the mountains. Imagine yourself there now. Let yourself really be there. Just leave all the discomfort and be in the mountains. See the trees and flowers. Watch the chipmunks playing. Smell the fresh air and the pine trees. Listen to the gentle wind. Listen to the running stream. Imagine yourself running or walking, if you like."

## Suggestions for Feelings Antithetical to Pain

- *Comfort.* "Recall a time when you felt very comfortable, very good. Now bring those good comfortable feelings into the present. Let your body feel comfortable here and now. You can let comfortable feelings fill your whole body and mind completely, until there is just no room for discomfort. You can be completely comfortable, and you can keep these good feelings for as long as you like."
- *Laughter.* "Laughing helps pain go away. Think of the funniest movie you ever saw or the funniest thing you ever did or your friend did. Each time you imagine laughing, your pain becomes less and less. You may find yourself really laughing and feeling very good."
- *Relaxation.* "Notice that *breathing out is relaxing.* And you can get more comfortable each time you breathe out. When you get more comfortable, the discomfort becomes less. Each time you breathe out –more and more comfortable" (see Kohen, 2017).

## Directing Attention to the Pain or Discomfort Itself

For various reasons, some children refuse or are unable to focus attention on anything but the experiences of pain. The therapist can utilize this behavior to the child's own advantage. By joining with the child and asking for a detailed description of the discomfort/pain, the therapist can offer subtle suggestions for change and relief.

## Distraction Techniques

- *Focus on unrelated material.* Young children often obtain some pain relief if the therapist tells a story, either in its original form or with ridiculous variations such as changing the characters (e.g., "Once upon a time there were three little wolves and a big bad pig") or their roles (e.g., "Once there was a wolf who cried, 'Boy! Boy!'"). Older children may be distracted by discussion of areas of interest such as sports or music.
- *Focus on the procedure or injury.* This method is especially useful for children for whom cognitive mastery is a major coping mechanism. The therapist asks the child to describe the injury in detail, how it occurred, how others reacted, and so on. In the case of a painful procedure, the therapist describes various instruments and asks the child to assist by holding instruments or bandages, counting sutures, or checking the time at various points.

- *Focus on the lesser of two evils.* If a child feels both pain and cold, the therapist can focus on the cold. If the child is having a spinal tap and also has an IV running, the therapist can focus on the IV.
- *Lighted globe.* "Imagine you are inside a lighted globe, and you can see yourself walking around on the inside of a map of your discomfort. Notice that discomfort very carefully. See it right now in a color you don't like. I'll ask you to check it again later. Notice what size it is. It might be the size of a grapefruit or a grape or a lemon. Even a pinhead has a size. We'll check the size again later. And notice the shape. What shape is it right now? And what is it saying to you now? How loud is it right now? Later we'll see if you can still hear it. Look again. What color is it now? That's interesting. It seems to be changing. I wonder how you did that. How small is it now? Can you change the size, too? Yes. You are really in charge there in that lighted globe. You are a good map maker. You can go wherever you want. Feel whatever you want. What shape is the discomfort now? Can you still hear it?"
- *Amnesia.* Constructive use of amnesia along with an explanation of how the body works is another way of distracting from a focus on discomfort. "I know you know that we discussed that discomfort is a signal to let you know that something was injured and, in the case of after an operation, to let you know that the tissues are now healing, so it's good to pay attention to that signal, but once you know about it and pay attention to it for a while, then you don't have to bother paying attention to it any more. In fact that discomfort is so new that your brain hardly knows it very well. In fact, your brain has much more experience with no pain or discomfort in that part of your body than it does with this [shoulder, abdomen, head, etc.]. So, I wonder if it would be okay with you to let your brain just forget to remember about this discomfort in between times that you remember to notice it and check the level? And, because it remembers so well what no discomfort feels like, it's easy then to forget to remember the discomfort that used to be there anyway, and in that way it can go a way that it doesn't have to disturb. It's funny how you can program that computer we call the brain to remember to forget about the bother or to forget to remember about it, or even to remember to forget to remember or to forget to remember to forget." In addition to the confusional suggestion for amnesia, these represent invitations to the patient to perceive his or her discomfort in a different way.
- *Trip around the body.* This is another metaphoric storytelling and reframing approach that is often very useful, particularly in a naturalistic, Ericksonian approach to pain control. "I knew this girl once who was only [pick an age slightly younger than the patient] years old and she liked to pretend she was so tiny that she could go inside of her own body and take a trip around the body. She sometimes pretended she was riding on a bike on the bones or the nerves and at other times pretended that she was in a boat traveling through the bloodstream. She visited different parts of the body. She went to the strong heart and watched how great it was pumping blood and over to the lungs to admire the way they were breathing so easily, and then she visited other places and took a repair kit along and just fixed things that weren't quite right." This could also be used in combination with the switches technique: "And she made her way all the way to that main computer we call the brain, and when she got there she saw all these lights and buttons and switches, and she found the one that said [shoulder, tummy, etc.], and she turned it down, sometimes partway down and sometimes all the way off so the hurt didn't bother her at all."
- *Time distortion and reframing.* Particularly useful with children with chronic or recurrent pain or with postoperative pain is teaching the use of time distortion. This can often be accomplished easily in a naturalistic and expectant fashion by appealing to the child's

(and parents') sense of experience in daily life and our routine perceptions of time: "Did you ever notice how when you're having a good time, like at a party or a sleepover or when playing with favorite friends that time seems to go fast? People even say that sometimes, don't they? They say things like, 'Whew, time flies when you're having fun!' Don't they? Right, and, of course, it doesn't really fly, but it sure seems like it, doesn't it? And it works the other way around, too, doesn't it? Like, if you're worrying about something or can't wait for something to begin or end, it seems like time goes soooo ... slooowly. And people talk about that, too. They say things like, 'Wow, this feels like it's taking forever, but I just looked at the clock and only 2 minutes have gone by. It seemed like an hour!' You can do the same with your discomfort, like just paying attention to it for 5 minutes every hour. Pay very close attention and notice what number it is on the bother scale, and keep track, especially noticing how it changes, getting better and better each time you measure it."

- *Confusion techniques.* Older children can benefit from a technique of focusing on breathing, then shifting focus to the area of discomfort, with emphasis on the fact that it is changing. Subsequently, the therapist can ask the child to focus on a piece of music or a scent (e.g., by bringing an open bottle of perfume or some other pleasant scent near the child's nose) and on the discomfort at the same time. The child will gradually learn that the perception of two stimuli fades as the attention is shifted to one.

## Reinforcement

We encourage – but do not demand – that our patients practice their skills in hypnotic pain control, using variations or new methods as they see fit. The more confident children are of their ability to use these skills, the more likely it is that they will use them whenever it is appropriate to do so. Other methods of reinforcement include selected use of recording self-hypnosis on a variety of devices; parents acting as therapeutic allies; group meetings; and communication with other patients who have successfully used hypnosis for pain control. After several practice sessions, the therapist can ask the child which type of relaxation or imagery exercise is most helpful. This can be recorded and placed over the child's favorite music, if he or she wishes, and made available to the child during procedures. The child can also be encouraged to record himself guiding himself through a relaxation exercise; this can also be placed over favorite music. Therapists should also encourage children who are skilled in pain control to help the therapist coach other children. This gives confidence to the child who is teaching and encourages the learner who can identify with that other child.

## Conclusion

Children can learn self-hypnosis to decrease or eliminate both affective and sensory aspects of pain. Functional magnetic resonance imaging (fMRI) studies have demonstrated that changes occur in the brain when hypnosis is used for pain control. Different areas of the brain are involved, depending on whether the discomfort is primarily affective or sensory. Teaching children hypnotic pain control must be based on the child's age, developmental stage, previous experiences with pain, and personal preferences. Children who use self-hypnosis successfully for pain control also enhance their sense of mastery and control. Because pain related to procedures or chronic pain can lead to posttraumatic stress disorders in children, it is important to provide all children with effective pain control interventions, including nonpharmacological interventions such as training in self-hypnosis.

## References


Accardi, M.C. & Milling, L.S. (2009). The effectiveness of hypnosis for reducing procedure-related pain in children and adolescents: a comprehensive methodological review. *Journal of Behavioral Medicine, 32*, 328–339.

Albunese, M.C., Duerden, E.G., Rainville, P., & Duncan, G.H. (2007). Memory traces of pain in human cortex. *Journal of Neuroscience, 27*, 4612–4620.

Anand, K. (1990). The biology of pain perception in newborn infants. In D. Tyler & E. Krane, Eds., *Advances in Pain Research and Therapy. Vol. 15. Pediatric Pain* (pp. 113–122). New York: Raven Press.

Anbar, R.D. (2001). Self-hypnosis for the treatment of functional abdominal pain in childhood. *Clinical Pediatrics, 40*, 447–451.

Barber, T.X. & Hahn, K.W. Jr. (1962). Physiological and subjective responses to pain producing stimulation under hypnotically-suggested and waking imagined "analgesia." *Journal of Abnormal and Social Psychology, 65*, 411–418.

Barnes, A.J. & Kohen, D.P. (2006). Clinical hypnosis as an effective adjunct in the care of pediatric in-patients. *Journal of Pediatrics, 149*, 563–565.

Birnie, K.A., Noel, M., Chamers, C.T., Uman, L.S., & Parker, J.A. (2018, October 4). Psychological interventions for needle-relate procedural pain and distress in children and adolescents. *Cochrane Database Systematic Reviews, 10*(10), CD005179.

Braid, J. (1960). *Neurypnology; or the Rationale of Nervous Sleep*. New York: Julian Press (original work published 1843; revised as *Braid on Hypnotism*, 1889).

Colville, G. (2008). The psychologic impact on children of admission to intensive care. *Pediatric Clinics of North America, 55*, 605–616.

Colville, G., Durkins, J., Hesketh, J., Bennett, V., Alcock, J., & Noyes, J. (2009). The impact on parents of a child's admission to intensive care: integration of qualitative findings from a cross-sectional study. *Intensive Critical Care Nursing, 25*, 72–79.

Colville, G., Kerry, S., & Pierce, C. (2008). Children's factual and delusional memories of intensive care. *American Journal of Respiratory and Critical Care Medicine, 177*, 976–982.

Crasilneck, H.B. & Hall, J.A. (1973). Clinical hypnosis in problems of pain. *American Journal of Clinical Hypnosis, 15*, 153–161.

Cyna, A.M., Tomkins, D., Maddock, T., & Barker, D. (2007). Brief hypnosis for severe needle phobia using switch-wire imagery in a 5-year-old. *Pediatric Anesthesia, 17*, 800–804.

Dahlquist, L.M., Gil, K.M., Armstrong, F.D., Ginsburg, A., & Jones, B. (1985). Behavioral management of children's distress during chemotherapy. *Journal of Behavior Therapy and Experimental Psychiatry, 16*, 325–329.

Delivet, H., Dugue, S., Ferrari,A., Postone, S., & Dahmani, S. (2018). Efficacy of self-hypnosis on quality of life for children with chronic pain syndrome. *International Journal of Clinical and Experimental Hypnosis, 66*(1), 43–55.

Dinges, D.F., Whitehouse, W.G., Orne, E.C., Bloom, P.B., Carlin, M.M., Bauer, N.K., & Gillen, K.A. (1997). Self-hypnosis training as an adjunctive treatment in the management of pain associated with sickle cell disease. *International Journal of Clinical and Experimental Hypnosis, 45*, 417–432.

Eland, J.M. & Anderson, J.E. (1977). The experience of pain in children. In A. Jacox, Ed., *Pain: A Source Book for Nurses and Other Health Professionals* (pp. 246–250). Boston, MA: Little, Brown and Company.

Erickson, C.J. (1991). Applications of cyberphysiologic techniques in pain management. *Pediatric Annals, 20*, 145–156.

Fitzgerald, M., Millard, C., & McIntosh, N. (1988). Hyperalgesia in premature infants. *Lancet, 1*, 292.

Fowler-Kerry, S. (1990). Adolescent oncology survivors' recollection of pain. In D. Tyler & E. Krane, Eds., *Advances in Pain Research and Therapy. Vol. 15. Pediatric Pain* (pp. 365–371). New York: Raven Press.

Gerik, S.M. (2005). Pain management in children: developmental considerations and mind–body therapies. *Southern Medical Journal, 98*, 295–302.

Goldstein, A. & Hilgard, E.R. (1975). Lack of influence of the morphine antagonist naloxone on hypnotic analgesia. *Proceedings of the National Academy of Sciences, 72*, 2041–2043.

Grant, J.A. & Rainville, P. (2005). Hypnosis and meditation: similar experiential changes and shared brain mechanisms. *Medical Hypotheses, 65*(3), 625–626.

Grant, J.A., Courtemanche, J., Duerden, E.G., Duncan, J.H., & Rainville P. (2010). Cortical thickness and pain sensitivity in zen meditators. *Emotion, 10*, 43–53.

Haslam, D.R. (1969). Age and the perception of pain. *Psychonomic Science, 15*, 86–87.

Hilgard, E.R. & Hilgard, J.R. (1975). *Hypnosis in the Relief of Pain*. Los Altos, CA: William Kaufman.

Hilgard, E.R. (1977). *Divided Consciousness: Multiple Controls in Human Thought and Action*. New York: John Wiley & Sons.

International Child Palliative Care Network (ISPCN). (2015). ISPCN pain assessment tool for children. Available at https://www.icpcn.org/icpcn-pain-assesssment-tool-for-children/

Jay, S.M., Ozolins, M., Elliott, C.H., & Caldwell, S. (1983). Assessment of children's distress during painful medical procedures. *Health Psychology, 2*, 133–147.

Jong, M.C., Boers, I., van Wietmarschen, H., Busch, M., Naafs, M.C., Kaspers, G.J.L., & Tissing, W.J.E. (2020). Development of an evidence-based decision aid on complementary and alternative medicine and pain for parents of children with cancer. *Support Care Cancer, 28*(5), 2415–2429.

Katz, E.R., Sharp, B., Kellerman, J., Marston, A.R., Hershman, J.M., & Siegel, S.E. (1982). Beta-endorphin immunoreactivity and acute behavioral distress in children with leukemia. *Journal of Nervous and Mental Disease, 170*, 72–77.

Kohen, D.P. (2017). The "3 and 6" hypnotic induction technique for children and adolescents. In M.P. Jensen, Ed., *The Art and Practice of Hypnotic Induction: Favorite Methods of Master Clinicians*. Kirkland, WA: Denny Creek Press. www.dennycreekpress.info

Kohen, D.P. & Zajac, R. (2007). Self-hypnosis training for headaches in children and adolescents. *Journal of Pediatrics, 150*, 635–639.

Kuttner, L. (1989). Management of young children's acute pain and anxiety during invasive medical procedures. *Pediatrician, 16*, 39–44.

Kuttner, L. (1991). Helpful strategies in working with preschool children in pediatric practice. *Pediatric Annals, 20*(3), 120–127.

Kuttner, L. (2010). *A Child in Pain: What Health Professionals Can Do to Help*. Bethel, CT: Crown House Publishing.

LeBaron, S. & Zeltzer, L. (1984). Assessment of acute pain and anxiety in children and adolescents by self-reports, observer reports, and a behavior checklist. *Journal of Consulting and Clinical Psychology, 52*, 729–738.

Liossi, C., White, P., & Hatira, P. (2006). Randomized clinical trial of local anesthetic versus a combination of local anesthetic with self-hypnosis in the management of pediatric procedure-related pain. *Health Psychology, 25*, 307–315.

Milling, L.S., Valentine, K.E., LaStimolo, M., Nett, A.M., & McCarley, H.S. (2021). Hypnosis and the alleviation of clinical pain: a comprehensive meta-analysis. *International Journal of Clinical and Experimental Hypnosis, 69*(3), 297–322.

Nunns, M., Mayhew, D., Ford, T., Rogers, M., Curie, C., Logan, S., & Moore, D. (2018). Effectiveness of nonpharmacological interventions to reduce procedural anxiety in children and adolescents undergoing treatment for cancer: a systematic review and meta-analysis. *Psychooncology, 27*(8), 1889–1899.

Olness, K. (1985). Hypnotherapy: a useful tool for busy pediatricians. *Contemporary Pediatrics*, 2, 66–78.

Olness, K. & Singher, L. (1989). Five year follow-up of 61 children taught cyber-physiologic strategies as adjunct management in cancer. *Topics in Pediatrics*, 7, 2–6.

Olness, K. & MacDonald, J. (1987). Headaches in children. *Pediatrics in Review, 8*, 307–311.

Petrie, A. (1967). *Individuality in Pain and Suffering*. Chicago: University of Chicago Press.

Rainville, P., Carrier, B., Hoffbauer, R.K., Bushnell, M.C., & Duncan, G.H. (2001). Dissociation of sensory and affective dimensions of pain using hypnotic modulation. *Pain, 82*, 159–171.

Rainville, P., Duncan, G.H., Price, D.D., Carrier, B., & Bushnell, M.C. (1997). Pain affect encoded in human anterior cingulate but not somatosensory cortex. *Science, 277*, 968–971.

Richardson, J., Smith, J.E., McCall, G., & Pilkington, K. (2006). Hypnosis for procedure-related pain and distress in pediatric cancer patients: a systematic review of effectiveness and methodology related to hypnosis interventions. *Journal of Pain and Symptom Management, 31*, 70–84.

Ross, D.M. & Ross, S.A. (1984). Childhood pain: the school-aged child's viewpoint. *Pain, 20*, 179–191.

Roy, M., Piche, M., Chen, J.I., Peretz, I., & Rainville, P. (2009). Cerebral and spinal modulation of pain by emotions. *Proceedings of the National Academy of Science, 106*, 20900–20905.

Russo, D. & Varni, J.W., Eds. (1982). *Behavioral Pediatrics: Research and Practice*. New York: Plenum Press.

Savedra, M.C., Tesler, M.D., Holzemer, W.L., & Ward, A. (1989). *Adolescent Pediatric Pain Tool (APPT) Preliminary User's Manual*. San Francisco, CA: University of California Press.

Schecter, N.L., Bernstein, B.A., Beck, A., Hart, L., & Sherzer, L. (1991). Individual differences in children's response to pain: role of temperament and parental characteristics. *Pediatrics*, *87*, 171–177.

Schecter, N.L., Berde, C.B., & Yaster, M., Eds. (2003). *Pain in Infants, Children, and Adolescents*, 2nd ed. Baltimore, MD: Lippincott Williams & Wilkins.

Stam, H.J. & Spanos, N.P. (1980). Experimental designs, expectancy effects, and hypnotic analgesia. *Journal of Abnormal Psychology*, *89*, 751–762.

Tome-Pires, C. & Miro, J. (2012). Hypnosis for the management of chronic and cancer procedure-related pain in children. *International Journal of Clinical and Experimental Hypnosis*, *60*(4), 432–457.

Tome-Pires, C., Sole, E., Racine, M., de la Vega, R., Castarlenas, E., Jensen, M.P., & Miro, J. (2016). Use of hypnotic techniques in children and adolescents with chronic pain: do the ages of patients or years of practice and theoretical orientation of clinicians matter? *International Journal of Clinical and Experimental Hypnosis*, *64*(4), 483–498.

US Department of Health and Human Services. (1992). *Acute Pain Management: Operative or Medical Procedures and Trauma*, Clinical Practice Guideline, AHCPR Pub. No. 92-0032. Rockville, MD: Agency for Health Care Policy and Research, US Public Health Service.

Varni, J.W. & Gilbert, A. (1982). Self-regulation of chronic arthritic pain and long-term analgesic dependence in a hemophiliac. *Rheumatology and Rehabilitation*, *22*, 171–174.

Varni, J.W., Katz, E.R., & Dash, J. (1982). Behavioral and neurochemical aspects of pediatric pain. In D.C. Russo & J.W. Varni, Eds., *Behavioral Pediatrics: Research and Practice*. New York: Plenum Press.

Varni, J.W., Thompson, K.L., & Hanson, V. (1987). The Varni–Thompson Pediatric Pain Questionnaire. I. Chronic musculoskeletal pain in juvenile rheumatoid arthritis. *Pain*, *28*, 27–38.

Vlieger, A.M., Menko-Frankenhuis, C., Wolfkamp, S.C., Tromp, E., & Benninga, M.A. (2007). Hypnotherapy for children with functional abdominal pain or irritable bowel syndrome: a randomized controlled trial. *Gastroenterology*, *133*(5), 1430–1436.

Wakeman, R.J. & Kaplan, J.Z. (1978). An experimental study of hypnosis in painful burns. *American Journal of Clinical Hypnosis*, *21*, 3–12.

West, N., Oakes, L., & Hinds, P.S. (1994). Measuring pain in pediatric oncology ICU patients. *Journal of Pediatric Oncology Nursing*, *11*, 64–68.

Wood, C. & Bioy, A. (2008). Hypnosis and pain in children. *Journal of Pain and Symptom Management*, *35*, 437–446.

Zeltzer, L., Dash, J., & Holland, J.P. (1979). Hypnotically induced pain control in sickle cell anemia. *Pediatrics*, *64*, 533–536.

# 13

# THERAPEUTIC HYPNOSIS FOR PEDIATRIC MEDICAL PROBLEMS

## Introduction

A growing body of clinical and research data attests to the effectiveness of therapeutic hypnosis applications in pediatric medicine (Anbar, 2007; Anbar & Hall, 2004; Barnes & Kohen, 2006; Bothe & Olness, 2007a, 2007b; Esparham & Dilts, 2019; Gillan, 2021; Hoekman et al., 2021; Jones, Culbert, & Kohen, 2009; Kohen, 2010a; Kohen & Ondich, 2004; Kohen & Zajac, 2007; Lee et al., 2021; Rutten et al., 2017; Sawni & Breuner, 2017; Sugarman, 2007; Wester & Sugarman, 2007).

In many instances, children can utilize their self-regulatory talents adjunctively to reduce or eliminate disease symptoms such as nausea or pain. Although clinical self-hypnosis may sometimes be a preferred primary therapeutic modality in certain conditions such as migraine or enuresis, currently it is more often a useful adjunct in modulating and moderating symptoms and effects of a wide variety of problems. As we develop more precision in making recommendations regarding self-hypnosis strategies, including timing, and as we learn more about the neurophysiologic correlates of the hypnotic experience (Acunzo, Oakley, & Terhune, 2021; Farahzadi & Kekecs, 2021; Houze, Streff, Piche, & Rainville, 2021; Raz, Keller, Norman, & Senechal, 2007), we may document the fact that specific disease processes may indeed be altered or even eliminated.

When children with medical problems successfully use therapeutic hypnosis skills, their expressions of victory and triumph are obvious and justified. They have less need for medications that, at best, are a nuisance and, at worst, may have harmful side effects such as stunting growth, damaging other body organs, causing hypoxia, and clouding consciousness. They spend less time in hospital wards and emergency rooms, and they suffer through fewer unpleasant medical procedures. They enjoy the physical and psychological benefits of normal activity. They move beyond the constricting role of the "sick one" in their families and develop a fuller sense of self based on a more balanced expression of needs and abilities. In every way, they are healthier.

For some children with chronic or life-threatening disease, therapeutic hypnosis accomplishments, and expectations for them, may be limited. These children often develop behavior disorders or experience severe anxiety and depression, usually associated with helplessness, hopelessness, and low self-esteem. Such difficulties may limit capacity for constructive fantasy and preclude the positive aspects of a doctor–patient relationship that seem to underlie successful use of hypnotherapeutic skills. Donald R., an adolescent boy with sickle cell anemia, initially seemed enthusiastic that learning self-hypnosis might allow better pain control and possibly reduce the

DOI: 10.4324/9781003243687-15

length of his frequent hospitalizations. He had good imagery skills and enjoyed hypnotic tennis games during which his pain and depression vanished; however, he could not overcome 16 years of being infantilized by his parents and living with the assumptions that the safest place was a hospital and that comfort came from narcotic drugs. Despite obvious relief from therapeutic hypnosis, he refused to use his skill in the absence of the therapist. As soon as she left his hospital room, he called the nurse to request more narcotics. Repeated efforts to help him met with this continued resistance, and the therapist eventually terminated visits.

There is much that we do not understand about the effects of chronic disease on perception and on the personality. One study, designed to investigate the relationships among perceived stress, self-esteem, and functional pain in adolescents with and without chronic disease found, unexpectedly, that patients with chronic disease scored significantly higher on self-esteem measures and lower on stress measures (Adams & Weaver, 1986). It has long been known that living through a critical situation gives one experience in facing later problems which also reduces the stress induced by such problems.

For some children, recent advances in medical management have allowed for cures to be achieved or for life and quality of life to be extended and improved, but new problems arise that challenge us to develop new therapeutic hypnosis approaches. Children who would have died a decade ago now live but have the added and new stress of having to cope with permanent disfigurement, with "survivor guilt" generated by the death of peers with the same illness, or with continuing pressure to feel deserving of having received an organ transplant at the risk of harming another person. We know relatively little about these problems of survival except that we can expect them to occur with increasing frequency unless therapeutic approaches that focus on prevention are developed. The possible role of clinical hypnosis as a preventive tool requires exploration.

Therapeutic methods that enhance a sense of mastery and competency are most likely to help children cope with medical problems and with the complications or effects of being cured. Children who successfully develop mastery skills may carry these skills into adulthood, becoming more able to cope effectively and reducing morbidity when illness occurs (Kohen, 2010a) and perhaps to prevent certain diseases. Therapeutic hypnosis interventions seem ideally suited to these ends.

The following discussion presents the applications of therapeutic hypnosis and self-hypnosis training for a wide variety of medical problems, based on the existing literature and on our own clinical experiences. There are many other medical problems in which clinical hypnosis might appropriately and analogously be expected to be useful, and we urge the reader to extrapolate from these examples to other problems accordingly.

## Allergies

### *Asthma*

Asthma affects more than 22 million Americans, including 6 million children; it is one of the most common chronic diseases of childhood. Asthma affects not only the child or adolescent patient but also their families and communities in terms of days lost from school and work, reduced quality of life, and preventable emergency department visits, hospitalizations, and deaths (National Asthma Education and Prevention Program Coordinating Committee et al., 2007). With a growing willingness to identify the problem of reactive airway disease as asthma in younger children, increasing numbers of preschool children carry the diagnosis of asthma and its attendant morbidity. In school children, asthma is the leading cause of time lost from school due to chronic disease. Nationally, 20–25% of school absenteeism is due to asthma, and an estimated 12 million days are spent in bed rest and 28 million days in restricted activities (Gevgen, Mullally, & Evans, 1988). Additional well-known morbidities include economic stress (physician and hospital visits, medications, laboratory studies) (Marion, Creer, & Reynolds, 1985; Sheffer, Bailey, Bleecker et al., 1991), time missed from school (Konig, 1978) and play (Francis, Krastins, & Levison, 1980), and negative effects on healthy, normal development such as maladaptive life styles (Leffert, 1980; Mattson, 1975). Many reports have focused on education-based, self-management programs (Bauchner, Howland, & Adair, 1988; Blessing-Moore, Fritz, & Lewiston, 1985; Carson, Council, & Schauer, 1991; Guevara, Wolf, Grum, & Clark, 2003; Hampel, Rudolph, Stachow, & Petermann, 2003; Hindi-Alexander, 1985; Kohen & Wynne, 1997; Rachelefsky & Siegel, 1985; Rachelefsky, Lewis, & de la Sota, 1985; Rakos, Grodek, & Mack, 1985; Smith et al., 2005; Wolf, Guevara, Grum, Clark, & Cates, 2003).

According to the 2007 National Asthma Education and Prevention Program Coordinating Committee report, asthma can best be understood and defined as follows:

> Asthma is a chronic inflammatory disorder of the airways in which many cells and cellular elements play a role: in particular, mast cells, eosinophils, neutrophils (especially in sudden onset, fatal exacerbations, occupational asthma, and patients who smoke), T lymphocytes, macrophages, and epithelial cells. In susceptible individuals this inflammation causes recurrent episodes of coughing (particularly at night or early in the morning), wheezing, breathlessness, and chest tightness. These episodes are usually associated with widespread but variable airflow obstruction that is often reversible either spontaneously or with treatment. (p. 9)

Limitation of airflow in asthma is caused by changes in the airway that are influenced by airway inflammation. In response to a variety of stimuli (e.g., irritants, allergens), bronchial smooth muscles contract and bronchoconstriction occurs, narrowing the airways. Airways of people with asthma are hyperreactive or hyperresponsive to stimuli, and as the disease becomes more persistent and inflammation more progressive, further narrowing of the airway occurs through hypersecretion of mucus, mucosal edema (swelling of the lining of the airway), and formation of mucus plugs. Different manifestations of asthma may have varying patterns of inflammation (such as varying intensity, cellular mediator pattern, or therapeutic response) (National Asthma Education and Prevention Program Coordinating Committee et al., 2007). Hormonal, autonomic nervous system, and neurotransmitter imbalances have been postulated as being involved. For example, Henderson and colleagues (1979) reported experiments in which patients with asthma were compared with normal controls and with patients who had allergic rhinitis. The pupils of the patients with asthma required significantly less phenylephrine to dilate than did the pupils of the other two groups. This difference suggests greater autonomic sensitivity or responsiveness in the patients with asthma.

Psychological factors have long been known to play a role in asthma. Though the nature, frequency, and evolution of this role has not been clearly defined, many children with asthma are described as anxious, shy, and dependent and may see themselves as passive victims of their disease (Anbar, 2017a, 2017b; Anbar & Sachdeva, 2011). They may be convinced, for example, that they must rely on medications for control of wheezing, and some with moderately severe asthma even conclude that a hospital is the only environment in which they can be safe. These children and adolescents will enter the emergency room dramatically and may not respond to drugs or psychological intervention until they are safely admitted and assured of remaining in the hospital.

The symptoms of asthma are powerful weapons, and children can use them consciously or unconsciously to control their families or to satisfy a variety of emotional needs (Anbar, 2003;

Anbar, 2017a, 2017b; Anbar & Sachdeva, 2011, Kohen, 1986b, 1997). Many clinicians have seen children stop wheezing within hours after being hospitalized, thus escaping from pressures and stressful and/or pathological interactions at home. Such observations may lead to recommendations for residential treatment, sometimes at a great distance from home. The problem with this approach is that, although patients may improve because of the separation, they eventually return to the same environment, with the likelihood of the vicious cycle beginning anew. It seems more effective in some cases to work with the child in the context of family treatment (Lehrer, 1998; Lehrer, Sargunaraj, & Hochron, 1992), perhaps including therapeutic hypnosis approaches for the entire family (Kohen, 1980a; Kohen & Wynne, 1997; Moore, 1980). At times, we encourage children to lead relaxation sessions with their parents, thus giving them the opportunity to exert a measure of control and influence with parents in a more constructive and positive way.

Other important psychological factors in asthma are expectation and suggestibility. Clinical observations of children and adults with asthma have demonstrated both increased and decreased wheezing in response to placebos coupled with appropriate suggestions. Laboratory studies have further documented this finding. Luparello, Leist, Lourie, and Sweet (1970) found that adults with asthma not only demonstrated increased airway resistance when given a placebo antigen but also reversed their bronchospasm when given a saline solution placebo. Thorne and Fisher (1978) found that adults with asthma experienced changes in physiological asthma, provided they were responsive to hypnotic induction. The same phenomena have been reported in children, based on both clinical observations (Reaney, Chang, & Olness, 1978) and laboratory research, including pulmonary function studies (Khan, Staerk, & Bonk, 1974). The latter study included 20 children with asthma, ages 8–13 years. Positive responses to hypnotically suggested asthma occurred in four children, all of whom scored high on the Barber Suggestibility Scale. Seven other high scorers, however, showed no change in pulmonary functions following the hypnotic suggestions. Moreover, some children reacted positively to sham allergens but not to hypnotic suggestion of bronchospasm, and *vice versa*. These data confirm our clinical impressions that psychological aspects of asthma are complex and that simplistic treatment approaches are likely to have a limited effect.

## Therapeutic Hypnosis Approaches to Childhood Asthma

Kohen (1986a, 1993, 1995b, 1997, 2000; Kohen & Wynne, 1997) noted that self-hypnosis is often helpful in the management of childhood asthma. It involves reduction of anxiety during acute episodes, early rapid abatement of wheezing, and reduction of frequency of wheezing episodes (Anbar, 2001, 2010), as well as reduction of functional morbidity such as school absences, improvement in personal sense of mastery, possible improvement in pulmonary function, and prevention of long-term morbidity.

Among the several reports of therapeutic hypnosis with children with asthma, most have positive results, but the actual methods used vary greatly from one study to another, making comparisons difficult. Treatment techniques have included hypnoanalytic and other insight-oriented methods, general ego-strengthening suggestions, relaxation training (Anbar, 2001, 2003; Chiang, Ma, Huang, Tseng, & Hsueh, 2009), teaching patients to increase and decrease wheezing, other suggestions aimed at enhancing the child's sense of control, training in self-hypnosis, and direct suggestions for symptom relief. Before reviewing this literature, we present three case reports representative of our current approaches to the problem. Generally, we emphasize increased mastery and control, and we urge patients to extend their hypnotic skills by training in self-hypnosis (Kohen, 1997). And even though we attempt to understand the underlying dynamics, insight-oriented techniques often play a relatively minor role. Careful assessment of individual adaptation and associated problems and needs is emphasized, however, because in selected cases, psychotherapy may be essential and integral to the evolution of change. The National Asthma Education and Prevention Program Coordinating Committee noted that their goal is "to help people with asthma control their asthma so that they can be active all day and sleep well at night." We agree and believe that the learning and practice of self-hypnosis facilitates achievement of this goal through symptom relief as well as through episode reduction and, in the process, through promotion of a sense of well-being and competency to both prevent and easily respond to modulate or eliminate future episodes of wheezing.

Sam M. was hospitalized at age 6 years for treatment of status asthmaticus. He had experienced multiple hospitalizations in another state for asthma, which had begun at age 4 years. He was hospitalized four times in rapid succession before being referred for help with clinical hypnosis. It was noted on the fourth admission that the patient "enjoys the hospital environment." There were significant family stresses, in that the parents had divorced approximately 1 year previously, the mother had a new baby by her second husband, and the parents were fighting over custody of Sam.

Sam was seen as an outpatient six times over a period of 6 weeks for therapeutic hypnosis. First, Sam and his family were given information about the disease, aided by drawings of the airway as an upside-down tree, with comparison of relaxed (dilated) and tight (constricted) branches. Sam was asked to prepare his own drawings of the bronchial tree with and without asthma, again to reinforce his knowledge and mastery of the situation. In hypnosis, he enjoyed visualizing himself on a flying blanket, going where he chose, in control, and loosening up his airways. He also visualized himself in the future, free of his asthma and enjoying an active game of football, his favorite sport. In between sessions, he was encouraged to practice self-hypnosis at home. It was noted during the third visit that he came in with active wheezing and a respiratory rate of 36 per minute over a 4-minute period. While in hypnosis, his respiratory rate reduced to 16 per minute, and wheezes were no longer heard on auscultation. A few minutes later, in the waiting room, he was heard to ask his mother if he could go home to play. She said that he would have to clean his room. Within 5 minutes, severe wheezing occurred that was again relieved via his self-hypnosis exercises. Shortly after treatment began, Sam's father noted that, while at home, he was able to "stop a bad attack in 20 minutes" using his self-hypnosis. Subsequently, he was seen approximately once a month for 6 months during which time, despite frequent acute episodes at home, he had no emergency room visits and no hospitalizations. Thirteen months after beginning therapeutic hypnosis, he was hospitalized and during his hospitalization he refused hypnosis. At this time, he seemed very upset over the conflict between his parents regarding his custody. His admission seemed to have been triggered by being grounded at home by his mother. He did not want to go home and repeatedly refused to practice his self-hypnosis. Subsequent follow-up was by telephone only. His father stated that the patient clearly could use his self-hypnosis and did so frequently; however, the family conflict remained unresolved. The parents refused a recommendation for psychotherapy.

Hugh N. was first seen for therapeutic hypnosis at age 7 years. His asthma had progressed to the point that he frequently had to stay home from school, and his pediatrician was about to begin steroid therapy. A cute redhead, Hugh's eyes sparkled at the idea of learning hypnotic skills. When he described his problem as not being able to get enough air into his lungs, the therapist explained that the problem in asthma is really not being able to get trapped air out of the lungs. Following good response to hypnosis initiation involving progressive relaxation and hand levitation, the therapist asked, "What color are your lungs today?" When Hugh said he didn't know what color his lungs were, the therapist – with a twinkle – told him to stop talking like a grownup and to answer the question. Grinning, Hugh said his lungs were green. Then the therapist said, "Good. Now what color is the air for you today?" Still grinning, Hugh said the air was orange.

The therapist then said, "Fine. Now take a nice deep breath. Watch that orange air go all the way down to the very bottom of your lungs until all you see is orange. Then breathe out and watch all the orange air come up so that your lungs are all green again, from top to bottom." After Hugh successfully used this imagery, the therapist remarked that she hadn't heard him wheeze and asked him to imagine a beginning acute episode of asthma. He produced a barely audible wheeze. The therapist said, "That's not much of a wheeze – can't you do better than that?" When Hugh wheezed more clearly, the therapist said, "Good. Now you have shown us that you really can control your wheezing. You can make it worse. Now control it the other way and make it go away." He did.

This conversation led to further discussion of mastery, following which Hugh was taught self-hypnosis. The therapist suggested that he practice the color exercises daily and that he also use his hypnotic talent at the first sign of any wheezing. In the office Hugh demonstrated his skills to his mother, and they agreed that he would be responsible for practice. One week later, Hugh's mother reported marked improvement, and treatment was terminated after three more sessions. About 1 year later, Hugh requested another appointment, stating that he had forgotten his skills and that his asthma was getting worse again. One therapeutic hypnosis review session was sufficient to put him back in control, and follow-up some months later revealed continuing gains. Steroids were never begun. In the initial sessions, Hugh's mother admitted that she feared he might die or get into serious trouble and that she knew she was overprotective toward him; however, she refused the therapist's suggestion that she obtain counseling or psychotherapy for herself. The family eventually moved away, out of state.

Gerald was first taught self-hypnosis when he was 9 years old. He had wheezing as an infant, which was first officially called asthma when he was 2 years old. One of two children of a hard-working single mother who smoked, Gerald was frequently ill with ear infections, colds, and other respiratory illnesses, many of which triggered acute episodes of wheezing. In the 3 years prior to learning hypnosis, he had been hospitalized on more than 10 occasions and had been to the emergency room almost monthly for acute wheezing. He was taught the anatomy and pathophysiology of asthma, with emphasis on the imagery of the lungs and airways as an upside-down tree and muscles around airways that can be looser or tighter. In hypnosis he was asked to imagine himself doing something he liked – such as playing basketball. He was then asked to notice the very first and earliest sign of wheezing beginning and to "let that be your signal to stop, do your self-hypnosis, picture your breathing tubes and let the muscles around them get loose, soft, floppy, relaxed, and comfortable so that all the air you need can get in and out." As this was reviewed and reinforced, Gerald agreed to practice once or twice daily even when he was feeling fine "so that your muscles can learn what to do at the right time in the right way, maybe even automatically," as well as practicing whenever he had wheezing. The frequency of acute episodes, emergency room visits, and hospitalizations decreased dramatically with the practice of this cue-controlled self-hypnosis.

Two years later, the therapist asked Gerald if he would make a videotape demonstration of his control of asthma with hypnosis. Considering its potential educational value, the clinician wondered about giving Gerald hypnotic suggestions to develop and then stop the wheezing. Having never done so in any prior clinical hypnosis sessions with Gerald or other patients, the clinician casually asked Gerald what he thought of that possibility as they walked to the room where their session was to be videotaped. Gerald responded with a look of skepticism. The clinician reassured him matter of factly that he didn't know if he'd suggest anything like that, but if he did that it didn't matter, offering the "waking," conversational suggestion "because you know how to get rid of wheezing when you need to anyway." A few minutes later, the interview and therapeutic hypnosis session began (Kohen, 1982). In the interview Gerald noted that since learning hypnosis he had not had to come to the emergency room that much and that if he got his wheezing he would "just practice." Like many children, his internal understanding of the hypnotic experience was clearer than his verbal explanation. He noted, "When I practice, I go to my room and just think. But before I do, I sit up there and think about what I'll be thinkin' about, and then when I practice I'll know what I'll be thinkin' about when I think about it." Gerald spontaneously suggested that the imagery be about "mountain climbing," supplying a wonderful metaphor for problem solving.

In the therapeutic hypnosis session that followed, the clinician offered many suggestions – both direct and indirect – for control of Gerald's asthma, including (1) making sure that the ropes for climbing were tied just right, not too loose and not too tight, "just like your climbing muscles and lung muscles"; (2) noticing that "each time you take a turn on the path while climbing that you get more and more relaxed and comfortable"; and (3) "noticing how proud you feel for what you are accomplishing." Suggestions were then given that he would notice coming near a cloud of thick, gray smoke while climbing and that the smoke made breathing more difficult. He began to cough, breathe more rapidly, and to wheeze. Suggestions for increasing awareness of this response resulted in more wheezing and increased respiratory rate that were then followed by calm suggestions to "walk right away from that cloud and notice how much easier it is to breathe." His respiratory rate slowed again, and the wheezing disappeared.

Following the therapeutic hypnosis session, Gerald alerted and was asked to describe what he had experienced. He reported that he had imagined climbing the mountain with a friend (though no such imagery had been suggested), and that they had "got a lot higher than half of it." He said that "when we got pretty high, I started wheezing, and I asked him what we should do, and he said we should rest, and while we were resting, I practiced, and in my practice I imagined that I was on this trip to Hawaii on this beach." The clinician was amazed at this wonderful imagery and asked, "So, while you were mountain climbing in your imagination you had *another* imagination, and while you were doing that what happened to your wheezing?" Gerald replied, "It got clear … it was kind of hard to do it, but I did it." His sense of pride was clearly evident, as was his awareness that the imagery used to accomplish success was his own. At the end of the interview, the clinician asked Gerald if he used his hypnosis for anything else, knowing that he had already solved his problems of nocturnal enuresis and nail biting with self-hypnosis. Gerald demurred talking about those but instead casually described how he doesn't feel any discomfort "… when a nurse "gives me a shot. It doesn't hurt. I kind of just notice it." Gerald agreed to make a sequel to his video someday.

More than 6 years later, at age 17 years, he called, needing a physical examination. The clinician had not seen him in over 2 years and asked if he would be willing to make another videotape. He agreed. In the video (Kohen, 1987), he reported the continued utility of his self-hypnosis, particularly for exercise-induced asthma, noting that he needed only a few minutes to get himself together after he started wheezing, for example, while playing basketball. He described multisensory techniques: "I picture my lungs upside down. I hear it, and when I hear it less, I know I'm better. And I feel it. You know, you can massage that mucus out of there." He then spontaneously described what we have speculated about and heard from other children: "The imagination, now it's automatic, it is … it's like it's built in" (Kohen, 1987). In discussing this with Gerald he reflected his own sense of changing understanding of hypnosis and self-hypnosis as he matured from a boy of 11 to a young adult of 17. He even said, "When I was younger, in doing my hypnosis I used to concentrate on sound. I hear it less and I know I'm getting better. … Now I still do that, *but* I can also tell from *feeling* it and *seeing* it in my imagination." Gerald's insights reflect the growth of his understanding and how he can use internal resources to develop comfort, relieving the asthma as well as the symptoms of anxiety and associated dyspnea. Anbar (2004), Anbar and Sachdeva (2011), and Anbar (2017a, 2017b) also described the value of hypnosis in helping dyspnea and other symptoms associated with asthma and other conditions.

## Results of Therapeutic Hypnosis with Children with Asthma

Review of research literature reveals that widely disparate clinical hypnosis techniques result in similar and sometimes dramatic improvement in asthma. Clearly, we don't yet understand the mechanisms of change. Possibilities include enhancement of mastery, reduction of anxiety that may have some physiological effect, direct effects in relaxing bronchial smooth muscle, changes in parental attitudes and behavior, and resolution of unconscious conflicts. In any study, it is important to realize that the postulated mechanisms of change, derived from theoretical positions and related technical approaches, may or may not actually be responsible for the observed and obviously improved medical status.

Diamond (1959) used hypnoanalytic techniques with 55 children with asthma who had no positive findings on skin testing or had not responded to vaccine therapy. Five children did not respond at all to hypnotic induction, and another ten achieved only a "modest response." Of the remaining 40 patients, all achieved complete remission of symptoms and remained symptom free during a 2- to 4-year follow-up period. These children reportedly experienced hypnotic age regression to the time of the first episode of asthma, associated with emotional trauma such as severe guilt or fear of loss of parental love. They then responded to insight-oriented approaches in which they reportedly no longer needed to use their asthma as a way of getting positive parental attention and developing feelings of emotional security.

Smith and Burns (1960) used direct hypnotic suggestions for immediate and progressive symptom relief with 25 children and adolescents with asthma ages 8–15 years. All responded satisfactorily to clinical hypnosis, and some claimed subjective improvement over the 4-week treatment period; however, repeated pulmonary function tests revealed no significant change in any of the children. The authors concluded that they had failed to demonstrate any value of hypnotic suggestion for improved pulmonary functions. We wonder whether the experimenters expected negative results and therefore may have communicated a subtle bias. We also wonder whether the "strongly suggested" relief was expressed, perhaps, in a very authoritarian way in this clinic, perhaps circumventing the children's egos and unwittingly supporting passivity.

Diego (1961) taught five boys with asthma, ages 11–13 years, to precipitate and stop acute episodes of asthma in hypnosis. He then gave them posthypnotic suggestions that they would be able to stop future such episodes by hypnotic relaxation. All five patients reported rapid subjective improvement, and four continued to improve over several months of follow-up. One boy relapsed after a month but improved again following a year of insight-oriented psychotherapy.

Years later, Aronoff, Aronoff, and Peck (1975) studied the efficacy of therapeutic hypnosis in aborting acute episodes of asthma in 17 children and adolescents, ages 6–17 years. Subjects were given direct hypnotic suggestions for chest relaxation, easy breathing, and reduction of wheezing. In most cases, they experienced immediate improvement, as measured both by pulmonary function tests and subjective reports. The authors noted that anxiety may aggravate asthma by stimulating the autonomic nervous system, and they speculated that "hypnosis, by promoting general relaxation, diminishes vagal stimulation and consequently diminishes release of mediators felt to be responsible for the bronchospasm" (Aronoff et al., 1975, p. 361). Though the method in this study is like that of Smith and Burns (1960), we suspect that the general approach may have been more permissive and ego supportive.

Collison (1975) reported a retrospective analysis of 121 patients with asthma managed with therapeutic hypnosis. This report included six patients under age 10 years and 39 under age 20 years.

Collison developed four categories of response: "excellent," when there was complete freedom from episodes of asthma without medication in the follow-up period; "good," when there was a reduction of acute episodes with continuation of medications; "poor," when there was less than 50% improvement in frequency of episodes or need for medication; and "nil," when there was no change from the pre-treatment assessment. Of the six youngest patients, four had excellent or good responses. Of 39 patients in the 11- to 20-year-old category, 32 had excellent or good responses. The older age groups, however, had significantly fewer satisfactory responses. Because the youngest groups also were most responsive to hypnotic induction, there was some question as to whether age or depth of trance would be a better predictor of success in a prospective study. Severity of disease was also an important variable. Patients whose asthma was not so severe as to require steroids generally responded best to hypnotherapy. Collison's techniques included suggestions for ego strengthening and for general relaxation, together with exploration of psychological factors related to the disease. He deliberately avoided direct suggestions for symptom removal, fearing that such suggestions might serve only to mask medical problems and ultimately have a harmful effect. He noted the inherent difficulties in retrospective analysis and the need for prospective studies that control the multiple variables involved.

Barbour (1980) reported preliminary results of the use of self-hypnosis in adolescents with asthma. A study of six patients over a 5-month period indicated that the use of self-hypnosis was associated with a reduction in the severity and frequency of acute episodes of asthma. Before self-hypnosis training, skin tests with local inhalant antigens done on four patients demonstrated positive reactions to 14 antigens; skin tests were positive for only seven antigens after 5 months of self-hypnosis. The same four patients also had skin testing done in a hypnotic state, and no reactivity to antigens occurred in any of the patients. This finding encourages the possibility that immune responses may be modified via appropriate uses of therapeutic hypnotic suggestion and that therapeutic hypnosis may not only reduce morbidity from asthma but also, in fact, be curative in certain patients.

Kohen (1986b, 1995b) reported a prospective study of 28 children with asthma who were randomized to control groups and a group who learned self-hypnosis techniques. Although there were no differences between the experimental and control groups with respect to pulmonary function tests from the initial to post-intervention periods, dramatic improvements were observed after 1 year and after 2 years of follow-up. There were dramatic improvements in Forced Expiratory Flow (FEF) 25–75% in five patients at 2 months. These correlated with evidence prior to the study that these children had previous experience with significant, spontaneous self-hypnosis. Future studies that control for this variable are essential.

Chiang and colleagues (2009) reported the results of a randomized controlled trial of relaxation breathing training on anxiety and asthma in children 6–14 years old in Taiwan with moderate to severe asthma. Selected from an outpatient clinic, patients were randomly assigned to an experimental group who received 30 minutes of training in a relaxation-breathing technique and a CD for home practice or to a control group. Both groups received training and education in an asthma self-management program. The relaxation training was classical Jacobsonian relaxation with progressive tensing and relaxing of muscles beginning at the feet and progressing upward, ending in the chest, neck, shoulders, and face. The children were taught to self-report the degree of relaxation on a relaxation visual analogue scale, and frontal electromyogram biofeedback was also employed. Beyond the use of the home CD, younger children were coached by parents, and researchers contacted patients weekly over the 12-week experimental period. Participants reported practicing an average of at least 30 minutes three times weekly over the 12 weeks. The results demonstrated that relaxation breathing combined with a self-management (education) program improved physiological indicators including peak expiratory flow rate (PEFR) and psychological indicators (anxiety), but comparable improvement was seen in the control group who did not have the relaxation breathing component. Notably, state anxiety was significantly lower for children in the experiment group than in the control group.

Although we do not recommend the use of therapeutic hypnosis in childhood asthma as a substitute for usual medications, we do believe that it can reduce the need for visits to emergency rooms, hospitalizations, and, in some children, the requirement for certain medications.

Hackman and colleagues (Hackman, Stern, & Gershwin, 2000) published a review of studies of hypnosis in asthma. In their tabulation and discussion of 20 studies published between 1960 and 1997, they identified 1,040 subjects between 2 and 80 years of age who had learned hypnosis for asthma. Studies are described and categorized by their degree of randomization and control as well as results, and the authors noted their exclusion of numerous case studies. In summarizing, they concluded that hypnosis was more effective in subjects more "susceptible" to hypnosis and that the duration of hypnosis may affect the results, and they suggested drawing a distinction between hypnosis and relaxation. They also concluded that the significant benefits reported in non-randomized and non-placebo-controlled studies suggest that hypnosis is a powerful technique for treating asthma; therefore, additional randomized trials are necessary to further explore and understand these benefits. Curiously, Hackman et al. also concluded that pharmaceutical products seem to work better and are more time effective than hypnosis. We think this is an erroneous conclusion (Kohen, 2000), particularly as we and others have observed that for some people the application of self-hypnosis even for the first time has been effective in resolving acute episodes of wheezing and as a deterrent to hospitalization (Anbar, 2010, 2017b; Kohen, 1986a, 2000). For some, it has been of sufficient value to obviate the need for any medication at all (Kohen, Colwell, Heimel, & Olness, 1984), and for most in our experience it has been a very welcome and effective addition to an overall treatment program geared to the goals outlined (Kohen, 1995b; National Asthma Education and Prevention Program Coordinating Committee et al., 2007).

Although we are not attempting a complete review of all psychological approaches to childhood asthma, we want to mention that several studies involving other forms of self-regulation, notably relaxation training (without mention of hypnosis *per se*) or biofeedback training have reported positive results (Feldman, 1976; Khan, 1977; Scherr & Crawford, 1978). The work of Kotses and colleagues (Kotses & Miller, 1987; Kotses et al., 1991) suggests that biofeedback (electromyographic facial biofeedback) as a method of producing relaxation in facial muscles improves some measures of pulmonary function in children with asthma and adults without asthma. In a clinical trial with 29 children with asthma, Kotses and colleagues (1991) compared the long-term effect of training to decrease facial muscle tension with training to hold it at the same level. Subjects showed improvement in some pulmonary function measurements, and those trained to decrease facial muscle tension also showed a greater improvement in their attitudes toward asthma and a reduction in anxiety, both of which may have also contributed to the observed changes in pulmonary function.

Spevack, Vost, Maheux, and Bestercezy (1978) reported that children with asthma responded well to training in "passive relaxation." We wonder about the extent to which these children may have been responding to unintended hypnotic suggestion, especially as some of the studies included training in progressive relaxation. As we have noted earlier, hypnosis can occur without any formal hypnotic invitation or initiation. At the same time, when studies purport to relate hypnotherapy to relief from asthma but fail to measure trance responsiveness, it is not clear that children who improve were actually in hypnosis. We have already seen (Khan et al., 1974) that some children with documented hypnotic talent do not respond to suggestions related to their disease. Clearly more research is required before we can untangle the possibilities in this complex area.

## Recurrent Hives

We have noted clinically that children suffering from recurrent generalized hives or massive reactions to bee stings have had fewer difficulties and more rapid recoveries when using adjunct therapeutic hypnotic suggestions. Suggestions given have included those for general relaxation, mastery, and imagery of the patient without the swellings. It is possible that the state induced by hypnosis does reduce the allergic response. It may be directly, through effects on a mediator of immune reactions, such as the mast cell (a cell which stores granules containing potent inflammatory and repair materials released upon injury to the organism), or indirectly, through reduction of heart rate, blood pressure, and respiratory rates. Preliminary studies of the effects of suggestions given under hypnosis on immune processes were conducted by Good (1981) in the late 1950s. Because of the important implications for patients with specific allergies and immunodeficiencies, these studies should be expanded and replicated (see also Chapter 18).

## Specific Allergies

Perloff and Spiegelman (1973) reported the use of therapeutic hypnosis in treating a 10-year-old girl's allergy to dogs. The child, acutely sensitive to dog dander but wishing to have a dog, was taught a visual desensitization while in hypnosis. Thereafter, her sensitivity to dog dander disappeared. Barbour's (1980) study with adolescents lends credibility to this clinical report.

Madrid and Barnes (1991) presented a case report of a successful single session therapeutic hypnosis intervention for a 12-year-old girl with a 7-year history of "stuffy and running nose continually … since she moved to the country." With the hypothesis that their technique triggered state-dependent memory, learning, and behavior, they suggested to the patient that when her body remembered how to heal itself and starts doing it her index finger would twitch and float in an ideomotor response. After several suggestions evoked no response, they noted, "Consider your nose is too small to be fighting off these pollens all by itself. You need to use the rest of your body to get involved in dealing with these irritants. Use your arms and chest and legs and stomach to handle these things. Your nose is so small and can't do it all." In response to this suggestion, the patient's finger twitched, and legs and torso jerked for 15 seconds. Reinforcing suggestions were offered that her body could remember how to do this. Her nose was clear after the session and remained clear at a 3-month follow-up.

An 11-year-old patient of ours, Sarah, had learned and applied self-hypnosis very effectively for management of her asthma, so much so that with the guidance of her allergist she was able to stop taking any medications and, instead, applied self-hypnosis whenever she had what became very infrequent episodes of minor wheezing. One day Sarah called from the lobby of the hospital and asked if she could come up to my office and talk. As there was room in the schedule that day, I was able to meet with her. Sarah said matter-of-factly, "Can hypnosis help with hay fever?" I asked her why she wanted to know, and she explained that even though her asthma was "tons better," that she continued to have "major problems" with runny nose and itchy red eyes for several months during pollen season. She then asked, "What are allergies, anyway?" I followed with a brief explanation of mast cells and how upon exposure to various antigens (such as pollens in the air) they release substances such as histamine into the bloodstream that ultimately cause the allergic reaction. A bright young lady, she said, "Histamine? Oh, is that why I sometimes take an "*anti*histamine to help the symptoms?" I, of course, answered, "Yes." She then inquired, "So, then all I really have to do with my hypnosis is keep the histamine inside the mast cells, and not let it go outside into the bloodstream?" Though surprised at this observation, I agreed. She said, "Thanks a lot!" and left.

Several months later her mother informed me that, despite the high pollen counts, Sarah's hay fever symptoms of allergic conjunctivitis and rhinitis had been so minimal as to require no medications. As we have noted with so many of our patients, we are unsure whether these results are a function of the self-hypnosis and its positive suggestions, the patient's positive expectations, self-confidence, an understanding of the physiology involved, the specific imagery, or some combination of all of these. Even though it may not matter at the clinical level, there is much research to be done to clarify the answer to these questions (see also Chapter 18).

## Cystic Fibrosis

Cystic fibrosis (CF) is the most common life-shortening autosomal recessive disease of Caucasians in the United States; it occurs in approximately 1 in 2,500 white live births and 1 in 17,000 black live births in the United States. In 1992, the median projected life expectancy for patients in the United States was 28 years; in 2000, it was 32 years; and by 2008 the figure had risen to a mean predicted age of survival of 37.4 years (Cystic Fibrosis Foundation, 2010).

Today, because of improved medical treatments and care, more than half of people with CF are age 18 or older. Many people with CF can expect to live healthy, fulfilling lives into their 30s, 40s, and beyond (Cystic Fibrosis Foundation 2022).

Over 95% of patients die of progressive respiratory failure. Now known to be caused by defects in a single gene on the long arm of chromosome 7, CF is characterized by chronic obstruction and infection of airways, maldigestion, and their consequences. Dysfunction of exocrine glands is responsible for a sometimes confusing and broad array of manifestations. It is the major cause of severe chronic lung disease of children and also causes most exocrine pancreatic insufficiency in early life. The current treatment of CF addresses delaying the consequences of organ dysfunction and failure rather than correcting the underlying defect. With identification of the gene for CF in 1989 and cloning of the DNA, it is hoped that gene therapy will provide a breakthrough in treatment, and research is ongoing.

In the meantime, those with CF require extensive therapy, including (1) dozens of pancreatic enzyme pills, (2) antibiotics, (3) nutritional supplements, (4) chest percussion by a respiratory therapist or a motorized, vibratory vest, and (5) aerosolized nebulizer medications. Clinic visits, hospitalizations, repeated pulmonary function tests, blood tests, and intravenous therapies round out the framework of management for the average youngster with CF, whose life is often functionally quite different from that of his or her peers. Physical activity may be limited both by the severity of lung disease and the rigorous schedule of daily treatments.

A 1994 pilot study explored the effects of self-hypnosis as a coping strategy for 12 children and teenagers with CF (Belsky & Khanna, 1994). The authors focused the hypnotic imagery on a theme of overall mastery of the effects of chronic illness and improvements in functioning, with specific suggestions for thinner mucus, clearer lungs, deeper breathing, and improved absorption of medication. Six children with CF in the experimental group (learning hypnosis) were studied along with six comparable youngsters with CF in the control group. Results supported the authors' hypothesis that self-hypnosis would be associated with well-being as measured by five standard psychological measures. On four of five measures, the change scores from the first to the second interview showed statistically significant differences between the group learning self-hypnosis and the control group. Significant differences were noted in (1) locus of control (Nowicki–Strickland Locus of Control for Children), with children who learned self-hypnosis reflecting more internality or sense of independence; (2) children's health locus of control (Parcel Children Health Locus of Control), with the experimental group showing a positive change in attitude about control; (3) Piers–Harris Self-Concept Scale; and (4) trait anxiety, with an increase in anxiety for the control group and a decrease in the experimental group. In addition, the experimental group could be distinguished from the control group by differences (improvements) in peak expiratory flow rate, a measurement of lung function. Although the authors noted the limitations of generalizability of this small-sample-size study, they have provided preliminary information that supports the value of self-hypnosis in enhancing psychological well-being and improving physiological functioning. Future studies can and should build upon this important research.

We have had the opportunity to work with an increasing number of children, adolescents, and young adults with CF. Each was referred for clinical hypnosis treatment to help with one or more problems associated with CF or its treatment (Kohen, 1994). Each has benefited definitively and sometimes dramatically from therapeutic hypnosis. Applications have included (1) pain control, including distraction, dissociation, switches to turn down or turn off pain, and amnesia for previous (painful) experiences; (2) anxiety control, via distraction or dissociation, relaxation, focused breathing, the jettison technique, and various forms of imagery; (3) taste control, through the switches technique and negative and positive hallucinations; (4) nausea control, through use of imagery, distraction, and dissociation; and (5) general control of disease, with suggestions for the use of imagery, future projection, and self-control. Case descriptions of successful utilization of therapeutic hypnosis with children and adolescents with CF are also discussed in Chapter 15, and details can be found in a recent publication (Friedrichsdorf & Kohen, 2018).

Although our patients have varied from 5 to 28 years of age and CF has played a unique role in each of their lives, some generalizations can be made from their collective experience. The application of hypnotic strategies to help modulate the uncertainty and anxiety that are hallmarks of chronic illness is perhaps its greatest value. Our clinical observations of this are strongly supported by Belsky and Khanna's (1994) work as described above. The ability to use hypnosis to reduce, manage, or eliminate the fear of loss of control has been markedly evident in the young people with whom we have worked. Anbar has also reported on this in several publications (Anbar, 2000b, 2001, 2017b).

Our experience was echoed by Anbar (2000b) in his case report of a 13-year-old young man who learned self-hypnosis to manage phlebotomy-associated pain and anxiety and later developed this competency in self-regulation to help himself fall asleep at night, to eliminate headaches, and to be generally more confident. Anbar's (2001) report of the efficacy of self-hypnosis to manage chronic dyspnea reinforces the application of self-hypnosis training for youth with CF. In his study of 49 patients with CF who learned self-hypnosis, Anbar (2000a) reported that 86% of patients considered hypnosis to be beneficial, notably to relax, to improve tolerance of medical procedures, to cope with headaches, and, for some, to improve adherence to therapies. Anbar (2010) also recently described the importance of hope for children with chronic illness and how hypnosis may contribute positively to hope.

In a paper, Delord et al. (2013) described a pilot study utilization medical hypnosis to assist in acclimating children to be able to cope with non-invasive positive pressure ventilation (NPPV) during sleep. One of the patients was a 13-year-old with CF who had end stage lung disease and severe dyspnea. Despite her respiratory failure and initial fear of the apparatus, she was able to use imagery in hypnosis successfully (imagining herself on a shopping tour) to dissociate from her fear and accept the non-invasive positive pressure ventilation. Within a few breaths she noticed relief and adhered easily to the NPPV (Delord et al., 2013). Although a cure for CF seems to be on the not too distant horizon, the knowledge that anxiety can be managed with the aid of hypnosis is a great comfort to those already in the end stages of this disease and suffering the anxiety associated with dyspnea, hypoxia, and associated sleep deprivation. The ability to take a measure of control of appetite, to modulate discomfort, and to exercise control of weight not only provides comfort but can also potentially add life to this as yet life-threatening disease. Details regarding specific therapeutic hypnosis approaches to various aspects of CF can be found in a recent publication (Anbar, 2017b).

No other references to the applications of hypnosis for children and youth with CF were identified between 2011 and 2021.

## Dermatological Problems

### *Itching, Scratching, and Picking*

Therapeutic hypnosis provides a useful adjunct in the management of many skin conditions, including atopic eczema, psoriasis, and acne. In these conditions, teaching of self-hypnosis may serve to reduce scratching or picking and therefore interrupt the vicious cycle of scratching and picking, discomfort, scratching and picking, exacerbation, and more discomfort. Suggestions that encourage general relaxation, a sense of mastery in controlling the disease progress, and images of coolness and wetness seem most helpful in these situations.

Mirvish (1978) reported a case history in which clinical therapeutic hypnosis led to relief of symptoms and improved behavior in a 10-year-old boy with chronic eczema. Olness (1977) reported a case of intractable itching in a 9-year-old boy hospitalized for evaluation of possible rheumatoid arthritis. The pediatric resident caring for the boy considered teaching the boy self-hypnosis but had not yet begun when a social worker came to request urgent help. The boy was, at that moment, clawing at himself frantically. Olness established that the social worker had good rapport with the boy and asked her to sit down with him and talk about something cool like a swimming pool or a lake. The social worker said, "He's afraid of water. In fact, he won't get in the bathtub here." Olness then suggested the concept of snow and ice and winter sports. An hour later, the social worker returned, elated. She had discovered that snow sliding was a great joy for this boy. They sat together, imagining a particular hill and its particular bumps, and they felt the snow spray as they slid down the hill. The incessant scratching stopped. Two days later, when a resident asked the patient's private physician about starting steroids, the physician, watching the boy racing down the hall, said, "He doesn't need them now. Since he started that self-hypnosis, he's doing fine." One might question whether or not formal clinical therapeutic hypnosis was used. Certainly, rapport with an interested and caring therapist, imagery, and suggestion of a feeling to counter pruritus all contributed to the successful outcome for this patient. This is very consistent with the utilization principle, i.e., the value of rapport leading to elucidation of the child's interests and helping him to *utilize his own favorite imagery/activity to* reduce/eliminate the troublesome symptoms.

As is true in conditions associated with uncomfortable symptoms, it is often helpful to teach self-hypnosis to children who itch and to recommend that they practice when they are comfortable in order to have more facility in self-control when symptoms recur. Often a simple playful suggestion (e.g., "Just picture the *itch switch* in your mind's imagination … and when you see it clearly … then … just … turn … it … down until it's turned off. That's right.") will suffice to empower the child to practice and develop control over the troubling symptom. Even without the necessity or benefit of a formal hypnotic invitation procedure, offering such a suggestion coupled with enthusiasm and positive expectancy may evoke a positive hypnotic response and outcome of reduced or eliminated itch. This Ericksonian approach has been effective on several occasions when during an interview or conversation a child has begun to scratch repeatedly, even incessantly, and complain of intense itching. Kohen has approached this with an abrupt change of focus and an appeal to both the obvious desire for change and the child's imaginative abilities: "Hey! You mean I never told you about the itching switch? You know, the one inside your mind? Just close your eyes and look at it … see what color it is … see what shape it is, and then, when you're ready, turn it off … 1 … 2 … 3 … CLICK!" Commonly the child opens his eyes and says, "It worked!" After a "high 5" congratulations we change the subject of conversation.

## Hyperhidrosis

Ambrose (1952) reported a case of a 13-year-old boy with excessive sweating who responded to therapeutic clinical hypnosis. The condition had begun at age 8, when the boy was evacuated during World War II. While hypnotically regressed to age 8, he remembered being beaten up by a gang of boys while on his way to his new school. The boy became quite tense when describing these events, which he also recalled out of trance. Following six visits, he had no further problems in control of sweating. Ambrose postulated that the clinical training in therapeutic hypnosis cut off the increased release of acetylcholine at the postganglionic nerves that had previously caused excessive sweating. At this time, this hypothesis has been neither confirmed nor denied, but studies of chemical mediations coincidental with clinical hypnosis are essential for comprehension of mechanisms involved in such dramatic resolution of autonomic response problems.

We saw an 8-year-old girl who was referred specifically for clinical therapeutic hypnosis for profuse sweating. As neither the referring pediatrician nor the consulting dermatologist was able to determine a successful therapy, they concluded that "hypnosis might be worth a try." Although the mother was concerned that in the future her daughter's profuse sweating would produce an offensive odor, the girl was already distraught at being teased for having wet hands and at reprimands from teachers for smearing or smudging her school papers. Indeed, during the first visit her hands literally dripped sweat when held out palms downward. During the initial interview and development of rapport, an imagery idea presented itself. As the history of the problem was being discussed, the patient became increasingly sad and soon began to cry, first slowly and then profusely. With comforting from her mother and the therapist, the tearfulness slowed and ceased, and the sadness lightened. She was reassured at the first visit that the therapist had some good ideas that would probably help her a lot. At the second visit she was taught self-hypnosis, and in the first trance she was asked to recall how in her mind the "faucets" for her tears had seemed to turn on all by themselves in response to her feelings and then equally quickly turned off "because somewhere in your mind they got the signal to turn off." She was asked to find the faucets for her sweat glands in her hands and to practice turning them down. After four biweekly visits for therapeutic hypnosis review, practice, and reinforcement, she and her mother reported "better than 50% improvement" and a sense of growing confidence; they decided no further follow-up was required.

## Warts

Warts are reported to respond to many interventions (Chandrasena, 1982). Left to its own devices, the half-life of a wart is about 1 year. Surman, Gottlieb, and Hackett (1972) reported the successful hypnotic treatment of a 9-year-old girl who had 31 warts on her hands and face that had failed to respond to four attempts at conventional treatment. She was told that first one side would be treated for five sessions and, if the warts went away, the other side would be treated. She chose her left hand and left side of her face for initial wart removal. Hypnotic invitation included eye closure, simulated stair descent, and hand levitation. The patient was then told she would feel a tingling sensation in all the warts on the left side. The left-sided warts began to disappear after the first session. By the fifth visit, she had lost 26 warts. After 3 months of follow-up, only two small warts remained.

Tasini and Hackett (1977) reported the use of therapeutic clinical hypnosis in three immunosuppressed children all of whom had developed numerous warts. Each of the patients had been repeatedly treated with standard wart regimens for several years prior to the successful application of clinical hypnosis. Hand levitation was used for initiation of hypnosis. The patients were asked to think of doing something they enjoyed and to relax more each time they breathed out. While in trance, the patients were told that the warts would feel dry, then turn brown, and fall off. Patients were seen for three to five sessions. Dramatic regression of warts began within a few weeks in each child, eventuating in complete disappearance. There was no evidence of recurrence in follow-ups that ranged from 4 to 8 months.

Following an appropriate initiation of hypnosis, one can ask children to give themselves the message that they are cutting off the food supply to the wart or warts. This suggestion may be included during a routine physical examination, and the child is asked to reinforce the suggestion twice daily at home. We recall cases in which warts were treated topically in routine office practice only to have patients return with wart recurrences. Since we have adopted clinical hypnosis as the primary mode of wart therapy, our patients have not required further topical chemicals.

In a report of 41 consecutive cases of warts treated with clinical hypnosis, Ewin (1992) described 11 prepubertal children (under 12 years of age) and 5 adolescents. Ten of the 11 children and 4 of the 5 adolescents were described as healing in response to direct hypnotic suggestion in hypnosis, with no focus on ongoing self-hypnosis. Children ranged from 6 to 12 years of age, and most required three visits or less. One child required six visits, and one required 12 visits. Clinical presentations and time to healing varied considerably; for example, one 7-year-old had one wart that was gone in 2 weeks, a 12-year-old had 7 warts that took 25 weeks to disappear, and the 32 warts of a 6-year-old who had only one visit were gone within 10 weeks. Ewin believes that daily attention via self-hypnosis detracts from natural healing processes and instead suggests hypnotically that the subconscious mind will heal the warts and that the patient should ignore the warts and get interested in other things. Compared to conventional treatment of warts, none of his child patients had any scars and none experienced recurrence of the warts.

In commenting on studies reporting disappearance of warts following the utilization of clinical hypnosis, Thomas (1979) emphasized the potential value of understanding what goes on when a wart disappears in association with hypnosis. He recommended further investigation in this area. Clawson and Swade (1975) speculated that the mechanism involved in wart removal via clinical hypnosis is the constriction of capillary sites to the warts. We participated in a multi-center study (seven clinical sites) of wart regression in children in which self-hypnosis (relaxation and imagery) treatment was compared to topical treatment and equal time interventions (Felt et al., 1998). Sixty-one children ages 6–12 years participated. Subjects selected one common (index) wart and had four visits over 8 weeks. At each visit, the total and index extremity wart number were counted, and a photo was taken of the index wart (with a centimeter ruler in the field) for subsequent measurement. At study entry (week 1) children all watched a 3-minute video prepared for the study and narrated by children describing warts and the study in general. While caretakers completed questionnaires about their children's health, wart history, and treatment, children completed a questionnaire about favorite activities and sensory preferences.

They were then randomly assigned to self-hypnosis (relaxation and mental imagery, or RMI), topical treatment with a salicylate agent, or equal time with the doctor without specific intervention. The hypnosis intervention group was instructed in how to relax and imagine doing something they enjoy. The children were then asked to imagine not feeing their warts anymore "so the warts will go away" and how nice their skin would look without the warts. The duration of the experience was 10–15 minutes. The session was audiotaped, and the children were asked to practice their RMI twice a day with the tape and to keep a written record of their practice. Subsequent visits were at weeks 2, 4, and 8, at which time the total number of warts, number on upper extremity, and size of the index wart were documented, and the practice of RMI (or review of the other intervention/non-intervention) took place. On average, total wart number decreased by 10% and the index wart area decreased by 20%, with no significant group differences during the first 8 weeks. Telephone follow-up was conducted 6–18 months from study entry. At phone follow-up there was a trend for more self-hypnosis and topical therapy subjects to report complete wart resolution ($p = 0.07$) compared to controls. We were surprised by the results, which showed no particular benefit in the short term, as this was in direct contrast to the case reports in the literature and our own experiences where self-hypnosis has resulted in dramatic short- and long-term improvement in wart regression (e.g., Goldstein, 2005; Kohen, Mann-Rinehart, Schmitz, & Wills, 1998; Lankton, 2007). We learned from this study that future investigations of wart regression in children would benefit from considering larger numbers of subjects per experimental group, tighter age range for children within each group, determination of age and duration of wart at study entry, longer direct follow-up, inclusion of different types of suggestions, and assessment of positive suggestion alone vs. self-hypnosis with home practice. Overall, the study suggested that, although there was no significant short-term benefit for self-hypnosis in this randomized controlled trial, longer term benefits for both self-hypnosis and topical treatment were suggested (Felt et al., 1998).

Whether the mechanism is vascular or immunological, it would seem that its understanding might relate eventually to treatment of other tumors and skin diseases. We address this further in Chapter 18 on Psychoneuroimmunology.

## *Diabetes*

Ratner and colleagues (Ratner, Gross, Casas, & Castells, 1990) reported a therapeutic hypnosis intervention with seven adolescents, ages 11–19 years. Six of them were followed for more than 6 months. Compliance improved according to the average hemoglobin A1c (HbA1c) and blood glucose levels. Each adolescent had three clinical hypnosis sessions with additional visits as needed. The psychological components of diabetes are well known (Ehrlich, 1974). Parents feel guilty about genetics and resent their lack of control. Family members are anxious about possible insulin reactions or episodes of ketoacidosis. Patients resent the intrusion of blood tests, diets, and drugs by injections. Some children develop fears over injections. The daily injection of insulin may become a *cause célèbre* in the family unit. Therapeutic hypnosis, presented in the context of patient mastery, can provide a solution for some of the difficulties. We have taught self-hypnosis to many children and adolescents with diabetes in individual and group sessions.

Paul B. was referred for clinical hypnosis to overcome his fear of needles when he was 6 years old. A year earlier, he had been diagnosed as having diabetes mellitus. Insulin injections were given for a few weeks and stopped as he entered the "honeymoon phase" of the disease. When insulin was required again nearly a year later, this naturally aggressive, active, and rather dominating child was crushed. He struggled to avoid injections, screamed throughout them, and was generally depressed. His mother, father, and younger brothers were upset, torn by their sympathy for Paul's predicament and their need to cooperate with the treatment regimen. When Paul was seen initially in the office, he sat sullenly next to his young, intelligent, and obviously concerned mother. He responded with interest when handed a 50¢ piece to hold but made no comment as his mother briefly described the onset of diabetes and Paul's fear of needles. The therapist said,

> I once knew a 5-year-old boy who had diabetes and was so mad that he had to have those shots every day. He was mad at his doctor and at his parents and at his brother, who didn't need to get the shots. But then he learned something that they didn't know, about how to handle needles himself. He knew, but his brother didn't.

Paul asked, "What was it?" The therapist answered, "It was a way to turn off switches between his skin and where the needle went in and his brain – except in the beginning I couldn't tell him that because he was too young to know what a brain was." "I know what a brain is," said Paul. "Do you know what a nerve is too?" "Yep," he said proudly. "Well, you're already way ahead of this younger kid." Paul then learned the coin technique of initiation of hypnosis, followed by favorite place imagery, suggestions about his switch system, and how he could use it. Throughout, the therapist stressed his ability, his control, and his choice to use his skill when he wished and to share with his family as he wished. At the conclusion of the first session, Paul was comfortable when touched with an insulin needle. He agreed to practice at home daily and to return in a week. His mother reported that injections no longer posed problems: "He turned off his switch before each one, and the rest of the family didn't know how he did it." Subsequently, Paul attended group sessions where he was a good teaching assistant and very helpful to children with similar problems.

It is possible that the use of therapeutic hypnosis to enhance mastery in children with diabetes, particularly as they approach adolescence, will indirectly affect morbidity from the disease. Children who are actively participating in their therapy may also be more likely to follow recommendations regarding urine testing, eating, and insulin with fewer complications and hospitalizations.

Wester and Sugarman (2007) noted the value of hypnosis in helping a child in ketoacidosis with newly diagnosed diabetes "turn down the pain switches" so needles wouldn't bother as much. In turn, her mother noted very positively that "this is going to make things much easier." Kuttner and Catchpole (2007) analogously described the value of hypnotic strategies in assisting both the child (only 20 months old) and parents in managing regular insulin injections in their overall adaptation to newly diagnosed diabetes.

A study of adult diabetes evaluated the effects of acute psychological stress on metabolic control (Kemmer et al., 1986). Those with diabetes and controls were subjected to the acute stresses of mental arithmetic and public speaking. Blood pressure rose, and plasma epinephrine and cortisol increased in all subjects, but there were no changes in blood glucose, free fatty acids, glucagon, or growth hormone. The authors acknowledged that laboratory-induced stress may not be representative of stressful life events, but they concluded that metabolic control in insulin-treated diabetic patients is not jeopardized by sudden, short-lived emotional arousal. The primary benefit of clinical hypnosis may be to enhance comfort for children who must suffer injections and to enhance compliance.

Since the publication of the fourth edition of this text, while a variety of health care publications have appeared in the literature, few have provided any new scientific information regarding the value of therapeutic hypnosis or closely aligned therapeutic strategies (imagery, relaxation) in modulating either the biologic markers of diabetes control (e.g., HbA1c) or the psychoemotional toll – or management of – the disease and its management. The well-known practice of employing multi-disciplinary teams to facilitate "best practices" for children and families with chronic illness is described by Gelder (2013) in a description of "optimising management through the care pathway." This is an interesting discussion of implementation of the "*Paediatric diabetes best practice tariff* in England" (Gelder, 2013) to facilitate an in-depth clinical assessment of psychosocial and physical health by the multidisciplinary team, most notably for inpatient children and adolescents with diabetes. Integrated in this discussion is recommendation for relaxation and guided imagery, and case descriptions are provided of a 3-year-old and a 15-year-old (Gelder, 2013). No data was provided, and we have not identified any follow-up reports regarding this program.

A bit more recently, Gelernter and colleagues (2015) reported their blinded randomized controlled trials (RCT) comparing the effects of auditory guided imagery ("AGI"), the equivalent of hypnosis, accompanied by background music, to background music alone in children with type

1 diabetes mellitus. Study participants were from 7 to 16 years of age and included a total of 13. In the "short phase" of the study participants were connected to a continuous glucose monitoring system for 5 days and the outcome measure was the change in interstitial glucose concentration (IGC). The mean IGC decreased in both the experimental (AGI) group and the control (background music only) while listening. In the "long phase" participants listened to the recording twice a week for 12 weeks, and the outcome measures were Quality of Life (QOL) and HbA1c. While the HbA1c decreased in both groups, the decrease in the experimental group was significant and not in the control group. The authors noted both optimism for AGI as a treatment and the need for further, larger research studies.

In 2016, a report from Greece described a pilot study of a 12-week intervention program including elements of: psychoeducation about stress, healthy lifestyle, diaphragmatic breathing, progressive muscle relaxation, guided imagery, cognitive restructuring, gratitude and health locus of control in children and adolescents with type 1 diabetes and their parents. Their hypothesis was that compared to controls the patients of the intervention group would have lower HbA1c levels and lower anxiety and depressive symptomatology following the intervention. Another hypothesis was that parents in the intervention group would have lower levels of perceived stress, anxiety and depressive symptoms, and a significant change in health beliefs compared to the control group. There were 32 patient-parent dyads assigned randomly to the intervention group ($n = 17$) and control group ($n = 15$). The HbA1c levels were recorded before and after the intervention. A significant reduction in HbA1c was observed in the children and adolescents in the experimental group compared to the control group ($p < 0.014$).

While to be sure this is a very positive result, the authors are clear in their recommendation for further research and notably for a larger sample. Moreover, not unlike many program protocols, no mention was made of any effort to somehow discriminate which individual or combination of components of the intervention were most instrumental in effecting the observed decrease in HbA1c levels (Panayi, Kanaka-Gantenbein, Darviri, & Chrousos, 2016).

Like so many conditions, diabetes care would benefit from a controlled study of application and efficacy of therapeutic hypnosis strategies, which we know have been clinically valuable to individual children and adolescents with diabetes. With the prevalence of type 2 diabetes in children increasing exponentially in the context of the rising prevalence of obesity in children, it would seem especially prudent to both study and therapeutically provide the availability of self-hypnosis training to facilitate preventive health maintenance and interdisciplinary care of diabetes in young people.

## Dysphagia

Dysphagia, or difficulty in swallowing, is more common in adults than in children, and its variety of organic causes can usually be easily discerned through careful history, physical examination, or radiological studies. In children, dysphagia is not uncommonly the result of psychological influences, including apparent conditioned responses in which dysphagia is associated with an acute illness or episode of physical or psychological trauma and then prolonged well after cessation or resolution of the original problem. These may include circumstances as common as difficulty in swallowing in association with tonsillitis (e.g., strep throat, infectious mononucleosis), with an injury, or with psychological trauma, such as forced oral sex in sexual abuse cases (see also Chapter 8 for discussion on hypnosis and child abuse).

Elinoff (1993) described the case of a 9-year-old girl who developed an inability to swallow rough-textured foods following an episode of feeling as though a nut in some ice cream had stuck in her throat. When she refused to eat anything except liquids and soft foods, her mother became worried about her nutritional status and increased the pressure on her daughter to eat, resulting in the emergence of a power struggle and further refusals to eat. Integrated into the routine of a busy family practice visit, the author offered a so-called "waking" hypnotic suggestion ("Did you ever watch water go over a waterfall?") and added ego-strengthening suggestions to the effect that food would become easier to swallow. Four days later the patient's symptoms had worsened, the mother had become increasingly insistent that the child needed better nutrition, and the patient had lost 5.5 pounds. Reinforcement of the same hypnotic imagery was accomplished through suggestions to remember that even as a baby she had known how to swallow and that all she needed to do was to let her body do what it already knew how to do, helping it by thinking about the waterfall each time she swallowed. Two days later she began to eat solid foods, and in follow-up 1 week later and 2 years later she remained symptom free with no recurrence.

LaGrone (1993) described a case of a 10-year-old boy who refused to take liquid medications for his reactive airway disease, because liquid medicines were for "little kids," but he had been unable to swallow pills for many years because they made him gag or vomit if he was able to swallow them. The pediatrician referred the patient for assistance in being able to take pills or capsules. After ascertaining the absence of any major intrapsychic problems, the therapist involved the child in a commitment to a plan including imagery and relaxation, self-monitoring, and self-regulation in the form of desensitization with direct suggestion and self-reinforcement. A ten-session desensitization with hypnosis treatment plan resulted in the child's ability to comfortably swallow pills and to maintain that comfort at 1-year follow-up.

Culbert and colleagues (Culbert, Kajander, Reaney, & Kohen, 1996) described several different cases in which hypnotic approaches were very successful when tailored to the individual needs of the child, in the context of the specificity of their problem and with imagery that was a good fit with their likes and dislikes and their level of maturation. We have seen many similar patients, and our experience concurs with these reports that the problems are common, usually easily amenable to resolution with therapeutic hypnosis, and rarely recur (see also Chapter 14, Surgery and Emergencies).

## Erythromelalgia

Chakravarty, Pharoah, Scott, and Barker (1992) described the case of an 18-year-old woman with a 4-week history of severe, constant burning pain in her hands and feet, which was unresponsive to usual analgesics and relieved only when immersed in ice water. Examination also revealed persistent hypertension (165–185/110–125), and within 3 days, her feet and hands had become hot, red, and swollen, typical of this unusual condition. Her pain was unresponsive to aspirin, paracetamol, nonsteroidal anti-inflammatory agents, beta-blockers, vasodilators, and tricyclic antidepressants. Psychiatric evaluation revealed no evidence to suggest conversion disorder. Therapeutic hypnosis suggestions included allowing the pain to flow out of the affected extremities, leaving normal sensation behind, and teaching self-hypnosis. The patient became pain free and remained so at 6-month follow-up. Her elevated blood pressure was controlled initially with medication that was discontinued after 2 weeks.

## Epistaxis

Edel (1959) reported the case of a 10-year-old boy who had been referred for reading difficulties. After eight sessions using therapeutic hypnosis, his reading problem disappeared, and he no longer required tutoring. Two months later, he was brought into the physician's office because of a severe nosebleed. The use of bilateral anterior nasal packs with vasoconstrictors was to no avail.

The physician gave instructions for posterior nasal packing and decided to add therapeutic hypnotic suggestions as an adjunct. He told the patient that he could stop the bleeding himself, that he should hold his head way back and relax. Within minutes, the bleeding stopped, and the boy breathed easily. When his head was placed forward, no blood spilled out. The next morning, the parents reported there had been no further bleeding. While this was reportedly successful, we note that it is not generally appropriate to advise patients with a nosebleed to tilt the head "way back," as mechanically that will allow blood from the nasopharynx to move down the throat into the stomach, where blood is an irritant and likely to cause vomiting, which would only complicate the anxiety associated with the nosebleed. Although this was a patient previously familiar with hypnosis, it would be reasonable to give similar suggestions for cessation of bleeding to any child with life-threatening bleeding from any source.

### *Hemophilia*

In Czarist Russia, the monk Rasputin used hypnosis to aid the hemophiliac Czarevitch in the control of bleeding. In the 1950s, therapeutic hypnosis was reported to be effective in control of bleeding and pain during dental surgery in those with hemophilia. LaBaw (1975) taught a group with hemophilia self-hypnosis and encouraged them to use this technique when faced with anxiety-provoking situations, particularly bleeding episodes. His 4-year study documented a significant reduction in the number of units of blood products required by ten adult and child patients who practiced self-hypnosis on a regular basis.

Gustke's pilot work (1973) suggested that some patients with hemophilia were able to increase factor VIII levels in association with therapeutic hypnotic suggestions; however, no controlled studies support the idea that clinical hypnosis consistently reduces bleeding in people with hemophilia. As routine adjunct therapy, therapeutic hypnotic suggestions may be as valuable for its enhancement of mastery as for what it can do to reduce pain, relieve anxiety, or reduce the frequency of bleeding episodes.

Olness and Agle (1981) reported group practice sessions for patients with hemophilia over 6 years and their families. Although individual practice sessions are available to the patients with hemophilia, most become comfortable and prefer the group format. Sessions last 1 hour. During the initial 10 minutes, patients share experiences, ask questions, and explain to newcomers. Thirty minutes of therapeutic hypnosis exercises include suggestions for general relaxation, pain control, and reduction of bleeding. Following this, adults are invited to participate in self-hypnosis exercises. Children join their parents if they wish to or go to another room for play or movement exercises with another clinician. In recent years, children have been offered the option of practice in thermal biofeedback. Graphic evidence of control of skin temperature seems to have encouraged many children to pursue their self-hypnosis exercises more regularly. A typical account of such a group session follows.

The boys participating in this group included J.K., who had taught his family to do relaxation exercises during the summer, and his mother was able, for the first time with his help, to have major dental work done without general anesthesia. T. was doing very well with his intravenous injections. One morning, while he was at the Art Institute, he experienced pain associated with the eruption of a molar. His mother was concerned that they would have to leave because T. was so miserable. She asked him to sit down and "turn off his switches," which he did promptly. He and his family were happy and comfortable during the rest of their visit. D.D., age 4 years, has been doing well in turning off his switches for IVs and has amazed the nursing staff. When we asked the children about the sort of imagery they were using, one child, J.K., reported that he imagined antique cars running about his bloodstream to stop bleeds, especially in his ankle; he said this was effective. K.K. imagined planes full of bombs of factor VIII that he dispatched to parts of his body that needed them, as well as a special glue that he named "Super-Clot" and squeezed out in bleeding areas. The group went through a review of the switch-off technique, a coin initiation of hypnosis also using favorite place imagery, and an exercise in which each child visualized a package containing a special gift for that child. The therapist guided the parents through a general relaxation using the image of a walk along a beach. The children also participated with their parents and expressed pleasure in the experience.

Over a 6-year period, these children with hemophilia decreased their average use of factor VIII replacement therapy. They also became more mobile due to less frequent use of splints and crutches, and fewer days were lost from school because of bleeding episodes. They also became older – and perhaps more careful about activities that might result in bleeding. Several moved from hospital to home administration of replacement therapy, and two had major surgery that required large amounts of replacement therapy over a short period.

It is our perception that younger children learn best from older children in the group setting. If not threatened by much individualized cajoling and attention, they seem to learn by osmosis. Some younger children (age 2–3 years) merely sit quietly, observing for one or two sessions without giving overt evidence of participation. Parents often report evidence of their learning at home before they show cooperation in the group sessions.

The children in these groups have provided many subjective reports of decreased bleeding; for example, Lanny L. said he awakened at midnight with a stiff arm. He turned off the bleeding, and his arm was fine by morning. His parents confirmed the report. Tom H., age 3 years, said he had a stiff arm (confirmed by his parents) but "I unstiffed my arm today." Parents involved in the hemophilia groups have reported perceived benefits for themselves associated with the relaxation exercises. Not only have they learned specific pain control techniques, which they have invoked during dental procedures or surgical experiences, but they also have found themselves calmer in stress situations related to the hemophilia. One father attributed reduction of his blood pressure (20 millimeters diastolic) over a period of several months to his regular practice of self-hypnosis. For his part, J.K. became a physical therapist and contacted one of us when he was 40 years old. He was married and had three children. He said that learning self-hypnosis was the single most useful thing he had learned in his life that he was in demand as a speaker to hemophilia groups around the United States, and that he recommended self-hypnosis to his families.

A pilot study (Ritterman, 1982) examined the use of adjunctive hypnotic techniques with families in which at least one member had hemophilia. Little systematic work has been done previously to introduce families to such techniques. This study used an open-systems approach model of hemophilia coupled with interviews to facilitate that introduction.

## Persistent Somatic Complaints

A guideline for therapists evaluating persistent somatic complaints in children and a questionnaire on this subject can be found in Appendixes F and B, respectively, in the fourth edition of this text.

## Gastrointestinal Disorders

### *Recurrent Abdominal Pain (RAP) aka Functional Abdominal Pain (FAP)*

Recurrent abdominal pain is a common symptom among pediatric patients and one for which organic causes are often not found (Apley, 1977; Berger, Honig, & Liebman, 1977; Dodge, 1976).

As a last resort, these patients are sometimes referred for therapeutic hypnosis to relieve symptoms. A typical case history follows.

Linda, age 15, was referred by a pediatrician for symptomatic relief from abdominal pain that had been present for 6 months. The pain was recurrent, intermittent, and not associated with any specific time of day or situation. The parents had divorced 2 years earlier, and both had remarried. The patient's mother had custody, and the patient visited her father and his new family on weekends. Evaluation had included numerous laboratory and radiological studies, the results of which were normal. The patient was losing weight, which increased uneasiness in the referring pediatrician who was concerned about an undetected malignancy. At the time of the first visit for clinical hypnosis, the patient and her mother were uneasy. They spoke very little to one another and demonstrated little affect. The patient was told that she would learn a self-hypnosis exercise that she could review at home if she wished. The patient indicated her wish to learn hypnosis but during the first effort to initiate hypnosis she responded mechanically. When she returned, she claimed to have practiced but said there was no improvement. During this session, she used hypnotic age regression to recall an event that she had enjoyed and in which she had felt in control, and she enhanced the feeling of joy and mastery by squeezing her right fist. She was then asked to become aware of things that were irritating her or worrying her and to decide if she could let go of any of them. Following this session, she spontaneously said that she felt better but did not reveal any of her possible concerns. She then refused a recommendation for psychotherapy. She said she would practice self-hypnosis at home and that she was feeling better. A week later, she left her mother's home and moved into her father's home. All symptoms abated; she gained weight and continued to come for follow-up appointments for review of therapeutic hypnosis over the next 2 years. Although she continued to refuse psychotherapy, she had no recurrence of abdominal pain and no indication of substitute symptoms.

Williams and Singh (1976) reported the case of an 11-year-old boy hospitalized for the third time in 16 months because of recurrent abdominal pain. The results of laboratory and x-ray studies were normal. Eighteen months earlier, he had undergone surgery to correct a right hydronephrosis. Subsequent recurrences of pain triggered gastrointestinal, neurological, and metabolic evaluations with normal results. There was a strong family history of abdominal disorders. After psychiatric evaluation, therapeutic clinical hypnosis was recommended. The boy was an excellent subject and, while in trance, repeated the following statements after the therapist: (1) "cooped-up feelings can cause tension," (2) "tension can cause physical pain," and (3) "by relaxing I can reduce tension and eliminate the pain." The patient reported the disappearance of pain during the exercise and was taught self-hypnosis to maintain his clinical improvement. In 20 months of follow-up, he had only one transient recurrence of abdominal pain, which was possibly due to gastroenteritis. The authors noted that this child, as is true of most with abdominal pain, no longer had any need to continue self-hypnosis exercises once the presenting symptom had resolved. We have also found this to be the case.

Marie was almost 11 years old when she was referred to us for chronic recurrent abdominal pain. She had experienced an onset of vague complaints of intermittent abdominal discomfort 10 months earlier. Like many with similar symptoms, she had been to her doctor and to several specialist consultants and had endured many laboratory and radiological studies before a large, benign ovarian cyst was identified and removed. She had a benign intraoperative and post-operative course and seemed to be back to normal for about 3 months, when she began to have abdominal pain again. Although her examinations and tests were normal, both she and her mother were reluctant to accept this in view of what they considered had been a misdiagnosis or at least a delayed diagnosis of the ovarian cyst months before. When the pain continued and she began to miss a lot of school, she was referred to us for "possible hypnosis." As with many youngsters with this problem, Marie had developed a well-organized belief system, the underpinnings of which included uncertainty and mistrust about physicians and an understandable fear that a not yet identified tumor could explain her symptoms.

In the context of Marie's fears and mistrust, we focused on developing rapport – slowly – and made the decision to avoid any formal statement about hypnosis. Following Erickson's dictum (1958) to "go with the patient," she was asked simply to monitor her discomfort (we never used the word "pain" even if she did) on a scale from 0 to 12, with 12 being the worst imaginable discomfort and 0 being none at all. She was asked to give herself a rating after school and at bedtime and to record these on a calendar. She continued to complain but began to attend school and appeared to feel better, although she continued to record, present, and discuss self-ratings of 11 or 11.5 for several weeks.

After the fourth or fifth visit, she was gently asked about the apparent discrepancy between how she appeared, how she reported she felt, and what she was able to do. She was asked to "please help me understand." She said she still had the pain, but she was "dealing with it better." Using her own language, it was suggested that perhaps she should also have a "deal with it" scale from 0 to 12 and could record that alongside the recordings of discomfort. This "conversational hypnotic suggestion" was readily accepted, and she really liked this idea, and the first week's recordings of "deal with it" ratings were all 8 or 9, while the discomfort ratings remained 11. Continued contact with her treating physicians revealed no positive tests or explanation for the problem and complaints of pain. The "deal with it" ratings began to drop weekly, and the pain ratings also began to move down. As the "deal with it" ratings reached 4 or 5 (i.e., the lower her self-ratings of "deal with it," the better she was doing = the easier it was to deal with it, the pain ratings dropped to 9 and sometimes 8). It was then, over 6 weeks into the therapeutic relationship, that the naturalistic hypnotic suggestion was offered: "It's interesting, isn't it, how the more you deal with it better, the less there is to deal with, and the less it bothers you?" Within 3 months, the "deal with it" ratings had dropped to 0, and the pain ratings decreased to 1 or 2 with no functional impairment. At our last session, she was given the posthypnotic waking suggestion that it was "good to know that your body will let you know when there's a problem, and in the meantime, you don't have to pay much attention to it at all." She agreed and remained pain free at 1-year follow-up.

Sokel, Devane, and Bentovim (1991) reported the successful use of hypnosis with 6 children, ages 7–14 years, who had recalcitrant recurrent abdominal pain. Each child had an extensive medical evaluation. The interval between onset of abdominal pain and referral for hypnosis ranged from 2 months to 6 years. Children were taught relaxation and guided mental imagery and were given suggestions for pain relief that were tailored to the age and interests of each child. Examples included a switch to turn down the pain, magic potions, and a pet animal that soothed away the pain. Each child was provided a recording of the session and instructed to practice daily with the tape and to use the self-hypnosis when he or she felt an episode of pain beginning. Each child was seen weekly for 3 weeks, and subsequently at 2-, 3-, and 6-month intervals. Children were able to resume normal activities within a mean period of 17.6 days (range, 5 days to 8 weeks). Our experiences are consistent with their description.

Increasingly, children with recurrent abdominal pain have been described as benefiting from hypnotic-like or therapeutic hypnosis strategies, including relaxation, biofeedback, and imagery. Many clinical reports and systematic reviews have appropriately emphasized the value of a holistic biopsychosocial approach to this common problem and highlighted the efficacy of hypnosis (Banez, 2008; Brent, Lobato, & LeLeiko, 2009; Bursch, 2008; Galili, Shaoul, & Mogilner, 2009; Masters, 2006; Whitfield & Shulman, 2009).

Since the fourth edition of our text, there have been many excellent randomized controlled studies and clinical reports published that scientifically validate the value of therapeutic hypnosis for the treatment of functional abdominal pain or pediatric irritable bowel syndrome or IBS (Gillan, 2021; Gottsegen 2011; Gulewitsch, Muller, Hautzinger, & Schlarb, 2013; Jong et al., 2018; Mahler, 2015; Rutten, Korterink, Venman, Benninga, & Tabbers, 2015; Rutten, Reitsma, Vlieger, & Benninga, 2013; Rutten et al., 2017; Vlieger, Rutten, Govers, Frankenhuis, & Benninga, 2012).

Writing in the *American Journal of Clinical Hypnosis* a general pediatrician (Gottsegen, 2011) published a thorough review of diagnostic considerations for Functional Abdominal Pain available at that time; and reviewed 57 studies in the pediatric literature within which psychological approaches (e.g., CBT) and guided imagery and hypnosis had the greatest proven efficacy for abdominal pain in children. Weydert, Ball, and Davis (2003) and later studies affirmed these findings. Gottsegen (2011) further discusses the clinical evidence for use of hypnosis for FAP and published descriptions of therapeutic hypnosis for FAP. The report closes with two examples of clinical cases: One was a 15-year-old young woman with a history of "stomach aches and diarrhea every time she ate" and a history of diagnosis of IBS. Following a careful history and development of rapport, a hypnotic strategy of favorite place imagery and relaxation was followed by training in use of self-hypnosis control of imagined pain "switches" to modulate discomfort. Though she reportedly declined the invitation to self-monitor pain and bowel movements with a symptom diary, she requested an audiotape recording of the hypnotic imagery and suggestions initially provided. Over several weeks time she practiced self-hypnosis and telephone follow-up revealed substantial decrease in severity and frequency of discomfort. The second case, a young 7-year-old boy had a 3-year history of functional abdominal pain and substantial food allergies with associated considerable anxiety about what to eat. He was described as an "apt student of self-hypnosis" who learned quickly and practiced daily. He improved rapidly with substantial decrease in anxiety by the second visit and dysphagia and abdominal pain having subsided by the third visit.

Drawing conclusions from these two cases, Gottsegen reinforced several important principles in treating children with FAP: (1) regular practice of self-hypnosis practice is important if not essential for its effectiveness; (2) pain or other symptom diaries may be important for research but should always be at the discretion of the patient; (3) access and utilization of vivid imagery often enhance efficacy (as with the 7 year old); (4) an added benefit of therapeutic hypnosis is that once it has been successful, e.g., with FAP, it may be easily applied to manage other problems (Gottsegen, 2011).

Having previously demonstrated that gut directed hypnosis is highly effective in the treatment of children with functional abdominal and IBS, Vlieger et al. (2012) proceeded to investigate the long-term effects of therapeutic hypnosis vs. standard medical treatment plus supportive therapy. All 52 participants of their previous RCT completed a standardized abdominal pain diary, scoring pain intensity and frequency. Additionally, the Children's Somatization Inventory and a general quality of life questionnaire were completed. Clinical remission was defined as over 80% improvement in pain scores as compared to baseline. Results showed that all 27 therapeutic hypnosis patients and 22 of 25 standard treatment patients participated. After a mean duration of 4.8 years follow-up, therapeutic hypnosis remained highly superior to conventional therapy with 68% of patients compared to 20% of standard care patients in remission after treatment ($p = 0.005$). Pain intensity and pain frequency scores at follow-up were 2.8 and 2.3, respectively, in the hypnosis group compared to 7.3 and 67.1 in the standard therapy group ($p < 0.01$). The authors concluded that the beneficial effects of gut directed therapeutic hypnosis are long lasting in children with FAP or IBS with over 2/3 still in remission almost 5 years after treatment, making it a highly valuable therapeutic option (Vlieger et al., 2012).

In a systematic review to assess efficacy of therapeutic hypnosis in pediatric FAP and IBS patients, Rutten et al. (2013) searched Medline, Embase, PsychINFO, Cumulative Index to

Nursing and Allied Health Literature databases and Cochrane Central Register of Controlled Trials for RCT in children with FAP or IBS, investigating efficacy of hypnosis on abdominal pain scores, quality of life, costs, and school absenteeism. They found three RCT's comparing hypnosis to a control treatment with sample sizes between 22 and 52 children. They concluded that the therapeutic effects of hypnosis appeared superior to standard medical care of children with FAP or IBS but that quantification of exact benefits was difficult at that time. They recommended more high-quality research and indeed went on to conduct many such additional studies and their research continues as discussed next.

Also in 2013 Gulewitsch and colleagues writing in the *European Journal of Pediatrics* (Gulewitsch, Muller, Hautzinger, & Schlarb, 2013) reported a RCT of a "brief hypnotherapeutic-behavioral intervention" for children with recurrent abdominal pain. Their study included 38 children ages 6–12 randomly assigned to a therapeutic hypnosis treatment (20) or a waiting list condition (18). Evaluating child-rated pain measures and pain related disability as well as parent completed measures of their children's pain and pain related disability, 11 of 20 children (55%) receiving therapeutic hypnosis showed over 80% improvement compared to only one child in the waiting list group (5.6%) who was characterized as a positive "responder." While noting the clear treatment success, the authors also acknowledged the limitation both of small sample size and follow-up limited to 3 months following the initiation of the intervention, and recommend both comparison with other active intervention(s) and longer follow-up.

In 2017 Rutten and colleagues (2017) the initiation of their comprehensive study of 260 children, ages 8–18 with IBS or FAP(S) according to Rome III criteria. This randomized controlled study compared the use of self-hypnosis exercises (performed by a qualified therapist with therapeutic hypnosis by means of CD recorded self-exercises at home in children with IBS or FAP(S)) with individual therapy by qualified therapists. Children were randomized to either six sessions of individualized therapeutic hypnosis by a qualified therapist over 3 months or therapeutic hypnosis through self-exercises at home with a CD for 3 months. Follow-up was 1 year. The therapeutic hypnosis interventions are described in detail and modeled after "the Manchester protocol for gut directed hypnosis and in the van Tilburg et al trial" (Ruttten et al., 2017).

In 2017, these investigators (Rutten et al., 2017) published the results of this seminal study, concluding that the long-term effectiveness of home-based therapeutic hypnosis with a CD of hypnosis for self-hypnosis practice at home is not inferior to individual therapeutic hypnosis provided by skilled therapists during in-person (clinic) visit. And, accordingly, that treatment with hypnosis utilizing a CD provides a significant important and attractive treatment option for children with FAP or IBS for whom individual clinic treatment is unavailable.

## *Functional Nausea*

In a recently published open access paper, Browne et al. (2021) treated 100 children and youth between 8 and 18 years with a main complaint of chronic nausea. They were formally diagnosed to have either functional nausea or functional dyspepsia. They were randomized to treatment with therapeutic hypnosis (five to six hypnosis sessions) or medication and supportive talks with their pediatrician. They were followed for 1 year. While both approaches were effective in reducing nausea symptoms in children, in those with functional nausea diagnosis therapeutic hypnosis was more effective than the standard, supportive talks treatment, both during and after the first 6 months of treatment. They concluded and recommend that both treatments, applied either separately or in combination, should be offered as option(s) to children with recurrent nausea (Browne et al., 2021).

### *Irritable Bowel Syndrome*

Whorwell, Prior, and Colgan (1987) reported on their experience with therapeutic hypnosis for 50 patients with severe, intractable irritable bowel syndrome (IBS). Their report does not indicate whether any children or adolescents were part of the cohort. They noted, however, that the response rate to therapeutic hypnosis was best among those under 50 years of age (100% experienced no relapse for 18 months after treatment with therapeutic hypnosis) compared to poor responses for those over 50 years of age (25%). Therapeutic hypnosis suggestions were directed toward control of intestinal smooth muscle.

Over the past 20 years increasing numbers of studies have documented the efficacy of therapeutic hypnosis in treating IBS, producing significant improvement not only in the cardinal symptoms of IBS (abdominal pain, bloating, distention, altered bowel patterns) but also in associated symptoms of emotional well-being, ability to attend work or school, and overall quality of life. Detailed analyses and reviews of these studies have been published by Tan, Hammond, and Gurrala (2005) and Whitehead (2006). Ongoing updates of published research on hypnosis for IBS are generously provided by Palsson (2010) on his public information website.

Weydert and colleagues conducted several studies on the effects of relaxation and imagery (hypnosis) in children with recurrent abdominal pain (Ball, Shapiro, Monheim, & Weydert, 2003; Ball & Weydert, 2003; Weydert et al., 2006). Ball et al. (2003) described a pilot study of ten children with recurrent abdominal pain who were evaluated by a pediatric gastroenterologist and then trained in relaxation and guided imagery over 4 weekly 50-minute sessions. Pain diaries completed at 0, 1, and 2 months indicated that the children experienced a 67% decrease in pain during treatment ($p < 0.001$), despite having been previously refractory to conventional treatment by their physician and pediatric gastroenterologist. Clearly hypnotic, the training was described as "learning to feel the difference between tense and relaxed muscles and using your imagination to tell your body what to do." Suggested imagery included picturing what their pain might look like and picturing what might get rid of or destroy the pain. In their later study, Weydert et al. (2006) enrolled 22 children with recurrent abdominal pain between the ages of 5 and 18 years in a randomized trial to learn breathing exercises alone or guided imagery with progressive muscle relaxation. Each group had 4 weekly sessions with a therapist, and the children recorded the numbers of days with pain, pain intensity, and missed activities due to pain at baseline and during the intervention. Children who learned guided imagery and relaxation (hypnosis) had a significantly greater decrease in the number of days with pain than those learning breathing exercises alone after 1 month (67% vs. 21%, $p = 0.05$) and 1 months (82% vs. 45%, $p < 0.01$). The hypnosis group also had fewer days of missed activities than the breathing exercise group at 1 month (85% vs. 15%, $p = 0.02$) and 2 months (95% vs. 77%, $p = 0.05$).

In a landmark study very significant to the care of children, Vlieger and colleagues (Vlieger, Menko-Frankenhuis, Wolfkamp, Tromp, & Benninga, 2007) conducted a randomized controlled trial in Amsterdam that compared the effectiveness of six sessions of therapeutic hypnosis over 12 weeks with results from standard medical therapy plus six sessions of supportive therapy in children with functional abdominal pain or IBS. Fifty-three children, 8–18 years old with functional abdominal pain (31) or IBS (22), were randomly assigned to treatment with either therapeutic hypnosis or the comparison treatment. Although pain scores decreased significantly in both groups from baseline to follow-up a year later, there was significantly greater reduction in pain in the therapeutic hypnosis group than in the comparison group. At the time of the 1-year follow-up, treatment was found to be successful in 85% of those treated with therapeutic hypnosis compared to 25% in the comparison group ($p < .001$).

Reproducing the efficacy of therapeutic hypnosis for abdominal pain, a recently conducted pilot study demonstrated the effectiveness of audiotaped guided imagery in reducing functional abdominal pain in children (van Tilburg et al., 2009). Thirty-four children, 6–15 years old with a diagnosis of functional abdominal pain, were randomly assigned to receive 2 months of standard medical care with or without guided imagery treatment. Those in the standard care group were also given audiotaped guided imagery after 2 months, and all were monitored for 6 months following guided imagery treatment. There were significantly more responders in the guided imagery treatment group (12/19 = 63.1%) compared to the medical-care-only group (4/15 = 26.7%, $p$ = .03). When the children in the standard medical treatment group later had imagery added to their treatment, a comparable number (8/13 = 61.5%) also became treatment responders. Most parents (85%) reported that their children were somewhat to markedly better after imagery treatment. In their assessment of the long-term effects (benefits) of guided imagery, the authors reported that at 6-month follow-up paired $t$-tests revealed no relapse of pain or disability and significant differences from the pre-treatment assessment to the 6-month follow-up evaluation. The authors concluded that audiotaped guided imagery was superior to standard medical care in reducing abdominal pain, disability, and medical visits and in improving quality of life in that treatment effects, as noted, were sustained over 6 months. Discussion appropriately considered similarities and differences between audiotaped guided imagery and individual therapist-administered guided imagery or hypnotherapy, noting that therapeutic gains were comparable between individual therapy and audio-recorded imagery and also noting that it can be expected that effects may be better and possibly longer lasting when treatment is individualized.

The paper by van Tilburg et al. (2009) includes a detailed description of the standardized guided imagery scripts that were recorded on CDs and tested for likeability with a 6-year-old boy and a boy and girl each 9 years old, and then with boys 6 and 11 years old and a girl 10 years old. None of these children was a later participant in the study. Each session included induction (initiation or invitation) imagery to produce relaxation, followed by imagery and suggestions for decreased discomfort and healing. In the first session, children were invited to imagine floating comfortable on a big puffy cloud and instructed to relax. Suggestions for decreasing discomfort included asking the child to "imagine a special object melting into one's hand like butter and making the hand shiny and warm." The children were then instructed "to place this hand on their belly, imagining the light and warmth spreading through their belly and making a protective barrier inside that does not let anything irritate the belly." In the second session, "progressive relaxation is introduced by the children imagining sitting in a gently rocking boat. Suggestions for decreased discomfort are … to imagine drinking a favorite drink to wash away discomfort, which leaves them feeling healthier and happier with each sip." In the third session, they "imagine sitting on a flying blanket and enjoying a flight to a mountaintop where they imagine the special object melting in their hand again. The light in the hand flashes and becomes stronger with every flash, so that the children have more power to decrease any pain or discomfort." Although we appreciate this effort at standardization for expediency and study purposes, we strongly believe that individualized, personally prepared and designed recordings are far preferable for individual patients, and we generally discourage the use of commercially available tapes or CDs because they obviously are not made for a given child and therefore cannot speak to that child's needs nearly as well as a personally focused recording tailored to the individual needs or preferences of the child.

Mahler (2015) reviewed her model of a "multi-factorial biopsychosocial model" and in our mind essential approach to the child with recurrent abdominal pain. Recognizing as a pediatric gastroenterologist that so-called standard or usual medical treatment rarely offers relief, in this review she characterizes abdominal pain syndromes as "disorders of bi-directional mind-brain-gut interactions"; and emphasizes the importance of a careful and clear diagnosis and education of the patient and family. Amplification of the essential ingredient of rapport with all patients precedes an appropriate elaboration of "techniques," imagery ideas, and examples which readers will find helpful (Mahler, 2015).

Also in 2015, Rutten and colleagues (2015) reviewed 24 RCTs of nonpharmacological treatment of functional abdominal pain disorders. These included 1,390 children (3–18 years old) and significant improvement of abdominal pain was reported after therapeutic hypnosis compared with standard care and/or wait-list control groups. Conclusions noted that while some evidence showed efficacy of therapeutic hypnosis, high-quality studies were said to be lacking.

Several years later, Abbott and colleagues (2018) published an extensive review which included treatment for recurrent abdominal pain in children as provided in 55 RCT's involving 3,572 children with RAP. Emphasizing the significant morbidity of RAP in noting that 4–25% of school-aged children complain of RAP sufficiently severe to interfere with daily activities, their review found that hypnotherapy, probiotic diets, and Cognitive Behavioral Therapy (CBT) were reported to reduce pain in the short term. With specific reference to the effectiveness of therapeutic hypnosis, four studies including 152 children were evaluated and therapeutic hypnosis was found significantly more effective in providing pain control compared to controls. As also noted earlier, long-term follow-up date from Vlieger et al. (2012) found 68% of the intervention (therapeutic hypnosis) group were symptom free after 5 years compared to only 20% in the control group ($p = 0.005$).

### *Inflammatory Bowel Disease*

We have utilized therapeutic hypnosis as an adjunct in management of children with ulcers, chronic hepatitis and varices, and inflammatory bowel disease (Crohn's disease, ulcerative colitis), with a focus on control of discomfort, ego strengthening, and imagery of both healthy mucosa (e.g., "Picture the lining of your intestines and see it in a smooth, healthy, pink color, just like the color and texture and healthy lining of your mouth and inside of your cheeks") and good health in general. A recent clinical report (Shaoul, Sukhotnik, & Mogilner, 2009) described success in the reduction of symptoms and a decrease in inflammatory markers with therapeutic hypnosis for children with inflammatory bowel disease. The authors emphasized the need for and importance of future controlled studies to assess the effects of hypnotherapy on morbidity and mortality in these diseases. It remains our impression that the enhancement of mastery and reduction of pain contribute to more rapid improvement in these patients (Keefer, Kiebles, Martinovich, Barrett and Palsson, 2013).

In 2013 Keefer and colleagues (Keefer, et al, 2013) described the value of "gut-directed hypnotherapy" in augmenting remission in quiescent ulcerative colitis. Very recently Lee and associates published a RCT pilot study on the utilization of clinical hypnosis for adolescents with pediatric Crohn's disease (Lee et al., 2021). Forty adolescents with Crohn's were randomized to a "hypnosis intervention" or a waitlist control group. The intervention was described as a single in-person clinical hypnosis session combined with education in self-hypnosis and recordings for home practice. Initial objectives of the study were to assess the impact of clinical hypnosis on quality of life, abdominal pain, and psychosocial measures, and disease activity compared with standard care. Of the 40 enrolled 50% were female; and 78% had inactive disease and 55% had abdominal pain. After intervention, significant improvements were noted in parent reported quality of life in the therapeutic hypnosis intervention group compared with the waiting list in total score ($p = 0.05$), social functioning ($p = 0.01$), and school functioning ($p = 0.04$). Curiously, however, patient-reported quality of life was unchanged. Abdominal pain severity significantly improved in the hypnosis group compared to controls ($p = 0.03$) and school absences decreased in significantly more intervention than control patients.

## Juvenile Rheumatoid Arthritis

Juvenile rheumatoid arthritis (JRA) is well known as a disease of exacerbations and remissions. Conventional treatment deprives the patient of many controls and may in itself trigger emotional problems. The loss of free movement associated with the disease process invariably leads to varying degrees of depression in children and family members. We often recommend therapeutic clinical hypnosis as an adjunct with these patients not only for relief of symptoms but also to enhance self-mastery and enable the patient to control as much of their therapy as possible. The complexities of psychogenic components of this disease are demonstrated in the following case history.

Mary F., a 10-year-old girl, came with her 12-year-old sister and mother to "learn hypnosis for pain control." Both girls had been diagnosed as having rheumatoid arthritis and eczema and were under the care of rheumatologists. They suffered intermittent pain, particularly in the knee and ankle joints, and they often missed school. In addition to the problems of arthritis and eczema, the 10-year-old girl was obese. She had attended one session of a group meeting for weight control but had refused to return. Mary said she had been taught some hypnosis by a 14-year-old friend. Her sister and mother also said they had used self-hypnosis exercises for general relaxation. When asked about her interests, the patient said she liked singing, painting, and handicrafts. Her favorite colors were blue and red. Her mother described her as very creative and added that she often wrote stories and poems for fun.

Following progressive relaxation exercises, Mary rapidly appeared comfortable. When she confirmed via ideomotor signals that she was ready to go on, she imagined herself in a favorite place, doing what she liked, enjoying the feeling of being comfortable. After 2 minutes, she appeared to be asleep. Then she became upset and began crying. The therapist told her she was safe, that she need not continue to feel upset, that she could leave her favorite place if she found it upsetting and come out of her hypnotic trance when she was ready. Almost immediately she stopped crying, opened her eyes, and said that her favorite place was in bed. She had fallen asleep, and she had this once or twice a week while sleeping – that is, a night terror. Her mother confirmed that she frequently had night terrors. The patient was asked to think about a scene in which she could be very comfortable without falling asleep and then to describe what it was when she returned for her next visit. Her 12-year-old sister went through the identical progressive relaxation and imagery exercise with no evidence of discomfort and subsequently demonstrated good evidence of pain control.

A follow-up appointment was made but not kept because of a death in the family. The sister required hospitalization, and she was able to use self-hypnosis and pain control suggestions very well. When Mary returned a month later, she explained that she wished to use imagining herself floating in water to begin her hypnosis, to focus on pain control and weight reduction. She seemed enthusiastic, did well in the therapeutic hypnosis session, and agreed to practice twice daily. Subsequently, she lost weight, demonstrated pain control, and returned for monthly group practice sessions for children with chronic pain problems.

This patient demonstrates some of the problems that can develop during therapeutic hypnosis. Although it is often appropriate to allow a child his or her own favorite place without having to reveal its whereabouts, it clearly would have been better to have known in this situation. Mary's choice of her bed as a favorite place suggests depression, which would also be consistent with her obesity and other chronic problems. An additional problem was the previous uncontrolled practice of self-hypnosis at home. This practice, while possibly leading to rapid initiation of self-hypnosis, may also have made her less responsive to hetero hypnosis. She did, however, seem to be highly motivated to have some personal part in her treatment and was very pleased with her subsequent excellent response.

Whether psychogenic components of JRA are causal or reflect the disease process and its treatment is not clearly understood. Much is known about immune factors and chemistries that reflect changes in those factors. One study (Domangue, Margolis, Lieberman, & Kaji, 1985) measured self-reported levels of pain, anxiety, and depression, as well as plasma levels of beta-endorphin, epinephrine, norepinephrine, dopamine, and serotonin, in 19 arthritis pain patients before and after hypnosis designed to produce pain reduction. Following therapeutic hypnosis clinically and statistically significant decreases in pain, anxiety, and depression were observed, in addition to increases in beta-endorphin-like immunoreactive material. The trigger for these changes, however, remains elusive (Russo & Varni, 1982).

Cioppa and Thai (1975) reported a fascinating account of a 10-year-old girl in whom JRA had been diagnosed by a rheumatologist. She responded minimally to large doses of salicylates and physical therapy. Prior to a trial of steroids, therapeutic clinical hypnosis was recommended. At the time of the first clinical hypnosis session, the patient was using a wheelchair and appeared severely depressed. The clinician teaching her self-hypnosis taught her ideomotor responses and asked, "Does some part of your mind know why you have arthritis?" The ideomotor response was in the affirmative and the patient appeared visibly upset. The clinician then gave her a general suggestion that her legs would feel better. The patient and her mother were upset by this approach and disconcerted that the session was held in the psychiatry department, as they did not believe that the arthritis had a psychological component. They did not want to return. That evening the girl spontaneously remarked that her legs felt different.

One month later, the patient could walk with difficulty, but deep depression persisted. The pediatrician asked that the child undergo a second therapeutic hypnosis session. The patient was told that she did not have to tell the therapist the problem as long as she knew what it was and as long as she was certain that it would quickly resolve itself if she really wanted it to resolve. She was given hypnotic suggestions that her joints would feel much better, that she would feel happier, and that she would be able to play with her friends soon. Four hours later, the patient rode her bicycle for the first time in 3 months. Ankle swelling and pain subsided rapidly over the next few days, and, for the first time in several months the patient could wear shoes. At that point, her depression began to lift. She was seen for three additional sessions. Improvements in her condition included being able to jump up and down with no pain, return of her sense of humor, and loss of fear of both injections and the hospital. Four months later, aspirin was stopped, and a 31-month follow-up revealed no recurrence of symptoms.

It was of interest that the hospital staff, at a follow-up conference, implied that the patient had not had JRA in the first place but merely a conversion reaction with concomitant laboratory findings suggestive of JRA. Prior to her remission, a conversion reaction had not been mentioned in the differential diagnosis. We have seen this phenomenon repeatedly among medical personnel who feel uncomfortable about "coincidental" cures that occur in conjunction with clinical hypnosis in "organic" disease.

Cioppa and Thai (1975) noted that a number of diseases could be considered to represent the conversion of a chronic tension state into an organically manifest disease state. Factors of spontaneous remission are poorly understood, although the writings of Norman Cousins (1976) have triggered much interest in the effects of attitude changes on remissions. Cioppa and Thai noted that, to be therapeutically effective, a reversal of attitude apparently must occur at a subconscious level. This may be brought about through the application of therapeutic hypnosis.

Walco, Varni, and Ilowite (1992) demonstrated the value of self-regulation strategies in 13 children between the ages of 4.5 and 16.9 years who had pauciarticular or systemic onset JRA. Baseline pain intensity and level of functional disability data were gathered for weeks prior to the patients being taught self-regulatory techniques that the authors described as "progressive muscle relaxation, guided imagery, and meditative breathing." The words "hypnosis" or "hypnotherapy" do not appear in this report. The authors, however, clearly describe hypnotic induction/initiation with muscle relaxation, meditative breathing (by saying the word "relax" to themselves upon exhalation), and therapeutic hypnotic suggestion in the form of guided imagery. The clearly defined aims here were to provide distraction through imagining a favorite place in which they had previously been pain free and to reinforce images that were metaphors for the children's sensory pain experience, with the intent to then alter the metaphor and thereby alter the perception of the discomfort. Practicing the techniques at home with the use of audiotapes was encouraged, and patients were seen weekly for eight visits.

Results showed substantial reduction of perceived pain intensity both short term and long term; follow-ups at 6 and 12 months demonstrated improved adaptive functioning. The authors correctly commented that conclusions from the data, although impressive, are limited by the absence of a placebo control group. Although there was no improvement in disease activity and no reduction of medication needs, the clear improvement in pain perception and in the concomitant functional status of the patients argues strongly for incorporating these self-regulation strategies as adjuncts to pharmacotherapy and other aspects of comprehensive care for children with JRA.

## Malignancies

Because cancer remains one of the leading causes of death in children, we have deferred discussion of studies of clinical hypnosis with terminal cancer patients to a separate chapter (Chapter 15) on palliative care and terminal illness. We want to emphasize here that since 1960 it is well known that there has been a dramatic increase in survivors of childhood cancers. Yet, although these children become free of disease, they often pay dearly in terms of psychological trauma resulting from diagnostic and treatment procedures and from the expectation of death. In addition, many have developed later learning and behavior problems associated with the very chemotherapeutic and radiation therapies designed and successfully applied to save their lives. These so-called *late effects* may include secondary or new cancers as well as the attendant emotional challenges for the patient and family. As with any chronic illness, clinicians utilizing hypnosis must remain informed and abreast of these issues and attend increasingly to these problems associated with prolonged life and survival.

The diagnosis of cancer in a child typically throws the entire family, extended family, and even their community into a state of disbelief, shock, and fear, followed by an urgency of medical tests, consultations, hospitalizations, and treatments often associated with unpleasant if not horrible side effects. If there is any single defining characteristic both early and in an ongoing fashion, it is uncertainty associated with the outcome of tests, choices of treatments, limitations or restrictions on activities, and alterations in short- and long-term plans. As such, the routines of daily life are stood on their proverbial heads, and navigating these uncertain waters is a daily challenge for the child-patient and those who care for and about them. Hypnotic approaches help children and families achieve mastery of both minutia and big-picture challenges, while respecting the varying defense mechanisms they have mobilized to protect themselves in the process. In a lovely discussion of Ericksonian hypnotic approaches with pediatric hematology–oncology patients and families, Jacobs and colleagues (Jacobs, Pelier, & Larkin, 1998) described the value of conversational hypnosis and informal strategies with this population. With rich clinical examples of children in different developmental stages, they noted the importance of careful attention to language and the importance of acknowledging and utilizing the natural hypnotic behavior that children move in and out of throughout their day. Their case vignettes serve as a wonderful model of how to find and utilize the hypnosis in the encounter.

It is also important that clinicians utilizing hypnosis consider themselves and their feelings and responses and that they re-examine their personal perspectives from time to time. Transference and countertransference problems can be particularly intense in a therapeutic relationship with a child with a life-threatening illness. Moreover, it is possible that clinicians' attitudes may affect morbidity and eventual therapeutic outcomes. Although this area is fraught with problems for the researcher, we hope to see answers take shape. Specifically, we wonder whether patients can use certain self-hypnotic strategies or techniques to facilitate biochemical, immunological, nutritional, and psychological interactions that lead to cures (see also Chapter 18).

## *Medical Procedures*

Clinical hypnosis approaches are very effective in helping children and adolescents prepare for, cope with, and tolerate the anxiety and discomfort associated with various medical procedures. Examples of effective hypnotic approaches to the common problem of needle phobia are described in Chapter 8. Here, we note some examples of effective application of hypnotic techniques for procedures as described in recently published literature.

Broome and her nursing colleagues (Broome, Lillis, McGahee, & Bates, 1992) described the effectiveness of imagery, relaxation, and distraction for 14 children receiving lumbar punctures (spinal taps) as part of their cancer treatment. Regular practice nightly and especially 3 nights prior to the next expected procedure were integral to the training in self-management. Although fear scores in children did not change, self-reports of pain ratings decreased significantly over time.

Green (1994) described the adjunctive value of guided visual imagery, relaxation, and therapeutic touch to the intensive-care management of a 17-year-old boy with muscular dystrophy and deteriorating respiratory status. The patient's ultimate acceptance of and coping with a tracheostomy seemed to be directly temporally related to the comfort he was able to achieve with the assistance of imagery and relaxation.

Marino (1994) described the effective use of therapeutic hypnosis strategies of imagery, relaxation, and joining with the patient to facilitate intensive care unit (ICU) extubation of a 12-year-old girl with severe asthma who had required 5 days of ventilator-assisted respiration. With shared imagery of their respective love of the beach, Marino's clinical hypnosis approach included elements of information giving (detailed description of the process of extubation and what could be expected), distraction and dissociation with post-hypnotic suggestion (i.e., she could go to her favorite beach during the extubation, a sure sign that she was getting better), and reframing (post-extubation cough described as a good sign of her improvement).

Pederson (1993) produced a videotape featuring four vignettes of children (actors) utilizing a variety of clinical hypnosis techniques (relaxation, favorite place imagery, dissociation, and pain switches) as an educational and research tool for children in a pediatric oncology clinic. Specific reference is made to the usefulness of these strategies for procedures, such as starting IVs, spinal taps, and bone marrow procedures.

In recent years, many clinicians have reported effective use of hypnosis and related techniques to assist children in coping with medical procedures, including immunizations, venipunctures, and laceration repairs, as well as during magnetic resonance imaging (MRI). Working in Australia, Cyna and colleagues (Cyna, Tomkins, Maddock, & Barker, 2007), described the value of conversational hypnosis with switch-wire imagery for a 5-year-old with Bruton's disease who required repeated IV placements. Because of severe needle phobia, he had previously received inhalational general anesthesia on 58 prior occasions for IV cannulation. When oral premedication and ketamine were unsatisfactory, hypnosis was considered, and he was able to experience painless venipuncture with cooperation, stillness, and no local anesthetic or other medication.

Gold and associates (Gold, Kim, Kant, Joseph, & Rizzo, 2006) reported on the effectiveness of a virtual reality imagery-distraction strategy for children requiring IV placement for magnetic resonance imaging and computed tomography. Ten children receiving standard treatment of topical anesthetic without distraction were compared to those receiving the same standard treatment plus virtual reality. There was a fourfold greater report of pain in the control condition, and those using the virtual reality showed significantly more child, parent, and nurse reported satisfaction with pain management. The authors concluded that virtual reality holds promise and that larger controlled studies would be an appropriate next step.

In adults with burns, Hoffman and Patterson (Hoffman, Patterson, & Carrougher, 2000; Hoffman, Patterson, Carrougher, & Sharar, 2001) have pioneered the use of virtual reality as a significant adjunct to pain management. Patterson continues to research the use of virtual reality and its relationship to hypnosis in the management of chronic pain (Patterson, 2010). A recent search on Google® Scholar revealed 51 citations regarding studies on virtual reality through the US National Institutes of Health, only 5 of which were related to children. Three studies that have been completed focused on (1) preoperative anxiety in pediatric reconstructive burn patients and the role of virtual reality hypnosis, (2) the usability of a virtual reality system in children with brain injury, and (3) the effects of interactive video game cycling on obese adolescent health. Two additional studies in progress are investigating combined biofeedback with virtual reality in the treatment of pediatric headache and virtual reality analgesia during pediatric physical therapy (http://clinicaltrials.gov).

Accardi and Milling (2009) conducted a comprehensive, methodologically informed review of studies of the effectiveness of hypnosis in the reduction of procedure-related pain in the pediatric population. An exhaustive review of PubMed and PsychINFO databases identified 13 studies between 1982 and 2006 that met specific criteria. The studies were required to use a between subjects or mixed-model design in which hypnosis was compared with a control condition or an alternative intervention in reducing the procedure-related discomfort of patients under age 19. Overall, the 13 studies reviewed involved 528 children between the ages of 3 and 19 years. Most of the studies involved children undergoing either bone marrow aspirations or lumbar punctures, or both (Hawkins, Liossi, Ewart, Hatira, & Kosmidis, 1998; Katz, Kellerman, & Ellenberg, 1987; Kuttner, Bowman, & Teasdale, 1988; Liossi & Hatira, 1999, 2003; Liossi, White, & Hatira, 2006; Wall & Womack, 1989; Zeltzer & LeBaron, 1982). Others included effects of hypnosis in modulation of other procedures or surgery (Butler, Symons, Henderson, Shortliffe, & Spiegel, 2005; Huth, Broome, & Good, 2004; Lambert, 1996; Lobe, 2006). In their analysis, Accardi and Milling found that hypnosis was consistently more effective than control conditions in alleviating discomfort associated with bone marrow aspirations, lumbar punctures, voiding cystourethrograms, the Nuss procedure, and postsurgical pain.

In 2013 Keefer and colleagues (Keefer, Kiebles, Martinovich, Barrett and Palsson, 2013) described the value of "gut-directed hypnotherapy" in augmenting remission in quiescent ulcerative colitis.

Iserson (1999) described the use of hypnosis in four children, 3–12 years old, who presented to the emergency room with forearm fractures. Two were Colles-type fractures (fracture of the distal radius and ulna at or near the wrist), and the other two were mid-forearm fractures with angulation. Hypnosis was the only sedation and analgesic utilized and was conducted by the emergency room physician while the orthopedist reduced the fracture and applied the cast. As the author noted, although the hypnotic suggestion was to sleep and not to feel pain and to not remember the pain or the process for reducing the fractures, upon observation, "All patients appeared awake at the time of the greatest amount of fracture manipulation (total time for reduction was 2–3 minutes) and seemed to experience pain" (Iserson, 1999, p. 55). Thereafter however, all went into a peaceful sleep state immediately following the reductions. About 2 hours later, all of the children, including the 3-year-old, said they had a broken bone, and they now had a cast, but none remembered how the cast was put on or any of the procedures in between, and all denied having any pain. These clinical experiences are consistent with our own observation of the efficacy of hypnotic approaches in pediatric emergencies (Kohen, 1986b).

Smart (1997), a clinical nurse specialist, investigated the value of guided imagery as compared to IV sedation in helping children relax to undergo magnetic resonance imaging (MRI). Twenty children between the ages of 4 and 8 years were randomly assigned to a control group (standard sedation) or to the experimental group, which listened to an imagery tape ("Magic Island") via headphones. Children unable to remain still and relax for the procedure were given IV sedation. Seven of the ten children listening to imagery remained still and calm for the MRI. Of the three who required sedation, one began the MRI fine and remained relaxed for 20 minutes before requiring sedation; the other two are described as having listened "only briefly." By contrast, only two of the ten in the control group were able to remain calm and did not require sedation.

Uman and colleagues (Uman, Chambers, McGrath, & Kisely, 2008) conducted a comprehensive review of 28 trials with 1951 child and adolescent participants. Most involved needle procedures for immunizations and injections. Even with what we would consider somewhat arbitrary distinction between imagery and hypnosis and other hypnotic-like interventions, this extensive review concluded that there is sufficient evidence to support the efficacy of distraction, hypnosis, and combined cognitive behavioral therapy in reducing pain and distress in children and adolescents undergoing needle procedures. Moreover, only distraction, hypnosis, and distraction plus suggestion were effective in reducing self-reported pain or distress.

In a recently published study, Berberich and Landman (2009) demonstrated the efficacy of a multifaceted distraction method designed to reduce injection-associated pain in school-aged children. While also demonstrating that high-quality research can be accomplished in a busy pediatric practice setting, this RCT in a California practice evaluated 41 children, 4–6 years old, who were given three standard pre-kindergarten immunizations. Twenty-one were randomly assigned to an office routine control group, and the other 20 received a multifaceted, discomfort-reducing intervention that included adding verbal suggestions of diminished sensation and a visual focusing activity to the use of a topical ethyl chloride spray. The distraction materials used included topical ethyl chloride, an improvised plastic multipronged arm gripper, and a vibrating instrument descending on the contralateral arm, thus providing the focusing task and visual distraction. With the use of patient and parent Faces Pain Scale–Revised scores and videotaped observation scores, the intervention group showed highly significant reductions in pain and discomfort compared with the control group (patient self-report, $p < .0013$; parent report, $p < .0002$; observation score, $p < .0001$).

In a recent report, Claude and associates (2016) described their effective use of hypnosis in radiotherapy as an alternative to general anesthesia for children requiring radiation for cancer.

More recently several studies have shown the value of therapeutic hypnosis for procedural anxiety. In 2013, Delord and colleagues in France published a pilot study to evaluate the efficacy of medical hypnosis with nine children with various causes for anticipatory anxiety as candidates for long-term non-invasive positive pressure ventilation (NPPV) (Delord et al., 2013). Seven of the nine children had anticipatory anxiety in association with prior and/or underlying conditions: two children had a tracheostomy since birth, two had prior maxillofacial surgery, two had dyspnea because of lung disease, one had morbid obesity with depression. The other two patients had obstructive sleep apnea and had failed standard initiation of NPPV. Hypnosis was started in all patients to facilitate acclimatization to the NPPV. A narrative description of the therapeutic hypnotic approaches notes the appropriate variety and tailoring of the hypnosis strategies to the age and development of the children, their personal histories and anxieties, and their personal imagery. Following a mean duration of 15 minutes (range = 10–30 minutes) first hypnosis session all of the patients accepted the interface and NPPV at the first session. A median of three sessions was required for an overnight NPPV acceptance (= over hours). All patients were able to sleep at least 4 hours with the ventilator the first night and at least 6 hours with NPPV after the third night, after which they were able to be discharged from the hospital. No further formal hypnosis was required at home. Long-term follow-up at 6 months was described as excellent with compliance of a median of 7.5 hours/night in eight of the nine patients (Delord et al., 2013).

Khirani and associates (Khirani, Kadlub, Delord, Picard, & Fauroux, 2013) published a case report of a 4-year-old boy who had severe obstructive sleep apnea due to complete nasal obstruction because of cherubism. With a history of anticipatory anxiety with numerous prior surgical procedures, medical hypnosis was proposed to facilitate non-invasive continuous positive pressure ventilation (CPAP). After three hypnosis sessions CPAP via an oral interface was readily accepted and resulted in resolution of his obstructive sleep apnea syndrome (Khirani et al., 2013).

In 2021, Kumari and colleagues (Kumari, Bahuguna, Garg, & Yeluri, 2021) published their study to evaluate and compare the efficacy of immersive virtual reality and non-immersive virtual reality distraction on perceived pain in children during intraoral injections for dental procedures. Two hundred children participated, randomized with 100 in the immersive virtual reality group and 100 in the non-immersive group. They were introduced to Oculus Go Standalone (www.oculus.com) and the treatment procedure. Group I subjects were given a hand controller and told they could choose to play one of two games (temple run or roller coaster game) and Group II children could watch cartoons of their choice. Preoperatively the anxiety scores on the Modified Dental Anxiety Scale (MCDAS) were similar in both groups but postoperatively the anxiety scores on the MCDAS were higher in the non-immersive group compared to the immersive. Analogous differences were found, i.e., higher anxiety on the VAS and Wong-Baker Faces Pain Rating Scale (WBFRS) scales in the non-immersive group compared to the immersive group. Significant differences were found in the immersive group, both in lower anxiety and in perception of less pain during intraoral injection. The investigators concluded that the virtual reality distraction technique is a valuable adjunct to traditional behavioral management strategies already available to pediatric dentists (Kumari et al., 2021).

In a systematic review and meta-analysis, Nunns and colleagues (2018) evaluated the effectiveness of non-pharmacological interventions to reduce procedural anxiety in children and youth receiving treatment for cancer. They concluded that hypnosis shows promise for treatment of children with cancer.

For completeness, we wish to mention the potential importance and value of music and music therapy in facilitating comfort for children during medical procedures. Although a detailed exploration of this topic and its relationship to therapeutic hypnosis is beyond the scope of this volume, interested readers may wish to review the work of Klassen and colleagues, who recently conducted a systematic review of randomized controlled trials (involving 1,513 subjects) of music for pain and anxiety for children undergoing medical procedures (Klassen, Liang, Tjosvold, Klassen, & Hartling, 2008), a randomized study conducted by Caprilli and colleagues (Caprilli, Anastasi, Grotto, Abeti, & Messeri, 2007), and the work of Dr. Deforia Lane (1994).

## Neurological Problems

Therapeutic hypnosis has been associated with the disappearance of migraine headaches, post-encephalitic headaches, tics, hiccups, cyclic vomiting, and urine retention. It has also been used as adjunct therapy to help children with seizures, chronic muscle disorders, Tourette's syndrome, or cerebral palsy and to facilitate rehabilitation for complex regional pain syndrome, previously known as reflex sympathetic dystrophy (RSD), as well as severe neurological injuries. Its use in children with attentional disorders was discussed in Chapter 11.

## Headaches

Headache in childhood and adolescence is almost ubiquitous. In an epidemiological study in Germany of more than 5,400 children and adolescents, 65% of children at the age of 14 years had experienced headache, and 10.5% suffered regularly from headache at least once a week (Kroner-Herwig, Morris, & Heinrich, 2004). The frequency of headaches in children is reported as ranging from 21% to 55%; the reported prevalence of juvenile migraines ranges from 5% to 10%. Headaches may be characterized as migraine headaches, muscle-contraction headaches (tension), or organic headaches (brain tumors, malformations, or encephalopathies). It is possible that some headaches characterized as migraines or muscle-contraction headaches belong in the organic category. Careful diagnostic evaluation is essential prior to recommendation for any treatment intervention, including therapeutic clinical hypnosis (Olness & MacDonald, 1987). In particular, the child should be examined with respect to blood pressure measurements, neurological status, presence or absence of purulent rhinorrhea, bruits of the head, dental abscesses, temporomandibular joint status, growth velocity, and skin lesions. Environmental toxins such as lead or carbon monoxide may cause headaches. Food allergies may trigger the migraine syndrome.

In the event that the diagnosis of tension or migraine headache is reasonably well established, the child may benefit substantially from training in self-hypnosis. A number of uncontrolled clinical studies (Andrasik, Blanchard, Edlund, & Rosenblum, 1982; Houts, 1982; Labbé & Williamson, 1983; Werder & Sargent, 1984) and one prospective controlled study (Olness, MacDonald, & Uden, 1987) have reported success in teaching child migraineurs self-regulation techniques for control of pain. In our prospective study, we compared propranolol, placebo, and self-hypnosis in the treatment of juvenile classic migraine. Children ages 6–12 years with classic migraine who had had no previous specific treatment were randomized into propranolol or placebo groups for a 3-month period and then crossed over to the other treatment for 3 months. After this 6-month medication trial, each child was taught self-hypnosis, and this was reinforced in five visits over 3 months. The entire study was completed by 28 children. The mean number of headaches per child for 3 months during the placebo period was 13.3 as compared with 14.9 during the propranolol and 5.8 during the self-hypnosis periods. Statistical analysis showed a significant association between decrease in frequency of headaches and self-hypnosis training. There was no significant change in subjective or objective measures of headache severity with either therapy.

Engel, Rapoff, and Pressman (1992) did a long-term follow-up on 17 of 20 original participants from a prospective control-group experimental design study with random assignment to autogenic relaxation, progressive relaxation, autogenic plus progressive relaxation, or wait-list control groups. Long-term follow-up data were obtained at an average of 51 months after treatment. The participants from the three treatment groups had significantly more headache-free days and less severe headaches compared to the control group. Of the 13 treated participants, 12 used relaxation training to relieve headaches, and seven reported practicing within the past month.

Osterhaus and colleagues (1993) evaluated the outcome of a combined behavioral therapy program in a school with adolescents, ages 12–19 years. The program included relaxation training, temperature biofeedback, and cognitive training. Each subject received four group sessions and four individual sessions. In the group session, information was given about pain, migraine, and pain-coping strategies. The subjects also practiced progressive relaxation, autogenic relaxation, self-hypnosis, and rational emotive therapy. The four individual sessions consisted of 40 minutes of peripheral temperature biofeedback. Subjects were asked to practice the relaxation and self-hypnosis twice daily and were followed for 7 months. A 41% decrease in migraine frequency was observed in the experimental group, which increased to 54% at the 7-month follow-up. The acquired capacity to raise finger temperature during biofeedback training and decreased state anxiety during the sessions were related to headache reduction after the training. Older children showed more reduction in headache duration than the younger children. The authors noted that they could not comment on the effect of the separate therapeutic strategies, although we would judge that each of the strategies, except for rational emotive therapy, involves self-hypnosis.

We have described the effectiveness of self-hypnosis training for headache in a retrospective review of 178 consecutive youths referred to our program for help with recurrent headaches between 1988 and 2001 (Kohen & Zajac, 2007). In this retrospective review, complete data were available on 144 patients in this self-selected and uncontrolled observation. All patients were taught self-hypnosis for self-regulation of headaches, and the intensity, frequency, and duration of headaches before, during, and after treatment were measured. Compared with self-reports before learning self-hypnosis. children and youth who learned self-hypnosis for recurrent headaches reported a reduction in frequency of headaches from 4.5 per week to 1.4 per week ($p < .01$), a reduction in intensity (on a scale from 0 to 12) from an average of 10.3–4.7 ($p < .01$), and a reduction in average duration from 23.6 hours to 3 hours ($p < 0.1$). In response to training in self-hypnosis, 25% of patients became headache free, and those who still had some headaches reported relative ease and speed of management with self-hypnosis skills, reflected in their reported overall reduced duration of headaches.

Trautmann and colleagues (Trautmann, Lackschewitz, & Kroner-Herwig, 2006) reported a meta-analysis of studies regarding psychological treatments of recurrent headache in children and adolescents. They reviewed 23 studies (1966–2004) that met the following inclusion criteria:

1. The study had to be a RCT that incorporated psychological treatments aimed at preventing migraine or recurrent tension-type headache episodes or reducing their intensity and duration, and the control condition had to include a waitlist or an active control group (e.g., placebo).
2. All subjects, including controls, had to have had at least two headache episodes per month before the study.
3. The studies had to be available in English or German.
4. Study participants had to be primarily children and adolescents with an average age of < 18 years.
5. The studies had to examine one or more of relaxation training, biofeedback or cognitive behavioral therapy, or combinations of these.
6. The number of subjects in each treatment or control group had to be $N \geq 4$.
7. Sufficient data had to be available to calculate effect sizes regarding headache frequency, duration, intensity, and medication.

This analysis defined relaxation techniques as including progressive muscle relaxation, autogenic training, and self-hypnosis, all of which we would consider to be hypnosis or hypnosis-like procedures. Likewise, we would also consider biofeedback procedures to all have hypnotic-like processes, and as discussed earlier, we agree that many if not most cognitive behavioral interventions often include elements of relaxation and imagery. Initially, 43 outcome studies were identified, and 20 were excluded for one or more reasons of not meeting the inclusion criteria noted above. The 23 studies comprised an overall sample of 935 children and adolescents and were performed in the United States (8), Canada (4), Germany (4), Sweden (5), the Netherlands (1), and Australia (1). The most frequently examined treatment was relaxation training (as defined above) in 16 studies, and the overall average age of participants was 12 years. In this important and careful analysis across studies, significantly more patients improved to a clinically relevant degree (i.e., ≥ 50% reduction in headache) in the treatment groups compared to the control/wait-list condition groups. Long-term stability was also confirmed, as the treatments analyzed led to improvement up to 1 year following treatment.

In a randomized controlled trial of college students with migraine headache ($N$ = 90) or tension headaches ($N$ = 51), D'Souza and associates (D'Souza, Lumley, Kraft, & Dooley, 2008) compared relaxation training to written emotional disclosure. Their intention was to compare the efficacy of interventions that reduce arousal and negative emotions, such as relaxation with interventions that may temporarily increase negative emotions (e.g., written emotional disclosure). As predicted, the relaxation training led to an immediate increase in calmness for both tension and migraine headache groups, and at 3-month follow-up the relaxation training led to greater reductions in headache frequency ($p$ = 0.04) and less headache disability ($p$ = 0.003) for the tension headache group compared to the control (written emotional disclosure) group. For the migraine headache group, the relaxation training was better than the control group only in pain severity but not on the other outcomes measured. The authors speculate that this difference was likely related to the fact that the relatively modest relaxation training intervention was limited to four brief 20-minute audiotape relaxation sessions without therapist contact and that migraine is a more challenging condition. Indeed, the relaxation training intervention included four sessions in which the participants sat in a comfortable chair in a private room and listened to different sections of an audiotape. Session 1 focused on active relaxation training for 14 muscle groups (cued and release); session 2 taught deep breathing and autogenic procedures; session 3 added vivid imagery and breathing techniques to differential relaxation; and session 4 integrated the previous skills. Participants were encouraged to practice at home and were given the standardized tape. No individual rapport, history review, or personalized training was provided.

Connelly and colleagues (Connelly, Rapoff, Thompson, & Connelly, 2006) introduced a different minimal-therapist contact intervention by evaluating "Headstrong," a pain management program on CD for children with recurrent headache. Children 7–12 years of age were randomly assigned to a wait-list control group (and continued with prescriptions and recommendations of their neurologist) or to the use of the "Headstrong" program, which they worked through on home computers for 4 weeks. Data were collected on daily headache activity and headache-related disability at baseline and up to 3 months after treatment. Children who used the "Headstrong" program ($N$ = 14) had improved headache frequency ($p < .01$), duration ($p < .01$), and severity ($p < .01$) compared to the control group. Although the article makes no mention of hypnosis or hypnotherapy, the description of the "Headstrong" program and its described components (i.e., "Module 1, Education; Module 2, Relaxation; Module 3, Coping; Module 4, Behavior) clearly represents a therapeutic hypnosis methodology. Module 1 provides a discussion of the types, prevalence, and diagnosis of headache. The four lessons provided in Module 2 are "Rationale for Relaxation," "How to Use Guided Imagery," "How to Use Deep Breathing," and "How to Use Progressive Muscle Relaxation." These critical ingredients of self-hypnosis are supplemented in lessons in Modules 3 and 4, which address thought changing, problem solving, positive and negative pain behaviors, and pain behavior management, all of which appropriately could be characterized as *utilization* in a therapeutic hypnosis framework. In discussion, the authors promote the promise of this apparent value-added standardized program that supplements regular medical care of the child with headache (Zimmern, 2017).

We would add that, although such standardized CDs, like standardized audiotapes, have potential value, such value is considerably enhanced when the programs have the ability to be personalized and, in some way, tailored to the individual needs and desires of the individual child. As a rule, therefore, although we do not quarrel with families who ask about audiotape programs or CDs (which they typically have already purchased), we preferentially offer to prepare personally developed audio CDs for our patients' use. Commonly, children and teens request these, are eager to participate in developing ideas for the content for their personal CDs and are very grateful to feel that they have their personal coach at home as needed.

The effectiveness of therapeutic hypnosis approaches in managing chronic daily headache in several adolescents was recently described (Kohen, 2009). Even adolescents who have had relentless and debilitating daily headaches for several years can learn self-hypnosis and effectively reduce or eliminate the substantial morbidity and suffering that have sadly become their maturation-impeding way of life. One of our patients, an accomplished poet at 17 years of age, wrote a lengthy poem reflecting his successful application of self-hypnosis. This poem is published in its entirety in the fourth edition of this text (Kohen & Olness, 2011, Chapter 13, pp. 290–294).

We recommend that children who have migraine or other forms of chronic headache learn self-hypnosis, if they are willing, as soon as possible after the diagnosis is made. Practically, training requires three or four visits and twice daily practice by the child for at least a month. Following the initial intense practice period, practice can gradually be reduced to once daily and then to twice weekly. As is true with respect to other chronic problems that benefit from some training in self-regulation of autonomic processes, it is essential that the child, not the parent, control practice. As computer game feedback programs appropriate to training in chronic pain syndromes become increasingly available, these should make regular home practice more appealing to most children.

Follow-up, by telephone, email, or letter, is important. Children who have biological bases for pain syndromes usually do far better in achieving the desired pain control than do children who have pain that is triggered primarily by emotional experiences. Therapists must be alert to the possibility that the biological basis for the syndrome has been missed or that a biological basis has developed for continuing headaches.

Based on a completed project (Kohen, 2010b), we now have evidence of the apparent enduring benefit of learning self-hypnosis for the management of headaches during childhood and adolescence. Following the retrospective review of our 178 consecutive patients with headaches trained in self-hypnosis, we conducted a mail survey of all these patients who we could find. We sought to ascertain their current status regarding headaches and to learn what we could about their attitudes and beliefs regarding self-hypnosis, both when they were having headaches and initially came to us for help and later, 9–20 years after their last clinical visits. We were able to locate 134 of the original 178 patients; of the 134 delivered surveys, 52 were returned complete. From 9 to 20 years after treatment, 85% (44/52) reported continued relief from self-hypnosis, 44% (23/52) reported decreased headache frequency, 31% (16/52) noted decreased severity, and well over half (29/52) reported that self-hypnosis reduced headache intensity. Many (26/52) emphasized the value of self-hypnosis to life stresses:

- *From an 18-year-old woman.* "I lay in my bed and put on my headphones to block out any noise. There's no specific music type, just whatever I feel like. I close my eyes and focus on the music. I skip around from image to image and let myself 'sink' into nowhere! … I have passed the self-hypnosis techniques to other friends who suffer from migraines. I just give them the basics and let them find a system that works for them."
- *From a 21-year-old woman who learned self-hypnosis when she was 8 years old.* "I usually practice before I go to bed at night. I use my tape that you made me 13 years ago. I use the imagery on the tape."
- *From a 24-year-old woman who learned self-hypnosis when she was 13 years old.* "Lay down in a dark room and close my eyes and picture myself standing on a beach in the sun. As I begin to walk down the beach there are numbers written in the sand beginning with whatever number my headache is currently at. I use my feet to erase the numbers. When I reach zero,

I sit or lay down on the beach and focus on what a pain-free head feels like. Usually, I fall asleep at this point. I use my scene now whenever I feel overwhelmed … even if it's not headache related. … I simply begin my numbers at the point of stress rather than my pain scale. I've also felt an aura coming on and used them to calm myself down into relaxation before a full aura starts. I am so grateful for teaching me how to deal with my migraines. I don't know how I would have survived them without his advice and 'coaching.' I am so happy and proud to say I've been migraine free for eleven years! Thank you for doing wonderful work!"

- *From a 16-year-old female.* "I imagine myself walking thru the woods. I do my self-hypnosis wherever I am when I need to do it. I listen to the air currents in the room, and I imagine that I'm chasing Magic (my uncle's dog) through the woods. When I catch the dog I know my headache is gone. I also use self-hypnosis when I'm really nervous. It helps me calm down so I can concentrate on whatever I need and am doing. Sometimes I use it when I am angry. It helps me calm down."
- *From a 28-year-old male.* "I pulled out the original imagery audio tapes made for me in our first visits together when I was 17, at the age of 23 so I could relearn how to make my body relax. For the last 4 years I have had very few actual migraine headaches, reduced the intensity of stress headaches, and learned to better manage stress in general, due in no small part to our sessions."
- *From a 25-year-old woman.* "I begin by sitting in my bed with some relaxing music playing softly. My eyes close and I begin to visualize a staircase. The staircase leads to a hot tub and after relaxing my hot tub leads me to a meadow and at the end is a pond with a seat. While at the pond I concentrate on relieving any pain I might have and completely relax. I use it daily to unwind after work or just a long day. I have also used it for sleep. I had a very complicated pregnancy and quite a bit of pain, and imagery helped me to control the pain. The pain never ceased but it was tolerable with the imagery. Not even medication helped it. I wanted to thank you for the wonderful gift you gave me. Mental imagery helped me through my very difficult pregnancy. Between kidney surgery and a 4-month migraine which no medication could help, imagery helped me to control pain to being manageable versus bedridden. I also used imagery on bed rest to help with my back pain. Again, I want to thank you for this gift and send my best wishes to you."

In children and adolescents, self-hypnosis is associated with significant improvement of headaches and with an enduring positive effect for many years following training. Along with the work of Kuttner (1998) in describing the lasting value of learning self-hypnosis in children with cancer, these results support our long-held clinical intuition of the common and spontaneous generalizability of self-hypnosis by young people to modulation of other problems in their lives.

The case of a 15-year-old young woman with severe chronic daily headache was presented in detail in a recent publication (Kohen & Kaiser, 2014). This adolescent's verbatim account of learning to manage, eliminate, and prevent headaches provides another example of the essential ingredients of rapport, individualizing language and allowing the patient to lead themselves where they wish to go (Kohen & Kaiser, 2014, pp. 88–89).

Recently, one of us (DPK) described the particular value of storytelling as integral to therapeutic hypnosis for children and youth with headaches (Kohen, 2016). This strategy, the "I knew this kid once who … ." is described in detail and reflected in case examples in two different recent publications (Kohen, 2016, 2018).

With the emergence of the "new" specialty of Integrative Medicine/Integrative Pediatrics Medicine over the past decade, increasing attention has been paid appropriately to the value of what had previously been relegated to "complementary and alternative medicine" and notably so in the context of the biopsychosocial model of health care of particular value in caring for children and families. The case was made for understanding that pediatric hypnosis was likely among the earliest approaches to embrace the concept of pediatric integrative medicine, and this is reflected in the article by Kaiser and colleagues in 2018 (Kaiser, Kohen, Brown, Kajander, & Barnes, 2018). Children and teens are described who learned and utilized therapeutic hypnosis as integrated variably with mindfulness meditation, biofeedback, acupuncture, yoga, as well as with timely utilization of medication and nutritional guidance.

Esparham and Dilts (2019) provide added detail to our understanding of the ways in which lifestyle approaches, dietary supplements, nutraceuticals, transcutaneous neurostimulation may be applied and added to psychological strategies and therapeutic hypnosis in the management of primary headache disorders (Esparham & Dilts, 2019).

## *Seizures*

Therapeutic hypnosis has been reported to be successful not only for psychogenic seizures (see Chapter 7) but also for seizures whose etiology is primarily organic (Puskarich et al., 1992). Crasilneck and Hall (1975) reviewed the literature concerning adults and concluded that "although the mechanism for such effect is not always clear, it may often be usefully conceptualized as a change in the balance of facilitating or inhibiting neural impulses" (pp. 205–206). They noted further that reported improvement of epilepsy after therapeutic hypnosis "may involve some change in the excitability of the cortex around the epileptogenic focus, although experimental validation of this hypothesis is lacking" (p. 206). Five case histories were reported in which children and adolescents with chronic seizure disorders responded well to a combination of psychotherapy and clinical hypnosis. They emphasized that uncontrolled seizures produce psychological trauma for any patient and that treatment that enables the patient and family to deal with this trauma more effectively might contribute to the breaking of a cycle of seizure-inducing psychophysiological activation.

We employed clinical therapeutic hypnosis with a patient who had nocturnal epilepsy and was unresponsive to conventional anticonvulsants. Although the patient had significant psychological problems and was being seen concurrently for psychotherapy, the fact that seizures occurred primarily during sleep suggests an organic basis for her epilepsy. We present the case in some detail to underscore the difficulty of understanding both etiology and treatment mechanisms.

Katie Q. was first referred for clinical hypnosis as adjunct management of nocturnal seizures at age 15.5 years. The patient had first developed seizure-like activity at age 12. She was hospitalized and found to have EEGs with abnormal foci in left anterior and frontal regions of the brain. She was treated with the then standard anticonvulsant medications, phenobarbital, and Dilantin™. During a subsequent hospitalization for seizure control, her EEG was found to be normal (a finding that does not rule out organic etiology) and medications were discontinued. Her "spells" continued, usually at night and rarely during the day. She would awaken with severe muscle spasms, lasting about 2 minutes, followed by the feeling of paralysis of all her body except her left arm and head. She frequently urinated and felt a loss of control. After many months' trials of anticonvulsants and psychiatric treatment, with little change in seizure control, the patient was referred for therapeutic hypnosis.

Katie was seen six times for clinical hypnosis treatment. During the first session, efforts were initially made to determine her hobbies, interests, and dislikes. She indicated a preference for rock and jazz music and enthusiasm about horseback riding, bicycle riding, and walks. The therapist went on to discuss sleep stages and how they are reflected in EEG patterns. Rapid eye movement (REM) and non-rapid eye movement (non-REM) sleep were discussed. Katie was told that it would be useful if her subconscious mind could give information to her about the stage during which the seizures were triggered (e.g., from medium to deep sleep or from light to medium sleep).

Hypnosis was achieved via eye fixation on one of many rings she had on her fingers. She then focused on breathing out and coordinating that with progressive relaxation. She was given the option of closing her eyes and visualizing numbers in sequence until she found a favorite place in her mind. She used a lifted finger to signal when she felt as though she were in a favorite place. She rapidly indicated she was there and was given the option of relaxing even more deeply by imagining she was horseback riding or bicycle riding in an area of her choosing. She chose horseback riding. She was asked to ride until she was so relaxed that her body recognized she could identify the sleep phase in which her seizures occurred. Although she appeared very relaxed, she did not, over a 10-minute period, give any further finger signals. Recognizing possible resistance, we suggested to her that perhaps she would need more practice before she was ready to obtain this information and that she should, nonetheless, program herself to turn off the trigger to the seizure as she was passing from one stage of sleep to another. She accepted this and, when out of the hypnotic trance, agreed that she would practice the exercise twice a day.

Two weeks later, Katie seemed eager to go into hypnosis. The hypnotic invitation was similar, and once again she was asked to continue relaxing until she was ready to identify the sleep phase in which her seizures occurred. Repeatedly, her right and left thumbs raised slightly, and after 12 minutes, the right pointer finger lifted. When asked if that was her "yes" finger, she again raised the right finger and signaled that the left pointer finger was "no." Further inquiry about sleep stages revealed no new information. The therapist reinforced the suggestion that, at an unconscious level, she had all the information she needed to control the seizures and that she could turn off the trigger as she passed from one sleep stage to another.

On the third visit, Katie seemed more relaxed than in any previous session and went through the initial invitation without verbal cues. After 5 minutes, she raised her right index finger, signaling that she was relaxed enough to program her autonomic nervous system to control body functions in a way that was good for her. The therapist said, "It's all right. If you wish to have pleasant dreams instead of seizures—to enjoy those dreams, let those dreams be satisfying and pleasant. When you control the seizures, you will be a stronger and happier person. Sunshine always follows rain." Following this session, Katie was relaxed and good humored and said she thought the time passed was 5 minutes instead of the actual 25 minutes.

In the month before beginning therapeutic hypnosis, Katie had 15 seizures. During the next month, there were only four seizures. Between the third and fourth sessions, Katie had two nocturnal seizures, possibly associated with anxiety concerning a planned 20-mile charity walk. At the fourth visit, the therapist added positive future imagery, asking Katie to imagine feelings of physical and emotional well-being at a future time when she was seizure free. She was then asked if she would be willing to determine her seizure aura. She agreed and went rapidly into a trance with very few verbal cues. She indicated with an ideomotor signal when she was prepared to determine the aura. After 5 minutes she opened her eyes, said it was "weird," and she didn't enjoy the part when she was getting information about her aura. She said she felt as though both legs were moving rapidly up and down. She said in the fifth session that she did not want to pursue the aura. She was taught a jettison technique after focusing on a happy memory amplified with a clenched fist. On coming out of trance, she said she had enjoyed this. Ability to jettison problems was reinforced in the sixth session. Subsequently she improved remarkably in school and home relationships. There were no further seizures over a 2-year follow-up.

### *Urine Retention*

Positive response was reported after a single session of therapeutic hypnosis in the case of a 10-year-old girl with psychogenic urinary retention. This followed a herpes zoster infection in her inguinal area and placement of a suprapubic cystostomy. Urinary infections followed and life-threatening sepsis was a possibility in this patient with compromised immunological defenses. The psychiatrist noted that this patient had been traumatized and terrified by numerous bodily invasions that deprived her of autonomous control of body functions. While she was in a trance state, he had her repeat the following statements out loud: (1) "when people are very scared and upset they stop making pee-pee"; (2) "by relaxing, I can overcome my scared and upset feelings"; and (3) "the sooner I can make pee-pee, the sooner they will take the tube out." The three points were written down on a card for the patient to review during self-hypnosis. Within a few hours, after this single session, she began voiding.

We have often written reminder affirmation statements for children to use during self-hypnosis. This may be important especially in children who have stronger visual than auditory images. The following case history concerns an adolescent patient with acute neurological handicaps, including urinary retention, who developed his own creative imagery to overcome the problems.

Neal C., age 17 years, was admitted to the hospital for the sixth time in relapse with Hodgkin's disease, stage IV-B. He was referred for clinical hypnosis to control severe back pain, headaches, and nausea. At the time of the initial therapeutic hypnosis session, he was pleasant and interested but complained of pain and anorexia. After some discussion about his interests, likes, dislikes, and habits, the therapist chose a method of invitation to hypnosis which was related to his interest in electronic circuitry. He imagined himself constructing a radio until he was ready to accept suggestions for relief of symptoms.

At the first visit, he was given hypnotic suggestions to recall a happy mealtime and enjoy feelings of pleasant hunger. At the conclusion of the first clinical hypnosis session, he volunteered that his headache was "almost gone," and he added, "Strange, now I feel hungry." Chemotherapy was begun on the following day. Although the patient had expressed prior fears about vomiting, no nausea or vomiting occurred. When seen 2 weeks later in outpatient follow-up, he reported having had no nausea or vomiting throughout the recent course of treatment. He also volunteered that he used self-hypnosis to enable him to easily sleep each night. At that visit, clinical self-hypnosis techniques reviewed included progressive relaxation and imagery of computer construction. It was recommended that the patient read Norman Cousins's article in the *New England Journal of Medicine* (1976) concerning personal mastery in the face of chronic illness.

Neal did well for 9 months until he was admitted to the hospital with severe neurological symptoms including diplopia, loss of balance, absent gag reflex, and urinary retention. Consultants in neurology and oncology were unable to explain the symptoms. Results of EEG studies, computerized tomography scans, analysis of spinal fluid, and other laboratory studies were normal. Because of the patient's inability to care for himself after a week of hospitalization, plans were under way for nursing home placement. Happily, the patient dramatically improved. His dictated account, requested from him on the day following his recovery, follows:

> Early afternoon the doctors came into my room and said that unless I improved in the next 48 hours they would begin an experimental drug called ARA-C in order to remove or help restore my double vision, dizziness, bladder control, balance, and gag reflexes. ARA-C was an experimental drug and both agreed that it didn't provide much hope, so that night I was going to try to program my own and restore all or release some of these reflexes.

The reflex that I missed most was stereo vision, and if I was going to have one eye covered in order that I would not get these headaches and nausea and see double, that was the first one I concentrated on. At 7 p.m. that night, I virtually closed off my room to the public, had a dose of Tylenol and laid back, uncovered my left eye, and looked at the ceiling at a cat poster, which had been put there a day earlier. This cat was going to be my object and the focus for the next 12 hours while I concentrated on obtaining my vision without the headaches, nausea, and dizziness and tried to regain control of my bladder.

The way I went about relaxing or restoring these functions was very simple. I simply lowered the head on the bed back to a comfortable position, opened both eyes, and immediately I would see two cats spread apart approximately 2 feet and they were throbbing and coming in and out at me. This was confusing, but with the Tylenol the headache was tolerable. I continued staring at the cat for a period of 10 to 15 minutes when I would have to shut both eyes in order to relax for a while because I could feel the headache coming on and felt that if I pushed it too far to begin with the headache might become unbearable, and I would give up. After resting my eyes for a period of 3 to 5 minutes, I would begin opening my eyes and again concentrate on the cat, trying to maintain a single image in my mind where there was two. I would think of a single cat, and sometimes the cats would be closer together and sometimes a little farther apart. To this method, I would go through over and over and whenever I needed a rest, I'd shut both eyes in order that they both would get the same effect.

After 3 or 4 hours I began to notice that the cat was a bit closer and maybe not throbbing as much, which was encouraging, and I would rest, and I would get my Tylenol in order to help relax and relieve the headache. After about 6 to 8 hours, at about 3:30 in the morning, I could maintain a single cat without really trying very hard, but the pulsating was still there, and I fell asleep for about 2 hours. At 6:30 that morning, I again was staring at the cat; this time it was much easier to maintain a single image, and the throbbing had virtually disappeared. The pain had subsided enough that the next day I did not take Tylenol at all, and the doctors, because of this, postponed the ARA-C another 24 hours.

Also during the night that I was concentrating on my cat, I was concentrating on bladder control. I had not been able to control my bladder for about 7 days. I thought that was another function that I would be able to return to myself. The way I went about doing that was as I concentrated on the cat I concentrated on having my bladder turned off, as an on-and-off faucet, and the faucet was turned all the way off. I felt that if I could keep the faucet "off for 12 hours and then turn it 'on' and concentrate just on going on after 12 hours, the bladder would have to be full of enough liquids that no matter what, it would go. This method proved effective except that when I turned the 'on' back, it took about 10 minutes for the first stream to flow. Once again, the doctors thought this was encouraging; therefore, they would let the drugs slip by for 1 more day.

I myself felt much happier and was in brighter spirits that day because I feel like I accomplished much more than I could have with the drug. All Saturday, with my stereo vision restored and not having to wear a patch and my partial bladder control restored, the main worry was having headaches, and there was still the gag reflex and more control of the bladder. I turned the bladder off in my mind and just concentrated that it was in the 'off' position for a full 12 hours before I'd even try to go. This proved to be effective, as this time when I let my mind turn the bladder 'on,' I went to the bathroom almost immediately. … [For] the gag reflex, I had no idea about how to go about getting this small reflex back.

> I had something I would try and that was just to imagine that every time I swallowed that swallowing is like a wave coming on an ocean, and this would go down my throat and when the wave would break it would hit my stomach. This I repeated over and over and over, and it seemed that that night that I was even able to swallow water. I just imagined a wave and that it would break on my stomach.
>
> Sunday morning, I continued to show improvement in all areas, and I believe the doctors were much happier. One doctor was finally smiling, and the other didn't come in. I had gotten control of most of my functions, more control, felt weak, unbalanced, unsteady with standing up, but this may be due to being in bed for a week straight. I was in much greater spirits, and I feel that I can have a quicker recovery rate, and Sunday afternoon my NG tube was removed, and I was able to swallow clear liquids on my own.
>
> Unfortunately, I will begin chemotherapy in another hour. I am very nervous. I will try to use relaxation. I feel that I can give better answers if I were posed questions as I am a terrible dictator. I've been very brief, and I have been unable to put into words exactly how, what, when, why, whatever happened."

Subsequently, the patient underwent 5 days of chemotherapy without difficulty and was discharged. Discharge diagnosis was Hodgkin's disease, stage IV-B now in partial remission, and acute brain syndrome, cause unknown. The patient remained in good health for 4 months. He then developed influenza complicated by pneumonia and died after 48 hours.

## *Vomiting*

Children are often referred to a clinician who utilizes hypnosis for help with management of nausea and vomiting associated with chemotherapy or with some perceived stressful situation such as going to school. It is essential to evaluate the problem in terms of what triggers nausea and vomiting in the child, how the family reacts, and how medical staff react. Vomiting is one of the most easily conditioned of reflexes. Presumed biological bases for nausea and vomiting include viral illnesses, allergies, chemotherapeutic agents, antibiotics, radiation therapy, and many metabolic disorders. The feeling of nausea or act of vomiting may be linked with environmental factors including persons, rooms, cars, buildings, colors, scents, songs, food, television programs, and so forth. The sight of a needle or of a medicine tray may induce vomiting.

Sokel and colleagues (Sokel, Devane, Bentovim, & Milla, 1990) reported an apparent example of such a conditioned response in a 9-year-old boy with vomiting. Previously well, this boy had been given a prescription for bisacodyl for treatment of constipation and developed nausea in association with this medication. When the medication was discontinued, the vomiting persisted, leading to school avoidance in the context of having already experienced bullying at school and of increased parental attention. Intractable vomiting persisted, occurring effortlessly 5–10 minutes after meals, resulting in a 15% weight loss, hospital admission, and extensive radiological and laboratory studies, all of which were normal. Weight loss was reversed, and vomiting reduced with nasojejunal feeding. He and his family had the vomiting explained to them as a reflex habit that could be treated with clinical hypnosis. He was taught self-hypnosis, including relaxation, guided imagery that incorporated his love of cooking and animals, and a story of a special garden in which he found ingredients with antiemetic powers to bake into a cake. Direct suggestions were given: "You feel your tummy becoming relaxed and comfortable so that when you eat you do not vomit." The suggestions were recorded on audiotape for him to listen to before meals. Privileges in the hospital were contingent upon success, and individual counseling was also provided. Symptom relief began immediately and progressed so that the patient was able to retain food for 20 minutes by the third day and until the next meal by the 11th day. Cessation of all vomiting was achieved by the 17th day. A week later he had a relapse when he also developed chicken pox, but vomiting was eliminated by 4 weeks with no recurrence at 12-month follow-up.

Chemotherapy-related nausea and vomiting are distressing for children. Drug noncompliance due to severe nausea and vomiting has been reported to be as high as 33% in children and 59% in adolescents (Smith, Trueworthy, Klopovich, Vats, & Snodgrass, 1984). Published studies have investigated the use of hypnosis as a behavioral intervention to ameliorate these side effects (Cotanch, Hockenberry, & Herman, 1985; Hockenberry & Cotanch, 1985). Cotanch et al. (1985) suggested that chemotherapy-related nausea and vomiting in children might be reduced and oral intake improved with the use of a behavioral intervention.

In 2017 Zimmern provided an interesting and useful review of the literature of the use of hypnosis in pediatric anesthesia and pediatric headaches (Zimmern, 2017).

Jacknow, Tschann, Link, and Boyce (1994) investigated the effectiveness of hypnosis in decreasing antiemetic usage in children with cancer experiencing chemotherapy-related nausea and vomiting. Twenty newly diagnosed cancer patients between 6 and 18 years old with no prior chemotherapy experience were randomized to receive either a standardized antiemetic medication or therapeutic hypnosis as a primary treatment for nausea and vomiting with the option of supplemental antiemetic medication on an as-needed basis. The study monitored nausea, vomiting, and antiemetic medication use during the first two courses of chemotherapy and anticipatory nausea and vomiting at 1–2 months and 4–6 months following diagnosis. Hypnosis training was conducted in two to three sessions during the initial chemotherapy courses. Hypnotic procedures were personalized to the developmental level of the child with an emphasis on active involvement of imagination. In the initial session, children were taught imagery incompatible with the sensation and experience of nausea and vomiting. If nausea and vomiting developed, they were later also given direct hypnotic suggestions and instruction, such as: "Find the vomiting control center and turn it down." During both the first and second courses of chemotherapy, children learning hypnosis used less antiemetic medication than those in the control group who had not learned hypnosis. In addition, at 1–2 months after diagnosis, patients in the hypnosis group experienced significantly less anticipatory nausea than those in the control group who had not learned hypnosis. This effect was not sustained, however, as at 4–6 months no further significant differences were identified for anticipatory nausea.

Prior to recommending an intervention, the therapist must assess the child's tolerance for procedures such as intravenous injections. He or she must learn exactly when the vomiting usually occurs. If it is associated with chemotherapy, can the environment be modified somehow? Do family members or members of the treatment team reinforce the expectancy of vomiting by asking, "Are you nauseated yet?" Do family members become anxious themselves just before the treatment? How long a wait does the child usually have in the clinic?

If vomiting is associated with a procedure, and needle phobia is present, the therapist should first address the issue of needle phobia. After several sessions of hetero-hypnosis, the therapist may make an audio-recording that can be listened to over headphones during procedures. Kuttner (1986, 1988, 1989) recommended that young children should be encouraged to focus on blowing out their breath slowly to relax and gain control during procedures. She also encouraged young children to blow bubbles when preparing for procedures (Kuttner, 1986, 1998; Kuttner & Catchpole, 2007).

Zeltzer, LeBaron, and Zeltzer (1984a, 1984b) studied nausea and vomiting in children who have cancer and recommended that therapists become familiar with a variety of interventions, including distracting techniques and more formal invitation techniques of hypnosis. Storytelling with appropriate metaphors was recommended by Zeltzer and colleagues as well as by Kuttner.

An image of a cool, moist wind such as that associated with skiing, tobogganing, or walking in gentle rain is one that may counteract the feeling of nausea.

Videos (tapes, DVDs) are available that demonstrate many of these approaches. The British Columbia Children's Hospital offers Dr. Kuttner's videotapes (DVD's), *No Fears, No Tears* (1986) and *No Fears, No Tears: 13 Years Later* (1998) through their website (http://bookstore.cw.bc.ca). Video games have also been used successfully to induce self-hypnosis for treatment of pediatric oncology patients experiencing acute psychological and physical reactions to chemotherapy, including nausea and vomiting (Kolko & Rickard-Figueroa, 1985). Access to video games resulted in a reduction of the number of anticipatory symptoms and a diminution in the adverse nature of the side effects.

Parents may be of great help in reinforcing self-hypnosis practice for children who have nausea and vomiting. For the younger child, parents may benefit from various resources of metaphors and meditations designed to help children and assist parents in developing their own creativity and storytelling to help children with various symptoms (Garth, 1991, 1992, 1997; Hudson, 2009; Reznick, 2009; Thomson, 2005, 2007). The following vignette illustrates the need to spend time in getting to know the child. Andrew, age 5 years, had experienced bone marrow transplantation and had not retained food for more than a month. He vomited whenever food was brought to his room.

Prior to his illness, he had enjoyed tricycle riding, playing with Transformers, and drawing. He had once lived in Florida and enjoyed seeing oranges on trees. He liked Michael Jackson's music. During the first visit, the therapist played with the Transformers and emphasized changes in Transformers and changes in people. She asked that hospital staff obtain a portable tape recorder and arrange to have Michael Jackson's songs played through the headphones a few minutes before meals were brought in. During the second visit, she asked Andrew to image a story of himself and his mother (he had often expressed fear that she would not return) going for a tricycle ride, going wherever they wished, enjoying what they were seeing, feeling, and hearing. They rode past orange groves. When they became hot and thirsty, they stopped to eat a big juicy orange. One hour after this session, Andrew ate a whole orange and did not vomit thereafter. His mother retold him the story of the trike ride many times.

## *Cyclic Vomiting*

We are unable to find any reports in the literature of clinical hypnosis for cyclic vomiting. We have worked with 20 of these patients, each of whom achieved some degree of symptom relief through learning self-hypnosis. In each case, however, we referred the patient to medical subspecialists for further evaluation, and eventually organic explanations for the vomiting were found. This is a reminder, especially in difficult and uncertain areas, that one should be wary of the grab-bag diagnosis of "psychogenic."

Karen I., age 10 years, was referred for therapeutic clinical hypnosis after 60 hospitalizations for rehydration necessitated by cyclic vomiting. She had previously undergone extensive evaluations and 1 year of psychotherapy. Shortly before the onset of the vomiting, 3 years earlier, she had been frightened by a description of the movie *The Exorcist*. Karen had been informed by one group of consultants that the symptom would resolve in puberty and that there was no cure. In the initial therapeutic hypnosis session, Karen was taught progressive relaxation and given general ego-strengthening suggestions. In subsequent sessions, she was given suggestions to counter nausea. Although she managed to abort her attacks when the therapist was present, she could not use self-hypnosis for this purpose, and the frequency of hospitalizations did not decrease. The therapist asked that she be evaluated by a pediatric neurologist and endocrinologist who, after 1 year of intricate testing, defined a urea cycle abnormality and found that the patient could eliminate the attacks by controlling her intake of protein. They tested their hypothesis by giving her a protein load and following the rise in her blood ammonia levels. Subsequently, she did well. Although self-hypnosis helped her symptomatically while the cause was being elucidated, it did not substitute for a thorough medical evaluation.

### Neurologically Mediated Intractable Reflexes

Both intractable hiccoughs and sneezing may be treated successfully with clinical hypnosis. Patients may be taught progressive relaxation and given diagrams of the involved reflex with suggestions to control the switch between the brain and the reflex. Daily reinforcement through self-hypnosis is recommended.

### Cerebral Palsy

Lazar (1977) described her treatment of a 12-year-old boy with athetoid cerebral palsy and mild mental retardation. After induction using imaginary television, treatment included observation of the self with relaxed and controlled hands, recall of previous relaxing experiences, suggestions designed to increase hand function, and focusing on feelings about independence and anger. Sessions were reinforced with cassette tapes. Although the boy reached only a light hypnotic state, he nonetheless achieved good results. His teachers noted improvement in his handwriting and in his ability to work in shop class. Lazar postulated that teaching such a patient self-hypnosis encourages independence and a sense of accomplishment, so important in people with disabilities. She suggested that therapeutic hypnosis might be most effective with these children if begun at an early age when there is the best chance of minimizing secondary emotional problems and maximizing motivation for optimal motor functioning.

Secter and Gelberd (1964) advocated hypnosis as a relaxant for patients with cerebral palsy. In a brief study of 12 children with cerebral palsy, they found that eight responded to hypnotic induction; intelligence levels of the children ranged from "subnormal" to normal.

A search of the past 20 years of literature on the use of hypnosis with young people with cerebral palsy yielded no controlled studies. The Department of Integrative Medicine at the University of Arizona (Mauersberger, Artz, Duncan, & Gurgevich, 2000) investigated a combination of biofeedback and hypnotherapy to assess children's ability to reduce muscle tone with the use of self-regulation. Electromyogram biofeedback was employed to measure muscle tension in two muscle groups before, during, and after hypnosis in four children with spastic quadriplegic cerebral palsy. Three of the four showed a very significant decrease in muscle tension during hypnosis and were able to reproduce self-hypnosis for relaxation during subsequent stressful situations. Two of the children also had athetoid movements, and each was able to better control these movements with the aid of hypnosis. One of us (DPK) had a 9-year-old patient with cerebral palsy who had a left hemiparesis, learned self-hypnosis very well, and was able to reproducibly demonstrate an improved, more stable gait (both walking and running) after practice of self-hypnosis. Not surprisingly, his effectiveness in modulating his limp was greater when his motivation was high and much less when his motivation was lower or when he was more tired, such as at the end of the day.

The successful use of therapeutic hypnosis in maximizing the performance of athletes encourages its trial in any problem involving muscle function. Rehearsal of correct movements mentally is associated with measurable changes in catecholamine responses (Landsberg & Young, 1978). The adjunct use of hypnosis would seem reasonable in rehabilitation following injuries and muscle disease.

## Complex Regional Pain Syndrome (Reflex Sympathetic Dystrophy)

One of our colleagues (Lewenstein, 1978, pers. comm.) shared with us the following case history; so far as we know, it is the first report of successful therapeutic hypnosis with reflex sympathetic dystrophy (RSD, now known as CRPS = Complex Regional Pain Syndrome). A 15-year-old girl felt something "snap" in her right knee while standing still on a basketball court. Subsequently, she developed pain in her right lower leg distal to the knee and involving the entire lower leg. The pain was described as maximal behind her leg and on the right sole. The entire lower leg distal to the midthigh turned purple. She obtained several medical consultations. Diagnoses of torn ligaments or thrombophlebitis were made. She was hospitalized and given anticoagulants. When x-rays and a venogram were normal, and she did not improve, she was transferred to another hospital for further evaluation and treatment.

On admission she was found to have a mottled, cool, right leg from the midthigh down, and she was unable or unwilling to bear weight on the right leg because of intense pain. There was circumferential hyperesthesia with pain on light touch in the lower leg and an area of numbness over the right thigh. Despite aggressive physical therapy with hydrotherapy, the patient did not improve. She was referred for therapeutic hypnosis 2 weeks after admission.

During the first clinical hypnosis session, she was asked to imagine a tree, with multiple branches, growing and blossoming in the spring sunlight. She was told that she could imagine the blood vessels in her legs as like the branches of the tree. She was told that the nerves and blood vessels to her legs had been confused at the time she injured her knee and that she could correct this problem by focusing on the imagery of the healthy tree in her self-hypnosis practice. Because she recognized that she had injured her right arm a few years ago and it had healed completely, it was likely that her right leg would also heal completely. The patient noted subjective improvement by the following day and walked without crutches 2 days later. The patient was seen every 2–3 days for an additional 10 days and was encouraged to continue self-hypnosis practice. She was discharged to home and was doing well 5 months later.

Successful therapeutic hypnosis treatment of eight children with reflex sympathetic dystrophy was later reported by one of us (Olness, 1990). We have since seen several patients with this complicated disorder. Although therapeutic hypnosis has been generally successful, this has consistently been within a context of the principles previously discussed in approaching children with chronic pain syndromes and comorbidity of any chronic illness. Beyond the essential ingredient of rapport, clinicians are reminded of the importance of helping the patient to carefully define the goals of self-hypnosis therapy and concurrently helping the patient to define the role of family members in the therapeutic process.

## Rehabilitation Following Central Nervous System Injury

Crasilneck and Hall (1970) reported the successful use of adjunctive therapeutic hypnosis in the treatment of a 10-year-old boy who suffered cerebral contusion, concussion, and edema following a 15-foot fall. Three and one-half months after the fall, he was discharged to home in a fetal position, with a fixed stare, no evidence of recognition, and no speech. He was also incontinent. The mother then requested a trial of clinical hypnosis. In the first session, the therapist told the patient that he could be helped if he could cooperate and then asked him to close his eyes. When the boy did not respond, the therapist gently closed his lids manually and gave him repeated suggestions that he could achieve [a state of] deep hypnosis. When he was thought to be in trance, he was told that he could get well and that he could communicate by blinking his eyes, once for "no" and twice for "yes." He immediately responded to questions with appropriate eye blinks. He was seen for therapeutic clinical hypnosis once weekly for a year. Each time, suggestions were made for return of essential functions. Gradually the patient improved, eventually redeveloping normal speech, ability to walk assisted, and ability to read normally. The authors postulated that the therapist's attitude and persistence, combined with the structured therapeutic hypnosis session, led to a changed expectation for recovery by the family and facilitated positive motivation and behavior change in the boy. This case also points out the importance of speaking to noncommunicating patients as if they are hearing and as if response is expected.

## *Tics and Tourette's Syndrome*

The prevalence of tic disorders in childhood is increasing (McCracken, 2000), and the prevalence of Tourette's syndrome is estimated to range from 3 to 8 per 1,000, with chronic motor tic disorders being even more common (Scahill, Williams, Schwab-Stone, Applegate, & Leckman, 2006). A complete review of Tourette's syndrome is beyond the scope of this work, but several important observations strongly support the utilization of, and continued evolution of research with, self-hypnosis, therapeutic hypnosis, and analogous forms of self-regulation training. Clinical symptoms of Tourette's syndrome, with its vocal and motor tics and often comorbid obsessive–compulsive behaviors, are commonly associated with socioemotional challenges. Despite increased public awareness through educational television and the presence of Tourette's specialists in many school districts, school children are often ridiculed because of their tics and may be viewed as more aggressive, more withdrawn, and less popular by peers and teachers alike (Woods & Marcks, 2005). Amidst the sparse literature regarding the impact of tics on quality of life, one study identified 59 children with a chronic tic disorder as generally having a lower quality of life than unaffected peers in most areas of function, including psychosocial distress from tics (Storch et al., 2007). It has been our experience, and that of others noted below, that learning self-hypnosis results in a significant reduction in tic behaviors and, in turn, a concomitant improvement in quality of life. For an up-to-date review of Tourette's syndrome, readers are encouraged to review the recently published work of Zinner and Coffey (2009).

Habit reversal training is often described as an effective behavioral therapy for the tics of Tourette's syndrome. Descriptions of habit reversal training include no mention of hypnosis, but relaxation training is seen as one of the integral pieces of this behavioral training, along with awareness training, self-monitoring, competing response training, and motivational techniques (Himle, Woods, Piacentini, & Walkup, 2006). None of the research or descriptions of habit reversal that we reviewed mentioned discriminating between the impact or value of one or the other of these components of habit reversal (Himle et al., 2006; Woods, Himle, & Conelea, 2006; Woods, Twohig, Flessner, & Roloff, 2003).

In a report by Kohen and Botts (1987), four children with Tourette's syndrome were referred for self-hypnosis training. Three were on haloperidol, and all were experiencing frequent tics, which were socially embarrassing and caused other children to avoid them. Three of the patients learned relaxation and mental imagery exercises on the first visit and demonstrated increased facility with home practice. Diminished frequency of tics was noticed almost immediately by both patients and their families. Improvement was sustained over time, with substantial reduction of medication in one child, cessation of medication in another, and no initiation of medication in the third. Later, an additional four children with Tourette's syndrome were taught self-hypnosis and demonstrated sustained success analogous to the patients described in this report. In each patient, the focus of therapeutic suggestion with imagery and relaxation was on the development of metaphors for control of tic behavior. Individualized to the favorite activities of each of the patients, these included, for example, the imagery of one child as quarterback of the football team (and his brain as quarterback of the muscles of his body) and another as playing the cello (making all the right movements at the right time in the right way as the metaphor for control of muscles).

Young and Montano (1988) described a hypnobehavioral approach in which three children were taught to utilize habit reversal and response prevention along with training in self-hypnosis for control of their tic behaviors. Prior to training in tic control, patients were taught increased awareness of tic behavior to help identify the tics that were most troubling to them and also to discriminate tic from other motoric behavior. This would also appear to be of value in helping children with this disorder to overcome the denial (of awareness) of the tic behavior commonly noted in Tourette's syndrome. Self-hypnosis training was provided at the same time, utilizing muscle relaxation and favorite activity imagery. Children were asked to notice in imagination the subjective urge or feeling that preceded their tic behaviors and to focus on this. The clinician determined the muscle response that competed with the tic behavior, and then, in trance, children were asked to select and apply either symptom prevention or habit reversal. Training in self-hypnosis and suggestions for daily practice and relapse-prevention training were also provided. The authors believe that self-hypnosis played multiple roles in their patients, including (1) increasing self-awareness, motivation, and concentration; (2) promoting self-confidence through self-selection of habit reversal or response prevention; (3) facilitating decreased tic behaviors; (4) modifying perceptions of tics and allowing the conceptualization of tics as within their control; and (5) reducing symptoms and development of mastery.

Culbertson (1989) described a four-step treatment model of therapeutic hypnosis that helped an adolescent male with Tourette's syndrome help himself over the course of nine treatment sessions in 6 months. In addition to classical Jacobsonian relaxation training, this adolescent was also taught finger-temperature biofeedback as a measure of degree of relaxation and as a metaphor for his own ability to create physiological control. Self-hypnosis training, favorite personal imagery, and use of audiotapes for reinforcement of practice are described as integral ingredients in management.

Kohen (1995a, 1995c) described in detail the successful application of indirect, Ericksonian strategies for more than 35 patients with Tourette's syndrome and the use of self-hypnosis as a coping strategy in Tourette's syndrome. These reports and the work of Young and Montano (1988), Kohen and Botts (1987), Culbertson (1989), and Zahm (1990) all provide narratives of hypnotic suggestions and verbalizations that were effective with their patients.

In a recent report, Ahmed and colleagues in Great Britain (Ahmed, Martinez, Yee, Cahill, & Besag, 2008) reported on 34 youth between the ages of 3.5 and 15 years (mean age was 10 years, 1 month) who had abnormal body movements. Thirteen of the 34 had tic disorders; among these, 2 had chronic motor disorders, 5 had Tourette's syndrome, and 5 had psychogenic movement disorder. All but one were described as having tics that intensified with stress and improved substantially with full relaxation or with distraction.

In a recent report, Lazarus and Klein (2010) described and demonstrated the very effective use of videotape biofeedback in conjunction with hypnosis to help children with Tourette's syndrome help themselves. In this methodology, now increasingly user-friendly and available to most clinicians, the child is videotaped during an interview, when tics or vocalizations are evident, when learning and doing hypnosis, when experiencing improvement, and, often, when the tic behavior disappears while in trance. Subsequently, when the children view the videos, they can see their tics and their disappearance, thus reinforcing the success and value of their newly acquired self-regulation skills.

The mechanism of these apparent positive results of self-hypnosis on Tourette's syndrome remains unknown, as is the precise biological nature of the disorder, which continues to be characterized as a complex neurobehavioral disorder. Is it successful solely because of the therapeutic value of relaxation techniques as an effective coping strategy? Does the attention of a sensitive therapist contribute to its success? Or do these techniques act in a similar way to haloperidol, improving and altering associated behaviors by evoking mediators that stimulate the blockage of dopamine receptors?

The research of Raz and colleagues (Raz, Keller, Norman, & Senechal, 2007) has contributed substantially to our understanding of not only Tourette's syndrome but also the value of hypnosis and ways in which it is effective. Raz examined hypnosis as a treatment for Tourette's syndrome and as a means of understanding its mechanisms. He noted that "during highly focused attention, patients calm down and tics disappear" and emphasized the importance, therefore, of elucidating the neural bases of these effects. As research proceeds on this problem, it seems prudent to consider self-hypnosis as a potentially useful adjunct early in the comprehensive evaluation and management of children with this disorder.

## Pelvic Examinations in Adolescent Girls

Kohen (1980b) reported the successful use of therapeutic clinical hypnosis to assist adolescent girls through their first pelvic examinations. The anxiety of this event can be reduced by gentle, sensitive physicians. The use of therapeutic hypnosis can foster a sense of competency and control in the teenager undergoing her first pelvic examination as well as reduction of anxiety prior to future similar examinations. Prior to the pelvic examination, the physician should allow the patient time to acknowledge her concerns and then express his or her willingness to help the patient be comfortable through the examination. It is explained to the patient that she can use her imagination to facilitate comfort. If she has previously stated that she enjoys skiing, for example, the physician suggests, "Go ahead and let yourself imagine that you're skiing" and continues to give suggestions for progressive relaxation. The physician of course must explain each part of the procedure as he or she also reinforces the suggestions of relaxation and comfort. A posthypnotic suggestion is given to relax even more easily and quickly during future pelvic examinations.

If patients have negative expectations based on uncomfortable previous examinations, the physician may ask, "Would it be okay if it doesn't bother you this time?" This question may represent the beginning of an indirect hypnotic suggestion and invitation, causing the patient to pause and reflect on the idea that there is in fact a choice in this matter. It is important that the therapist understand how the patient believes things will be different or better because of therapeutic hypnosis. The teenager must be reminded of her own skills and responsibility for success in achieving comfort and control. Time spent in adding therapeutic hypnosis as an adjunct to pelvic examinations makes it possible to perform better examinations more quickly, thus saving time in the long run.

Sand-Jecklin (2008) reported the value of what she calls the "color breathwork relaxation method" for helping adolescent and young adult women through a gynecologic examination. Each of her patients was taught breathing focused relaxation and encouraged to imagine a favorite "place of peace." They were invited to imagine that the room was filled with the color peach, to breathe in the color, and to exhale any remaining tension. Measurements before and after demonstrated significant decreases in heart rate, systolic and diastolic blood pressure, and self-rated anxiety after practicing the technique.

## Sports Medicine

Morgan (1980) reviewed potential applications of hypnosis in sports medicine research and practice. Appropriate uses of hypnosis in this area include management of excessive pre-competition anxiety and analysis of factors involved in slumps, long periods when athletes inexplicably perform well below previous levels. Athletes may become aware of errors in body movement that they do not recognize in their usual cognitive state. In some cases, hypnosis may properly be used to help an injured athlete perform, but the therapist must be keenly aware of the signal value of pain and must not put the athlete in a situation where he or she is likely to become further disabled. Facilitation of performance by hypnosis should be attempted only when such an approach is not contraindicated at a medical, physiological, or psychological level. Morgan concluded that evidence for positive effects of hypnosis on muscle strength and endurance is equivocal, although negative hypnotic suggestions often result in performance decrement. These findings lead us to question the validity of the many popular books that state that imagery and relaxation exercises – possibly involving hypnosis – can enhance performance in individual sports such as tennis and skiing (Gallwey, 1974; Gallwey & Kriegel, 1977). Certainly, attempts to "psych up" an athlete to perform at record-breaking levels are not likely to be helpful and may be dangerous. Morgan further reported that hypnotically suggested exercise alters cardiac rate, respiration rate, total ventilation, oxygen consumption, and cardiac output in the non-exercise state. Observed metabolic changes often approximate responses reported for actual exercise. The application of this finding to actual performance, however, is unclear.

Liggett (2000) studied the value of hypnosis as a performance aid for athletes by comparing the intensity of imagery with and without hypnosis. The study involved 14 athletes, 6 females and 8 males. Four participants were distance runners, ages 26, 30, 33, and 39 years; three were gymnasts, ages 12, 14, and 15 years; two were soccer players, 17 and 26 years; one was a 22-year-old mountain biker; one was a 30-year-old rugby player; one was an 18-year-old tennis player; and one was an 18-year-old who played water polo. All were proficient enough in their sport to compete at regional, intercollegiate, or interscholastic levels. They were asked to vividly imagine themselves in four separate situations in their own particular sport: (1) practicing alone, (2) practicing with others, (3) watching a teammate, and (4) participating in a competition. For each situation, they rated the subjective clarity or intensity of the imagery on four dimensions:

1. *Visual.* How vividly did you see yourself doing this activity?
2. *Auditory.* How clearly did you hear the sounds of doing this activity?
3. *Kinesthetic.* How well did you feel yourself making the movements?
4. *Affective.* How clearly were you aware of your mood?

The rating scale was from 1 = no image present to 5 = an extremely clear, vivid image. For each of these situations, scores were obtained for imaging in a trance and four more out of trance. Results indicated that participants reported that the imagery under hypnosis was more intense for each dimension and for each situation. No significant difference was observed with regard to whether the imagery was done first with or without hypnosis. There was no consideration or analysis of the relationship of the study results to actual or eventual performance, although the author concluded that the study supports the use of imagery to enhance sports performance, specifically imagery enhanced by the hypnotic state.

Others have examined whether the use of internal imagery can measurably affect performance outcome. Olsson and colleagues in Sweden (Olsson, Jonsson, & Nyberg, 2008) reported on a study of 24 high jumpers recruited from a national track and field high school, 13 males and 11 females with a mean age of 19.3 years (varying from 16 to 29 years of age). The final sample included ten athletes in the motor group and nine in the motor plus imagery group. In the control (motor) group, participants met individually for 12 sessions over a 6-week period. The purpose of the study was to examine whether internal imagery would enhance high jumping performance after 6 weeks of intervention. The intervention phase was based on studies on physical training in which 6 weeks of practice led to positive effects on motor performance, in this case high jumping. The high jumping instruction for internal imagery, clearly hypnotic, was as follows:

> Imagine that you are running toward the bar in a calm pace. At the curve you are slightly leaning inward from the bar. In the last two steps the legs run past the body, and you lean slightly backward. In the take-off you plant the whole foot, you feel that the knee is straight, and you lean away from the bar. The lead leg bends and is parallel with the bar. The arms help you up. The take-off foot leaves the ground; you rotate so that your back is against the bar. You pull your heels toward your head so your back bends. You push your hip up and lean your head back and pull your legs over the bar. You land on the pit and you made the jump.

In each session participants did imagery for 1.5 minutes followed by 30 seconds of rest and then another 1.5 minutes. In the experiment, each group performed a pre-test series of jumps, followed by the intervention, followed by another series of jumps. All were recorded on video. Both the control and experimental group showed positive trends on all measured variables, although none was statistically significant, except that the experimental group had a 50% greater gain in bar clearance than did the control group, suggesting that the internal imagery training program helped to improve this component of the high jump, considered to be a critical component of high jumping.

Newmark and Bogacki (2005) briefly described their experience with relaxation, imagery, and hypnosis in sport psychiatry, providing several brief clinical vignettes. Our clinical experience in using hypnotherapy for sports problems has been primarily focused on its use for pre-performance anxiety. Jane P., age 11 years, was referred because she had severe anxiety for several days prior to solo ice-skating competition, and this was adversely affecting her performances. She had been skating since the age of 4 and had competed many times with no difficulty until 6 months prior to referral. After discussion of her interests, likes, and dislikes, she entered a hypnotic state easily by imagining herself reading a favorite story. She was taught ideomotor signals and asked if she would be willing to review past skating competitions. When she readily agreed, the therapist asked her to regress to competitions at age 8, 9, and 10 years. She had positive recollections of the earlier competitions but recalled an unpleasant comment from a peer at the latest competition, after which her excessive anxiety began. While still in hypnosis, she was asked if she would be willing to get rid of this comment that was still bothering her. When she agreed, she was given the option of sending the comment off in the distance via pony express, airplane, or train. She chose the pony express and let the horse gallop into the distance until she could no longer see it. Following this, she was asked to focus on the image of herself successfully completing the next competition, doing well, and feeling pleased with her performance and her control. She then practiced self-hypnosis once daily until the next competition. She was calm and happy thereafter, did well in her next public performance, and called the therapist to express her pleasure.

Elaine, age 13 years, was regarded by her tennis coach and family as an exceptional tennis player. She first learned to hold a racket at the age of 4 and had progressed to competition on a national level. She said that she enjoyed tennis and competition until she had an experience that was followed by hyperventilation. It happened on a practice day; she had been playing well, and many players, including adults, had asked to play with her. The temperature was 90°F, with 30% humidity. She became so absorbed in play that she forgot to eat lunch and had only a few drinks during the day. Not surprisingly, she developed signs of heat exhaustion, including rapid breathing. By the time her parents realized that she had overdone it, she was hyperventilating and required medical attention. Subsequently, she began to hyperventilate before every tennis game;

she found that she was playing poorly and did not enjoy playing. She was referred for evaluation and possible hypnotherapy.

Elaine chatted openly with the therapist about whether or not this symptom might keep her out of a game she no longer enjoyed. Her parents had asked the same question. Elaine said that she enjoyed many activities, but that tennis had been her favorite. Following a discussion of body response to stress, she learned a progressive relaxation exercise, which she practiced twice daily. A week later, I asked her to add a focus on a favorite safe place. I then asked her a variety of questions to which she responded with ideomotor signals; a few of the questions probed her wish to play tennis. Her responses were immediate and positive. I added a rehearsal of a tennis game while she was relaxed and asked her to review this twice daily. She returned to tennis a week later and experienced no hyperventilation. Six months later, she won her divisional championship.

In his book *Peak Performance* (1985), Garfield reviewed Russian approaches to improving the performance of athletes by training them in self-hypnosis. In his assessment of the steps involved in this approach, Garfield (1985) noted voluntary relaxation, mental rehearsal, disciplined imagination, poise, and letting go. These steps are entirely consistent with hypnotherapeutic approaches in focusing intensely on imagination and feeling. It is essential that the athlete establish a mental picture of the desired outcome, rehearse the feeling of attaining that outcome, and, at the time of performance, just let it happen.

Although no research data in the English literature documents children actually improving their proficiency in specific sports by means of self-hypnosis, this seems a reasonable proposition. In the meantime, until this area is studied further, it is appropriate to teach self-hypnosis for the reduction of performance anxiety.

## General Recommendations

In a paper on therapeutic hypnosis with pediatric cancer patients, Olness (1981) made several recommendations to therapists who work in this area. Because these recommendations are applicable to many pediatric medical problems, we have adapted them here:

- Child healthcare professionals should be encouraged to learn and use self-hypnosis for themselves. Proper use of this modality can lead to the reduction of personal stress, which is an inevitable factor in working with children who have medical problems. The heightened ego receptivity of the hypnotic state (Fromm, 1977) may also facilitate creativity in considering diagnostic issues and developing treatment plans. In some cases, healthcare professionals can participate in group sessions with patients and their families (e.g., groups for children with cancer, hemophilia, asthma). The shared experiences may be of benefit to all.
- Clinicians utilizing therapeutic hypnosis must be willing to spend time with child patients, getting to know them as individuals and planning treatment accordingly. Standardized, scripted, or canned approaches are likely to fail, given the fact that there is no such thing as a standard patient.
- When therapeutic clinical hypnosis may be appropriate for a medical problem, children should be exposed to this possibility as soon after diagnosis as possible. Progress tends to be slower among children who have developed secondary emotional problems or who have well-established negative conditioned reflexes from months or years of accumulated fears of procedures and drugs.
- Therapeutic hypnosis teaching and reinforcement sessions should occur frequently during the first weeks of diagnosis, and children should be encouraged to practice on their own. Children with chronic illnesses should be invited to attend group practice sessions on a

monthly or twice-monthly basis to avoid loss of hypnotic skills during long symptom-free or medication-free periods.

- Every clinical hypnosis session should enhance the child's sense of mastery and should be conducted at the child's speed. Practice efforts of children should be facilitated, not coerced or mandated.
- The effects of parental attitudes and mental health status on the evolution of childhood diseases must be considered carefully, and techniques must be developed to meet parental mental health needs. Parents and siblings can be encouraged to learn self-hypnosis and to participate in group sessions.
- For children who are discouraged or uncertain of their hypnotic skills, the use of thermal biofeedback and other forms of biofeedback – with visual or auditory proof of control over physiological processes – should be considered as an adjunct.

## Conclusion

Therapeutic clinical hypnosis is useful as a primary or adjunctive tool in the management of a wide range of childhood medical problems. It is of particular value in the enhancement of mastery in children who have chronic diseases, especially if the focus is on early intervention and prevention. For many medical problems, several different hypnotherapeutic approaches have been reported to be successful. More prospective studies and randomized controlled trials are necessary to determine which approaches are most successful and to assess the particular value of hypnotherapy in relation to other kinds of treatment. Long-term follow-up studies of children with hypnotic skills (e.g., Kohen, 2010a) will allow us to note enhancement or waning of those skills as well as possible relationships to ability to cope with medical problems in adulthood.

## References

Abbott, R.A., Martin, A.E., Newlove-Delgado, T.V., Bethel, A., Whear, R.S., Thompson Coon, J., & Logan, S. (2018). Recurrent abdominal pain in children: summary evidence from 3 systematic reviews of treatment effectiveness. *Journal of Pediatric Gastroenterology and Nutrition, 67*(1), 23–33.

Accardi, M.C. & Milling, L.S. (2009). The effectiveness of hypnosis for reducing procedure-related pain in children and adolescents: a comprehensive methodological review. *Journal of Behavioral Medicine, 32*, 328–339.

Acunzo, D.J., Oakley, D.A., & Terhune, D.B. (2021). The neurochemistry of hypnotic suggestion. *American Journal of Clinical Hypnosis, 63*(4), 355–371.

Adams, J.A. & Weaver, S.J. (1986). Self-esteem and perceived stress in young adolescents with chronic disease: unexpected findings. *Journal of Adolescent Health Care, 7*, 173–177.

Ahmed, M.A.S., Martinez, A., Yee, A., Cahill, D., & Besag, F.M.C. (2008). Psychogenic and organic movement disorders in children. *Developmental Medicine & Child Neurology, 50*, 300–304.

Ambrose, G. (1952). Nervous control of sweating. *Lancet, 1*, 926.

Anbar, R.D. (2007). User friendly hypnosis as an adjunct for treatment of habit cough: a case report. *American Journal of Clinical Hypnosis, 50*(2), 171–175.

Anbar, R.D. & Sachdeva, S. (2011). Treatment of psychological factors in a child with difficult asthma: a case report. *The American Journal of Clinical Hypnosis, 54*(4), 47–55.

Anbar, R.D. (2010). Adding hypnosis to the therapeutic toolbox of pediatric respiratory care. *Pediatric Asthma, Allergy & Immunology, 20*(20), 1–6.

Anbar, R. (2017a). Asthma (Chapter 15). In G.R. Elkins, Ed., *Handbook of Medical and Psychological Hypnosis: Foundations, Applications, and Professional Issues* (pp. 161–168). Springer Publishing Company. (English language)

Anbar, R. (2017b). Cystic fibrosis (Chapter 20). In G.R. Elkins, Ed., *Handbook of Medical and Psychological Hypnosis: Foundations, Applications, and Professional Issues* (pp. 199–204). Springer Publishing Company. (English language)

Anbar, R.D. (2000a). Self-hypnosis for patients with cystic fibrosis. *Pediatric Pulmonology, 30*, 461–465.

Anbar, R.D. (2000b). Hypnosis, Theodore Roosevelt, and the patient with cystic fibrosis. *Pediatrics, 106*(2), 339–342.

Anbar, R.D. (2001). Self-hypnosis for the management of chronic dyspnea in pediatric patients. *Pediatrics, 107*(2), E21.

Anbar, R.D. (2003). Self-hypnosis for anxiety associated with severe asthma: a case report. *BMC Pediatrics, 3*(1), 7.

Anbar, R.D. (2004). Stressors associated with dyspnea in childhood: patients' insights and a case report. *American Journal of Clinical Hypnosis, 47*(2), 93–101.

Anbar, R.D. & Hall, H.R. (2004). Childhood habit cough treated with self-hypnosis. *Journal of Pediatrics, 144*, 213–217.

Andrasik, F., Blanchard, E.B., Edlund, S.B., & Rosenblum, E.L. (1982). Autogenic feedback in the treatment of two children with migraine headache. *Child and Family Behavioral Therapy, 4*, 13–23.

Apley, J. (1977). Psychosomatic aspects of gastrointestinal problems in children. *Clinics in Gastroenterology, 6*, 311–320.

Aronoff, G.M., Aronoff, S., & Peck, L.W. (1975). Hypnotherapy in the treatment of bronchial asthma. *Annals of Allergy, 34*, 356–362.

Ball, T.M., Shapiro, D.E., Monheim, C.J., & Weydert, J.A. (2003). A pilot study of the use of guided imagery for the treatment of recurrent abdominal pain in children. *Clinical Pediatrics, 42*, 527–532.

Ball, T.M. & Weydert, J.A. (2003). Methodological challengers to treatment trials for recurrent abdominal pain in children. *Archives of Pediatrics and Adolescent Medicine, 157*, 1121–1127.

Banez, G.A. (2008). Chronic abdominal pain in children: what to do following the medical evaluation. *Current Opinion in Pediatrics, 20*, 571–575.

Barbour, J. (1980). Medigrams: self hypnosis and asthma. *American Family Physician, 21*, 173.

Barnes, A.J. & Kohen, D.P. (2006). Clinical hypnosis as an effective adjunct in the care of pediatric inpatients. *Journal of Pediatrics, 149*, 563–565.

Bauchner, H.C., Howland, J., & Adair, R. (1988). The impact of pediatric asthma education on morbidity: assessing the evidence [abstract]. *American Journal of Diseases of Children, 142*(4), 398–399.

Belsky, J. & Khanna, P. (1994). The effects of self-hypnosis for children with cystic fibrosis: a pilot study. *American Journal of Clinical Hypnosis, 36*, 282–292.

Berberich, F.R. & Landman, Z. (2009). Reducing immunization discomfort in 4- to 6-year-old children: a randomized clinical trial. *Pediatrics, 124*(2), e203–e209.

Berger, H.G., Honig, P.J., & Liebman, R. (1977). Recurrent abdominal pain: gaining control of the symptom. *American Journal of Diseases of Children, 131*, 1340–1344.

Blessing-Moore, J., Fritz, G.K., & Lewiston, N.J. (1985). Self-management programs for childhood asthma: a review. *Chest, 87*(1), 107S–110S.

Bothe, D. & Olness, K. (2007a). Anxiety among youth. Part I. *Contemporary Pediatrics, 24*, 58–63.

Bothe, D. & Olness, K. (2007b). Anxiety among youth. Part II. *Contemporary Pediatrics, 24*, 82–89.

Brent, M., Lobato, D., & LeLeiko, N. (2009). Psychological treatments for pediatric functional gastrointestinal disorders. *Journal of Pediatric Gastroenterology and Nutrition, 48*(1), 13–21.

Broome, M.E., Lillis, P.P., McGahee, T.W., & Bates, T. (1992). The use of distraction and imagery with children during painful procedures. *Oncology Nursing Forum, 19*, 499–502.

Browne, P.D., de Bruijn, C.M.A., Speksdijder, E.M., den Hollander, B., van Wering, H.M., Wessels, M.M.S., Groenweg, M., Goede, J., Frankenhuis C., Tromp, E., Benninga, M.A., & Vlieger, A.M. (2021, October 27). Skills or pills: randomized trial comparing hypnotherapy to medical treatment in children with functional nausea. *Clinical Gastroenterology and Hepatology. S1542-3565(21)01142-3*. doi: 10.1016/j.cgh.2021.10.029. Online ahead of print

Bursch, B. (2008). Psychological/cognitive behavioral treatment of childhood functional abdominal pain and irritable bowel syndrome. *Journal of Pediatric Gastroenterology and Nutrition, 47*(5), 706–707.

Butler, L.D., Symons, B.K., Henderson, S., Shortliffe, L.D., & Spiegel, D. (2005). Hypnosis reduces distress and duration of an invasive medical procedure for children. *Pediatrics, 115*, 77–85.

Caprilli, S., Anastasi, F., Grotto, R.P.L., Abeti, M.S., & Messeri, A. (2007). Interactive music as a treatment for pain and stress in children during venipuncture: a randomized prospective study. *Journal of Developmental and Behavioral Pediatrics, 28*, 399–403.

Carson, D.K., Council, J.R., & Schauer, R.W. (1991). The effectiveness of a family asthma program for children and parents. *Children's Health Care, 20*(2), 114–119.

Chakravarty, K., Pharoah, P.D.P., Scott, D.G.I., & Barker, S. (1992). Erythromelalgia: the role of hypnotherapy. *Postgraduate Medical Journal, 68*, 44–46.

Chandrasena, R. (1982). Hypnosis in the treatment of viral warts. *Psychiatric Journal of the University of Ottawa, 7*, 135–137.

Chiang, L.C., Ma, W.F., Huang, J.L., Tseng, L.F., & Hsueh, K.C. (2009). Effect of relaxation-breathing training on anxiety and asthma signs/symptoms of children with moderate-to-severe asthma: a randomized controlled trial. *International Journal of Nursing Studies, 46*, 1061–1070.

Cioppa, F.J. & Thai, A.D. (1975). Hypnotherapy in a case of juvenile rheumatoid arthritis. *American Journal of Clinical Hypnosis, 18*, 105–110.

Claude, L., Morelle, M., Mancini, S. Duncan, A., Sebban H., Carrie C., & Marec-Barard (2016). Use of hypnosis in radiotherapy as an alternative to general anesthesia in pediatric radiation oncology. *Bulletin du Cancer, 1013*(11), 921–927. (Fr.)

Clawson, T.A. Jr. & Swade, R.H. (1975). The hypnotic control of blood flow and pain: the cure of warts and the potential for the use of hypnosis in the treatment of cancer. *American Journal of Clinical Hypnosis, 17*, 160–169.

Collison, D.R. (1975). Which asthmatic patients should be treated by hypnotherapy? *Medical Journal of Australia, 1*(25), 776–781.

Connelly, M., Rapoff, M.A., Thompson, N., & Connelly, W. (2006). Headstrong: a pilot study of a CD-ROM intervention for recurrent pediatric headache. *Journal of Pediatric Psychology, 31*(7), 737–747.

Cotanch, P.H., Hockenberry, M., & Herman, S. (1985). Self-hypnosis as antiemetic therapy in children receiving chemotherapy. *Oncology Nursing Forum, 12*, 41–46.

Cousins, N. (1976). Anatomy of an illness (as perceived by the patient). *New England Journal of Medicine, 295*, 1458–1463.

Crasilneck, H.B. & Hall, J.A. (1970). The use of hypnosis in the rehabilitation of complicated vascular and post-traumatic neurological patients. *International Journal of Clinical and Experimental Hypnosis, 28*, 145–159.

Crasilneck, H.B. & Hall, J.A. (1975). *Clinical Hypnosis: Principles and Applications*. New York: Grune & Stratton.

Culbert, T.P., Kajander, R., Reaney, J., & Kohen, D.P. (1996). Uses of hypnosis and biofeedback for children with dysphagia. *Journal of Developmental and Behavioral Pediatrics, 17*(5), 335–334.

Culbertson, F.M. (1989). A four-step hypnotherapy model for Gilles de la Tourette's syndrome. *American Journal of Clinical Hypnosis, 31*(4), 252–256.

Cyna, A.M., Tomkins, D., Maddock, T., & Barker, D. (2007). Brief hypnosis for severe needle phobia using switch-wire imagery in a 5-year-old. *Pediatric Anesthesia, 17*, 800–804.

Cystic Fibrosis Foundation. (2010). *Frequently asked questions*. www.cff.org/aboutcf/faqs/

Cystic Fibrosis Foundation. (2022). www.cff.org, accessed 1.6.2022.

Delord, V., Khirani, S., Rairez, A., Joseph, E.L., Gambier, C. Belson, M., Gajan, F., Fauroux, B. (2013). Medical hypnosis as a tool to acclimatize children to noninvasive positive pressure ventilation: a pilot study. *Chest, 144*, 87–91.

Diamond, H.H. (1959). Hypnosis in children: the complete cure of forty cases of asthma. *American Journal of Clinical Hypnosis, 1*, 124–129.

Diego, R.V. (1961). Hypnosis in the treatment of the asthmatic child. *Bulletin of the Tulane Medical Society, 20*, 307–313.

Dodge, J.A. (1976). Recurrent abdominal pain in children. *British Medical Journal, 1*, 385–387.

Domangue, B.B., Margolis, C.G., Lieberman, D., & Kaji, H. (1985). Biochemical correlates of hypnoanalgesia in arthritic pain patients. *Journal of Clinical Psychiatry, 46*, 235–238.

D'Souza, P.J., Lumley, M.A., Kraft, C.A., & Dooley, J.A. (2008). Relaxation training and written emotional disclosure for tension or migraine headaches: a randomized controlled trial. *Annals of Behavioral Medicine, 36*, 21–32.

Edel, J.W. (1959). Nosebleed controlled by hypnosis. *American Journal of Clinical Hypnosis, 2*, 89–90.

Ehrlich, R.M. (1974). Diabetes mellitus in childhood. *Pediatric Clinics of North America, 21*, 871–884.

Elinoff, V. (1993). Remission of dysphagia in a 9 year old treated in a family practice office setting. *American Journal of Clinical Hypnosis, 35*, 205–208.

Engel, J.M., Rapoff, M.A., & Pressman, A.R. (1992). Long-term follow-up of relaxation training for pediatric headache disorders. *Headache, 32*, 152–156.
Erickson, M.H. (1958). Pediatric hypnotherapy. *American Journal of Clinical Hypnosis, 1*, 25–29.
Esparham, A.E. & Dilts, J.J. (2019). Integrative management of pediatric primary headaches. *Pediatric Annals, 48*(6), e231–e235.
Ewin, D. (1992). Hypnotherapy for warts (verruca vulgaris): 41 consecutive cases with 33 cures. *American Journal of Clinical Hypnosis, 35*(1), 1–10.
Farahzadi, Y. & Kekecs, Z. (2021). Towards a multi-brain framework for hypnosis: a review of quantitative methods. *American Journal of Clinical Hypnosis, 63*(4), 389–403.
Feldman, G.M. (1976). The effect of biofeedback training on respiratory resistance of asthmatic children. *Psychosomatic Medicine, 38*, 27–34.
Felt, B.T., Berman, B., Broffman, G., Coury, D., Dattner, A., French, G., Hall, H., Kohen, D.P., Schmidt, W., Young, M.H., & Olness, K. (1998). Wart regression in children: comparison of relaxation-imagery to topical treatment and equal time interventions. *American Journal of Clinical Hypnosis, 41*(2), 130–138.
Francis, P.W.J., Krastins, I.R.B., & Levison, H. (1980). Oral and inhaled salbutamol in the prevention of exercise induced bronchospasm. *Pediatrics, 66*, 103–108.
Friedrichsdorf, S.J. & Kohen, D.P. (2018). Integration of hypnosis into pediatric palliative care. *Annals of Palliative Medicine*, 7(1), 136–150. 10.21037/apm.2017.05.02
Fromm, E. (1977). An ego-psychological theory of altered states of consciousness. *International Journal of Clinical and Experimental Hypnosis, 25*, 372–387.
Galili, O., Shaoul, R., & Mogilner, J. (2009). Treatment of chronic recurrent abdominal pain: laparoscopy or hypnosis? *Journal of Laparoendoscopic & Advanced Surgical Techniques, 19*(1), 93–96.
Gallwey, W.T. (1974). *The Inner Game of Tennis.* New York: Random House.
Gallwey, W.T. & Kriegel, B. (1977). *Inner Skiing.* New York: Random House.
Garfield, C. (1985). *Peak Performance.* New York: Warner.
Garth, M. (1991). *Starbright: Meditations for Children.* New York: HarperCollins.
Garth, M. (1992). *Moonbeam: A Book of Meditations for Children.* San Francisco, CA: HarperOne.
Garth, M. (1997). *Earthlight: New Meditations for Children.* San Francisco, CA: HarperOne.
Gelder, C. (2013). Diabetes in children and young people: optimising management throughout the care pathway. *Journal of Diabetes Nursing, 17*(8), 294–300.
Gelernter, R., Lavi, G., Yanai, L., Brooks, R., Bar, Y., Bistrizer, Z., & Rachmiel, M. (2015). Effect of auditory guided imagery on glucose levels and on glycemic control in children with type 1 diabetes mellitus. *Journal of Pediatric Endocrinology and Metabolism.* 10.1515/jpem-2015-0150
Gevgen, P.J., Mullally, D.I., & Evans, R. III (1988). National survey of prevalence of asthma among children in the United States 1976-1980. *Pediatrics*, 81(1), 1–7.
Gillan, C. (2021). Review article: the effectiveness of group and self-help hypnotherapy for irritable bowel syndrome and the implications for improving patients' choice and access to treatment. *Alimentary Pharmacology & Therapeutics, 54*(11-12), 1389–1404.
Gold, J.I., Kim, S.H., Kant, A.J., Joseph, M.H., & Rizzo, A. (2006). Effectiveness of virtual reality for pediatric pain distraction during IV placement. *CyberPsychology & Behavior, 9*(2), 207–212.
Goldstein, R.H. (2005). Successful repeated hypnotic treatment of warts in the same individual: a case report. *American Journal of Clinical Hypnosis, 47*(4), 259–264.
Good, R.A. (1981). Foreword: interactions of the body's major networks. In R. Ader, Ed., *Psychoneuroimmunology* (pp. xviii–xix). New York: Academic Press.
Gottsegen, D. (2011). Hypnosis for functional abdominal pain. *American Journal of Clinical Hypnosis, 54*, 56–69. 10.1080.00029157.20911.575964
Green, L. (1994). Touch and visualization to facilitate a therapeutic relationship in an intensive care unit—a personal experience. *Intensive and Critical Care Nursing, 10*, 51–57.
Guevara, J.P., Wolf, F.M., Grum, C.M., & Clark, N.M. (2003). Effects of educational interventions for self-management of asthma in children and adolescents: systematic review and meta-analysis. *British Medical Journal, 14*, 1308–1309.
Gulewitsch, M.D., Muller, J., Hautzinger, M., & Schlarb, A.A. (2013). Brief hypnotherapeutic behavioral intervention for functional abdominal pain and irritable bowel syndrome in childhood: a randomized controlled trial. *European Journal of Pediatrics, 172*(8), 1043–1051.

Gustke, S.S. (1973). Alterations in in vitro coagulation during hypnosis in hemophiliacs, paper presented at the annual meeting of the American Society of Clinical Hypnosis, Toronto.

Hackman, R.M., Stern, J.S., & Gershwin, M.E. (2000). Hypnosis and asthma: a critical review. *Journal of Asthma, 37*(1), 1–15.

Hampel, P., Rudolph, H., Stachow, R., & Petermann, F. (2003). Multimodal patient education program with stress management for childhood and adolescent asthma. *Patient Education and Counseling, 49*, 59–66.

Hawkins, P.J., Liossi, C., Ewart, B.W., Hatira, P., & Kosmidis, V.H. (1998). Hypnosis in the alleviation of procedure-related pain and distress in paediatric oncology patients. *Contemporary Hypnosis, 15*, 199–207.

Henderson, W.R., Shelhamer, J.H., Reingold, D.B., Smith, L.J., Evan, R., & Kaliber, M. (1979). Alpha-adrenergic hyper-responsiveness in asthma: analysis of vascular and pupillary responses. *New England Journal of Medicine, 300*, 642–647.

Himle, M.B., Woods, D.W., Piacentini, J.C., & Walkup, J.T. (2006). Brief review of habit reversal training for Tourette syndrome. *Journal of Child Neurology, 21*, 719–725.

Hindi-Alexander, M.C. (1985). Decision-making in asthma self-management. *Chest, 87*(1, Suppl.), 100S–102S.

Hockenberry, M. & Cotanch, P. (1985). Hypnosis as adjuvant antiemetic therapy in childhood cancer. *Nursing Clinics of North America, 20*, 105–107.

Hoekman, D.R., Vlieger, A.M., Stokkers, P.C., Mahhmod, N., Rietdijk, S., de Boer, N.K., de Meij, T.G., Frankenhuis, C., D'Haens, G.R., & Benninga, M.A. (2021). Hypnotherapy for irritable bowel syndrome-type symptoms in patients with quiescent inflammatory bowel disease: a randomized, controlled trial. *Journal of Crohn's & Colitis, 15*(7), 1106–1113.

Hoffman, H.G., Patterson, D.R., & Carrougher, G.J. (2000). Use of virtual reality for adjunctive treatment of adult burn pain during physical therapy: a controlled study. *The Clinical Journal of Pain, 16*(3), 244–250.

Hoffman, H.G., Patterson, D.R., Carrougher, G.J., & Sharar, S.R. (2001). Effectiveness of virtual reality-based pain control with multiple treatments. *The Clinical Journal of Pain, 17*(3), 229–235.

Houts, A.C. (1982). Relaxation and thermal feedback of childhood migraine headache: a case study. *American Journal of Clinical Biofeedback, 5*, 154–157. http://clinicaltrials.gov

Houze, B., Streff, A., Piche, M., & Rainville, P. (2021). Spinal and supraspinal modulation of pain responses by hypnosis, suggestions, and distraction. *American Journal of Clinical Hypnosis, 63*(4), 329–354.

Hudson, L. (2009). *Scripts and Strategies in Hypnotherapy with Children: For Young People Aged 5 to 15*. Bethel, CT: Crown House Publishing.

Huth, M.M., Broome, M.E., & Good, M. (2004). Imagery reduces children's post-operative pain. *Pain, 110*, 439–448.

Iserson, K.V. (1999). Hypnosis for pediatric fracture reduction. *The Journal of Emergency Medicine, 17*(1), 53–56.

Jacknow, D.S., Tschann, J.M., Link, M.P., & Boyce, W.T. (1994). Hypnosis in the prevention of chemotherapy-related nausea and vomiting in children: a prospective study. *Journal of Developmental & Behavioral Pediatrics, 15*(4), 258–264.

Jacobs, E., Pelier, E., & Larkin, D. (1998). Ericksonian hypnosis and approaches with pediatric hematology oncology patients. *American Journal of Clinical Hypnosis, 41*(2), 139–154.

Jones, M.B., Culbert, T.P., & Kohen, D.P. (2009). Pediatric pain management [audiotape and transcript]. *AAP Pediatric Update: An Approved System for Continuing Medical Education, 30*(6), 1–10.

Jong, M.C., Boers, I., van Wietmarschen, H.A., Tromp, E., Busari, J.O., Wennekes, R., Snoeck, I., Bekhof, J., & Vlieger, A.M. (2019). Hypnotherapy or transcendental meditation versus progressive muscle relaxation exercises in the treatment of children with primary headaches: a multi-centre, pragmatic, randomised clinical study. *European Journal of Pediatrics*, 178, 147-154. 10.1007/s00431-0183270-3

Kaiser, P., Kohen, D.P., Brown, M.L., Kajander, R.L., & Barnes, A.J. (2018). Integrating pediatric hypnosis with complementary modalities: clinical perspectives on personalized treatment. *Children, 5*(108), 1–25. 10.3390/children5080108

Katz, E.R., Kellerman, J., & Ellenberg, L. (1987). Hypnosis in the reduction of acute pain and distress in children with cancer. *Journal of Pediatric Psychology, 12*, 379–394.

Keefer, L., Taft, T.H., Kiebles, J.L., Martinovich, Z., Barrett, T.A., & Palsson, O.S. (2013). Gut-directed hypnotherapy significantly augments clinical remission in quiescent ulcerative colitis. *Alimentary Pharmacology & Therapeutics, 38*, 761–771.

Kemmer, F.W., Bisping, R., Steingruber, H.J., Baar, H., Hardtmann, F., Schlaghecke, R., & Berger, M. (1986). Psychological stress and metabolic control in patients with type I diabetes mellitus. *New England Journal of Medicine, 314*, 1078–1084.

Khan, A.U. (1977). Effectiveness of biofeedback and counterconditioning in the treatment of bronchial asthma. *Journal of Psychosomatic Research, 21*, 97–104.

Khan, A.U., Staerk, M., & Bonk, C. (1974). Hypnotic suggestibility compared with other methods of isolating emotionally-prone asthmatic children. *American Journal of Clinical Hypnosis, 17*, 50–53.

Khirani, S., Kadlub Nk Delord, V., Picard, A., & Fauroux, B. (2013). Nocturnal mouthpiece ventilation and medical hypnosis to treat severe obstructive sleep apnea in a child with cherubism. *Pediatric Pulmonology, 48*(9), 927–929.

Klassen, J., Liang, Y., Tjosvold, L., Klassen, T.P., & Hartling, L. (2008). Music for pain and anxiety in children undergoing medical procedures: A systematic review of randomized controlled trials. *Ambulatory Pediatrics, 8*(2), 117–128.

Kohen, D.P. (1980a). Hypnotherapy in a child with asthma. Videotape presented at the annual meeting of the ambulatory pediatric association, San Antonio, TX.

Kohen, D.P. (1980b). Relaxation–mental imagery (hypnosis) and pelvic examinations in adolescents. *Journal of Behavioral and Developmental Pediatrics, 1*, 180–186.

Kohen, D.P. (1982). Use of relaxation/mental imagery in an 11.5-year-old boy with asthma. Videotape presented at the annual meeting of the American Society of Clinical Hypnosis, Denver, CO.

Kohen, D.P. (1986a). The value of relaxation/mental imagery (self-hypnosis) to the management of children with asthma: a cyberphysiologic approach. *Topics in Pediatrics, 4*(1), 11–18.

Kohen, D.P. (1986b). Applications of relaxation/mental imagery (self-hypnosis) in pediatric emergencies. *International Journal of Clinical and Experimental Hypnosis, 34*(4), 283–294.

Kohen, D.P. (1987). Use of relaxation/mental imagery in a 17 year old boy with asthma. Videotape presented to the Society for Behavioral Pediatrics, Anaheim, CA.

Kohen, D.P. (1993). Entspannung und mentales Vorstellungstraining (Selbsthypnose) als Hilfe zur Selbshilfe fur Kinder mit Asthma [Helping children with asthma help themselves with relaxation/mental imagery (self-hypnosis)]. In S. Mrochen, K.L. Holtz, & B. Trenkle, Eds., *Die Pupille des Bettnassers: Hypnotherapeutische Arbeit mit Kindern und Jugendlichen [The Eye in the Middle of the Crater: On Child Hypnosis]* (pp. 212–235). Heidelberg: Carl Auer.

Kohen, D.P. (1994). Self-regulation by children and adolescents with cystic fibrosis: applications of relaxation/mental imagery (self-hypnosis). Paper presented at the annual meeting of the American Society of Clinical Hypnosis, Philadelphia, PA.

Kohen, D.P. (1995a). Ericksonian communication and hypnotic strategies in the management of tics and Tourette syndrome in children and adolescents. In S.R. Lankton & J.K. Zeig, Eds., *Ericksonian Monographs No. 10: Difficult Contexts for Therapy* (pp. 117–142). New York: Brunner/Mazel.

Kohen, D.P. (1995b). Relaxation/mental imagery (self-hypnosis) for childhood asthma: Behavioral outcomes in a prospective, controlled study. *Hypnos—Swedish Journal of Hypnosis in Psychotherapy and Psychosomatic Medicine and the Journal of the European Society of Hypnosis in Psychotherapy and Psychosomatic Medicine, 22*, 132–144.

Kohen, D.P. (1995c). Coping with the stress of Tourette syndrome in children and adolescents: use of self-hypnosis techniques. *Australian Journal of Clinical and Experimental Hypnosis, 23*, 145–157.

Kohen, D.P. (1997). Teaching children with asthma to help themselves with relaxation mental imagery (self-hypnosis). In W.J. Matthews & J.H. Edgette, Eds., *Current Thinking and Research in Brief Therapy: Solutions, Strategies, Narratives* (pp. 169–191). New York: Brunner/Mazel.

Kohen, D.P. (2000). Hypnosis in the treatment of asthma. *The Integrative Medicine Consult, 2*(6), 61–62.

Kohen, D.P. (2009). Application of hypnosis for chronic daily headache in adolescents. Paper presented at XVIII International Congress, Hypnosis and Neuroscience: Clinical Implications of the New Mind–Body Paradigms, Rome, Italy, September 22–27.

Kohen, D.P. (2010a). A pediatric perspective on mind–body medicine. In T.P. Culbert & K. Olness, Eds., *Integrative Pediatrics* (pp. 267–301). New York: Oxford University Press.

Kohen, D.P. (2010b). Long term follow-up of self-hypnosis training for recurrent headaches: what the children say. *International Journal of Clinical and Experimental Hypnosis, 58*(4), 417–432.

Kohen, D.P. (2016). Headaches – children (Chapter 27). In Elkins, Ed., *Handbook of Medical and Psychological Hypnosis: Foundations, Applications, and Professional Issues* (pp. 259–271). Springer Publishing Company, New York.

Kohen, D.P. (2018). So, what am I supposed to do about these headaches that keep coming?! (Chapter 14). In M.P. Jensen, Ed., *Hypnotic Techniques for Chronic Pain Management: Favorite Methods of Master Clinicians Denny* (pp. 277–299). Kirkland: Creek Press. www.dennycreekpress.info

Kohen, D.P. & Botts, P. (1987). Relaxation-imagery (self-hypnosis) in Tourette syndrome: experience with four children. *American Journal of Clinical Hypnosis, 29*(4), 227–237.

Kohen, D.P., Colwell, S.O., Heimel, A., & Olness, K.N. (1984). The use of relaxation/mental imagery (self-hypnosis) in the management of 505 pediatric behavioral encounters. *Journal of Developmental and Behavioral Pediatrics, 5*(1), 21–25.

Kohen, D.P. & Kaiser, P. (2014). Clinical hypnosis with children and adolescents – What? Why? How?: origins, applications, and efficacy. *Children, I,* 74–98. 10.3390children1020074

Kohen, D.P., Mann-Rinehart, P., Schmitz, D., & Wills, L. (1998). Using hypnosis to help deaf children help themselves: report of two cases. *American Journal of Clinical Hypnosis, 40,* 288–296.

Kohen, D.P. & Olness, K. (2011). *Hypnosis & Hypnotherapy with Children,*4th ed. New York: Routledge – Taylor and Francis Group.

Kohen, D.P. & Ondich, S. (2004). Children's self-regulation of cardiovascular function with relaxation/mental imagery (self-hypnosis): report of a controlled study. *Hypnos: The Journal of European Society of Hypnosis in Psychotherapy and Psychosomatic Medicine, 31*(2), 61–74.

Kohen, D.P. & Wynne, E. (1997). Applying hypnosis in a preschool family asthma education program: uses of storytelling, imagery, and relaxation. *American Journal of Clinical Hypnosis, 39,* 2–14.

Kohen, D.P. & Zajac, R. (2007). Self-hypnosis training for headaches in children and adolescents. *Journal of Pediatrics, 150,* 635–639.

Kolko, D.J. & Rickard-Figueroa, J.L. (1985). Effects of video games on the adverse corollaries of chemotherapy in pediatric oncology patients: a single-case analysis. *Journal of Counseling and Clinical Psychology, S3,* 223–228.

Konig, P. (1978). Pharmacologic management of childhood asthma. *Advances in Asthma and Allergy, 5*(3), 58–65.

Kotses, H., Harver, A., Segreto, J., Glaus, K.D., Creer, T.L., & Young, G.A. (1991). Long term effects of biofeedback-induced facial relaxation on measures of asthma severity in children. *Biofeedback and Self-Regulation, 16,* 1–22.

Kotses, H. & Miller, D.J. (1987). The effects of changes in facial muscle tension on respiratory resistance. *Biological Psychology, 25,* 211–219.

Kroner-Herwig, B., Morris, K., & Heinrich, M. (2004). New epidemiological facts on headache in children and adolescents. Paper presented at the German Pain Congress, Leipzig, Germany.

Kumari, S., Bahuguna, R., Garg, N., & Yeluri, R. (2021). Immersive and non-immersive virtual reality distraction on pain perception to intraoral injections. *Journal of Clinical Pediatric Dentistry, 45*(6), 380–394.

Kuttner, L. Director/Producer. (1986). *No Fears, No Tears: Children with Cancer Coping with Pain.* DVD available from BC Children's Hospital (http://bookstore.cw.bc.ca; 1-800-331-1533, ext. 3).

Kuttner, L. (1988). Favorite stories: a hypnotic pain reduction technique for children in acute pain. *American Journal of Clinical Hypnosis, 30*(4), 289–295.

Kuttner, L. (1989). Management of young children's acute pain and anxiety during invasive medical procedures. *Pediatrician, 16,* 39–44.

Kuttner, L. Director/Producer. (1998). *No Fears, No Tears: 13 Years Later.* DVD available from BC Children's Hospital (http://bookstore.cw.bc.ca; 1-800-331-1533, ext. 3).

Kuttner, L., Bowman, M., & Teasdale, M. (1988). Psychological treatment of distress, pain, and anxiety for young children with cancer. *Journal of Developmental and Behavioral Pediatrics, 9,* 374–381.

Kuttner, L. & Catchpole, R.E.H. (2007). Developmental considerations: hypnosis with children. In W.C. Wester II & L.I. Sugarman, Eds., *Therapeutic Hypnosis with Children and Adolescents* (pp. 25–44). Bethel, CT: Crown House Publishing.

LaBaw, W.L. (1975). Autohypnosis in hemophilia. *Haematologia, 9,* 103–110.

Labbé, E.E. & Williamson, D.A. (1983). Temperature biofeedback in the treatment of children with migraine headaches. *Journal of Pediatric Psychology, 8,* 317–326.

LaGrone, R. (1993). Hypnobehavioral therapy to reduce gag and emesis with a 10-year-old pill swallower. *American Journal of Clinical Hypnosis, 36*(2), 132–136.
Lambert, S.A. (1996). The effects of hypnosis/guided imagery on the postoperative course of children. *Journal of Developmental and Behavioral Pediatrics, 17*, 307–310.
Landsberg, L. & Young, J.B. (1978). Fasting, feeding, and regulation of the sympathetic nervous system. *New England Journal of Medicine, 198*, 1293–1301.
Lane, D. (1994). *Music as Medicine: Deforia Lane's Life of Music, Healing, and Faith.* Grand Rapids, MI: Zondervan Publishing House.
Lankton, S. (2007). Psychotherapeutic intervention for numerous and large viral warts with adjunctive hypnosis: a case study. *American Journal of Clinical Hypnosis, 49*(3), 211–218.
Lazar, B.S. (1977). Hypnotic imagery as a tool in working with a cerebral palsied child. *International Journal of Clinical and Experimental Hypnosis, 25*, 78–87.
Lazarus, J. & Klein, S.K. (2010). Nonpharmacological treatment of tics in Tourette syndrome adding videotape training to self-hypnosis. *Journal of Developmental and Behavioral Pediatrics, 31*(6), 498–504.
Lee, A., Moulton, D., Mckernan, L., Russell, A., Slaughter, J.C., Acra, S., & Walker, L. (2021). Clinical hypnosis in pediatric Crohn's disease: a randomized controlled pilot study. *Journal of Pediatric Gastroenterology and Nutrition, 72*(3), e63–e70.
Leffert, F. (1980). The management of acute severe asthma. *Journal of Pediatrics, 96*, 1–12.
Lehrer, P.M. (1998). Emotionally triggered asthma: a review of research literature and some hypotheses for self-regulation therapies. *Applied Psychophysiology and Biofeedback, 23*, 13–41.
Lehrer, P.M., Sargunaraj, D., & Hochron, S. (1992). Psychological approaches to the treatment of asthma. *Journal of Consulting and Clinical Psychology, 60*(4), 639–643.
Lewenstein, L.N. (1978). Personal communication.
Liggett, D.R. (2000). Enhancing imagery through hypnosis: a performance aid for athletes. *American Journal of Clinical Hypnosis, 43*(2), 149–157.
Liossi, C. & Hatira, P. (1999). Clinical hypnosis versus cognitive behavioral training for pain management with pediatric cancer patients undergoing bone marrow aspirations. *The International Journal of Clinical and Experimental Hypnosis, 47*, 104–116.
Liossi, C. & Hatira, P. (2003). Clinical hypnosis in the alleviation of procedure-related pain in pediatric oncology patients. *The International Journal of Clinical and Experimental Hypnosis, 51*, 4–28.
Liossi, C., White, P., & Hatira, P. (2006). Randomized clinical trial of local anesthetic versus a combination of local anesthetic with self-hypnosis in the management of pediatric procedure-related pain. *Health Psychology, 25*, 307–315.
Lobe, T.E. (2006). Perioperative hypnosis reduces hospitalization on patients undergoing the Nuss procedure for pectus excavatum. *Journal of Laparoendoscopic & Advanced Surgical Techniques, Part A, 16*, 639–642.
Luparello, T., Leist, N., Lourie, C.H., & Sweet, P. (1970). Interaction of psychologic stimuli and pharmacologic agents on airway reactivity in asthmatic subjects. *Psychosomatic Medicine, 32*, 509–513.
Madrid, A.D. & Barnes, S.H. (1991). A hypnotic protocol for eliciting physical changes through suggestions of biochemical responses. *American Journal of Clinical Hypnosis, 34*(2), 122–128.
Mahler, T. (2015). Education and hypnosis for treatment of functional gastrointestinal disorders (FGIDs) in pediatrics. *American Journal of Clinical Hypnosis, 58*(1), 115–128
Marino, R.V. (1994). Facilitation of extubation with physician-assisted cyber-physiologic ventilatory stabilization: common sense, compassion, and sensitivity really enhance outcomes! *Archives of Pediatrics and Adolescent Medicine, 148*, 545.
Marion, R.J., Creer, T.L., & Reynolds, R.V.C. (1985). Direct and indirect costs associated with the management of childhood asthma. *Annals of Allergy, 54*, 31–34.
Masters, K.S. (2006). Recurrent abdominal pain, medical intervention, and biofeedback: what happened to the biopsychosocial model? *Applied Psychophysiology and Biofeedback, 31*(2), 155–165.
Mattson, A. (1975). Psychologic aspects of childhood asthma. *Pediatric Clinics of North America, 22*(1), 77–89.
Mauersberger, K., Artz, K., Duncan, B., & Gurgevich, S. (2000). Can children with spastic cerebral palsy use self-hypnosis to reduce muscle tone? A preliminary study. *Integrative Medicine, 2*, 93–96.
McCracken, J. (2000). Tic disorders. In H. Kaplan & B. Sadock, Eds., *Comprehensive Textbook of Psychiatry*, 7th ed. (pp. 2711–2719). Philadelphia, PA: Lippincott Williams & Wilkins.

Mirvish, I. (1978). Hypnotherapy for the child with chronic eczema: a case report. *South African Medical Journal, 54*, 410–412.

Moore, C.L. (1980). Hypnotherapy with parents of asthmatic children. Paper presented at the annual meeting of the American Society of Clinical Hypnosis, Minneapolis, MN.

Morgan, W.P. (1980). Hypnosis and sports medicine. In G.D. Burrows & L. Dennerstein, Eds., *Handbook of Hypnosis and Psychosomatic Medicine*. New York: Elsevier/ North-Holland Biomedical Press.

National Asthma Education and Prevention Program Coordinating Committee, Third Expert Panel on the Management of Asthma, National Heart, Lung, and Blood Institute, and American Institutes for Research. (2007). *National Asthma Education and Prevention Program Expert Panel Report 3: Guidelines for the Diagnosis and Management of Asthma, NIH Publ.* No. 08-5846. Washington, DC: U.S. Department of Health and Human Services National Institutes of Health.

Newmark, T.S. & Bogacki, D.F. (2005). The use of relaxation, hypnosis, and imagery in sport psychiatry. *Clinics in Sports Medicine, 24*, 973–977.

Nunns, M., Mayhew, D., Ford, T., Rogers, M., Curle, C., Logan, S., & Moore, D. (2018). Effectiveness of non-pharmacological interventions to reduce procedural anxiety in children and adolescents undergoing treatment for cancer: a systematic review and meta-analysis. *Psychooncology, 8*, 1889–1899.

Olness, K. (1977). In-service hypnosis education in a children's hospital. *American Journal of Clinical Hypnosis, 20*, 80–83.

Olness, K. (1981). Imagery (self-hypnosis) as adjunct care in childhood cancer: clinical experience with 25 patients. *American Journal of Pediatric Hematology/Oncology, 3*, 313–321.

Olness, K. (1990). Pediatric psychoneuroimmunology: hypnosis as a possible mediator—potentials and problems. In R. Van Dyck et al., Eds., *Hypnosis: Current Theory, Research, and Practice* (pp. 71–81). Amsterdam: Free University Press.

Olness, K. & Agle, D. (1981). *The Enhancement of Mastery in the Child with Hemophilia, via Imagery-Relaxation Exercises (Self-Hypnosis) and Biofeedback Techniques*. New York: National Hemophilia Association.

Olness, K. & MacDonald, J. (1987). Headaches in children. *Pediatrics in Review, 8*, 307–311.

Olness, K., MacDonald, J., & Uden, D. (1987). A prospective study comparing self-hypnosis, propranolol, and placebo in management of juvenile migraine. *Pediatrics, 79*, 593–597.

Olsson, C.J., Jonsson, B., & Nyberg, L. (2008). Internal imagery training in active high jumpers. *Scandinavian Journal of Psychology, 49*, 133–140.

Osterhaus, S.O.L., Passchier, J., van der Helm-Hylkema, H., de Jong, K.T., Orlebeke, J.F., de Grauw, A.J.C., & Dekker, P.H. (1993). Effects ofbehavioral psychophysiological treatment on schoolchildren with migraine in a nonclinical setting: predictors and process variables. *Journal of Pediatric Psychology, 18*(6),697–715.

Palsson, O.S. (2010). *Overview of published research to date on hypnosis for IBS.* http://www.ibshypnosis.com/IBSresearch.html

Panayi, L., Kanaka-Gantenbein, C., Darviri, C., & Chrousos, G.P. (2016). Stress management and health promotion through family intervention improves metabolic control in children and adolescents with type I diabetes. *European Society for Paediatric Endocrinology Abstracts 86: RFC5.8.*

Patterson, D.R. (2010). Hypnosis and pain. Paper presented at the 52nd Annual Workshops and Scientific Program, American Society of Clinical Hypnosis, Nashville, TN.

Pederson, C. (1993). *Ways to Feel Comfortable [videotape and booklet]*. Minneapolis, MN: University of Minnesota, School of Nursing.

Perloff, M.M. & Spiegelman, J. (1973). Hypnosis in the treatment of a child's allergy to dogs. *American Journal of Clinical Hypnosis, 15*, 269–272.

Puskarich, C.A., Whitman, S., Dell, J., Hughes, J.R., Rosen, A.J., & Hermann, B.P. (1992). Controlled examination of effects of progressive relaxation training on seizure reduction. *Epilepsia, 33*(4), 675–680.

Rachelefsky, G.S., Lewis, C.E., & de la Sota, A. (1985). ACT (asthma care training) for kids: a childhood asthma self-management program. *Chest, 87*(1, Suppl.), 98S–100S.

Rachelefsky, G.S. & Siegel, S. (1985). Asthma in infants and children-treatment of childhood asthma, Part II. *Journal of Allergy and Clinical Immunology, 76*(3), 409–425.

Rakos, R.F., Grodek, M.V., & Mack, K.K. (1985). The impact of a self-administered behavioral intervention program in pediatric asthma. *Journal of Psychosomatic Research, 29*(1), 101–108.

Ratner, H., Gross, L., Casas, J., & Castells, S. (1990). A hypnotherapeutic approach to the improvement of compliance in adolescent diabetes. *American Journal of Clinical Hypnosis, 32*, 154–159.

Raz, A., Keller, S., Norman, K., & Senechal, D. (2007). Elucidating Tourette's syndrome: perspectives from hypnosis, attention and self-regulation. *American Journal of Clinical Hypnosis*, *49*(4), 289–309.

Reaney, J., Chang, P., & Olness, K. (1978). The use of relaxation and visual imagery in children with asthma. *Proceedings of the Ambulatory Pediatric Association*, p. 28.

Reznick, C. (2009). *The Power of Your Child's Imagination: How to Transform Stress and Anxiety into Joy and Success*. New York: Penguin Group.

Ritterman, M.K. (1982). Hemophilia in context: adjunctive hypnosis for families with a hemophiliac member. *Family Practice*, *21*, 469–476.

Russo, D. & Varni, J.W., Eds. (1982). *Behavioral Pediatrics: Research and Practice*. New York: Plenum Press.

Rutten, J.M., Reitsma, J.B., Vlieger, A.M., & Benninga, M.A. (2013, April). Gut-directed hypnotherapy for functional abdominal pain or irritable bowel syndrome in children: a systematic review. *Archives of Disease Childhood*, *98*(4), 252–257.

Rutten, J.M.T., Vlieger, A.M., Frankenhuis, C., George, E.K., Groeneweg, M., Norbruis, O.F., Tjon, A., Ten, W., van Wering, H.M., Dijkgraaf, M.G.W., Merkus, M.P., & Benninga, M.A. (2017). Home-based hypnotherapy self-exercises vs individual hypnotherapy with a therapist for treatment of pediatric irritable bowel syndrome, functional abdominal pain, or functional abdominal pain syndrome: a randomized clinical trial. *JAMA Pediatrics*, *171*(5), 470–477.

Rutten, J.M.T.M., Korterink, J.J., Venman, L.M.A.J., Benninga, M.A., & Tabbers, M.M. (2015). Nonpharmacologic treatment of functional abdominal pain disorders: a systematic review. *Pediatrics*, *135*(3), 522–535. 10.1542/peds.2014-2123

Sand-Jecklin, K. (2008). Patient anxiety levels related to gynecologic examinations: use of the color breathwork relaxation method. *Archives of Psychiatric Nursing*, *212*(4), 240–242.

Sawni, A. & Breuner, C.C. (2017). Clinical hypnosis, an effective mind-body modality for adolescents with behavioral and physical complaints. *Children*, *4*, 19. doi: 10.3390/children4040019

Scahill, L., Williams, S., Schwab-Stone, M., Applegate, J., & Leckman, J.F. (2006). Disruptive behavior problems in a community sample of children with tic disorders. *Advances in Neurology*, *99*, 184–190.

Scherr, M.S. & Crawford, P.L. (1978). Three-year evaluation of biofeedback techniques in the treatment of children with chronic asthma in a summer camp environment. *Annals of Allergy*, *41*, 288–292.

Secter, I.I. & Gelberd, M.B. (1964). Hypnosis as a relaxant for the cerebral palsied patient. *American Journal of Clinical Hypnosis*, *6*, 364–365.

Shaoul, R., Sukhotnik, I., & Mogilner, J. (2009). Hypnosis as an adjuvant treatment for children with inflammatory bowel disease. *Journal of Developmental & Behavioral Pediatrics*, *30*(3), 268.

Sheffer, A.L., Bailey, W.C., Bleecker, E. R. et al. (1991). Guidelines for the diagnosis and management of asthma: National Heart, Lung and Blood Institute, National Asthma Education Program expert panel report. *Journal of Allergy and Clinical Immunology*, 8(Suppl), 425–534.

Smart, G. (1997). Helping children relax during magnetic resonance imaging. *The American Journal of Maternal/Child Nursing*, *22*, 237–241.

Smith, J.M. & Burns, C.L.C. (1960). The treatment of asthmatic children by hypnotic suggestion. *British Journal of Diseases of the Chest*, *54*, 78–81.

Smith, J.R., Mugford, M., Holland, R., Candy, B., Noble, M.J., Harrison, B.D.W., Koutantji, M., Upton, C., & Harvey, I. (2005). A systematic review to examine the impact of psycho-educational interventions on health outcomes and costs in adults and children with difficult asthma. *Health Technology Assessment*, *9*(23), 1–182.

Smith, S.D., Trueworthy, R.C., Klopovich, P.M., Vats, T.S., & Snodgrass, W. (1984). Management of children with isolated testicular leukemia. *Cancer*, *54*, 2854–2858.

Sokel, B.S., Devane, S.P., & Bentovim, A. (1991). Getting better with honor: individualized relaxation/self-hypnosis techniques for control of recalcitrant abdominal pain in children. *Family Systems Medicine*, *9*, 83–91.

Sokel, B.S., Devane, S.P., Bentovim, A., & Milla, P.J. (1990). Self-hypnotherapeutic treatment of habitual reflex vomiting. *Archives of Disease in Childhood*, *65*, 627–628.

Spevack, M., Vost, M., Maheux, V., & Bestercezy, A. (1978). Group passive relaxation exercises in asthma. *Pediatric News*, *12*, 14.

Storch, E.A., Merlo, L.J., Lack, C., Milsom, V.A., Geffken, G.R., Goodman, W.K., & Murphy, T.K. (2007). Quality of life in youth with Tourette's syndrome and chronic tic disorder. *Journal of Clinical Child & Adolescent Psychology*, *36*(2), 217–227.

Sugarman, L.I. (1997/2007). *Hypnosis in Pediatric Practice: Imaginative Medicine in Action [video and instructional manual]*. Bethel, CT: Crown House Publishing.
Surman, O.S., Gottlieb, S.K., & Hackett, T.P. (1972). Hypnotic treatment of a child with warts. *American Journal of Clinical Hypnosis, 15*, 12–14.
Tan, G., Hammond, D.C., & Gurrala, J. (2005). Hypnosis and irritable bowel syndrome: a review of efficacy and mechanism of action. *American Journal of Clinical Hypnosis, 47*(3), 161–178.
Tasini, M.F. & Hackett, T.P. (1977). Hypnosis in the treatment of warts in immunodeficient children. *American Journal of Clinical Hypnosis, 19*, 152–154.
Thomas, L. (1979). *The Medusa and the Snail*. New York: Viking Press.
Thomson, L. (2005). *Harry the Hypno-potamus: Metaphorical Tales for the Treatment of Children*. Bethel, CT: Crown House Publishing.
Thomson, L. (2007). Hypnosis for children with elimination disorders. In W.C. Wester II & L.I. Sugarman, Eds., *Therapeutic Hypnosis with Children and Adolescents* (pp. 387–416). Bethel, CT: Crown House Publishing.
Thorne, D.E. & Fisher, A.G. (1978). Hypnotically suggested asthma. *International Journal of Clinical and Experimental Hypnosis, 26*, 92–103.
Trautmann, E., Lackschewitz, H., & Kroner-Herwig, B. (2006). Psychological treatment of recurrent headache in children and adolescents: a meta-analysis. *Cephalalgia, 26*, 1411–1426.
Uman, L.S., Chambers, C.T., McGrath, P.J., & Kisely, S. (2008). A systematic review of randomized controlled trials examining psychological interventions for needle-related procedural pain and distress in children and adolescents: An abbreviated Cochrane Review. *Journal of Pediatric Psychology*, 33, 842–854.
van Tilburg, M.A.L., Chitkara, D.K., Palsson, O.S., Turner, M., Blois-Martin, N., Ulshen, M., & Whitehead, W.E. (2009). Audio-recorded guided imagery treatment reduces functional abdominal pain in children: a pilot study. *Pediatrics, 124*, e890–e897.
Vlieger, A.M., Menko-Frankenhuis, C., Wolfkamp, S.C., Tromp, E., & Benninga, M.A. (2007). Hypnotherapy for children with functional abdominal pain or irritable bowel syndrome: a randomized controlled trial. *Gastroenterology, 133*(5), 1430–1436.
Vlieger, A.M., Rutten, J.M., Govers, A.M., Frankenhuis, C., Benninga, M.A. (2012). Long-term follow-up of gut-directed hypnotherapy vs. standard care in children with functional abdominal pain or irritable bowel syndrome. *American Journal of Gastroenterology, 107*(4), 627–631
Walco, G.A., Varni, J.W., & Ilowite, N.T. (1992). Cognitive–behavioral pain management in children with juvenile rheumatoid arthritis. *Pediatrics, 89*(6), 1075–1079.
Wall, V.J. & Womack, W. (1989). Hypnotic versus active cognitive strategies for alleviation of procedural distress in pediatric oncology patients. *The American Journal of Clinical Hypnosis, 31*, 181–191.
Werder, D.S. & Sargent, J.D. (1984). A study of childhood headache using biofeedback as a treatment alternative. *Headache, 24*, 122–126.
Wester, W.C. & Sugarman, L.I., Eds. (2007). *Therapeutic Hypnosis with Children and Adolescents*. Bethel, CT: Crown House Publishing.
Weydert, J.A., Ball, T.M., & Davis, S. (2003). Systematic review of treatments for recurrent abdominal pain. *Pediatrics, 111*(1), e1–e11. doi: 10.1542/peds.111.1e1
Weydert, J.A., Shapiro, D.E., Acra, S.A., Monheim, C.J., Chambers, A.S., & Ball, T.M. (2006). Evaluation of guided imagery as treatment for recurrent abdominal pain in children: a randomized controlled trial. *BMC Pediatrics, 6*, 29.
Whitehead, W.E. (2006). Hypnosis for irritable bowel syndrome: the empirical evidence of therapeutic effects. *International Journal of Clinical and Experimental Hypnosis, 54*(1), 7–20.
Whitfield, K.L. & Shulman, R.J. (2009). Treatment options for functional gastrointestinal disorders: from empiric to complementary approaches. *Pediatric Annals, 38*(5), 288–294.
Whorwell, P.J., Prior, A., & Colgan, S.M. (1987). Hypnotherapy in severe irritable bowel syndrome: further experience. *Gut, 28*, 423–425.
Williams, D.T. & Singh, M. (1976). Hypnosis as a facilitating therapeutic adjunct in child psychiatry. *Journal of the American Academy of Child Psychiatry, 15*, 326–342.
Wolf, F.M., Guevara, J.P., Grum, C.M., Clark, N.M., & Cates, C.J. (2003). Educational interventions for asthma in children. *The Cochrane Database Systematic Review*, Issue 1, Article No. CD000326.

Woods, D.W., Himle, M.B., & Conelea, C.A. (2006). Behavior therapy; other interventions for tic disorders. *Advances in Neurology, 99*, 234–240.

Woods, D.W. & Marcks, B.A. (2005). Controlled evaluation of an educational intervention used to modify peer attitudes and behavior toward persons with Tourette's syndrome. *Behavior Modification, 29*, 900–912.

Woods, D.W., Twohig, M.P., Flessner, C.A., & Roloff, C.A. (2003). Treatment of vocal tics in children with Tourette syndrome: investigating the efficacy of habit reversal. *Journal of Applied Behavior Analysis, 36*, 109–112.

Young, M. H., & Montano, R. J. (1988). A New Hypnobehavioral Method for the Treatment of Children with Tourette's Disorder. *American Journal of Clinical Hypnosis*, 31, 97–106. 10.1080/00029157.1988.10402875.

Zahm, D.N. (1990). Hypnosis in the treatment of Tourette syndrome. In C.D. Hammond, Ed., *Handbook of Hypnotic Suggestions and Metaphors* (pp. 501–502). New York: W.W. Norton.

Zeltzer, L. & LeBaron, S. (1982). Hypnosis and nonhypnotic techniques for reduction of pain and anxiety during painful procedures in children and adolescents with cancer. *Behavioral Pediatrics, 101*, 1032–1035.

Zeltzer, L., LeBaron, S., & Zeltzer, P.M. (1984a). The effectiveness of behavioral intervention for reducing nausea and vomiting in children and adolescents receiving chemotherapy. *Journal of Clinical Oncology, 2*, 683–690.

Zeltzer, L., LeBaron, S., & Zeltzer, P.M. (1984b). Paradoxical effects of prophylactic phenothiazine antiemetics in children receiving chemotherapy. *Journal of Clinical Oncology, 2*, 936–940.

Zimmern, V. (2017). Uses of hypnosis in pediatric anesthesia and pediatric headaches: a literature review [Thesis, Collections: UT Southwestern Medical School]. https://hdl,handle.net/2152.5.4767

Zinner, S.H. & Coffey, B.J. (2009). Developmental and behavioral disorders grown up: Tourette's disorder. *Journal of Developmental and Behavioral Pediatrics, 30*(6), 560–573.

# 14

# HYPNOTIC APPROACHES FOR PEDIATRIC SURGERY, ANESTHESIA, AND EMERGENCIES

## Introduction

The use of hypnosis as the sole anesthetic in major surgery is quite rare, probably because of the relative safety and convenience of chemical anesthetics. Hypnosis has been used infrequently for this purpose with adults (Hammond, 2008; Kroger & DeLee, 1957; Levitan & Harbaugh, 1992; Rausch, 1980; Wangensteen, 1962; Winkelstein & Levinson, 1959; see also Chapter 10). We know of no similar published accounts with children since the 19th-century work of Braid and Elliotson in England.

Hypnosis is useful in pediatric surgery for facilitating emergency room procedures, preoperative comfort, induction of anesthesia, and postoperative comfort and cooperation (Kohen, 2001a; Lambert, 1996; Lobe, 2007; Vagnoli, Bettini, & Amore, 2019). It is also used very effectively for a variety of minor surgical procedures in such areas as burn therapy and dentistry (Sabherwal, Kaira, Tvagi, Khatri, & Srivastava, 2021). We know of no instances in which pediatric surgical patients have used hypnosis inappropriately to mask symptoms, such as pain, when awareness is necessary for prompt diagnosis and treatment, although we have heard fears to the contrary. We remind our patients to give themselves suggestions that are in the best interests of their body and good health to offset the possibility that the signal value of symptoms will be ignored. The following case history is an example of a child's ability to use good judgment in applying hypnotic skills.

Joe T., age 10 years, came into the emergency room with severe periumbilical pain and a history of preceding nausea and vomiting. He also had a history of migraine headaches, for which he had successfully learned to use self-hypnosis. While in the emergency room, awaiting the surgery consultant, he was clearly uncomfortable. Nursing staff reassured him, saying he could probably have a medication for pain following the surgeon's visit. The surgeon made the diagnosis of appendicitis and scheduled the patient for surgery within the hour. When offered preoperative analgesics, the patient refused, saying, "It's going to be fixed, so now I can turn off my switch." He visibly relaxed and was comfortable until induction of general anesthesia. Following surgery, the patient used self-hypnosis to counteract pain and nausea and to facilitate healing.

DOI: 10.4324/9781003243687-16

## Emergency Situations

### *Modifying Attitudes*

If hypnosis is going to be successful during pediatric emergency room procedures, one must realize that children bring more to the situation than a laceration or fracture. They bring their own feelings, mixed in unknown ways with attitudes of parents, teachers, and others who have witnessed the current crisis or discussed previous crises with them (Brunnquell & Kohen, 1991). Kelly (1976) observed that fear, pain, and guilt are characteristic of virtually every emergency situation. There is fear of the process of the accident or problem and its outcome, as well as fear of losing control. Pain may include recall of past pain coupled with whatever the current sensation is and anticipation of future pain. Guilt may be real or conditioned by family or friends. In a study of children's emergency room visits, Alpert (1975) concluded that the majority of them had psychogenic antecedents – for example, a death in the family, a family quarrel, a move, or a serious illness in a parent. Emergency room staff should consider such possibilities, even though the reason for admission is, on the surface, clearly an accident. Increasingly, mainstream journals have begun to focus on these essential ingredients of all emergency situations, emphasizing the importance of using age and developmentally appropriate language and preparation for procedures, the value of parental presence, and the use of "nonpharmacologic techniques such as relaxation, distraction, and imagery" (Kennedy & Luhmann, 1999).

Successful hypnosis is also dependent on the attitudes of the emergency room staff; that is, if the staff expects a negative experience for all concerned, then negative suggestions will almost guarantee fulfillment of those negative expectations. The spontaneous immediate appearance or use of a restraint conveys an expectation that the child is going to resist and will require restraint. Likewise, requiring parents to leave the scene of repair conveys an expectation that they cannot be of help or, worse, that their presence will be detrimental to the child. When properly prepared, however, most parents can reinforce suggestions not only in the emergency room but also later at home. Allowing them to observe the induction of hypnosis and the procedure may be relaxing, desensitizing, and a good learning experience for them. There are exceptions, but most parents can be helpful in emergencies that involve children. Therapists gain more by expecting parents to be helpful and supportive than by expecting them to make procedures more difficult.

### *Modifying the Child's Experience*

Neither the nurse nor the treating physician, nor any other individual clinician who may be guiding the hypnosis, usually has much time to get to know a child who comes to the emergency room. The situation often precludes opportunities to explain hypnosis and to determine the value of several different induction techniques the way one might ordinarily proceed in a nonemergency situation; however, these circumstances do not rule out the use of hypnosis or of hypnotic language, strategies, and techniques without any formal induction. Precisely because of the emergency, children are often highly motivated to respond to positive suggestions and may indeed be in a spontaneous hypnotic state, albeit a negative one, narrowly focused on the reason for their emergency visit (e.g., the injured part, their bleeding, their difficulty breathing).

Sometimes direct or indirect hypnotic suggestions can be given before a child even reaches the emergency room. If a parent makes a preliminary telephone call, the doctor can suggest specific phrases that might be helpful. One of us (KO) found such techniques helpful when her daughter cut her forehead while being chased through the house by her sister. When the child felt the blood on her face, she started screaming. Her mother's first comment was, "What beautiful, healthy red blood you have. Let's go into the bathroom to get a better look at it." The child immediately stopped screaming. As she left for the emergency room, she leaned out the car window and yelled at her sister, "I have strong, healthy blood. Mama said so."

When the physician first greets the child in the emergency room it is important to convey understanding of the situation and its attendant feelings. One might say, "It's scary to come to a new place like this and to have that kind of cut. It's been bleeding a lot, and it might bleed a little bit more." The reference to "that" cut rather than "your" cut reflects the use of dissociative language and represents an invitation to the child to dissociate and thereby create potential for more comfort. The awareness that a child (or adult) in an emergency is commonly in a spontaneous hypnotic state allows the clinician to thoughtfully and spontaneously utilize hypnotic language and hypnotic suggestion naturalistically just as though a more formal invitation had taken place. As the doctor acknowledges the child's reality, the child is that much more ready to accept other statements and follow subsequent suggestions. When emergency room staff acknowledges to themselves that people (patients) in these situations of acute injury, pain, or anxiety are often already in a hypnotic state, then they give themselves the ability to approach the child hypnotically, finding the hypnosis in the encounter, and offering at once acknowledgment of the reality, reassurances of comfort, and positive expectancy suggestions for improvement. Thus, in addition to saying, "It's bleeding a lot, and it might bleed some more," the physician might also add the very positive and Ericksonian suggestion that "it will keep right on bleeding until it stops … soon" (Kohen, 2001a).

Erickson (1958) pointed out the value of commenting on certain aspects of the child's reality in order to turn apparently negative behavior to advantage; for example, one can comment that a child's tears are beautiful or that loud yelling reveals very healthy lungs. Although children need reassurance, vague statements that everything is going to be all right are usually of little value. A clearer, more specific comment may allow the child to be more hopeful that the current situation will change. The doctor who says, "I wonder if it will stop bleeding in 1 minute or 2 or 4?" not only suggests hope but also arouses curiosity that modifies anxiety and enhances cooperation. Compare this approach with the negative implications of saying, "I've got to try to stop this bleeding. Now you just have to be still."

After gaining rapport, the physician must explain what will happen to the child and how and when it will happen. Here, again, current approaches are often at variance with successful use of hypnotic techniques. For example, in the name of honest and full disclosure, it may be common to hear people tell a child, "This [procedure, cleaning, IV, needle-stick] is going to hurt." For two reasons, we believe that physicians may have become dishonest in their efforts to be honest with children. First, it is difficult, if not impossible, to predict the extent to which a child will experience the sensory and suffering components of any sort of pain. Second, children, as much as or more so than adults, can use various techniques to reduce their pain, and so-called honest statements about feeling pain may limit the child's creativity by imposing negative expectations. At the same time, one should not tell a child, "It won't hurt," for such a remark can undermine credibility and trust, both now and in the future. Erickson (1958) found the middle ground with comments such as, "Now, this could hurt a lot, but I think maybe you can stop a lot of the hurt or maybe all of it." Or, one might say, "This might hurt some, but it just may not bother you very much. Some people say this feels like pressure, some like a kitty scratching, some like a baby chick pecking, some like buzzing. I wonder what it will feel like for you?" Here, the child's curiosity is again aroused and willingness to cooperate is enhanced. In general, we find it quite useful to wonder aloud with our young patients and their families, not only in emergencies but also in most clinical encounters, with the clear therapeutic intent of empowering their own creativity and development of approaches and solutions. Thus, phrases such as "I wonder how few sutures you may need?" or "I wonder how soon those headaches will be totally gone?" or "I wonder what you'll have to eat for supper tonight?" imply success and positive outcomes without being directive or prescriptive.

A pediatric intern at The Johns Hopkins Hospital had the following experience, which demonstrates how therapeutic hypnosis can be used in emergency situations (K.A. Torjesen, pers. comm.). A 12-year-old girl was referred to the emergency room by her pediatrician for x-rays of her neck because she had not eaten solid foods for 3 weeks. She had choked while eating a strawberry and thereafter was convinced that she would choke and die if she ate any solids. She had lost 15 pounds. She was able to take clear liquids but, during the past few days, even this had become difficult. She had no previous similar episodes, and her general health had been excellent. Detailed family history suggested that her home life was normal and that she was a happy child. Physical examination revealed no abnormalities except that she appeared thin. Lateral neck x-rays revealed no abnormalities. Following the examination, the intern discussed the history and findings with the emergency room physician, who recommended that the family make an appointment with psychiatry. The intern, who had taken courses in pediatric clinical hypnosis and who had used self-hypnosis herself, spoke with the family about the psychiatry appointment. They agreed, but she noticed that the girl looked disappointed. She proceeded to draw diagrams for the girl of the esophagus, trachea, and epiglottis to explain to her that they were separate tubes and that normally choking did not occur. On impulse, she said,

> I have something you can practice before you go to bed tonight and tomorrow morning that may help you help yourself. It is easy to understand why you have this problem, because you became very frightened when you choked. You then worried about swallowing solid foods. As the days went by you developed a habit of not being able to swallow solids. You can reverse the habit by using your imagination. Would you like to learn how?

The girl was enthusiastic.

The intern told her to imagine herself in a comfortable, favorite place. She was instructed that when she felt very comfortable and relaxed she should imagine she was eating her favorite foods and that swallowing was easy and smooth and comfortable. The parents immediately noted that the intern had given a hypnotic suggestion but said they agreed with this approach. On the following day, the pediatric intern was busy in the clinic when her beeper went off. She was told that a family was waiting in the emergency room to see her. She found her patient eagerly waiting for her and the parents beaming. The patient threw her arms around the intern and said she had been able to eat solids the very next morning. The family had returned to keep the appointment with psychiatry, but there seemed little need for an additional consultation at that time. It is noteworthy that part of the treatment included demystification – in this case, an explanation of the swallowing process (see also Chapter 13). Puskar and Mumford (1990) described the value of cognitive mastery along with hypnosis in a 16-year-old boy whose treatment included looking in a mirror (at a scalp laceration) as part of the process of hypnosis easing the emergency room experience. We have found that such explanations and demystification are often important, integral parts of the hypnosis process.

Some children benefit from distraction. Others, for whom cognitive mastery is a major coping mechanism, prefer to watch every detail of a procedure. The physician can ask whether the child wants to learn about how doctors treat injuries or prefers to engage in some other enjoyable activity. Either way, the child achieves dissociation from pain. Gardner (1978) reported a case in which a 4-year-old chose to play with his cat and cheerfully described his play while the pediatrician placed four sutures in a thigh laceration without any anesthetic. In such cases, the physician might say, "Thank you for telling me what you would like to be doing. Go ahead and imagine you're doing it. I'll fix this while you're doing your favorite thing. You can help me by telling me what you're doing now." Many children readily accept these indirect suggestions for control and cooperation.

For the child who wants careful descriptions of the treatment, one can use relatively soothing words. Thus, injection of local anesthetic may be "a squeezing feeling." Antiseptic solution may be "cool or cold." A fractured arm or leg may be "like a block of wood." Burns can feel "more and more cool and comfortable." Children can be asked to time the procedure, to count stitches, to estimate blood loss, to hold bandages or instruments – generally to help in such a way as to enhance mastery, minimize anxiety, and indirectly reduce discomfort.

Distraction may be used in the context of cognitive mastery by asking the child to observe body parts that are not involved in the injury. If the injury involves the left knee, for example, the physician might also check the right knee carefully and say, "How does your *right* knee feel? Is it warm? Is there pressure here? Keep feeling that and please tell me if the feeling changes." Direct techniques for pain control, as described in Chapter 10, may also be used. It may also be helpful to include suggestions to stop bleeding (e.g., "It's bled enough. It would be okay to stop bleeding now"), to send fighter cells to take away germs, and to start healing immediately. Post-procedure suggestions should focus on ego strengthening, comfort, easy cooperation with future procedures (e.g., bandage changes, suture removal), and rapid healing.

Andolsek and Novik (1980) reported successful use of hypnosis for emergency treatment of two 3-year-old and two 4-year-old children. Procedures included suturing lacerations, treatment of a hematoma underneath a fingernail, and incision and drainage of a thumb abscess. Trance states were induced by encouraging the child to pick a topic of conversation and to focus on the most vivid sensory details of the chosen topic. Goals were to direct attention away from fears and to give the children a feeling of control over a potentially traumatic situation. Parents were encouraged to reinforce the positive suggestions. Following the procedures, the children and parents were encouraged to express their feelings about the experience.

Santer (1990) conducted a randomized controlled study of "formal communication techniques," including mental imagery instructions, as an adjunct to injected local anesthetic in a pediatric emergency room. Fifteen experimental and ten control children and their guardians did not differ in scores of behavioral distress, subjective pain, or anxiety. Children ranged from 6 to 16 years old. Ten children in the experimental and three in the control group reported using mental imagery during the procedure. Children who used imagery were significantly younger than those who did not ($p < 0.05$). Guardians were with children throughout the procedures. Five, including two parents of control children, were especially helpful to their children, suggesting focus on imagery and encouraging their children with words and touch. One mother of a 7-year-old in the experimental group, when the child decompensated and the physician insisted on forcibly restraining the child, offered the child a trip to McDonald's on the way home. When she began chanting "two all-beef patties ..." the child joined in and repeated the chant and held still. The repair was completed quickly. Three guardians were known to have bribed their children, and two yelled at their children. Santer concludes that the attitude and communications of guardians are important variables in these types of studies and that some guardians communicated in a way that was the equivalent of a hypnotic induction, whereas others counteracted the therapist's communication efforts.

Kohen (1986) reported six cases in which hypnosis techniques were helpful to children in an emergency room; in five of the cases, the children had no prior knowledge of either the therapist or hypnosis. Kohen facilitated relaxation and comfort for these children by allowing them to use their inherent imagery skills. Two of the children, grade-school-age boys, imagined that they were playing football during suturing procedures. A teenage girl imagined herself dancing during the diagnostic procedures prior to an appendectomy. In the case of a 12-year-old boy who was having a severe gastrointestinal hemorrhage, Kohen was asked to help when the boy resisted insertion of a nasogastric tube. The boy appeared to go into a spontaneous trance and responded quickly to an explanation of the diagnostic and treatment procedures, assurance that the blood dripping in through the IV was "running in to replace what you threw up," a request to breathe in good feelings and breathe out bad feelings, and the suggestion to turn off the switch to the nose and mouth to let the tube slide easily into the food tube. The tube slid in easily. Two boys in the emergency room with acute asthma achieved comfort by focusing on the images of what they would like to be doing rather than being in the emergency room. One imagined himself riding his bike, and the other imagined himself playing basketball. The excellent emergency room physician spontaneously meets the challenge to establish rapport quickly with a stranger while at the same time conducting a diagnostic assessment and developing an approach to treatment. In such situations, Kohen said, "It seems most prudent and efficient to simply 'do' hypnosis, rather than to engage in lengthy explanatory discussions which in another setting might be appropriate."

Bierman (1989) similarly described three children who came to the emergency department: a 7-year-old boy with multiple abrasions after a bicycle accident, a 12-year-old girl with a scalp laceration, and a 9-year-old boy with asthma and needle phobia. In each case, the quick establishment of rapport, suggestions for favorite activity imagery for distraction and trance, and both direct and indirect hypnotic suggestions were successful in alleviating discomfort and allowing treatment to proceed easily.

### *Preoperative Visits*

In the last decade there has been an appropriate – perhaps long overdue – focus on thoughtful preparation of children for surgery. Attention to the environment, behavioral approaches of staff, and presence or absence of parents in the pre-anesthetic room have been explored with particular focus on understanding and managing anxiety before surgery (Kain & Caldwell-Andrews, 2005; Lobe, 2007). Arnon, Hanan, and Mogliner (2018) described the effect of a hypnotic-based animated video on stress and pain reduction in pediatric surgery. The video, originally in Hebrew and also translated into Arabic, was titled "Flying Carpet Magical Journey." Thirty children, ages 3–16 years, watched the video one time prior to surgery for either undescended testes or umbilical/inguinal hernias. Results showed a statistically significant reduction in both anxiety and pain.

When a child is admitted to the hospital for surgery, a child health professional usually has time to get to know the patient and, it is hoped, to help coordinate attitudes and approaches of the family and the various hospital staff involved in the case. It is indeed unfortunate when a hypnosis is taught to help a child develop positive attitudes toward surgery only to be sabotaged by the negative suggestions of someone else, albeit well-meaning, who may have had a previous unpleasant surgical experience. It is sometimes helpful to warn children of this possibility and to suggest that they can remember positive images even if someone else suggests something to the contrary. If possible, all members of the treatment team should focus on mastery, reinforcing the concept that the child can be an active participant in the treatment process (Kohen, 2001a; Lobe, 2007).

In many hospitals, children and families may take a preoperative tour of the operating and recovery rooms or are encouraged to see short movies or engage in puppet plays describing events that will occur before, during, and after surgery. A clinician using hypnosis may use imagery techniques to facilitate good adaptation through rehearsal in fantasy. Because hypnosis does not involve any standardized equipment, it may be especially useful in dealing with individual surgical problems and psychological needs. Amputation of a limb, for example, is one kind of experience following an accident and an entirely different kind of experience following the discovery of a malignant tumor.

In general, hypnosis suggestions may focus on calmness and comfort, the "surprisingly" easy return of normal body functions, and rapid healing. Because many children fear death as a result of anesthesia or surgery, imagery concerning the immediate and long-term future is important. A sample set of useful suggestions follows:

> You know the nurses who get food for you and fix your bed. You know the doctor who will do the operation. He is helping, too. I'd like to teach you a way of helping us and helping you. You can help yourself get better faster, and no one else can do that as well as you. You can learn how to help yourself faster than grown-ups can. … You have learned many ways to control your body. You know how to use your muscles to walk, to write, to eat, to ride a bicycle. Now you can ride a bicycle without thinking about how you do it. You taught yourself, so it became automatic.
>
> You keep many parts of your body running automatically. Your food enters your stomach and then your blood and goes to all parts of your body. Your heart beats strongly to push that food around. You breathe in good pure oxygen that your body needs. You're doing it right now. Hardly without even thinking about it much, you just keep all those automatic systems moving smoothly and easily, the same way you ride your bicycle or the same way you write your name. You can do the same things after your operation. Your body can automatically remember nice hungry feelings, and you can enjoy your favorite foods. I wonder what the first thing you will want to eat will be? And your body can remember how to feel comfortable … how to move and walk … how to relax your bowel and bladder when you need to go to the bathroom … how to enjoy playing with toys and games. The doctors and nurses can help you as much as you need, and you can help yourself. Soon you will be well enough to go home. What is the first thing you want to do when you get home? Good. Think about that now.

Mary was born with sacral agenesis. When she was quite young her legs, which were nonfunctional, were amputated so the bone could be put in a bone bank to be periodically harvested later for successive orthopedic operative spine-lengthening procedures. As she would explain to others, in this way Mary could suddenly grow 5–6 inches all at once (in surgery) every couple of years. Having learned hypnosis for pain control when she was a young child, Mary called when she was about 13 years old with a special request for help. She explained that in a month or two she would be having her next spine-lengthening operation. While she was a little nervous in general, she was most concerned from previous surgery about being "so hungry" postoperatively and not being permitted to eat until her intestinal tract had started working again after the operation. She knew that the use of morphine for postoperative pain control contributed to slowing down her intestinal motility, and she had already decided that she would be able to eat sooner if she had no morphine. She asked me to lobby on her behalf with her spine surgeon and the nursing staff that she not have to have morphine or codeine unless she asked for it. She asked to review hypnosis suggestions for pain control, hunger, and return of normal gastrointestinal function. She assured me, her parents, her surgeon, and the nursing staff that she would take care of her discomfort (with self-hypnosis), and that they should simply make sure they had some food available for her to eat! After two hypnosis review sessions a month apart (the second a week before surgery), Mary underwent an uneventful 5- to 6-hour operation to lengthen her spine. Postoperatively she used self-hypnosis and acetaminophen for control of discomfort and ate supper 4 hours after her operation. She was very proud.

Although the focus is on positive suggestions, we are careful not to suggest that the child must deny appropriate feelings of anxiety, depression, or anger. In the course of therapeutic interviews, we listen carefully for evidence of these feelings in conversation, play, hypnotic fantasy, and reports of dreams. Then we help the child recognize and integrate the feelings, both in the context of supportive counseling and via self-hypnosis. Calipel and colleagues (Calipel, Lucas-Polomeni, Wodey, & Ecoffey, 2005) examined the efficacy of hypnosis for anxiety and perioperative behavioral problems in comparison to standard preoperative medication with midazolam. Fifty children between the ages of 2 and 11 years were randomized to receive either hypnosis instead of premedication or oral midazolam (0.5 mg/kg) 30 minutes prior to surgery. On a preoperative anxiety scale and a behavioral questionnaire, the groups showed no significant differences. The number of children who were anxious during face-mask induction of anesthesia was significantly less in the hypnosis group compared to the midazolam group (39% vs. 68%, $p < 0.05$). Additionally, hypnosis was found to reduce behavioral disorders (aggressiveness to authority, fear of separation, general anxiety) during the first 2 postoperative weeks compared to midazolam. The authors concluded that hypnosis was, in effect, more anxiolytic than midazolam.

Our experience has been similarly quite positive, as reflected in the case of Cory, an 8-year-old boy with cerebral palsy who required repeated surgical procedures to relieve some of the spasticity in his legs to facilitate easier walking with his walker. Cory was very anxious even when thinking and talking about prior surgeries, and his mother asked if self-hypnosis could help him prepare for the next surgical procedure. Cory also had some cognitive delays and was more like a 6-year-old developmentally. A charming boy who loved to tell jokes, he learned self-hypnosis quickly. Suggestions were offered in the context of his own language and understanding of what was planned to be done during surgery, along with medical play using an anesthesia mask, which in prior experience had been a major trigger to Cory's extreme anxiety. In the interest of being able to rehearse at home for a week before the surgery, the last hypnosis session before surgery was videotaped and he was given a copy to view at home; his mother could provide reinforcement as needed, although she was not present during the videotaping. A description of the video follows (Kohen, 2001a):

> "[I came over] to get ready for my surgery next week so I won't have to be so scared." He showed his right thigh above the knee where "they'll open this incision and take out the hardware – plates and screws – which are in there (right thigh) and … then they'll put the phenol in, in my spine, to help relax my muscles … to walk better." As he then began to focus on the anesthesia mask, we began to playfully make references to the mask as having various favorite aromas associated with it. He moved the mask toward my face and, joining with him as part of the hypnotic rapport, I said "Wow, ummmmmm, you know what that smells like TODAY? It smells like chocolate cake!" Then he took it away and put it back on himself. When I asked, "What do YOU have" and he said "banana" and then moved through a series of other foods, including macaroni and cheese, chocolate cake, etc. He shifted and began to recline, asking, "Then what happens?" I told him, "Just find that switch in your mind that turns off the hurt to this hand or arm or that one and then 1–2–3, cllliccccckkkk! Off, no bother!" In response, he was in a fixed-gaze-stare, quiet, still mode. He then said, "They said they'll put the IV in after I'm asleep!" When I began to move the mask away, he pulled it back. I asked him to "run the tape on fast forward now in your mind and see yourself waking up in the recovery room, stretching and opening your eyes [until this suggestion, he was in trance with eyelid flutter, slowing of respiratory rate, and stillness] and see your Mom there smiling, and the nurses, and I don't know who else, and then Mom tells you how proud she is and guess how YOU feel?" He said, "HUNGRY!"

We have also described several other case examples (Kohen, 2001b). Mackenzie and Frawley (2007), working in Melbourne, Australia, described the effective application of preoperative hypnosis to help a child with substantial anticipatory nausea and vomiting. Their patient was a 6-year-old boy who had esophageal atresia repair in the newborn period followed by repeated esophageal dilatations (bouginage) every 6–8 weeks. Indeed, this youngster had 21 procedures in his first year of life and thereafter 74 balloon esophageal dilatations at 6- to 8-week intervals. He had substantial postoperative nausea and vomiting despite both prophylactic and therapeutic anti-emetics, and about a year prior to hypnosis intervention he developed anticipatory nausea and vomiting just before beginning the 3-hour journey from his home to the hospital. After first being taught about his disorder and mind–body connections with anatomical drawings, he was taught relaxation and mental imagery. Switch techniques were taught for turning on chewing and turning off gagging and turning on good feelings in the tummy. He began to improve dramatically. Tapes of his favorite music were added to suggestions for feelings incompatible with vomiting (e.g., thirst and hunger). After only four training visits, he improved substantially and after two subsequent visits he experienced no further anticipatory nausea or vomiting; by the following year, postoperative nausea and vomiting also disappeared.

Tusek and colleagues (Tusek, Church, & Fazio, 1997) studied 130 patients undergoing elective colorectal surgical procedures, randomly assigning them to routine perioperative care and to a guided imagery (hypnosis) group who listened to guided imagery tapes for 3 days before surgery, during anesthesia, intraoperatively, in the recovery area, and for 6 days after surgery. Participants were from 17 to 70 years old; although the median age was 40 years, information is included here to highlight the definitive results achieved. Patients in the imagery group experienced considerably less preoperative and postoperative anxiety and pain and required almost 50% less narcotic medications.

Vagnoli and colleagues (2019) randomized 60 children, ages 6–12 years, to preoperative training in relaxation imagery or to usual care. They described the experimental group as receiving instruction in deep breathing to achieve body relaxation and focus on the imagery of sights, sounds, smells, and taste in a favorite place. The last component was described as return to reality. The experimental group had less anxiety and less postoperative pain ($p<.001$).

For completeness we recommend that readers explore *Patient Sedation Without Medication*, by Drs. Elvira Lang and Laser (2009). This very accessible volume is a guide to procedural hypnosis via rapid rapport and quick hypnotic techniques and evolved from the authors' 16 years of research with rigorous prospective randomized studies with over 700 patients. Although their work is almost exclusively with adult patients, many of the suggestions – especially regarding rapport development and therapeutic language – are compatible with our clinical experiences and recommendations. Readers will likely find many ideas easily adaptable to work with children and adolescents.

## Intraoperative and Postoperative Hypnosis

It is well known that patients who approach surgery with a high degree of fear and agitation require larger amounts of chemical anesthesia, thus increasing the risks of complications. Their postoperative course is also likely to be more difficult from both a surgical and a psychological perspective. As anesthesiologists have come to appreciate the significance of the preoperative psychological state in pediatric surgical patients, they have made efforts to allay fears of general anesthesia by use of such techniques as stroking, storytelling, or rubbing a pleasant scent of strawberries, perfume, or bubble gum inside the inhalation mask. Although many anesthesiologists have had no formal training in hypnosis, they may use the analogy of a space trip, talking to the child about a space mask and about breathing special air like astronauts.

Since the 1950s, several reports have been published regarding the use of hypnosis with children as an adjunct to chemical anesthesia (Antitch, 1967; Betcher, 1960; Cullen, 1958; Daniels, 1962; Hopayian, 1984; Marmer, 1959; Scott, 1969). These reports describe several advantages of hypnosis and of the resulting alliance between the child and the anesthesiologist. By becoming more active participants, children cope better with the psychological trauma of surgery. They adjust more easily to the hospital environment and formulate more positive attitudes about the hospital experience. Preoperative sedation can be reduced or omitted altogether; this is particularly valuable for children who respond to partial clouding of consciousness by becoming more agitated rather than less so. With the child in hypnosis, it is easier to induce general anesthesia, and it is often possible to reduce the amount given. Many anesthesiologists note a smoother course both during surgery and in the postoperative phase.

The techniques of hypnotic invitation used by anesthesiologists vary appropriately with the age of the child. With infants and very young children, a soothing voice is sufficient even if the child does not understand the words (Cullen, 1958). Techniques reported for older children include storytelling, television games, suggestions for eye heaviness and sleep, eye fixation, and progressive relaxation. Some anesthesiologists give suggestions for postoperative comfort and return of normal body functions during the operative procedure. Simple suggestions may encourage the child to shift from negative to positive attitudes about the healing process; for example, one might say, "The sensations you have in the area of the incision are reminders that healing is taking place in that area." These suggestions may be aided if the child has, preoperatively, seen a drawing or diagram that explains the procedure. Some authors (e.g., Cheek, 1959) believe that anesthetized patients may hear comments in the operating room and respond accordingly to intended or unintended suggestions. Others (e.g., Trustman, Dubovsky, & Titley, 1977) have found methodological flaws in studies on this topic and have questioned the validity of the conclusions. In any case, it seems reasonable to be guided by the dictum that operating room staff members should not say anything they do not want the patient to hear.

Bensen (1971) reported the use of postanesthetic hypnosis in surgical patients in the recovery room. This report included 30 children and adolescents after tonsillectomy and one 11-year-old boy after circumcision. Among 16 children ages 5–12 years, only one child needed pain medication during the first day after tonsillectomy. Of the 14 older patients, ages 12–18 years, 3 required one dose of analgesic prescription a few hours postoperatively. The author pointed out the need for a reliable and accurate laboratory method to assess and measure the effectiveness of posthypnotic suggestion. Recently, a randomized controlled trial examined the effects of intraoperative therapeutic suggestions in children during general anesthesia for tonsillectomy and adenoidectomy (Fortier et al., 2010). Sixty-seven children received standardized general anesthesia and were randomly assigned to one of three interventions administered during general anesthesia. One group heard standard operating room noise (through headphones attached to an empty CD player to ensure blinding of anesthesiologists to group assignment). A "story" control group listened to a repeated recording of their mother's voice reading a neutral story written by the researchers and designed not to interfere with suggestions made on the therapeutic recording for the experimental group. The experimental (therapeutic suggestion group) listened to a repeated recording of their mother's voice reading a script with positive suggestions of good appetite and wellness. Elements included guided imagery to promote relaxation and suggestions such as "your body feels very, very relaxed … you can smell your favorite food" to increase gastrointestinal comfort. The therapeutic suggestion group had 27 children; the story group, 20; and the control group, 19. Results showed that, despite a statistically significant decrease in nausea and increase in appetite over the 3 postanesthetic days ($p < 0.001$), this main effect of time was across groups, and no difference between groups or a group effect was observed. Children in all groups experienced similar rates and severity of nausea and vomiting in the recovery room and at home and similar rates of improvement of appetite.

It is unfortunate that anesthesiologists often do not continue their postoperative visits beyond the recovery room. A child can benefit from frequent reinforcement of positive suggestions following surgery. A audio recording can be helpful in this regard, as can reinforcement by well-trained nurses or parents (Olness, 1977).

Gaal, Goldsmith, and Needs (1980) reported a controlled pilot study of the effect of hypnotic suggestion on expressions of anxiety and pain in a group of ten children, ages 5–10 years, undergoing tonsillectomy. No child had previous experience with either hospitalization or surgery. Each child met with the experimenter before surgery, at which time the experimenter answered questions truthfully and engaged in pleasant conversation designed to put the child at ease. In the 10 minutes immediately prior to surgery, the experimenter continued in the same way with the control group, asking about interests, hobbies, favorite television programs, and so on. For the experimental group, this 10-minute period was devoted to a hypnosis invitation, using a television game/visual imagery technique with suggestions for strenuous activity followed by fatigue, relaxation, and desire to sleep. After induction of anesthesia, the experimental group received tape-recorded suggestions for postoperative feelings of calm, comfort, ease of swallowing, and trust; the control group heard a tape-recorded nonsense story. Assessment of anxiety was made by independent observers who did not know to which group each child belonged. Anxiety was rated by behavioral indicators such as level of motor activity, tearfulness, verbalization of fear, and physical resistance. There were no differences between experimental and control subjects prior to the preinduction conversation; both groups were relatively calm and cooperative. After surgery was completed, the control group was significantly more anxious ($p = .05$). The experimental group was as calm as at the first measure of anxiety. Postsurgical intergroup comparisons showed the controls to be significantly more anxious and uncooperative than the experimental subjects ($p = .01$). Assessment of postoperative pain was based on the children's own reports and on their needs for chemical analgesics. Both measures showed significant differences between the two groups; that is, children in the experimental group complained less frequently and of less severe pain, and they required only one-fifth as much analgesic medication as the controls.

A multidisciplinary pain management intervention offered to children and families of children receiving liver transplants evaluated 27 children: 13 historical controls and 14 interventions (Sharek et al., 2006). No differences were found in mean pediatric intensive care unit (PICU) postoperative length of stay, total postoperative length of stay, time to extubation, total cost, or opioid use. Experimental group patients had a significant decrease in mean pain scores between postoperative day 0 and 6 ($p = 0.04$) and a decrease in mean parental pain perception scores ($p = 0.001$). The experimental group intervention had several components including substantial preoperative education, a package of nonpharmacologic postoperative pain management interventions (prominent among which were hypnosis and guided imagery), and standard postoperative pharmacological pain regimen. Given the multiple components and the small sample size, no effort was made to discern which ingredients had relatively more or less effect in producing the positive outcome.

In China, researchers asked parents of children undergoing surgery what nonpharmacological methods they used for their children's postoperative pain relief (He, Polkki, Pietila, & Vehvilainen-Julkunen, 2006). A sample of 206 parents (97 fathers, 109 mothers) was identified whose children, 6–12 years old, had undergone surgery in one of the 12 wards of 5 hospitals in Fujian Province in China. Questionnaires were distributed and completed postoperatively, 1–2 days prior to discharge. The most commonly used methods were parental presence (93%), touch (90%), and comforting/reassurance (84%). Among the cognitive behavioral methods, 80% of parents reported use of imagery, 62% relaxation, and 37% "breathing technique."

Lobe (2006) reported success with the use of hypnosis to reduce the postoperative hospital stay in patients (12–18 years old) undergoing the Nuss procedure for pectus excavatum chest wall deformity. Ten patients had the Nuss procedure; of these, five were managed with the standard treatment of an epidural catheter for pain management and five were taught self-hypnosis for postoperative pain management in one or two brief sessions. Patients in the hypnosis group spent an average of 2.8 days in the hospital compared to 4.6 days in the non-hypnosis group ($p < 0.01$). Manworeen and colleagues (2018) reported a study of 53 adolescents who had the Nuss procedure. Twenty-four received preoperative self-hypnosis training. They reported lower mean pain scores ($p = .0028$) and used less morphine equivalents/hour over time compared to the adolescents who did not receive self-hypnosis training.

Gaal's report (Gaal, Goldsmith, & Needs, 1980) and Fortier's controlled trial (Fortier et al., 2010) do not help us discern whether it is best to utilize hypnotic suggestions with pediatric surgical patients before, during, or after surgery or at all of these times. Further, one cannot be certain if the patient responds best to deliberate positive suggestions or to the absence of negative suggestions, such as, "I'll bet this kid is going to vomit a lot." Until additional studies clarify these issues, we are confident in our guidance that what works best for children is a thoughtful, sensitive, kind conversation that focuses on education and rapport in the context of the individual child and family and their personal history, finding the hypnosis in the encounter, and offering empowering suggestions for comfort and control. Controlled studies could clarify these issues.

## Plastic Surgery

Few articles can be found in the literature that deal specifically with the use of hypnosis in plastic surgery, although many reports have been published on the value of hypnosis in conditions encountered by plastic surgeons, who are concerned (as are all surgeons) with pain and the anxiety generated by it. Studies by Wiggins and Brown (1968) and Kelsey and Barron (1958) reported on induction of a cataleptic state to aid in immobilization of patients or their extremities during pedicle graft procedures. Scott and Holbrook (1981) used hypnosis to aid in the selection of patients for cosmetic surgery. Many studies have been made on the use of hypnosis in treating pain, but hypnotic techniques have not been studied extensively as a routine adjunct to the use of local anesthesia.

A study by Tucker and Virnelli (1985) stated that, "Hypnosis can usually produce effective relaxation and frequently allow actual enjoyment of the experience of undergoing a surgical procedure" (p. 141). The authors had used hypnosis since 1976 with both their pediatric and adult plastic surgery patients; they employed both formal induction and informal or indirect techniques, which became part of the routine daily management of these patients. They noted that, "Formal induction is used on hundreds of patients as an adjunct to local anesthesia; it has also been used to obtain hypno-anesthesia for removal of lesions without chemical anesthesia" (p. 142). They also found hypnosis sessions to be useful in decreasing anxiety and apprehension about upcoming procedures.

## Dermatologic Surgery

Pelaez Perez, Sanchez Casado, Quintana Diaz, Benhaiem, and Escriba Alepuz (2021) in Spain evaluated the effectiveness of hypnoanalgesia in pediatric dermatological surgery. They performed a prospective, longitudinal, observational study of 65 children, ages 5–16 years. Thirty-three were taught hypnosis and 32 experienced distraction via a digital tablet on which a cartoon or a music video was played. Authors described the hypnosis as helping the child create a safe place and to concentrate on his interior world. In the operating room the child chose between inhalational induction of a nitrous oxide and oxygen mixture and intravenous induction. Propofol was given and the surgeon also injected lidocaine local anesthesia prior to extraction of the skin lesions. There was a significant reduction of the intraoperative propofol dose in the hypnosis group and the stay in postoperative recovery was statistically shorter for children in the hypnosis group. The requirement for postoperative analgesia was much lower in the hypnosis group. Authors emphasized the importance of allowing the child to take part in their own medical care by using their own self-regulation resources.

## *Burns*

Children who are severely burned face multiple problems: pain, fear, depression, anorexia, insomnia, physical disability, itching, and cold. They also must deal with significant changes in body image and with reactions from other people in the hospital and at home. These problems can produce a vicious cycle of pain, anxiety, depression, anorexia, and poor healing secondary to inadequate nutrition, more grafting, and more pain.

Bernstein (1963, 1965) and LaBaw (1973) published clinical case reports describing the successful use of hypnosis for several of these problems, especially pain, anxiety, and anorexia. Wakeman and Kaplan (1978) reported a controlled prospective study in which patients, ages 7–70 years, who learned hypnosis used significantly lower percentages of maximum allowable analgesics as compared to controls who received supportive psychotherapy. Among the patients who used hypnosis, the youngest group, ages 7–18 years, used significantly fewer analgesics than did two adult groups, ages 19–30 and 31–70 years. In addition to suggestions for pain control, these patients were also given suggestions for general ego strengthening, improved body image, and ability to cope effectively after discharge from the hospital. Chester and colleagues (2018) conducted a randomized controlled trial to investigate whether hypnosis decreases pain, anxiety, and stress and accelerates wound healing in children undergoing burn wound procedures. Children 4–16 years were randomly assigned to a hypnosis or a standard care group. 27 children were taught hypnosis and 35 received standard care. Authors concluded that hypnosis may be effective for decreasing pre procedural anxiety and heart rate but not for reducing pain intensity or accelerating wound healing.

In our work with burned patients, we prefer to begin hypnosis on the first day of admission, before the patient has been negatively sensitized to whirlpool therapy or debridements or is lethargic from narcotics. It is especially true with burned patients that suggestions must be individualized and revised from day to day to keep pace with the child's changing condition and perceptions. We explain our approach to other members of the burn team and encourage them to reinforce specific hypnotic suggestions. In addition to suggestions for symptom relief, we sometimes give suggestions that the child can use hypnosis to facilitate healing directly. As yet, no data support our hypothesis, but we think it is reasonable, in light of other indications, to believe that children can successfully use hypnosis for treatment of dermatological problems (Mirvish, 1978; Tasini & Hackett, 1977) and that they can control their peripheral temperatures and, presumably, blood flow to extremities (Dikel & Olness, 1980).

The following case report is an example of our approach with burned patients. In this case, the problem was pain and poor cooperation during whirlpool therapy. Tammy S., age 4, was hospitalized with second-degree burns on her chest, sustained when a pot of coffee overturned on her at home. One week later, she was referred for hypnosis to control her discomfort during whirlpool therapy. She was a bright, active child who related well to hospital staff, except during whirlpool baths. Initially, the child psychologist sat by Tammy's bed and looked at drawings she had made that morning.

Tammy explained the figures in the drawings, including a girl with a bandaged chest. That provided the entry for discussion of her burns. She seemed relieved when the therapist said her burns were getting better every day and wondered if she had decided what she would do first when she got home. Then the therapist said she knew Tammy did not like whirlpool baths, and she could teach her what to do so they would not bother her. She added that she knew Tammy could learn easily and that she would need to practice her skills regularly. Leaving the decision to the child, the therapist played a game with her and then left with the comment that she would return when Tammy asked to learn these new skills. As she walked down the hospital corridor, Tammy came running after: "When will you teach me?" "Whenever you're ready." "Now."

In the office visit that immediately followed, trance was induced using eye fixation on a coin. The therapist then explained about nerves and how they carry feelings of cold, wet, warm, burning, sticky, soft, and many other feelings to her head. She was then taught the switch-off technique for pain control. She seemed very pleased at the conclusion of the session. When the therapist asked if she could go with Tammy for her whirlpool therapy the next day, the child agreed. She reviewed the hypnotic procedures and turned off the switch for her chest until the whirlpool therapy was over. In complete contrast to the previous day, she did not struggle, kick, scream, or cry. The nurse's notes said, "She tolerated the whirlpool therapy well." On the following day, Tammy said she did not need the therapist to show her how to turn off her switches, and she did well. On the third day, she was discharged.

In a pilot study of hypnosis and pain in patients with severe burns, Van der Does, Van Dyck, and Spijker (1988) included two adolescents in their group of eight patients. Both successfully applied self-hypnosis for pain control, finding distraction and relaxation particularly important components of their (self-) hypnotic procedure.

It is often inappropriate to use tape-recorded hypnotic suggestions for burned children in the early phases of treatment when problems are changing from day to day and even from hour to hour. A tape may be very useful in the later stages of treatment, however, when the child's condition is stable and problems are more predictable, at least for a few days at a time. The following material is a transcript of a tape-recording made for an 11-year-old burned patient several years ago when the therapist was going to be out of town for 4 days. Suggestions covered a variety of problems on which the child was then working. Wording was quite flexible as it was expected that the child might use the tape at any time of day or night, with or without other patients present. We have made no changes from the original transcript except to alter the child's name. If we were to make such a tape today, we would omit the word "try" in the suggestions, as this suggests the possibility of failure. The patient, however, reported no problems, saying she listened to the tape nine times during the therapist's absence and found it helpful in a variety of ways.

> Hi, Sherry. This is the tape recording that I told you I would make, and while you're getting ready to listen to it, try to get yourself in as comfortable a position as you can. Just fix your bed or wherever you are so that you are as comfortable as you can be. And then just as we have done before, think about the ways and the many, many times we have helped you get more and more relaxed. That's what we are going to do on this tape. We are going to think about helping you relax more and more. And we are going to think about the many positive things, the many things you can do now that you couldn't do before. How much better you are now, than you were before, knowing that you are getting better and better. You are getting well.
>
> So, try to make yourself just as comfortable as you possibly can and just listen to my voice on this tape. You can put the earphone, the ear plugs in your ears if you like, or you can just

listen without them, whichever feels more comfortable. And just try to imagine me there with you, imagine me sitting close to you. If you close your eyes and think very hard you can almost see a picture of me in your mind. You can hear my voice more and more clearly, almost as if I were there. And it will be almost as if I am there. Even though I am away for a little while, you know I am thinking of you. You know I still want you to get well. You know how very much I like you. You and I are pretty good friends. Sometimes we can get mad at each other, but we both know that's okay, and we can still be very good friends. And now as you have this picture of me in your mind, more and more clear, just let your whole body begin to relax, listening to everything I say. First, think about your head relaxing and your face, beginning at the very top of your head, and your forehead relaxing, and your eyes feeling very relaxed and maybe a little heavy, and if you feel like closing your eyes, you can do that. And your whole face feeling very relaxed and very comfortable. And think of your neck feeling very relaxed and very comfortable; your neck is going to get well. You have had grafting on your neck, and it is going to get better and better. So any worries you have about it, you can just let them go, knowing it's going to get better. And your shoulders can become more and more relaxed, and your arms and hands. Put your hands in a nice comfortable position. Your right hand and left hand. And think a minute about your hands, how much better they are, how much more you can do with your hands. Opening your mail, feeding yourself, making pizza in OT. So very many things – writing. And each day there will be more and more things you can do. More and more, so that your hands can feel very comfortable now and very relaxed, and you can feel better. And let those very nice feelings go down and down deeper and deeper through your whole body. And down and down through your legs, and all the way down through your feet, knowing that your legs and your feet are getting better too.

All of you is getting well little by little. And I want you to think of that thought that you are getting better. And every time that thought begins to slip away from you, you can catch it with your mind and bring it back, bring it back. Just like we focus a camera, you can focus your mind on that idea. Focus that thought. You are getting better, more and more safe, more and more deeply relaxed, through your whole body now.

And we know that there are times when you have some pain or some itching somewhere. And we don't like that, but we know that it is going to happen from time to time. But we also know that more and more you can control the pain and the itching, because you can let the pain or itching, whenever it begins, be like a signal for you to relax deeper and deeper down and down until comfortable feelings fill you up more and more. And there is no room left for bad feelings or scary feelings, or painful feelings. Whenever there is any pain or itching, it will be like a signal for you to focus and bring into your mind those nice relaxed feelings, immediately and completely until you are deeper and deeper relaxed, and comfortable feelings fill your whole body and your whole mind. And you know that more and more you can control any kind of feeling. Letting the scary feelings and the pain and the itching drift away, and letting the comfortable feelings fill you more and more. Fill you more and more with comfortable feelings, until there is no room left for any other kind of feelings.

And you know that this is getting to be more and more automatic; it happens without your even thinking about it. So that more and more you are able to sleep, you are able to sleep as much as you need to. And you may find that when it's time to go to sleep at night, you just let those relaxed and comfortable feelings just come to you closer and closer. Filling you

> more and more because you know you are getting better. So, you will have a good night's sleep, when it's time to go to sleep. And just as you will be able to sleep as much as you need to, you will also have nice hungry feelings and enjoy the things you eat. And just as you will find that more and more you're interested in getting up and doing things. All the activities on the ward, you will like those activities more and more. Because you will be able to do them more and more. So, you can sleep, you can eat, you can do all the activities, but most important, you can let yourself know you are getting better, because you deserve to get better. You're a good person, Sherry. You have worked very hard to get well.
>
> And we will continue to work. When I see you, we will work more, as much as you need. And you will listen to this tape, Sherry, as much as you need to, as much as you want to. It will be just up to you how much you listen to it. But when you do, you may find more and more each time that you can let yourself become very relaxed. Just as if I'm there talking to you. Feeling very safe, and very good. Knowing that if you need any medication for pain or itching, you can ask the nurses for it. But knowing that more and more you are getting to be able to control these problems yourself. And each time you listen to this tape, just as we practiced together, you will be more and more able to relax deeper and deeper. So that the pain and the itching and all the scary feelings will drift away, and you will have comfortable feelings, more and more.
>
> Now I am going to count up to five, and as I count, you can get just as alert as you would like to. If you want to, you can get very alert, and then you can do whatever would be good to do. Whether it's getting up, or eating or doing some activity, or just drifting off to sleep. Whatever would be good for you to do now, you can do. You can get as alert as you like, as much as you need to as I count to five. So that if there are activities you want to do, or things like eating, or getting up, you'll be very wide awake. But if you want to go to sleep, you can be nice and relaxed, and drift off to sleep. Even if you wake up, you can stay nice and relaxed, but you'll be wide awake. I'm going to count now, and when I get up to five, you can turn off the tape recorder, by pushing where the little square is, and that will turn off the tape recorder. Now I am going to count one … two … three … four … five … feeling very good, feeling very good, and I'll see you soon. Turn off the tape now.

Burned patients who have had extensive practice in using hypnosis often develop considerable confidence in their abilities. Betcher (1960) capitalized on this confidence in his work with a 10-year-old girl who had suffered third-degree burns and had used hypnosis successfully for dressing changes. Six months later, the child was readmitted for surgery to release severe flexion contractures of her neck that had forced her chin onto the sternum with complete inability to extend the head. Initially, it was planned to do the operation under general anesthesia; however, the position of the child's head combined with the depressive effect of the chemical agent had compromised her respiration to such an extent that she rapidly became cyanotic. The surgery was canceled, and it was decided to reschedule it later using hypnosis as the major anesthetic agent until the contractures were released. Betcher gave the following account of the second surgical attempt:

> Two weeks later the child was readmitted a few days before surgery. The patient and her parents were given an explanation of the method of anesthesia and since they were familiar with its use for the changing of the painful dressings during her first admission, they agreed readily. Two rehearsal sessions were performed on the days prior to surgery. Suggestions were given that her left arm was becoming numb. When the numbness was complete, she was to place it across her neck for transference of the numbness. Complete analgesia to

> pinprick was achieved at each session. The operation was rehearsed step by step using a blunt instrument and demonstrating how the surgeon would do the procedure. No premedication was given to the patient. On the operative day, the patient practiced hypnosis in her room and taken to the operating room. After the patient was placed on the operating table, suggestions were given for numbness in her left hand that was transferred to her neck.
>
> During the preparation by the surgeon, constant reassurances were given to reinforce the numbness in the region of the neck. Although analgesia to pinprick was complete, the patient began to whimper softly at the incision of the scalpel. The face had been covered by the sterile drapes since the operative area was from the mandible to the sternum. This draping was utilized to fashion a tent over the face and an anesthetic tube was placed in this area to allow the gases to flow over her face. The analgesia proved sufficient to allow the surgeon to proceed without any objection from the child. As soon as the neck was opened wide, the anesthetic mask was attached to the tubing and was applied to the face. Total chemical anesthesia was then produced. It was simple to introduce an endotracheal tube with the head now fully extended. The surgeon then completed the necessary surgery including skin grafting in two and a half hours. Only small increments of cyclopropane anesthesia were necessary for the smooth conduct of the anesthesia. Since posthypnotic suggestions had been given, the postoperative period was completely without discomfort even though the child was placed in a plaster of Paris shell from the head to the waist.

Soltani and colleagues (2018) described a randomized controlled trial of virtual reality to help distract patients from high levels of pain during burn wound care. This student included 39 participants of whom several were adolescents. Virtual reality reduced pain during range of motion exercises. As a uniquely attention-capturing medium, virtual reality shares certain characteristics of hypnosis, notably evoking dissociation via immersion in multisensory imagery. Hoffman and colleagues (Hoffman, Doctor, Patterson, Carrougher, & Furness, 2000) described this application in two adolescent males with severe burns. Both boys reflected substantial drops in pain intensity during wound care aided by virtual reality that they had not been able to achieve with traditional opioid analgesia. Steele and colleagues (2003) also reported the effectiveness of virtual reality in facilitating physiotherapy postoperatively adolescent with cerebral palsy unable to tolerate pharmacotherapy. We look forward to studies with children that examine the value of this innovative and exciting hypnotic–biofeedback tool for other forms of childhood pain and distress.

## Dentistry

Bernick (1972) reported a variety of applications of hypnosis in children's dentistry, including (1) raising the pain threshold, (2) reducing the resistance to local anesthesia, (3) assisting in the adaptation to orthodontic appliances, (4) reducing the gag impulse during taking impressions or x-rays and during general operative dentistry, (5) relieving general apprehension, (6) breaking habit patterns for thumbsucking and myofunctional problems, (7) motivating the child and parents to accept treatment and to improve oral hygiene, (8) relaxing facial muscles, (9) controlling saliva and capillary hemorrhage, (10) maintaining patient comfort in long procedures, and (11) as a premedication for general anesthesia.

Both Bernick (1972) and Shaw (1959) emphasized the importance of using nonhypnotic suggestion to help the child perceive the dental experience in a positive way. They suggest positive and pleasant communications from parents and dental office staff, getting to know the child's interests, allowing the child to experiment with various instruments, modeling behavior, behavior shaping, and giving careful explanations at a level the child can understand.

Pediatric dental patients respond to a variety of hypnotic techniques to achieve pain control. Bernick (1972) used glove anesthesia with a 13-year-old boy who had developed a morbid fear of injections. This child relied on hypnosis as the sole anesthetic agent for several dental visits. In later visits, he used hypnosis to facilitate acceptance of injections of local anesthetic for more extensive work. Shaw (1959) reported his use of the switch technique, in which the child is asked in hypnosis to turn off pain switches to various parts of the mouth. He also described other methods, including glove anesthesia and direct suggestions for numbness. All these methods may be used with or without additional local anesthesia, depending on the child's needs.

Neiburger (1976, 1978) reviewed patient reactions to dental prophylaxis for 150 children, ages 3–12 years, with and without waking suggestions that they would experience a tickling feeling and would want to laugh during the procedure. He found that the children were more cooperative when these sensory confusion suggestions were used than when no suggestions were given.

Hypnosis has been particularly helpful in controlling bleeding in patients with hemophilia who require dental work (Lucas, 1965). The mechanism by which bleeding is controlled is not yet understood, although Lucas emphasized the factor of emotional stress.

Crasilneck and Hall (1985) used hypnosis to help a 10-year-old boy overcome extreme apprehension about dentistry. Therapeutic procedures included abreaction of past dental trauma and posthypnotic suggestions for feelings of relaxation and well-being during future dental work. The boy subsequently remained calm and cooperative during several visits for extensive dental work.

Thompson (1963) reported the use of hypnosis with a 12-year-old girl who had a hysterical fear of dentistry. Suggestions focused on this child's ability to let go of fears that belonged to earlier experiences. Thompson heightened motivation for treatment with the "three crystal balls" technique, in which the child was asked to imagine her teeth (1) in their present state, (2) in the future without dental correction, and (3) in the future with dental correction. She then focused on the third image. Although the child achieved only a light hypnotic state, she did become sufficiently cooperative for dental work to be accomplished.

Heitkemper, Layne, and Sullivan (1993) reported a study of 45 children 8–11 years old about to undergo local anesthesia and either restoration or extraction of teeth. After three measures of anxiety were obtained while the children waited in the waiting room, they were randomly assigned to one of three audiotaped treatment groups: (1) paced respiration, (2) cognitive coping, and (3) placebo tape, controlled for expectations and experimenter contact. The paced respiration tape told the children that the tape helped children relax and then gave suggestions for imagery of walking down steps and becoming progressively relaxed while rhythmically slowing respirations to eight times per minute. The cognitive coping tape told the children that the tape helped reduce discomfort associated with dentistry by allowing thinking different things and by imagining an injection as pressure, numbness, or tickling. The third condition was presented by the authors as a placebo control, but the tape provided another version of imagery and relaxation: "This story may be an interesting way to pass the time while waiting for the dentist and might help your discomfort and also may help you relax and feel more at ease in the dentist's chair." On a measure of expected discomfort, the placebo, or story with no particular guidance for how to use positive suggestions, was significantly less believable.

Both treatment conditions (both hypnosis in our opinion) showed a reduction in anxiety on two measures, but the children's experience of pain was not affected by either of the approaches. The authors speculated that this was a function of excellent local anesthesia, which "left little pain to reduce." Although the authors do not identify their interventions as hypnotherapeutic *per se*, their descriptions clearly depict hypnotic suggestions. We wonder if the inclusion or addition of specific pain reduction or pain control hypnotic suggestions in one of the conditions might have provided better discrimination between the techniques described. Such distinction may be particularly important, as the authors concluded that "expected discomfort may be the most important part of dental pain, so expectations might well be the focus of such treatments."

Peretz and colleagues described a variety of effective hypnosis approaches for children and adolescents with dental anxiety, including confusional suggestions for an extremely anxious 13-year-old who required extensive dental restorations (Peretz, 1996a), the successful use of hypnosis in an 11-year-old boy with anxiety and claustrophobia (Peretz, 1996b), and reframing as a strategy (Peretz & Gluck, 1999). They also reported their experience evaluating the effects of suggestion before and during administration of local anesthetic in 80 children between the ages of 3 and 16 (Peretz & Bimstein, 2000). Wolf, Kellerhoff, Schmierer, Schmierer, and Halsbnd (2021) reported the successful use of hypnosis with a 4-year-old boy who had dental caries. The boy was asked to raise his "magic arm" and he kept it raised during the 16-minute dental procedure, which was videotaped. The dentist also played a CD titled "the tooth jungle tale" (English translation).

Ramirez-Carrasco, Butron-Tellez Giron, Sanchez-Armass, and Pierdant-Perez (2017) provided hypnosis to child dental patients via headphones. They described a three-minute progressive muscle relaxation followed by a 5-minute deepening procedure to increase the patients' focus, absorption and concentration. Patients were asked to visualize a safe and special garden with a fountain in the middles. They were told the fountain water would make their mouth numb and relaxed so they would feel completely comfortable and relaxed while the dentist "made their teeth feel better." They were asked to raise their right arm when their mouth had gone completely numb. Heart rates were lower in experimental group.

Sabherwal and colleagues (2021) conducted a randomized control trial of 60 children, ages 8–12 years who were undergoing primary molar extractions. They were randomly allocated to three groups hypnosis, progressive muscle relaxation and controls. Heart rates showed a statistically significant drop in the hypnosis and progressive relaxation group. Pain levels and analgesic requirements were much lower in the hypnosis and progressive relaxation groups. This is not surprising because progressive relaxation practice leads to hypnosis.

We have taught self-hypnosis to, and prepared audio recordings for, many children with dental anxiety in whom expected discomfort seemed to be the most important consideration. As in most children and circumstances, the imagery, relaxation, and pain control strategies for these children seem to be most effective when constructed and offered in the context of their individual experiences, personal style, and desired outcome.

As this brief review indicates, there has been a growing awareness of the positive value of hypnosis in pediatric dentistry; however, a survey of dental practice reported that only 2% of general dentists and 6% of pediatric dentists said that they utilized hypnosis in their dental practices (McKnight-Hanes, Myers, Dushku, & Davis, 1993). The survey included responses from 663 general dentists and 475 pediatric dentists, a response rate of 39% to a once-mailed random survey to 3,000 dentists. By contrast, all pediatric dentists and 96% of general dentists reported using tell-show-do techniques and voice control strategies as behavioral management approaches with children. These behavioral strategies, which may well contain elements of hypnosis approaches, are not described in further detail. We speculate that in view of these dentists' awareness and acknowledgment of these other behavioral strategies, that their use of hypnotic techniques is probably higher than the self-reported 2% and 6%. Nonetheless, we hope that more dentists and their assistants will seek out training in hypnosis for the benefit of their patients.

## Ophthalmology

Browning, Quinn, and Crasilneck (1958) compared nine children treated with hypnosis for suppression amblyopia with ten children who did not learn hypnosis. In hypnosis, the nine children were told that they would be able to see clearly with the amblyopic eye. Immediately following the hypnosis sessions, eight of the nine experimental subjects improved in near vision compared with only one of the control group who received "non-hypnotic persuasion techniques." Distance vision was unchanged in both groups. A few days following hypnosis, some of the experimental subjects regressed in near vision. This led the authors to question whether emotional factors might play a role in suppression amblyopia. At a 3-year follow-up (Smith, Crasilneck, & Browning, 1961), eight of the nine experimental subjects showed regression, although not always to the original prehypnotic level. A second hypnosis session produced improvement in near vision in six of these subjects, again suggesting a functional component in suppression amblyopia.

Look, Choy, and Kelly (1965) published a case report of a girl who had undergone unsuccessful surgery for strabismus at age 22 months. In spite of orthoptic training for several years, at age 12 the patient had no binocular fusion. Hypnosis training was then begun. Over the next 5 months, her visual acuity without glasses became normal and binocular fusion was developed. Orthoptic training and hypnosis continued regularly, and her gains were maintained over 3 years. This success suggests that long-term hypnosis is necessary to maintain gains as is generally true of all methods used to treat suppression amblyopia.

Williams and Singh (1976) reported the use of hypnosis in an 8-year-old girl with hysterical amblyopia. Two hypnosis sessions over a 3-day period resulted in full restoration of vision with no recurrence of symptoms in 14 months of follow-up. Olness and Gardner (1978) reported the successful use of hypnosis to facilitate comfortable insertion of contact lenses in a 2-year-old boy. When this patient developed bilateral cataracts, he and his mother were faced with two surgical procedures, followed by having to adjust to contact lenses in addition to glasses. The patient's mother sought anticipatory hypnosis training for herself and her son to allow them to cooperate with each other when she inserted the contact lenses. In two sessions of hypnosis, the mother and child learned imagery techniques in which they associated the contact lenses with feelings of quietness, gentleness, and mastery. The boy participated in the imagery exercise and, although he sometimes engaged in anticipatory fretting, he never had to be held down. His participation in this experience allowed him the opportunity to make a positive growth experience out of a potentially traumatic situation.

Lewenstein (1978) used hypnosis as the sole anesthetic with two children, ages 6 and 11 years, for postoperative evaluation and adjustment of sutures placed in the extraocular muscles during strabismus operations. Accurate adjustment is possible only when the patient is fully alert and cooperative. In one child, measurement of ocular alignment in hypnosis revealed that no further adjustments were necessary after initial surgery. In the other child, examination aided by hypnosis revealed that the initial correction was inadequate; adjustment was made while the child remained in hypnosis, thus obviating the need for reoperation under general anesthesia.

## Neurosurgery

In some neurosurgical procedures it is important to have the patient conscious and cooperative so the surgeon can make decisions concerning ablative procedures. Crasilneck, McCranie, and Jenkins (1956) reported the use of hypnosis, combined only with local anesthesia, in a 14-year-old girl who was having an epileptogenic focus removed from her cortex. The patient was having two or three seizures daily, in spite of anticonvulsant medications, since a head injury 4.5 years earlier.

She underwent four hypnosis sessions prior to surgery before undergoing a 9-hour neurosurgical procedure. She remained cooperative and was comfortable throughout except for mild pain while the dura was separated from bone. Of special interest is the fact that she alerted from trance twice when the hippocampal region was stimulated.

## Orthopedics

Jones (1977) reported the use of hypnosis as an adjunct to the anesthetic protocol in 23 children, ages 11–16 years, undergoing the Harrington procedure for idiopathic scoliosis. This procedure involves the operative placement of one or two metal rods for correction of the spinal curve. A risk of paraplegia exists. If the patient can be awakened during the surgery to demonstrate voluntary motor ability, the surgical team can check for the complication of paralysis and achieve immediate decompression if necessary. Patients in this study were seen by the anesthesiologist daily for 1 week prior to surgery. Hypnosis was explained and induced several times. The sequence of events in the operating room was rehearsed in hypnosis, and the patients were also taught self-hypnosis for relief of postoperative symptoms, especially secondary muscle spasm. About 4 hours after the beginning of surgery, the depth of chemical anesthesia was lightened to the point where the patients could blink their eyes on command. The patients were then asked to bend their toes and ankles. If they did so easily, they were reassured and anesthetized again. Postoperatively, the prearranged signals for relaxation were begun as soon as the patients began to awaken. A general decrease in the need for postoperative analgesics, increased cast tolerance, and decreased nausea were observed postoperatively.

Hypnosis can be useful before the application of splints and casts and during the recovery period for relief of muscle spasm and for preparation for cast removal and reestablishment of normal movement. It can also be useful in the postoperative period following amputation. Two representative case histories follow.

Mark C., an obese 8-year-old boy, suffered a fractured femur while playing football in a neighborhood lot. Following operative reduction, he was placed on oral codeine for treatment of the pain associated with quadriceps spasm. Three days later, he had developed nausea as a side effect of codeine, and his frequent vomiting episodes necessitated complicated bed changes (he was in traction) and more discomfort. He had also developed constipation as a side effect of the codeine, and defecation in his bedridden position became exceedingly difficult. At this point, he was referred to learn self-hypnosis.

We asked Mark if he would be willing to make himself feel better without the medicine, and he agreed immediately. When asked what he would prefer to be doing rather than being in the hospital bed, he said he would like to be riding a bicycle down a hill. We asked him to imagine himself doing that, and he quickly entered a hypnosis. We taught him the concept of nerves and central switches and encouraged him to find his own switches and turn them off for the area of the femur. We also gave suggestions for rapid healing and restoration of normal body functions. These suggestions were reinforced daily for 1 week. He had no further complaints nor requirement for codeine, and he was very pleased with his personal success. Following discharge, we asked Mark to practice visualizing normal leg motion in walking and running in preparation for removal of his cast. Rehabilitation was accomplished rapidly, and the patient again was pleased with his participation in therapy.

Nancy S., age 11 years, developed pain in her right leg. Bone biopsy revealed a Ewing's sarcoma, and amputation above the knee was performed. She was first seen in the recovery room where suggestions were given for comfort and normal sensations of hunger. Following return to her room, she experienced no vomiting and requested only oral medication for pain. On the first postoperative day, she was somewhat depressed. She asked to do hypnosis before attempting to move from her bed to a chair. She said she wanted to imagine taking a nap at home. After the therapist assisted her with this imagery, she moved to the chair and then back to bed with only minimal discomfort. The next morning, she was markedly depressed and expressed fear of pain during a physical therapy session scheduled later in the day. She consented to using hypnotic imagery to facilitate ambulation but involved herself only half-heartedly. In physical therapy, she was markedly anxious and cooperated poorly; however, the therapist continued to give informal suggestions for an easy return of ambulation. The third day, Nancy was in better spirits and stood up with the aid of parallel bars. The staff gave much praise for each bit of improvement. By the fifth postoperative day she was walking easily with crutches, clearly proud of her independence. The surgery and physical therapy staffs were very impressed with her progress. She was discharged 2 days later. This patient demonstrates the fact that significant depression and anxiety may interfere with optimal response to hypnosis but that, nonetheless, hypnotic suggestion may have a positive delayed effect, especially if other staff members approach the patient positively.

As noted in detail in Chapter 13, Iserson (1999) described the successful use of hypnosis for reduction of angulated forearm fractures in four children for whom no other form of analgesia was available.

## Otolaryngology

There are few reports of specific applications of hypnosis to otolaryngological problems in children. Edel (1959) reported the case of a severe nosebleed controlled by hypnosis (see Chapter 13), and Bensen (1971) noted the successful use of hypnosis in children and adolescents following tonsillectomy. The following reports describe successful hypnosis used to overcome otolaryngological problems.

Susan, age 10 years, had been unable to swallow solid foods for 6 months. She had lost approximately 5 pounds. The parents and patient recognized that the problem began when the patient witnessed her grandmother choke at the dinner table. The grandmother had no untoward sequelae, but the child was frightened of swallowing solids thereafter. Results of otolaryngological evaluation were normal. We told Susan that she could learn a method to solve the problem herself if she wished. Trance was achieved via the coin induction method, and the patient appeared very comfortable while focusing on a favorite place where she could enjoy being happy, comfortable, and safe. We taught her ideomotor signals, and she was asked, while still in trance, if she would like to solve her problem of eating. When her response was immediately positive, we proceeded to ask her to recall a happy meal prior to the frightening event, to remember her favorite foods, how good they tasted, how easy it was to swallow them. When the patient seemed comfortable with this, we suggested she imagine the same menu in a future meal, enjoying eating, tasting, and swallowing, knowing she was in control of swallowing and that she had solved the problem herself. General suggestions were given for relaxation, feeling better than before, and finding it easy to review the exercise at home. The patient went home and immediately ate her first complete dinner in 6 months without difficulty. One-year follow-up revealed no recurrences.

Charlie Y., age 24 months, had a history of chronic ear infections and had been restrained numerous times on a mummy board for examination and treatment. Hypnosis was requested when his anxiety increased to the point that he began crying as soon as he walked through the clinic door. He was seen for three hypnosis sessions during which suggestions for comfort and ease were given as he played with toys and participated in mock ear examinations, alternately taking the role of doctor and patient. Clinic staff agreed to discontinue use of the mummy board. At the end of 3 weeks, his anxiety was markedly reduced, and he cooperated easily with subsequent ear examinations. This little boy's mother was a nurse, who prompted the referral by insisting that there had to be a better way. Many parents are not as assertive. We hope to see surgical staff members make increasing use of techniques that minimize anxiety in their young patients. We also hope to see decreasing use of physical constraints which are bound to increase anxiety in children.

## References

Alpert, J.J. (1975). Accidental stresses: stressful accidents [audiotape]. *Pediatric Audio Digest Foundation, 219*(2).

Andolsek, K. & Novik, B. (1980). Procedures in family practice: use of hypnosis with children. *Journal of Family Practice, 10*, 503–507.

Antitch, J.L.S. (1967). The use of hypnosis in pediatric anesthesia. *Journal of the American Society of Psychosomatic Dentistry and Medicine, 14*, 70–75.

Arnon, Z., Hanan, H., & Mogliner, J. (2018). The effect of a hypnotic-based animated video on stress and pain reduction in pediatric surgery. *International Journal of Clinical and Experimental Hypnosis, 66*(2), 123–133.

Bensen, V.B. (1971). One hundred cases of post-anesthetic suggestion in the recovery room. *American Journal of Clinical Hypnosis, 14*, 9–15.

Bernick, S.M. (1972). Relaxation, suggestion, and hypnosis in dentistry: what the pediatrician should know about children's dentistry. *Clinical Pediatrics, 11*, 72–75.

Bernstein, N.R. (1963). Management of burned children with the aid of hypnosis. *Journal of Child Psychology and Psychiatry, 4*, 93–98.

Bernstein, N.R. (1965). Observations on the use of hypnosis with burned children on a pediatric ward. *International Journal of Clinical and Experimental Hypnosis, 13*, 1–10.

Betcher, A.M. (1960). Hypnosis as an adjunct in anesthesiology. *New York State Journal of Medicine, 60*, 816–822.

Bierman, S.F. (1989). Hypnosis in the emergency department. *American Journal of Emergency Medicine, 7*, 238–242.

Browning, C.W., Quinn, L.H., & Crasilneck, H.B. (1958). The use of hypnosis in suppressing amblyopia of children. *American Journal of Ophthalmology, 46*, 53–67.

Brunnquell, D. & Kohen, D.P. (1991). Emotions in emergencies: what we know, what we can do. *Children's Health Care (Journal of the Association for the Care of Children's Health), 20*(4), 240–247.

Calipel, S., Lucas-Polomeni, M., Wodey, E., & Ecoffey, C. (2005). Premedication in children: hypnosis vs. midazolam. *Pediatric Anesthesia, 15*, 275–281.

Cheek, D.B. (1959). Unconscious perception of meaningful sounds during surgical anesthesia as revealed under hypnosis. *American Journal of Clinical Hypnosis, 1*, 101–113.

Chester, S.J., Tyack, Z., DeYoung, A., Kipping, B., Griffin, B., Stockton, K., Ware, R.S., Zhang, X. , & Kimble, R.M. (2018). Efficacy of hypnosis on pain, wound-healing, anxiety and stress in children with acute burn injuries: a randomized controlled trial. *Pain, 159*(9), 1790–1801.

Crasilneck, H.B. & Hall, J.A. (1985). *Clinical Hypnosis: Principles and Applications*, 2nd ed. New York: Grune & Stratton.

Crasilneck, H.B., McCranie, E.J., & Jenkins, M.T. (1956). Special indications for hypnosis as a method of anesthesia. *Journal of the American Medical Association, 162*, 1606–1608.

Cullen, S.C. (1958). Current comment and case reports: hypno-induction techniques in pediatric anesthesia. *Anesthesiology, 19*, 279–281.

Daniels, E. (1962). The hypnotic approach in anesthesia for children. *American Journal of Clinical Hypnosis, 4*, 244–248.

Dikel, W. & Olness, K. (1980). Self-hypnosis, biofeedback, and voluntary peripheral temperature control in children. *Pediatrics, 66*, 335–340.

Edel, J.W. (1959). Nosebleed controlled by hypnosis. *American Journal of Clinical Hypnosis, 2*, 89–90.

Erickson, M.H. (1958). Pediatric hypnotherapy. *American Journal of Clinical Hypnosis, 1*, 25–29.

Fortier, M.A., Weinberg, M., Vitulano, L.A., Chorney, J.M., Martin, S.R., & Kain, Z.N. (2010). Effects of therapeutic suggestion in children undergoing general anesthesia: a randomized controlled trial. *Pediatric Anesthesia, 20*, 90–99.

Gaal, J.M., Goldsmith, L., & Needs, R.E. (1980). The use of hypnosis, as an adjunct to anesthesia, to reduce pre- and post-operative anxiety in children. Paper presented at the annual meeting of the American Society of Clinical Hypnosis, Minneapolis, MN.
Gardner, G.G. (1978). The use of hypnotherapy in a pediatric setting. In E. Gellert, Ed., *Psychosocial Aspects of Pediatric Care*. New York: Grune & Stratton.
Hammond, D.C. (2008). Hypnosis as sole anesthesia for major surgeries: historical & contemporary perspectives. *American Journal of Clinical Hypnosis, 51(2)*, 101–121.
He, H., Polkki, T., Pietila, A., & Vehvilainen-Julkunen, K. (2006). Chinese parents' use of non-pharmacological methods in children's postoperative pain relief. *Scandinavian Journal of Caring Science, 20*, 2–9.
Heitkemper, T., Layne, C., & Sullivan, D.M. (1993). Brief treatment of children's dental pain and anxiety. *Perceptual and Motor Skills, 76*, 192–194.
Hoffman, H.G., Doctor, J.N., Patterson, D.R., Carrougher, G.J., & Furness, T.A. (2000). Virtual reality as an adjunctive pain control during burn wound care in adolescent patients. *Pain, 85*, 305–309.
Hopayian, R. (1984). A brief technique of hypnoanesthesia for children in a casualty department. *Anaesthesia, 39*, 1139–1141.
Iserson, K.V. (1999). Hypnosis for pediatric fracture reduction. *The Journal of Emergency Medicine, 17*(1), 53–56.
Jones, C.W. (1977). Hypnosis and spinal fusion by Harrington instrumentation. *American Journal of Clinical Hypnosis, 19*, 155–157.
Kain, Z.N. & Caldwell-Andrews, A.A. (2005). Preoperative psychological preparation of the child for surgery: an update. *Anesthesiology Clinics of North America, 23*, 597–614.
Kelsey, D. & Barron, J.N. (1958). Maintenance of posture by hypnotic suggestion in patients undergoing plastic surgery. *British Medical Journal, 1*, 756.
Kelly, L.J. (1976). Hypnosis and children in the Emergency Department. Paper presented at the annual meeting of the American Society of Clinical Hypnosis, Chicago, IL.
Kennedy, R.M. & Luhmann, J.D. (1999). The "ouchless emergency department" getting closer: advances in decreasing distress during painful procedures in the emergency department. *Pediatric Clinics of North America, 46*(*6*), 1215–1247.
Kohen, D.P. (1986). Applications of relaxation/mental imagery (self-hypnosis) in pediatric emergencies. *International Journal of Clinical and Experimental Hypnosis, 34*(*4*), 283–294.
Kohen, D.P. (2001a). Hypnosis for children in anesthesiology and surgery. In L.E. Fredericks, Ed., *The Use of Hypnosis in Surgery and Anesthesiology: Psychological Preparation of the Surgical Patient* (pp. 138–162). Springfield, IL: Charles C. Thomas.
Kohen, D.P. (2001b). *Anticipatory anxiety for orthopedic surgery in 8 year old with cerebral palsy* [videotape]. Minneapolis, MN: Behavioral Pediatrics Program, University of Minnesota.
Kroger, W.S. & DeLee, S.T. (1957). Use of hypnoanesthesia for cesarean section and hysterectomy. *Journal of the American Medical Association, 163*, 442–444.
LaBaw, W.L. (1973). Adjunctive trance therapy with severely burned children. *International Journal of Child Psychotherapy, 2*, 80–92.
Lambert, S.A. (1996). The effects of hypnosis/guided imagery on the postoperative course of children. *Journal of Developmental and Behavioral Pediatrics, 17*, 307–310.
Lang, E. & Laser, E. (2009). *Patient Sedation Without Medication*. Boston, MA: Elvira V. Lang, M.D.
Levitan, A.A. & Harbaugh, T.E. (1992). Hypnotizability and hypnoanalgesia: hypnotizability of patients using hypnoanalgesia during surgery. *American Journal of Clinical Hypnosis, 34*(*4*), 223–226.
Lewenstein, L.N. (1978). Hypnosis as an anesthetic in pediatric ophthalmology. *Anesthesiology, 49*, 144–145.
Lobe, T.E. (2006). Perioperative hypnosis reduces hospitalization on patients undergoing the Nuss procedure for pectus excavatum. *Journal of Laparoendoscopic & Advanced Surgical Techniques, Part A, 16*, 639–642.
Lobe, T.E. (2007). Perioperative hypnosis. In W.C. Wester II & L.I. Sugarman, Eds., *Therapeutic Hypnosis with Children and Adolescents* (pp. 333–355). Bethel, CT: Crown House Publishing.
Look, Y.K., Choy, D.C., & Kelly, J.M. Jr. (1965). Hypnotherapy in strabismus. *American Journal of Clinical Hypnosis*, 7, 335–341.
Lucas, O.N. (1965). Dental Extractions in the Hemophiliac: Control of the Emotional Factors by Hypnosis. *American Journal of Clinical Hypnosis*, 7, 301–307. 10.1080/00029157.1965.10402436.

Mackenzie, A. & Frawley, G.P. (2007). Preoperative hypnotherapy in the management of a child with anticipatory nausea and vomiting. *Anaesthesia and Intensive Care, 35*, 784–787.
Manworren, R.C.B., Anderson, M.N., & Girard, E.D. (2018). Postoperative pain: outcomes after Nuss procedures: comparison of epidural analgesia, continuous infusion of local anesthetic, and peroperative self-hypnosis training. *Journal of Laparoendoscopic & Advanced Surgical Techniques, 28*(10), 1234–1242.
Marmer, M.J. (1959). Hypnosis as an adjunct to anesthesia in children. *American Journal of Diseases of Children, 97*, 314–317.
McKnight-Hanes, C., Myers, D.R., Dushku, J.C., & Davis, H.C. (1993). The use of behavior management techniques by dentists across practitioner type, age, and geographic region. *Pediatric Dentistry, 15*(4), 267–271.
Mirvish, I. (1978). Hypnotherapy for the child with chronic eczema: a case report. *South African Medical Journal, 54*, 410–412.
Neiburger, E.J. (1976). Waking hypnosis through sensory confusion: 302 cases of dental prophylaxis. *Journal of the American Society of Psychosomatic Dentistry and Medicine, 23*, 88–98.
Neiburger, E.J. (1978). Child response to suggestion: study of age, sex, time, and income levels during dental care. *Journal of Dentistry for Children, 45*, 396–402.
Olness, K. (1977). In-service Hypnosis Education in a Children's Hospital. *American Journal of Clinical Hypnosis*, 20, 80–83. 10.1080/00029157.1977.10403904.
Olness, K. & Gardner, G.G. (1978). Some guidelines for uses of hypnotherapy in pediatrics. *Pediatrics*, 62, 228–233.
Pelaez Perez, J.M., Sanchez Casado, M., Quintana Diaz, M., Benhaiem, J.M., & Escriba Alepuz, F.J. (2021). Effectiveness of hypnoanalgesia in paediatric dermatological surgery. *Children, 8*(12), 1195. 10.3390/children8121195
Peretz, B. (1996a). Confusion as a technique to induce hypnosis in a severely anxious pediatric dental patient. *The Journal of Clinical Pediatric Dentistry, 21*, 27–30.
Peretz, B. (1996b). Relaxation and hypnosis in pediatric dental patients. *The Journal of Clinical Pediatric Dentistry, 20*, 205–207.
Peretz, B. & Bimstein, E. (2000). The use of imagery suggestions during administration of local anesthetic in pediatric dental patients. *Journal of Dentistry for Children, 67*(4), 263–267.
Peretz, B. & Gluck, G.M. (1999). Reframing: reappraising an old behavioral technique. *The Journal of Clinical Pediatric Dentistry, 23*, 103–105.
Puskar, K.R. & Mumford, K. (1990). The healing power. *Nursing Times, 86*(33), 50–52.
Ramirez-Carrasco, A., Butron-Tellez Giron, C., Sanchez-Armass, O., & Pierdant-Perez, M. (2017). Effectiveness of hypnosis in combination with conventional techniques of behavior management in anxiety/pain reduction during dental anesthetic infiltration. *Pain Research & Management, 2017*, 1434015. 10.1155/20171434015
Rausch, V. (1980). Cholecystectomy with self-hypnosis. *American Journal of Clinical Hypnosis, 22*, 124–129.
Sabherwal, P., Kaira, N., Tvagi, R., Khatri, A., & Srivastava, S. (2021). Hypnosis and progressive muscle relaxation for anxiolysis and pain control during extraction procedure in 8-12 year old children: a randomized control trial. *European Archives of Paediatric Dentistry, 22*, 823–832.
Santer, L. (1990). Imagery use during laceration repair in children. Paper presented at the 41st Annual Scientific Meeting of the Society for Clinical and Experimental Hypnosis, Tucson, AZ.
Scott, D.L. (1969). Hypnosis as an aid to anesthesia in children. *Anesthesia, 24*, 643–644.
Scott, D.L. & Holbrook, L.A. (1981). Hypnotic psychotherapy and cosmetic surgery. *British Journal of Plastic Surgery, 34*, 478.
Sharek, P.J., Wayman, K., Strichartz, D., Sentivany-Collins, S., Good, J., Esquivel, C., Brown, M., & Cox, K. (2006). Improved pain management in pediatric postoperative liver transplant patients using parental education and non-pharmacologic interventions. *Pediatric Transplantation, 10*, 172–177.
Shaw, S.I. (1959). A survey of the management of children in hypnodontia. *American Journal of Clinical Hypnosis, 1*, 155–162.
Smith, G.G., Crasilneck, H.B., & Browning, C.W. (1961). A follow-up study of suppression amblyopia in children previously subjected to hypnotherapy. *American Journal of Ophthalmology, 52*, 690–693.

Soltani, M., Drever. S.A., Hoffman, H.G., Sharar, S.R., Wiechman, S.A., Jensen, M.P., & Patterson, D.R. (2018). Virtual reality analgesia for burn joint flexibility: a randomized controlled trial. *Rehabilitation Psychology*, 63, 487–494.

Steele, E., Grimmer, K., Thomas, B., Mulley, B., Fulton, I., & Hoffman, H. (2003). Virtual reality as a pediatric pain modulation technique: a case study. *Cyberpsychology & Behavior*, *6*(6), 633–638.

Tasini, M.F. & Hackett, T.P. (1977). Hypnosis in the treatment of warts in immunodeficient children. *American Journal of Clinical Hypnosis*, *19*, 152–154.

Thompson, K.F. (1963). A rationale for suggestion in dentistry. *American Journal of Clinical Hypnosis*, *5*, 181–186.

Trustman, R., Dubovsky, S., & Titley, R. (1977). Auditory perception during general anesthesia: myth or fact? *International Journal of Clinical and Experimental Hypnosis*, *25*, 88–105.

Tucker, K.R. & Virnelli, F.R. (1985). The use of hypnosis as a tool in plastic surgery. *Plastic and Reconstructive Surgery*, *76*, 140–146.

Tusek, D., Church, J.M., & Fazio, V.W. (1997). Guided imagery as a coping strategy for perioperative patients. *AORN Journal*, *66*, 644–649.

Vagnoli, L., Bettini, A., Amore, E., DeMasi, S., & Messeri, A. (2019). Relaxation-guided imagery reduces perioperative anxiety and pain in children: a randomized study. *European Journal of Pediatrics*, *178*, 913–921.

Van der Does, A.J.W., Van Dyck, R., & Spijker, R.E. (1988). Hypnosis and pain in patients with severe burns: a pilot study. *Burns*, *14*(5), 399–404.

Wakeman, R.J. & Kaplan, J.Z. (1978). An experimental study of hypnosis in painful burns. *American Journal of Clinical Hypnosis*, *21*, 3–12.

Wangensteen, O.H. (1962). New operative techniques in intestinal obstructions. *Wisconsin Medical Journal*, *62*, 159–169.

Wiggins, S.L. & Brown, C.W. (1968). Hypnosis with two pedicle graft cases. *International Journal of Clinical and Experimental Hypnosis*, *16*, 215.

Williams, D.T., & Singh, M. (1976). Hypnosis as a Facilitating Therapeutic Adjunct in Child Psychiatry. *Journal of the American Academy of Child Psychiatry*, 15, 326–342. 10.1016/s0002-7138(09)61491-6.

Winkelstein, L.B., & Levinson, J. (1959). Fulminating pre-eclampsia with cesarean section performed under hypnosis. *American Journal of Obstetrics and Gynecology*, 78, 420–423. 10.1016/0002-9378(59)90195-4.

Wolf, T.G., Kellerhoff, K.N., Schmierer, A., Schmierer, G., & Halsbnd, U. (2021). Caries treatment in a four-year-old boy using hypnosis-a case report. *American Journal of Clinical Hypnosis*, *63*(3), 217–228.

# 15

# VALUE OF HYPNOSIS IN PEDIATRIC PALLIATIVE CARE, GRIEF, AND BEREAVEMENT

## Introduction

Much has been learned and written about the process of grief and bereavement in children since Kübler-Ross (1969, 1974) first described the stages of grief and the mourning process. To even note the myriad of references available for parents, clinicians, and especially for children to help with the navigation of the grief and bereavement process is well beyond the scope of this book. We refer, therefore, to some of our favorite books and stories that have been helpful to children and families (Grollman, 1991; Miles, 1971; Viorst, 1971; White, 1952).

It seems clear that grief in its many forms is ubiquitous; therefore, child health clinicians must be mindful of when to consider that a diagnosis of grief (bereavement) response may be appropriate in a child or adolescent. Any change in a child's behavior may be a reflection of the sadness, anger, helplessness, fear (e.g., of the future, of his or her own safety), sense of responsibility (guilt), or confusion the child feels over some loss, whether that loss represents the death of a loved one or a pet, or is the symbolic, and almost equally or even more profound, loss felt in the common experiences of divorce of parents, move to a new home or school, move of a best friend, or disappointment in experiencing an unexpected outcome.

In the experience of their grief, children, like adults, respond in a highly individualized fashion, as well as according to their level of development and concomitant degree of understanding of death. Their reactions are also to some degree, but not always, reflections of the way in which those in their lives and families experience grief. Symptoms, therefore, may include:

- *Somatic complaints*. Headache, abdominal pain, limb pain, vomiting, recurrence or exacerbation of existing problems (e.g., enuresis, encopresis, asthma)
- *Sleep disturbances*. Inability or fear of going to sleep, nightmares, trouble staying asleep, exacerbation of existing parasomnias (e.g., night terrors, sleepwalking)
- *Eating disturbances*. Increase or decrease in appetite, exacerbation of existing problems
- *Disruptive behaviors*. Tantrums, oppositional behavior, angry outbursts
- *Sad behaviors*. Withdrawal, weepiness, etc.
- *School problems*. Disinterest, school refusal, avoidance or phobia, deterioration in performance
- *Anxiety*. Increase in separation anxiety, performance anxiety, etc.
- *Habit problems*. Development or exacerbation of tics, twitches, or other habits

DOI: 10.4324/9781003243687-17

## Approaches That Work

In the context of rapport and review of the history, clinicians must acknowledge and validate the helplessness, emptiness, anger, and whatever other feelings are expressed in order to help the child and family begin to acknowledge and then move toward understanding the nature of their grief and bereavement, particularly as a process extending over time. This allows for the setting of a tone in which one can offer and teach strategies to both children and their families that they may use to help themselves in accepting the sadness and associated feelings, as well as the intensity of those feelings – however normal such feelings are. To do so effectively requires that we as clinicians begin, as always, with ourselves, i.e., allowing ourselves to become aware of our own feelings and their intensity; and to attend appropriately to the powerful feelings of transference and countertransference we know are integral to effective therapy.

## Naturalistic Uses of Hypnotic Language and Therapeutic Hypnosis Strategies

Not unlike children or adults in an emergency situation (see Chapter 14), people who are grieving – and especially in the early, acute stages of grief and mourning – are often in a spontaneously altered state of awareness, i.e., a spontaneous hypnotic trance, and are narrowly focused on the loved one (or other loss) who is gone and/or on their own sadness, worry, aloneness, and confusion. Also, as with patients in emergencies with acute, severe pain, the spontaneous trance of acute grief is, in a sense, a "negative" trance, narrowly focused and cycling negatively on the feelings of sadness, helplessness, self-recriminations, and, in turn, on what may be considered an anticipated and relentless continued sense of sadness, loneliness, and helplessness. Awareness of these states as analogous to spontaneous trance behavior will allow the clinician not only to observe other characteristics of trance in children who are grieving – such as spontaneous regression – but also to approach helping such children through the application of therapeutic hypnosis suggestions and self-hypnosis strategies. Recognizing and finding the hypnosis in the encounter – as so often noted in this volume – is therefore integral and critical to an effective process.

We find it useful to invite the patient to talk about how his or her grief is experienced now as compared to when the loss occurred. Such inquiry is framed hypnotically to convey the expectancy that, in fact, the grief feelings now are *not* quite the same as they were before, even if the loss is very recent. This sets the tone and implies that in the future (e.g., next week, next month), further change, comfort, acclimation, and accommodation can and will come. This approach seems to be effective to normalize and validate grief and to begin to move from that posture to one that is better, easier, and ultimately healthier as needed. This naturalistic, therapeutic hypnotic communication is often easily accomplished by following Erickson's (1958) dictum to "follow the child." Such following and joining may occur by saying something such as: "What have you *noticed* about how you have been feeling since your [friend, grandmother, brother, uncle, cousin] died?" Hypnotic characteristics of such an inquiry include the implicit compliment to the patient that the therapist believes that he or she *has been able to notice feelings* and the expectancy and comfort in the invitation to share those feelings.

Recognition of the spontaneous hypnotic state might allow for simple history taking to take place through invitations for spontaneous waking hypnotic regression – for example, "Would you tell me about the funeral?" or "Would it be okay to share anything about the funeral with me?" This provides the opportunity for the child to make the decision to talk about where the funeral took place, what it was like, what was going through their mind at the time, et al. With the expression, or revivification of the effect of the moment, the therapist can, again, offer suggestions for *progress through implication* – for example, "And, since then, *notice now how things have changed*?" Such invitations for reframing help people to acknowledge that, as awful as they feel, things are, in fact, moving forward, and they are coping okay. If they happen to be stuck and do not feel as though they are moving forward, the hypnotic strategy of future projection may be useful; thus:

> Now, take a look in your mind a month or two or three *into the future*. See a calendar on the side of your inner mind and notice when it is. … That's good. … And notice how things are *starting to be different* and to improve. I don't know how much, maybe a lot, or a little, or in between, but you can notice, and the more you notice it the way it can be, then it will, when you're ready, because *you can create it this way* using the strength of your inner mind and memories.

As noted, integration of education and information about the normalcy, length, and see-saw nature of the bereavement process with hypnotic approaches and suggestions will often serve the child and family very well. These also set the tone for offering additional suggestions about how to cope even more as time goes on.

It may be useful to invite the grieving child or adolescent, in his or her spontaneous trance behavior, to consider "What can you say to that person right now in your imagination? You know he [or she] will always be with you, within your mind … and you can talk to him [or her] right now?" The clinician/therapist can help the patient protect his or her privacy and reinforce the patient's sense of control by adding a permissive suggestion to choose to keep these images confidential; thus:

> And you can have a conversation now in your inside mind. … Take your time … hear yourself and hear them … as long and as short as you need … and notice the feelings … and you can tell me what you noticed in this conversation, or you can keep it private because you know you are in charge of your imagination.

In addition to the ego strengthening presented, this is another way of offering permission for people to do what they may have already been doing in their mind and may even have been wondering or thinking that it in some way was wrong, bad, morbid, or confusing. As such, what had been potentially a disturbing, confusing, or recurrent and bothersome thought, can be re-framed in this manner as something that not only is normal but is also useful; and "a good way that you are taking care of yourself, and allowing yourself to *remember the way you want*."

Shifting the same concept to focus on future orientation, the therapist might then add:

> It's good to know that you can always talk to Grandma [or whoever has died] in your imagination this way – because you know her so well and you both love each other [note present tense] so much you'll probably even be able to hear her voice and her love in your inner mind when you do it this way. That's really a good thing to know.

Sometimes, children or adolescents may admit that they can't get the loved one out of their mind and are confused by the ambivalence of wanting the images of that person to stay and yet wanting the sadness and helplessness to go away. Direct permission to have both of these feelings and some guidelines for how to do that hypnotically may be useful, for example:

> Each hour [or 2 hours or 4 hours, or every night at bedtime] it would be really good to really picture [the person] in your mind for about 1 or 5 or 10 minutes (how long do you

> think would be good?), and when you do that, really enjoy remembering a conversation you had, a place you went, something you did together, and just notice all the wonderful things about them and you and that time – the sounds, the smells, the tastes, feelings – and then, before it's over for this time [this puts definitive closure on it hypnotically], remind [the person] and yourself that you'll be together again in your mind again tomorrow [or in a few hours, etc.] at the same time, for a similar or different and special time together in your mind. As time goes on you may both discover that you want to have more time in between such connections, but for, now every *however often* is just right for you … .

A 13-year-old boy, Jay L., was referred to one of us (DK) by a family therapist for medical evaluation and hypnosis for the problem of panic attacks that had been occurring nightly for 4 months, beginning the night before school began in the fall (Kohen, 1995). As the history unfolded at the first visit, a sad story of multiple grief experiences was revealed. The family had recently moved to the city from their home of many years, 4 hours away. Jay was angry and sad about leaving his home and especially missed his friends. The added stress of starting a new school seemed at first to explain the timing of the panic attacks. A closer examination of the symptoms, however, indicated that the panic attacks were occurring as he was awakening, usually within an hour of going to sleep. He would awake "in a panic" and confused, running around angrily, frightened, and experiencing subsequent amnesia. A more likely diagnosis seemed to be night terror disorder, with the stress of change, grief, and loss seemingly a trigger for the night terror behavior (see also Chapter 8). It was then noted in the history that the reason for moving was for the family to be able to be physically closer to Jay's father, who had recently completed a prison term for sexually abusing Jay's stepsister and was now completing his therapy while living in a group home in the city. Jay's sense of loss of – and ambivalence toward – his father and the loss of his stepsister (now out of the home) was obvious and added to the rapidly growing list of reasons for Jay to be grieving.

With three quarters of the first hour visit gone, Jay's mother abruptly became sad and explained, through emerging tears, that Jay had been very close with his maternal grandmother, who had died 5 years before, and that he missed her very much. As Jay's mother spoke of this, Jay, too, began to cry quietly. His father noted that Jay always preferred to stay in the car when they visited the grandmother's grave. Jay's spontaneous trance behavior was evident, with his stillness in his chair, slowing of his respiratory rate, tears, and a far-away look in his eyes. Acknowledging his sadness and his love for his grandmother, I asked him if he had a picture of her. He said he did not. At my request, the mother agreed to give Jay a picture of his grandmother that day. When Jay returned for follow-up 5 days later, he reported, and his family confirmed, that the nightly panic attacks or night terrors had abruptly stopped the night after our first visit. Again, in a spontaneous trance, Jay observed curiously, "Isn't it odd that my panicky stuff stopped the very same night I got my picture of Grandma?" Jay's grief therapy, with therapeutic hypnosis as one integral component, continued.

## The Uses of Therapeutic Hypnosis in Palliative Care and with Dying Children

It is virtually impossible to be certain that that therapeutic hypnosis *per se* is the source of positive clinical results; however, especially in cases of dying children, it has often been demonstrated that so-called usual or ordinary forms of reassurance and counseling, medications, and other traditional therapies have failed. Therefore, even without many controlled studies, and usually in the absence of any formal measures of ability to enter the hypnotic state, we are inclined to believe that that therapeutic hypnosis is indeed valuable for many who suffer terminal illness.

In the years since the previous edition of this text continued widespread growth has occurred in the provision of palliative care – first among adults, with the growth of hospice availability in many communities, and more recently with the accelerating growth of pediatric palliative care. Therapeutic hypnosis has been applied in palliative care for adults for over 25 years, commonly for terminally ill cancer patients (Finlay & Jones, 1996; Liossi & White, 2001). In their study with terminally ill adult cancer patients, Liossi and White (2001) demonstrated that patients in the hypnosis group had significantly better overall quality of life and lower levels of anxiety and depression as compared to the standard care group.

In working with chronically and terminally ill adolescents, Harper (1999) reflected the philosophy that weaves its way throughout our text in his description of a developmentally focused and individualized hypnotherapeutic intervention for youth as they navigate the challenges of the end of life. The treatment – applied in a personalized fashion to the psychological and physical discomfort associated with conditions including end-stage renal disease, cancer, organ transplant, and HIV disease – focuses on the use of metaphors for controlling and distancing from discomfort. Himelstein (2006) described pediatric palliative care (PPC) as being "about helping children and families to live to their fullest while facing complex medical conditions."

In this spirit, Fenton has noted "If one thinks of palliative care in the truest sense as a specialty that deals with both life-threatening and life-changing conditions, then Tourette Syndrome or a habit cough so pervasive that the child can't go to school are well within the purview of palliative care" (Fenton, 2019, personal communication).

Family-centered pediatric palliative care is the art and science of improving quality of life, attending to suffering, and assisting with medical decision-making for children with life-threatening conditions. Himelstein outlined and described 15 basic principles of pediatric palliative care as an interdisciplinary practice and elucidated a structure and function differentiating palliative care from hospice. Writing about the global need for palliative care for children, Connor, Downing, and Marston (2017) note that at least 20 million children around the world would benefit from PPC annually and over 8 million would need specialized PPC services (Connor et al., 2017). Kuttner and Friedrichsdorf amplified this in 2014 describing hypnosis applications for children and their families. (Kuttner & Friedrichsdorf, 2014)

Detailed descriptions and discussions of palliative care programs are beyond the scope of this volume but can be found in the work of Himelstein at the Children's Hospital of Wisconsin in Milwaukee (Himelstein, 2006). Duncan and colleagues at the Dana–Farber Cancer Institute and Children's Hospital, Boston (Duncan, Spengler, & Wolfe, 2007), the Pain and Palliative Care Program at Children's Hospitals and Clinics of Minnesota and at the Pediatric Advanced Care Team at the Children's Hospital of Philadelphia (Friedrichsdorf & Kang, 2007; Friedrichsdorf, Remke, Symnalla, Gibbon, & Chrastek, 2007; McSherry, Kehoe, Carroll, Kang, & Rourke, 2007), and the Royal Children's Hospital in Melbourne, Australia (Heath et al., 2010). Research priorities in pediatric palliative care have been examined and carefully articulated by a large collaborative group (Steele et al., 2008).

Most recently Friedrichsdorf and Kohen (2018) have published a review of PPC and the value and significance of attending to distressing symptoms at the end of life in children. Hypnosis is described in detail as a valued elemental approach to providing this care (Friedrichsdorf & Kohen, 2018).

In 2019, Gregoire and associates published a report of their pilot study of a group intervention assessing the acceptability and feasibility of combining self-care and hypnosis for children with cancer and their parents, and a quasi-experimental protocol aimed at assessing the efficacy of this intervention to improve quality of life, distress, fatigue, and coping. Results of the pilot study showed that the intervention was feasible and perceived positively by participants (Gregoire, Chantrain, Faymonville, Marini, & Bragard, 2019).

## Modification of Symptoms and By-products of the Disease and Treatment

A unique and timely study was conducted by Weekly, Walker, Beck, Akers & Weaver, (2018) in searching smartphone application platforms for apps relevant to calming, relaxation, and mindfulness for pediatric and adolescent patients. Twenty-two apps were identified and 16 were included in the final analysis. Seventy-five percent (12 of 16) featured a relaxation approach, soothing images (8 of 16) and guided breathing techniques. The major targeted symptoms were mood and sleep patterns. The apps target specific coping mechanisms such as calming music (44%) calming words (44%) mindfulness approach (38%), meditation (38%) and others. A team of six reviewers representing palliative care, psychology, child life, and nursing systematically reviewed apps in full. Several apps were determined to be most compelling by the study team: notably those with creative relational use of calming technology for children, e.g. Kindoma – *Kindoma Drawtime, version 2.7 Kindoma Inc, Palo Alto CA, 2017* or apps which allow a parent to read a bedtime story to a child from a distance. Other apps are referenced which allow for a speaker version in which a parent and child can breathe together to foster a relaxation approach (Weekly et al., 2018). Given that the vast majority of children, parents, and especially adolescents have a smartphone, clinicians are advised to consider this adjunctive option as a hypnosis or certainly hypnotic-like addition to palliative care.

Reports from several centers agree that therapeutic hypnosis can be valuable – sometimes in very dramatic ways – for a vast array of physical and psychological problems that arise in children with terminal illness (LeBaron & Zeltzer, 1985; Olness & Hall, 1985; Olness & Singher, 1989; Reaney, 1994). Crasilneck and Hall (1973, 1975) described their work with two boys, 4 and 8 years old, one with inoperable brain cancer and the other with leukemia. The specific problems treated included severe pain, poor tolerance of medical procedures, generalized anxiety, fear of dying, depression, insomnia, anorexia, and behavioral difficulties. Each of the boys went into deep hypnosis and responded very well to direct suggestions for symptom relief after one session. The younger boy was seen daily the first month, then three times weekly until his death the first week of the third month of clinical therapeutic hypnosis. The older child achieved rapid remission of his leukemia and was to be seen when necessary for further reinforcement of hypnosis. At the time of the report, this boy was successfully using self-hypnosis for therapeutic procedures. O'Connell (1985) described the use of hypnosis in several cases of terminal illness in which patients were taught self-hypnosis to ease pain and remain able to function with minds unclouded by medication. The hypnotic state was described as "a natural state, similar if not identical to the mental state of artists during creative periods and students during boring lectures" (p. 122).

As therapeutic hypnosis has become much more widely used with children who have cancer, such clinical observations are now common. Three research studies have reported results for a series of patients that have added to our understanding and brought out some of the complex issues not yet understood in the area of symptom relief. LaBaw, Holton, Tewell, and Eccles (1975) utilized adjunctive hypnosis, in both group and individual sessions, with 27 pediatric cancer patients, ages 4–20 years. In addition to the specific problems treated by Crasilneck and Hall (1975), this study reported successful modification of nosebleeds and of vomiting associated with chemotherapy. The results were presented in the form of brief clinical vignettes for 12 of the children, said to be representative of the group as a whole. Based on these 12 descriptions, we have classified the responses to therapeutic hypnosis as follows: none or minimal, three children; moderate, three children; good, six children. The authors did not draw conclusions as to which types of symptoms were most amenable to treatment. In this small group of 12, successful response to clinical hypnosis did not appear to be clearly related to age or sex, though there was a tendency for girls to respond better than boys. The authors noted that reasons for difficulty in using hypnosis or self-hypnosis included excessive dependency needs, extreme anxiety or pain, defensive passivity, and lack of parental support (LaBaw et al., 1975).

Hilgard and Morgan (1978) reported their use of hypnosis for modification of specific problems – chiefly pain and anxiety – in 34 pediatric cancer patients, ages 4–19 years. Seven other children were offered hypnosis but refused this treatment modality. The children's ability to use hypnosis for symptom relief was associated with age, score on the Stanford Hypnotic Clinical Scale for Children (SHCS-C), anxiety level, and nature of the problem.

Olness (1981) taught self-hypnosis for symptom relief to 21 pediatric cancer patients from a group of 25 consecutive referrals; three children and one set of parents refused this treatment modality. The age range at referral was 3–18 years. Symptom relief was defined as a reduction in pain associated with such procedures as intravenous injections, spinal taps, and bone marrow aspirates or a reduction in anorexia, nausea, or vomiting associated with radiation or chemotherapy. Specific indicators of improvement included reduction in analgesic or antinausea medication. Of the 21 patients taught self-hypnosis, 12 were referred at the time of initial diagnosis. These 12 all demonstrated substantial symptom relief. Of nine patients first trained during relapse, seven demonstrated substantial symptom relief. Among the other patients, a 3-year-old had only one practice session, and a 4-year-old was referred on the day of his death. Children who practiced most regularly obtained the most consistent relief. Benefits accrued about equally to both younger (5–11) and older (12–18) children, but the younger children achieved symptom control more quickly, in an average of two sessions as compared to four sessions for the older children.

It is difficult to make meaningful comparison of these three studies. In the first two, about half of the patients achieved significant symptom relief following therapeutic hypnosis. In Olness' study, the success rate was 90%. In the LaBaw et al. (1975) study, girls seemed to fare better than boys; the other two studies did not report sex differences. Hilgard and Morgan found that children 4–6 years old responded poorly as compared to older children, but Olness found no such difference. Hilgard and Morgan noted that the younger children had the most severe anxiety about major medical procedures, a finding like that of Katz, Kellerman, and Siegel (1980). It is not clear whether Olness treated anxiety in her young patients differently or whether they were less anxious. Hilgard and Morgan found different success rates according to the nature of the problem, but Olness' report does not permit this kind of comparison. Olness stressed the value of regular practice and early referral; the other studies did not comment on these issues. In two studies, the patients were trained from the beginning to use self-hypnotic techniques; Hilgard and Morgan encouraged self-hypnosis but apparently not to the same extent. Only Hilgard and Morgan used any formal measure of ability to achieve hypnosis and found two patients whose low scores on the SHCS-C suggested that their symptom improvement was due to factors other than hypnosis. We do not know how many similar cases were included in the other studies.

In all three studies, we do not know whether or how the results are related to the fact that the patients all suffered from cancer. Would the results be different for children suffering other kinds of life-threatening illness, or from chronic illnesses that are not life threatening? Or, are these data representative of pediatric patients as a whole? In short, we are unable to explain the available data in any truly satisfactory way. We urge researchers to continue an increasing focus on controlled clinical trials in which identical research protocols are used simultaneously at several medical centers.

While there has been a plethora of reports regarding pediatric palliative care since the publication of the fourth edition of this text, precious few make any mention of pediatric hypnosis beyond those already referenced here (or below) and no additional randomized controlled studies have been identified in an Internet search via Google Scholar. The interested reader may wish to explore one or more of several books that have been published in recent years which describe the uses of hypnosis in pain and/or palliative care across the age span, but which do not add to our knowledge in hypnosis for pediatric palliative care and are beyond the scope of this text (Brugnoli, 2015; Hain, Goldman, Rapoport, & Meiring 2021).

## Modification of the Disease Process

The idea that physiological and psychological processes are intertwined goes back many centuries. More recent reports document the association of psychological factors with a variety of children's diseases, including cancer (Greene & Miller, 1958; Jacobs & Charles, 1980). Because these are retrospective studies, the data are very difficult to interpret. For example, Jacobs and Charles (1980) emphasized that their review of life-stress events for children with cancer and with other illnesses must be interpreted only as contextual and not as causal. They also noted that a given event, such as parental divorce or change of residence, might be very stressful for one child but have little impact on another. Other important variables cited included the availability of social supports and the child's habitual coping skills. None of these factors has been adequately studied. Although we agree with the conclusion by Jacobs and Charles (1980) that the role of psychological factors as antecedents of childhood cancer remains a matter of conjecture, we also agree with their conclusion that there is a possibility that childhood cancer is a complex psychobiological phenomenon.

If psychological factors play a role in the development of cancer, then it is conceivable that psychological treatment might also affect the course and ultimate outcome of the disease. Recently, there has been a great deal of interest, especially in the press, in the possibility of using certain imagery techniques – which we would put in the general category of self-hypnosis – to affect the course of potentially terminal diseases, especially cancer. The technique consists of asking a patient to visualize some process in which cancer cells are destroyed and to focus on images of physical health and general well-being. The process is both appealing and benign to cancer patients, and some who have used it have gone on to make a good recovery from their disease with the aid of more traditional forms of treatment. The data are comprised of anecdotal reports, and prospective studies documenting causal relationships between these healing imagery techniques and positive therapeutic outcomes are lacking. Yet, despite the lack of any supporting scientific data, desperate cancer patients are increasingly asking their physicians for treatment by imagery techniques. These requests come not only from adult patients but also from pediatric cancer patients and their families. Particularly in a context of palliative care programs, such requests are both appropriate, and increasingly being met with a variety of therapeutic hypnosis interventions.

We respond to requests for imagery therapy; in the same way we respond to requests for other experimental forms of treatment. We tell our patients the nature of the available data, noting that, although we have no good scientific evidence that the method can affect the course of cancer, there is also no good evidence that it cannot do so. We say that the treatment has no known harmful effects, provided patients continue with other prescribed treatment such as radiation or chemotherapy. Further, although the treatment may have no effect on tumor growth, its use may have benefit in other ways. Patients who focus on positive ideation may become more hopeful, more motivated to get adequate nourishment and exercise, and more able to relax and get adequate rest. In such instances, patients can improve the quality of their lives even in the face of continued tumor growth.

For these reasons, we have provided [hypnotic] imagery therapy to patients who requested it and who have continued to show interest after hearing our cautionary remarks. Some have died; others continue to use the method with enthusiasm. Until further data are available, we will continue to use this approach to hypnotic imagery with patients who request it, always in the context of scientific integrity and modesty.

An example of the imagery method to combat cancer is cited from Olness' (1981) report of her work with cancer patients. A 13-year-old boy described his cancer cells as black knights lined up for attack, but they were smaller, weaker, and fewer in number than his healthy white blood cells, depicted as white knights. The white knights continually chopped up the black knights with daggers. The drugs were vicious beasts who supported the white knights in their attack. This patient thought about his imagery several times daily for 6 years. He was alive and well 35 years later.

Another of our patients was a 17-year-old boy who requested imagery therapy 4 years after losing an arm to cancer. He was well for 3 years after diagnosis and had achieved national ranking as a downhill skier with a disability. When he then developed multiple lung metastases, he underwent vigorous chemotherapy and began hypnotic imagery therapy several months later. He visualized himself in a downhill slalom race, increasing his feelings of love, safety, strength, health, and competence as he passed each flag on the course. Then he visualized feelings of physical, mental, and spiritual well-being held tightly in his hand and absorbed into his entire body. He enthusiastically practiced these and related techniques at least twice daily. His metastases disappeared, but he later suffered another relapse. He died about a year after beginning imagery therapy, having survived more than 5 years since initial diagnosis.

### *Modification of Patient's Ability to Respond with Mastery in the Dying Process*

There comes a time in the lives of some terminally ill children when it is clear to them that they will inevitably die because of their disease. The possibility and even the probability of dying have been stated directly by several of our young patients. One 4-year-old boy with leukemia said to his therapist, "Leukemia is a bad disease, and you could die from it." "Die?" "Yes, you just lie there and never wake up and you can't do anything anymore and then you are just bones." Another 4-year-old boy, who was losing his life-long battle against chronic granulomatous disease, said simply to his mother, "Mommy, I'm going to die."

Although denial is a common and frequently adaptive defense mechanism for children with life-threatening illness, as well as for their families and their doctors (LaBaw et al., 1975), it is also true that most of these children have quite an accurate understanding of their chances for survival. Families and doctors – more often than they would like to admit – are tempted to impose their own need for denial on the child, creating a maladaptive conspiracy of silence in which the child must bear the burden of dying alone; for example, a 12-year-old girl with a recently diagnosed inoperable brainstem tumor told her psychologist that she knew she would eventually die. When asked if she had talked about dying with her parents, she replied, "Oh, no. It would upset them too much."

Gardner (1977) outlined four basic rights of dying children. First is the right to know the truth about the probable outcome of their illness. Because most children have already figured it out for themselves, it would be more accurate to say "affirm the truth" rather than to imply that these children are learning it for the first time. Second is the right to share thoughts about dying – not just the probability of death but the many questions that follow: Does it hurt to die? Are your parents with you when they bury you? What do you wear when you get buried? If they bury you down in the ground, how do you get up to heaven? Third is the right to live as full and normal a life as possible, truly to live until they die. Fourth is the right to participate in the process of dying, to have input concerning whether treatment should be continued or stopped, to state a preference for dying in the hospital or at home, and so on. Not all children choose to exercise these rights, but we believe the option of choosing should be available to them.

We have found that therapeutic hypnosis can sometimes facilitate the process in which dying children exercise their rights. The mechanisms are occasionally direct – that is, interviewing the dying child in hypnosis concerning his or her problems. Much more often, therapeutic clinical hypnosis facilitates these goals indirectly. In such cases, the terminally ill child is usually first referred for therapeutic clinical hypnosis for some sort of specific symptomatic relief. A positive transference develops between the child and the therapist. In the context of a safe and trusting alliance, the child becomes more able to exercise his or her rights, usually with full parental support. After achieving initial symptom relief with the aid of hypnotic suggestion therapy, much of the work toward the larger goals of solving problems rather than enduring them may be done in the waking state, with clinical hypnosis utilized adjunctively as needed. Several case vignettes illustrate these direct and indirect processes.

D.M. Markowitz (pers. comm.) described to us his clinical hypnosis work with an intelligent adolescent boy on the day of his death from leukemia. In a waking interview the previous day, the boy had said he wanted to "write a will." He wanted to state what he would like done with some of his personal belongings, and he wanted to give some advice to his parents concerning how they should deal with their lives after his death. Unfortunately, he went into a coma before making the will. The following day, the clinician went to the boy's home, where he lay unconscious, and repeated a hypnotic induction (invitation) that he had used successfully on earlier occasions. He reminded the boy of his previously stated wish and told him that, if making a will was still important to him, he could become more alert, open his eyes, and dictate his thoughts to the therapist. In 90 seconds, the boy opened his eyes, and he then dictated to the therapist for nearly 2 hours, giving his skis to his father, his guitar to his sister, and so on. He then talked with his family for another 45 minutes, following which he relapsed into coma and died 3 hours later.

Becky S. was a 7-year-old girl in the end stages of cystic fibrosis, who was initially referred to us for clinical hypnosis to improve her tolerance of painful medical procedures such as fingersticks and tests of arterial blood gases. She achieved better pain control after one therapeutic hypnosis session and proudly told the therapist the next day that she had pricked her own finger. Some weeks later, during her terminal hospitalization, she complained to the therapist of diffuse anxiety, dizziness, and double vision. Recognizing the symptoms of hypoxia and noting the results of a recent blood-gas evaluation, the therapist asked the ward nurse whether the child could be given higher levels of oxygen. The nurse replied that the child was getting maximal oxygen through the nasal prongs she was using. She could get additional oxygen if she would use an oxygen mask instead of the nasal prongs, but she had refused suggestions from nurses and doctors that she wear a mask, apparently because she was afraid to have her face covered. The therapist returned to Becky's room and offered the same explanation and suggestion previously given by others. Becky immediately accepted the mask. The increased oxygen eliminated her hypoxic symptoms and allowed her to spend the evening cheerfully talking and playing with her family. It seemed that the context of the therapeutic hypnosis relationship allowed this child to make more constructive decisions about her own treatment. Working with an adolescent with cystic fibrosis, Anbar and Murthy (2010) described the effective use of hypnosis to re-establish hope in an adolescent with cystic fibrosis who was awaiting lung transportation.

LaClave and Blix (1989) described a case history of a 6-year-old girl with malignant astrocytoma who had severe vomiting. Therapeutic hypnosis was successful in resolving the vomiting, thus allowing chemotherapy to continue, and clinical hypnosis was also utilized for pain and anxiety. Despite significant neurological problems, the patient used audiotapes of clinical hypnosis sessions and was able to use visual imagery very effectively to create drawings reflecting her awareness and acceptance of dying. She used her hypnosis tapes effectively until she lapsed into a coma and later died.

Reaney (1994) described the inspiring story of Tommy, a young boy with immune deficiency and an overwhelming fungal infection, and the creative applications of hypnotherapeutic techniques he and his family learned and used to ease their experience of Tommy's dying. Kinesthetic therapeutic hypnosis images were especially important for Tommy. His favorite was the flying "home bed" that allowed him to dissociate from the intensive care unit; it provided a sense of safety and reduced the anxiety that had increased as illness led to blindness in the last weeks of life. In addition to teaching pain and anxiety control with switch imagery and rocking, the therapist integrated his own and the family's strong spiritual and religious beliefs into the therapeutic hypnotic suggestions by preparing audiotapes of personalized spiritual songs and hymns for Tommy. This sensitive and creative use of auditory imagery was a source of comfort and strength for Tommy and his family before, during, and after his death.

Joanne, 17 years old, was in end-stage respiratory failure from cystic fibrosis when her family arranged the trip to Europe that she had always wanted. Though the trip was shortened by increasing respiratory difficulty, she was able to enjoy more than a week of sightseeing, which she and her family thought was exhilarating. After the trip was cut short, she was immediately hospitalized. Within a few days, she expressed the decision that she have no further treatment and was ready to die. Even though some members of the healthcare team thought she might benefit from "resting" on a ventilator for a few days, she declined, and her family respected her wishes. She did not wish to suffer, however, and, though I had never previously met her I was asked to consult to see if hypnosis could help her relax during her last hours or days.

When I (DK) came to see her, the room was dark except for slight backlighting at the head of Joanne's bed. Her sister and mother sat quietly in chairs at the side and foot of the bed. When I introduced myself, they indicated they knew I'd be coming and said that I should just proceed as though they weren't there, and they continued their respective reading with their backs to me and Joanne. As I approached the right side of Joanne's bed, she seemed oblivious to me as she lay motionless in her bed, severely air hungry with an oxygen hood over her head, her face puffy and with an expression that exuded stress, fatigue, sadness, and helplessness. I touched her right hand gently as I said her name and told her mine. She turned so she could see me and opened her eyes. I asked if she knew I was coming, and she said she did. Her shortness of breath permitted no more than two or three words per breath. I told her that I needed to know one or two things and that after that she didn't need to talk except in her imagination, and I would do the talking. She smiled. I told her I heard she'd just been to Europe. At first, she smiled and then tears appeared as she told me the trip had to be cut short. This was quickly reframed to at once acknowledge that and to shift to asking what her favorite part of the trip had been. Slowly she told me of the beauty of the mountains of Switzerland. Recognizing her spontaneous state of hypnosis, I asked her if it would be okay to just be there in Switzerland and not be here. She smiled and closed her eyes. Multisensory imagery suggestions were offered to deepen the trance, and suggestions were given for being able to be totally there, knowing that everything here was being taken care of by her doctors and nurses and family and friends. Assurances of safety and comfort and not being alone were given as she was given explicit suggestions to be there as long and as much as she needed and wanted to. Her respiratory rate slowed and breathing became less labored. Over Joanne's next and final two days, the family did not permit any further therapeutic hypnosis visits as they gathered to say good-bye. Though there had been only this single formal or "official" clinical hypnosis session, Joanne's nurses reported that they reinforced suggestions of dissociation and comfort and that her last hours seemed easier as a result.

Remke (2005) and Russell and Smart (2007) added their clinical experience to our understanding of finding the hypnosis in the encounter – that is, using hypnosis and spontaneous imagery to help provide comfort at the end of life. Russell and Smart described their effective use of imagery to relieve spasms, control pain, enhance comfort during the repeated insertion of nasogastric tubes, improve sleep, and reduce anxiety in four children: a 12-year-old boy with a brain tumor, a 5-year-old girl in respite care, a 15-year-old with severe spasms, and a 13-year-old boy receiving end-of-life care.

Steven T., a 10-year-old boy, also in the end stages of cystic fibrosis, was referred to us for hypnosis because of depression and decreased tolerance of medical procedures, including postural drainage and intravenous infusions. He would resist and cry, asking the medical staff members why they continued these painful treatments when they knew as well as he did that he was going to die anyway. In the first clinical hypnosis session, Steven quickly learned self-hypnosis to control pain and to decrease his anxiety about being unable to get enough air during postural drainage treatments that resulted in prolonged and violent coughing. He was also able to clarify that he really did want continued treatment, because he wanted to live as long as possible, and he asked that the nurses ignore his pleas when his frustration resulted in "temper tantrum" behavior. He immediately developed a strong positive alliance with the therapist. His mother concurrently responded well to brief counseling from the therapist and to more extensive therapy from her social worker.

In a later, nonhypnotic psychotherapy session, Steven openly discussed his concerns about dying, especially his awareness that vigorous antibiotic therapy was no longer producing significant improvement in his pulmonary status. The therapist introduced a "life and death" game in an effort to modify the boy's increasing obsession with dying. Outlining a "life circle" and a "death circle" on a sheet of white paper, the therapist showed Steven two crayons, red and green, stating that life was to be represented by the color green and death by the color red. She then affirmed that treatment was of decreasing value and sometime soon would be of no value at all. She stressed that someday the doctors would have no more "life" (treatment) to give Steven and could offer him [only] a relatively comfortable death, with medications as needed for pain or anxiety. She then removed the green crayon, illustrating the problem. Steven said he still wanted life, and he asked for the green crayon so that he could color the life circle green. The therapist reminded him that she had no more green to give him, and she challenged him to create green by himself. Steven quickly saw that his only option at this point in the game was to color the death circle red. As he worked at the task, the therapist encouraged him to look at death, to acknowledge death. Then, using the principle of complementary colors, the therapist asked Steven to look again at the life circle. It turned green before his eyes.

Both amazed and amused, Steven saw conceptually as well as graphically, that he could take some responsibility for his own experience by acknowledging death and then setting it aside to create a more enjoyable life. He proceeded to arrange a pre-birthday party for himself in the hospital, instead of continuing to worry that he might not live another month until his 11th birthday. This being successful, he arranged a second pre-birthday party when he went to visit relatives. Then, on his actual birthday, he enjoyed still a third party.

In many other ways, Steven created life for himself. Shortly before he died, he made a new contract with hospital staff to the effect that he could refuse postural drainage if he wished and have narcotic medication when he requested it, all knowing that this was now his terminal hospitalization. Supported by his family, he spent his last days relating to them and to the hospital staff members, for many of whom he had become a favorite patient. On the night before he died, he requested and fully enjoyed a special dinner sent in from a local restaurant. For Steven, the initial use of strategic clinical hypnosis seemed to facilitate this dying child's ability to exercise all four of his basic rights. To a large extent he shifted his approach to the task of dying from helpless frustration to mastery and control.

In a recent publication (Friedrichsdorf & Kohen, 2018), I (DK) described three cases of children and teens with cystic fibrosis whom I had the privilege to know and from whom I had the good fortune to learn so much about living and dying. As I was preparing to begin writing the manuscript and case descriptions, I realized that it was now obvious to me that their stories could best be told by them, and not so much by me. Accordingly in addition to my copious notes about who had said what to whom at each visit, I asked that they write about their experiences with their cystic fibrosis and the details of how they utilized hypnosis to provide them with the comfort that they wanted and needed. In updating this chapter, I just reviewed their words again and was reminded of the depth of our clinical relationships; and of the mixture of joy and sadness as I recall the sense of wonder and faith I continue to have in the power and creativity of the human spirit. Rather than attempt to abstract any of the three stories, I invite the reader to obtain this manuscript and get to know them through their own words (Friedrichsdorf & Kohen, 2018).

## *Therapeutic Hypnosis in the Broadest Context of Experience*

Recent developments in holistic medicine and palliative care have substantially changed the way we treat children with life-threatening illness. Rather than directing efforts only at the disease process, we now appropriately emphasize the need for simultaneous attention to the physical, psychological, and spiritual needs of the patient and the family and the involved community (Booth, 2020; Friedrichsdorf et al., 2007; Himelstein, 2006; Whittam, 1993).

As compared with the narrower area of symptom relief, it is even more difficult to assess the precise or specific value of therapeutic clinical hypnosis in palliative care medicine. We can speculate that clinical hypnosis may have an impact on several interrelated areas. For the child, it can [help to] provide (1) symptom relief; (2) decreased anxiety, depression, passivity, and helplessness; (3) enhanced ego functions, especially feelings of safety, trust, hope, autonomy, competence, initiative, humor, reality testing, self-esteem, dignity, and grace; and (4) increased ability to relate positively to others in age-appropriate ways. For the family, it can provide (1) reduced feelings of anxiety and impotence; (2) increased ability to relate to the child and to offer comfort and reassurance, rather than to engage in defensive withdrawal; (3) increased ability to make constructive use of community resources such as friends and clergy; and (4) increased ability to deal creatively with the loss of a child, using the grief process in the service of personal growth. For the community, it can instill (1) increased responsiveness to the greater receptivity of the child and the family, (2) increased awareness of the value of such responsiveness, and (3) offer the opportunity for participation in healing (e.g., prayer circles, "Caring Bridge" participation (www.caringbridge.com).

Every one of these areas affects all others, each making its own contribution, perhaps including enhancing the child's ability to use therapeutic hypnosis, thus coming full circle in a complex set of causal relationships. Although the formal use of clinical hypnosis may appear to serve limited functions, it can interact with other resources of the child, the family, and the community to facilitate growth and mastery, and as such utilizing emotional upheaval in the service of attaining higher levels of ego integration.

We do not mean to overvalue the role of therapeutic clinical hypnosis but rather to recognize an entire spectrum of possible actions and reactions in the total experience of a dying child who uses this treatment modality. In the context of perceiving therapeutic hypnosis as one resource among many, each affecting the others in the broadest context of experience, we refer the reader to the third edition of this text for a detailed accounting of the previously published story of the child, David

(Gardner, 1976; Olness & Kohen, 1996). The authors again express their appreciation to David's parents for their assistance in the preparation of the material in the third edition and especially for their permission to include excerpts of a family tape recording.

At the 37th Annual Workshops in Clinical Hypnosis of the Minnesota Society of Clinical Hypnosis and Department of Pediatrics, University of Minnesota, Dr. Leora Kuttner presented a highly informative and profoundly inspiring 2-day advanced pediatric hypnosis workshop entitled "Embracing Life: Using Hypnosis During Palliative Care and Bereavement." Amidst all of the wonderful teaching and experiential learning, several salient features stand out. Kuttner (2008) taught that hypnosis has the potential to help at the end of life by working with paradox, by developing personal metaphor, by sustaining and promoting hope, by curtailing uncertainty and fear, by playing with possibilities, by envisioning optimal outcomes, by revealing personal truths, and by motivating to complete unfinished business. She suggested that we understand that clinical therapeutic hypnosis is in fact different at the end of life. Kuttner noted that spontaneous trance states occur when death nears, and children become quieter, more withdrawn, dissociated, and "spacey"; patients often report spontaneous vivid trance or dream experiences about their impending journey; and physiological changes may restrict the options available for hypnotic invitation (induction) or intensifying the trance in conventional ways (e.g., motor, energy, or breathing compromises). Kuttner also teaches us through her award-winning documentary, *Making Every Moment Count* (Kuttner, 2003). This film embodies the foregoing principles of palliative care and the ways in which caregivers, family, and patients alike use both spontaneous and planned, rehearsed self-hypnosis to facilitate comfort, not only for the dying but also for the bereaved.

Deutsch (2009), in an advanced pediatric hypnosis workshop at the 51st Annual Workshops of the American Society of Clinical Hypnosis, viewed and discussed an inspiring videotape of family therapeutic hypnosis for and with a dying child and her parents. Evident in the moving video were the clinician (Deutsch) joining with the child to help her find and use her spontaneous hypnosis, going with her to sometimes pace and sometimes lead, and then the poignant joining with the bereaved mother, reflecting hypnosis in the encounter facilitating her grieving process.

## Conclusion

Although therapeutic hypnosis seems to be valuable for many children with life-threatening illness and for their families, in some instances it is of limited value or none at all. Some children and parents simply refuse this treatment modality. Other children eagerly embark on learning hypnotic skills only to fail, for known and unknown reasons. Still other children respond well to therapeutic clinical hypnosis intervention for one purpose but not for another, or they respond well at one time and poorly at another. We still have a great deal to learn about potential uses of clinical hypnosis with dying children. How do we help them maximize their use of hypnotic talent? What are the limits of the possible uses of therapeutic hypnosis? How can we best facilitate the interaction of clinical hypnosis with many other forms of integrative pediatric medicine, surgical, and psychological treatment?

Child health professionals who utilize clinical hypnosis with dying children must also consider issues related to their own involvement. The therapeutic hypnosis relationship is characterized by more intense emotional responses, not only in the patient but also in the therapist. When working with dying children, the active clinician must be able to deal with his or her own reactions to loss and with the emotional stress of personal involvement, combining human caring with professional objectivity in such a way that the result is positive not only for the child and the family but also for the therapist. A paper on bereavement by Penson, Green, Chabner, and Lynch (2002) does not mention imagery or hypnosis as it presents a dialogue among caregivers regarding vignettes of two different deaths in their center. The manuscript ends, however, with the following:

> Grief for loss is an inevitable part of everyone's life. People cope, or fail to cope, in diverse ways. Bereavement may be one of the hardest tasks for health professionals confronted with the limitations of our endeavors. Medical staff have a responsibility to provide grieving families with support and care; care that goes beyond the death. A compassionate response helps both those who suffer and those who care.

Kuttner (2007) summarized that hypnosis helps develop personal metaphors that can "(1) transform anxiety, pain, uncertainty, and despair; (2) work with the paradox of living fully until one dies; (3) sustain hope; and (4) maximize opportunities and possibilities" (p. 464). We believe that therapeutic clinical hypnosis is one means through which both those who suffer and those who care can indeed be helped. In Kuttner's workshop (2008), an experiential exercise drawn from the work of Kearney (1996) gives the caregiver a taste of the near-death/dying process through hypnotic imagery. This powerful experience, along with viewing our colleagues' wonderful work on video (Deutsch, 2009; Kuttner, 2003), can go a long way toward developing the compassionate response described.

## References


Anbar, R.D. & Murthy, V.V. (2010). Reestablishment of hope as an intervention for a patient with cystic fibrosis awaiting lung transplantation. *The Journal of Alternative and Complementary Medicine, 16*(9), 1007–1010.

Booth, S. (2020). Hypnosis in a specialist palliative care setting – enhancing personalized care for difficult symptoms and situations. *Palliative Care and Social Practice, 14*, 1–11.

Brugnoli, M.P. (2015). *Clinical Hypnosis in Pain Therapy and Palliative Care: A Handbook of Techniques for Improving the Patient's Physical and Psychological Well-Being*. Springfield, IL: Charles C. Thomas Publisher Caring Bridge. www.caringbridge.com

Connor, S.R., Downing, J., & Marston, J. (2017). Estimating the global needs for pediatric palliative care for children: a cross-sectional analysis. *Journal of Pain and Symptom Management, 53*, 171–177.

Crasilneck, H.B. & Hall, J.A. (1973). Clinical hypnosis in problems of pain. *American Journal of Clinical Hypnosis, 15*, 153–161.

Crasilneck, H.B. & Hall, J.A. (1975). *Clinical Hypnosis: Principles and Applications*. New York: Grune & Stratton.

Deutsch, R. (2009). Helping kids and family members help themselves with hypnosis: coping with life-threatening, palliative and end-of-life experiences. *Videotape and Presentation to Advanced Pediatric Hypnosis Workshop, 51st Annual Workshops*. Boston, MA: American Society of Clinical Hypnosis.

Duncan, J., Spengler, E., & Wolfe, J. (2007). Providing pediatric palliative care: pact in action. *MCN: The American Journal of Maternal/Child Nursing, 32*, 279–287.

Erickson, M.H. (1958). Pediatric hypnotherapy. *American Journal of Clinical Hypnosis, 1*, 25–29.

Fenton, L.J. (2019). Clinical hypnosis and hypnotic language in pediatric palliative care. *NHPCO Pediatric E-Journal, 56*, 42–45.

Finlay, I.G. & Jones, O.L. (1996). Hypnotherapy in palliative care. *Journal of the Royal Society of Medicine, 89*, 493–496.

Friedrichsdorf, S.J. & Kang, T.I. (2007). The management of pain in children with life-limiting illnesses. *Pediatric Clinics of North America, 54*, 645–672.

Friedrichsdorf, S.J. & Kohen, D.P. (2018). Integration of hypnosis into pediatric palliative care. *Annals of Palliative Medicine*, 7(1), 136–150. 10.21037/apm.2017.05.02

Friedrichsdorf, S.J., Remke, S., Symnalla, B., Gibbon, C., & Chrastek, J. (2007). Developing a pain and palliative care programme at a U.S. children's hospital. *International Journal of Palliative Nursing, 13*, 534–542.

Gardner, G.G. (1976). Childhood, death, and human dignity: hypnotherapy for David. *International Journal of Clinical and Experimental Hypnosis*, *24*, 122–139.
Gardner, G.G. (1977). The rights of dying children: some personal reflections. *Psychotherapy Bulletin*, *10*, 20–23.
Greene, W.A. Jr. & Miller, G. (1958). Psychological factors and reticuloen-dothelial disease. IV. Observations on a group of children and adolescents with leukemias: an interpretation of disease development. *Psychosomatic Medicine*, *10*, 124–144.
Gregoire, C., Chantrain, C., Faymonville, M.-E., Marini, J., & Bragard, I. (2019). A hypnosis based group intervention to improve quality of life in children with cancer and their parents. *International Journal of Clinical and Experimental Hypnosis*, *67*(2), 117–135.
Grollman, E. (1991). *Talking about Death: A Dialogue between Parent and Child*. Boston: Beacon Press.
Hain, R., Goldman, A., Rapoport, A., & Meiring, M. (Eds). (2021). *Oxford Textbook Palliative Care for Children*, 3rd ed. Oxford, UK: Oxford University Press.
Harper, G.W. (1999). A developmentally sensitive approach to clinical hypnosis for chronically and terminally ill adolescents. *American Journal of Clinical Hypnosis*, *42*, 50–60.
Heath, J.A., Clarke, N.E., Donath, S.M., McCarthy, M., Anderson, V.A., & Wolfe, J. (2010). Symptoms and suffering at the end of life in children with cancer: an Australian perspective. *Medical Journal of Australia*, *192*, 71–75.
Hilgard, J.R. & Morgan, A.H. (1978). Treatment of anxiety and pain in childhood cancer through hypnosis. In F.H. Frankel & H.S. Zamansky, Eds., *Hypnosis at Its Bicentennial: Selected Papers*. New York: Plenum Press.
Himelstein, B.P. (2006). Palliative care for infants, children, adolescents, and their families. *Journal of Palliative Medicine*, *1*, 163–181. 10.1089/jpm.2006.9.163
Jacobs, T.J. & Charles, E. (1980). Life events and the occurrence of cancer in children. *Psychosomatic Medicine*, *42*, 11–24.
Katz, E.R., Kellerman, J., & Siegel, S.E. (1980). Behavioral distress in children with cancer undergoing medical procedures: developmental considerations. *Journal of Consulting and Clinical Psychology*, *48*, 356–365.
Kearney, M. (1996). *Mortally Wounded: Stories of Soul Pain Death & Healing*. New York: Scribner.
Kohen, D.P. (1995). Childhood grief and mourning: applications of hypnotherapy. Paper presented at the Annual Workshops of the Minnesota Society of Clinical Hypnosis, Minneapolis, MN.
Kübler-Ross, E. (1969). *On Death and Dying*. New York: Macmillan.
Kübler-Ross, E. (1974). *Questions and Answers on Death and Dying*. New York: Macmillan.
Kuttner, L. Director/Producer. (2003). *Making Every Moment Count*, 38-minute documentary available from The National Film Board of Canada (1-800-267-7710; 1-800-542-2164).
Kuttner, L. (2007). Hypnosis and palliative care. In W.C. Wester II and L.I. Sugarman, Eds., *Therapeutic Hypnosis with Children and Adolescents* (pp. 453–466). Bethel, CT: Crown House Publishing.
Kuttner, L. (2008). *Embracing Life: Using Hypnosis during Palliative Care and Bereavement*. Presented at 2-day Advanced Workshop 37th Annual Workshops in Clinical Hypnosis, Minnesota Society of Clinical Hypnosis and Department of Pediatrics, University of Minnesota.
Kuttner, L. & Friedrichsdorf, S.J. (2014). Hypnosis and palliative care for children and their families (Chapter 20). In L.I. Sugarman and W.C. Wester II, Eds., *Therapeutic Hypnosis with Children and Adolescents*. UK: Crowne House Publishers.
LaBaw, W.L., Holton, C., Tewell, K., & Eccles, D. (1975). The use of self-hypnosis by children with cancer. *American Journal of Clinical Hypnosis*, *17*, 223–238.
LaClave, L. & Blix, S. (1989). Hypnosis in the management of symptoms in a young girl with malignant astrocytoma: a challenge to the therapist. *International Journal of Clinical and Experimental Hypnosis*, *37*(1), 6–14.
LeBaron, S. & Zeltzer, L. (1985). The role of imagery in the treatment of dying children and adolescents. *Journal of Developmental Behavioral Pediatrics*, *6*, 252–258.
Liossi, C. & White, P. (2001). Efficacy of clinical hypnosis in the enhancement of quality of life of terminally ill cancer patients. *Contemporary Hypnosis*, *18*, 145–160.
Markowitz, D.M. (1980). *Personal communication*.
McSherry, M., Kehoe, K., Carroll, J.M., Kang, T.I., & Rourke, M.T. (2007). Psychosocial and spiritual needs of children living with a life-limiting illness. *Pediatric Clinics of North America*, *54*, 609–629.

Miles, M. (1971). *Annie and the Old One*. Boston, MA: Little, Brown.
O'Connell, S. (1985). Hypnosis in terminal care: discussion paper. *Journal of the Royal Society of Medicine*, *78*, 122–125.
Olness, K. (1981). Imagery (self-hypnosis) as adjunct care in childhood cancer: clinical experience with 25 patients. *American Journal of Pediatric Hematology/Oncology*, *3*, 313–321.
Olness, K. & Hall, M. (1985). Behavioral considerations in leukemia management. In C. Pochedley, Ed., *Acute Lymphoid Leukemia in Children*. New York: Masson Publishing.
Olness, K. & Kohen, D.P. (1996). *Hypnosis and Hypnotherapy with Children*,3rd ed. New York: The Guilford Press.
Olness, K. & Singher, L. (1989). Five-year follow-up of 61 children taught cyber-physiologic strategies as adjunct management in cancer. *Topics in Pediatrics*, 7, 2–6.
Penson, R., Green, K., Chabner, B., & Lynch, T. (2002). When does the responsibility of our care end: bereavement? *Oncologist*, 7(3), 251–258.
Reaney, J. (1994). Tommy's blankets and flying bed: hypnosis and a dying child. Paper presented at the Asia-Pacific Congress of Hypnosis, Cairns, North Queensland, Australia.
Remke, S. (2005). Using spontaneous imagery with children at end of life to promote comfort. *Biofeedback*, *33*(2), 58–62.
Russell, C. & Smart, S. (2007). Guided imagery and distraction therapy in pediatric hospice care. *Pediatric Nursing*, *19*, 24–25.
Steele, R., Bosma, H., Johnston, M., Cadell, S., Davies, B., Siden, H., & Straatman, L. (2008). Research priorities in pediatric palliative care: a Delphi study. *Journal of Palliative Care*, *24*, 229–239.
Viorst, J. (1971). *The Tenth Good Thing about Barney*. New York: Atheneum.
Weekly, T., Walker, N., Beck, J., Akers, S., & Weaver, M. (2018). A review of apps for calming, relaxation, and mindfulness interventions for pediatric palliative care patients. *Children*, *5*(2), 16. Special Issue Pediatric Palliative Care (/journal/children/special_issues/palliative_care) 10.3390/children5020016
White, E.B. (1952). *Charlotte's Web*. New York: HarperCollins.
Whittam, E.H. (1993). Terminal care of the dying child: psychosocial implications of care. *Cancer*, *71*, 3450–3462.

# 16

# BIOFEEDBACK, OTHER MIND–BODY INTERVENTIONS, AND HYPNOSIS WITH CHILDREN

## Introduction

Biofeedback is a useful form of adjunctive therapy for many biobehavioral problems in children and adolescents (Moss, Cyr, & Culbert, 2005). *Biofeedback* refers to information about specific physiological responses in humans. The child or adolescent can observe this information and practice changing his or her thinking to effect a desired change in the response. A blood pressure monitor, an oral thermometer, or a bathroom scale are examples of biofeedback instruments.

The study of biofeedback began when Miller (1969) described operant conditioning of autonomic nervous system functions such as heart rate, blood pressure, intestinal motility, urine production rate, and gastric and peripheral blood flow in the curarized rat (Schwartz & Olson, 2003). Subsequently, a great deal of optimism led to predictions that humans, via self-monitoring devices, would be able to self-regulate many autonomic functions. Hundreds of studies have documented that certain types of biofeedback are useful for certain clinical problems (Basmajian, 1989; Brown, 1974; Olton & Noonberg, 1980); however, several studies using false biofeedback have been associated with positive clinical results (Andrasik & Holroyd, 1980; Mullinix, Norton, Hack, & Fishman, 1978). Smith (1991) noted that, "The application of biofeedback may be useful in many clinical conditions, although there appear to be few conditions in which biofeedback is demonstrably superior to other behavioral techniques, such as relaxation training, hypnosis, or meditation."

It is noteworthy that training manuals provided with biofeedback equipment invariably state that relaxation imagery or therapeutic hypnosis should be used in the training process. Although it is useful in certain clinical conditions (e.g., Raynaud's disease, hypertension) to receive immediate feedback of peripheral temperature or blood pressure, long-term improvement related to biofeedback does require home practice of self-hypnosis-type exercises. Although reductions in costs and computerization of biofeedback devices now make it possible for many families to purchase the equipment for home use, having biofeedback equipment available will change nothing unless active, regular mental rehearsals are employed. A number of prospective, controlled studies with children naïve to therapeutic hypnosis or biofeedback have documented their ability to intentionally change a number of autonomic responses. A study by Dikel and Olness (1980) documented the ability of children to increase and decrease peripheral temperature with a few minutes of mental effort. Other studies include documentation that children can intentionally change auditory evoked potentials

DOI: 10.4324/9781003243687-18

(Hogan, MacDonald, & Olness, 1985), tissue oxygen measures (Olness & Conroy, 1985), blood pressure (Kohen & Ondich, 2004), electrodermal activity (Olness & Rusin, 1990), and muscle responses, including anorectal function (Olness, McParland, & Piper, 1980).

Lee and Olness (1995) demonstrated that intentional changes in imagery are associated with measurable changes in physiological responses such as heart rate, peripheral temperature, and electrodermal activity, although children may not be receiving any direct feedback. This is consistent with the work of Wang and Morgan (1992), who found that athletes demonstrate changes in physiological measures when they are imagining a sports activity that are equivalent to those when they are actually participating in the sport. The magnitude may relate to genetics or unrecognized conditioning experiences. It may prove to be important clinically to know how children respond physiologically to ordinary changes in thinking; for example, if thinking of something active such as riding a bicycle causes blood pressure to increase, it might be useful to coach a child (with biofeedback) to reverse this response.

## Clinical Applications with Children

We use biofeedback very often in the course of teaching self-hypnosis. It provides an excellent teaching device to help children understand that, by changing their thinking process, they cause changes in their body and that they can be in control of that. The use of appealing biofeedback can help a child to concentrate attention and focus, to cultivate self-awareness, to increase the internal locus of control, and to learn conditioned relaxation. Emphasis on the child's mastery and coping ability is the central theme in hypnosis, and this is facilitated by adjunctive biofeedback. We use biofeedback often when the clinical problem has no relationship to the specific type of feedback – for example, temperature feedback or electrodermal activity for enuresis. In such situations, the biofeedback response functions (we believe) as a metaphor for the concept that concentration on mental imagery can effect physiological change.

We find that monitoring multiple autonomic responses concurrently gives us useful information about the child. Although there are no standards for autonomic measures such as electromyographic, electrodermal, or peripheral temperature changes in children, we note that children seem to have an autonomic "fingerprint" or "stress profile." This is consistent with the studies of infants by Kagan (1994). Some children show extremely labile responses in all measures, some show lability in the heart rate but not in electrodermal activity, and others have autonomic measures that are very stable. Children have also been shown to vary in immunological reactivity. Inasmuch as immune cells have numerous receptors for neurotransmitters associated with autonomic responses, it is possible that other autonomic measures may be surrogate measures for immune reactivity. We hope that further studies of these autonomic "fingerprints" will be done because such information may be relevant to diagnosis and treatment procedures in hospitals or clinics, to prevention programs, to the anticipatory guidance provided by pediatricians, to how one prepares a child for a new situation such as the beginning of school, or to coaching and teaching strategies for a given child.

Biofeedback programs for children have been established in many hospitals and clinics. A biofeedback-assisted relaxation training (BART) program for children was established in the gastroenterology section at Children's Mercy Hospitals and Clinics in 2004 (Grayson, 2009). The program included autogenic training, progressive muscle relaxation, diaphragmatic breathing strategies, guided imagery, visualization, and "special place" techniques. The wording of the relaxation exercises was modified for two age groups: 8–12 years and 13–18 years. It is noteworthy that the techniques are the same ones that are used in teaching children self-hypnosis. The program at Children's Mercy Hospitals and Clinics involved weekly sessions for the first month and every other week for an additional 2 months. Biofeedback modalities include surface electromyography, peripheral skin temperature, and skin conductance. A stress profile is established during the first biofeedback session. Christie (2009) described the integration of biofeedback into a pediatric neuroscience department in Texas. Children and adolescents may receive biofeedback for conditions such as migraine, tension-type headaches, Tourette's syndrome, anxiety, pain, pseudoseizures, insomnia, and complex regional pain syndrome (CRPS). Biofeedback and hypnosis are also used to prepare children for surgery such as deep brain stimulation for children with dystonia. This program emphasizes that children learn to take control of their symptoms.

## Biofeedback Equipment

We designed and developed a mind–body machine, a biofeedback unit that reflected electrodermal activity and had a touch screen. It was located in the Cleveland Health Science Museum for 10 years and was used by thousands of school children who enjoyed the opportunity to make the animal of their choice smile (Bear, Fish, Dinosaur, Tiger) when they relaxed.

Biofeedback equipment can be very simple and inexpensive. Various types of small liquid crystal monitors, such as Biodots®, and stress testing cards that vary color with surface temperature changes, are available and may be given to children to take home to aid their self-hypnosis practice. These small units change color to reflect temperature changes, which is appealing to children. They can be applied to fingers, hands, or wrists and provide feedback during therapy or throughout the day. One manufacturer is StressStop.com.

Thought Technology (http://www.thought-technology.com) began developing simple biofeedback instruments in the 1970s and is now one of the leading companies in biofeedback. Its ProComp hardware systems vary in complexity and can be used for research or clinical work. They provide platforms for many new applications with the capacity to monitor multiple physiologic responses concurrently. Applications change or are updated frequently but include games that appeal to children, including those focused on neurofeedback. Some of these games allow children choose a particular character to move around the computer screen, such as a race car driver, a spy flying a stealth plane, a submarine in a secret mission, a clown fish, or a super hero. Thought technology still sells two of its early products (GSR/Temp (provides auditory feedback) and GSR2/Temp (adds visual feedback). The product includes relaxation instructions, is very portable and can be adapted to provision of computer feedback as we did with the mind body machine.

HeartMath® (www.heartmath.com) offers biofeedback programs that are appealing to both adults and children. The emWavePro system for Mac or Windows monitors heart-rate variability and gives children the opportunity to choose among a balloon traveling over a beautiful landscape, a rainbow that flows from the upper computer screen down to a pot of gold which then spills out coins, or a nature scene that fills with color and animals as the child relaxes. A child's performance can be saved from practice session to practice session, so children can see their progress if they wish. The software can be installed on small laptops, and the emWave2 standalone unit can fit in a pocket, so both products are portable and easy to use. Inner Balance is the newer program monitoring heart rate variability for use with Android and iPhones and available with both Bluetooth and wired systems. A child psychiatrist, knowledgeable of language and culture in Kosovo, took a small laptop with the Heart Math program to help children who had posttraumatic stress disorder after the war. She noted that the Freeze-Framer was the most helpful intervention she had for these traumatized children. It gave them the sense of personal control that they so much needed.

Bio-Medical Instruments (carries a wide variety of biofeedback and neurofeedback equipment and software, some of which is appealing to children. We have found that games enhance initial interest but that children will later request a new game. Some of the computer biofeedback programs provide the option of printing out a summary of the child's performance. Phone apps such as Inner Balance record performance and provide the learner with graphs that compare sessions. This has appeal for older children who enjoy comparing their performance from one practice session to another. Culbert (2017) has noted that technology-assisted relaxation devices have been designed to harness the same power, absorption, and fun of the electronic games children so much enjoy, but for health reasons rather than strictly entertainment. The Association for Applied Psychophysiology and Biofeedback (www.aapb.org) is the best central source for obtaining more information about education in biofeedback for health professionals.

The following sections provide examples of how biofeedback can be used clinically. They are not intended to be all inclusive.

## Migraine

Many controlled studies have documented the efficacy of nonpharmacological methods, including hypnosis and biofeedback, in the management of juvenile migraine (Burke & Andrasik, 1989; Olness, MacDonald, & Uden, 1987; Osterhaus et al., 1993; Smith, Womack, & Pertik, 1987). Nonetheless, children continue to receive medications that have not been adequately studied. When offering nonpharmacological methods to children with migraine, we may offer hypnosis alone or a combination of hypnosis and biofeedback. We are unaware of any specific mechanism by which learning to increase peripheral temperature or electrodermal activity or heart rate will interrupt the cascade of internal events that end with a migraine headache. Nonetheless, many children with migraine enjoy recognizing that they are intentionally changing various autonomic parameters. Inasmuch as migraine is a biological disorder and the triggers for symptoms may be multiple, it is possible that the regular practice of self-hypnosis with an emphasis on relaxation may prevent some internal physiological response that sets off the symptom cascade. This may be true for other chronic conditions such as asthma, hemophilia, or sickle cell disease.

Koechlin and colleagues reported a network meta-analysis on nonpharmacological interventions for pediatric migraine (Koechlin et al., 2021). They reviewed 12 studies including 576 subjects and concluded that biofeedback, relaxation, psychological treatments, and psychological placebos were significantly more effective than waiting list with effect sizes between SMD = 1.14 for long-term psychological placebos to SMD = 1.44 for short-term self-administered treatments.

Osterhaus and colleagues (1993) reported on combined behavioral therapy for school children with migraine. This included relaxation training defined as progressive relaxation, autogenic relaxation, and relaxation based on self-hypnosis. It also included temperature feedback and rational emotive therapy to reduce tension. Each of 32 children was seen eight times, four times in individual and four times in group therapy. They observed a rise in finger temperature during each successive biofeedback session (from 1.3 to 2.9°C). Undoubtedly, this reflected success in relaxation practice, for this phenomenon is evident in children doing self-hypnosis practice regardless of the presenting problem. Because side effects from pharmacologic prevention of migraine may be significant, we believe that nonpharmacological methods are treatments of choice. We recommend that all children with migraine have the opportunity to learn self-hypnosis with biofeedback. The biofeedback experience gives the child recognition of the connection between changes in thinking and changes in body responses and also enhances the child's sense of personal mastery.

## Complex Regional Pain Syndrome

This pain disorder is diagnosed by taking a detailed history and doing a careful physical examination. Most children report some injury before the onset of the typical symptoms. Children and adolescents with this problem often have significant peripheral temperature differentials between the affected and non-affected extremities. Sympathetic and parasympathetic signals are irregular or abnormal, causing the uncomfortable symptoms of edema, pain, and sometimes numbness. Pain is often described as tingling, burning, or electric shock-like. We have reported eight children and adolescents who responded well to training in self-hypnosis with biofeedback (Olness, 1990). As they practiced temperature control and observed their ability to achieve this, they gained more confidence that they could participate in their own treatment. Children with complex regional pain syndrome (CRPS) also benefit from intense physical therapy to prevent muscle wasting.

Thomson reported a case history of a 17-year-old girl with CRPS that developed after a field hockey injury (Thomson, 2022). After four years of limited success with treatments including occupational and physical therapy and steroids, she was referred for hypnosis. CRPS impacted every area of her life. She had to give up sports and dancing and could not tolerate car trips due to the vibration. After only four sessions of hypnosis she had nearly complete resolution of her symptoms. Thomas taught her age regression to remember her skills prior to the injury and then to imagine a time in the future with symptoms resolved. We recommend that all children with this problem be referred early for a trial of hypnosis with or without biofeedback.

## Raynaud's Disease

Raynaud's disease is another disorder of imbalance between sympathetic and parasympathetic nervous system tone resulting in vasoconstriction and cold extremities. Again, skin temperature feedback provides direct proof to the child or adolescent that he or she is succeeding in increasing peripheral temperature. The use of inexpensive, portable monitors such as GSR/Temp or Biodots is especially useful as an adjunct to the home practice of self-hypnosis for this problem.

## Cerebral Palsy

A study of 19 young people (8–18 years old) who completed 4-weeks training with a home-based video game controlled by their electromyographic responses found moderate improvement in body function measures. Seventy-four percent of participants reached their self-identified practice goals (MacIntosh, Desailly, Vignais, Vigneron, & Biddiss, 2020). There are also clinical reports of children with cerebral palsy who reduce symptoms with self-hypnosis practice (Mauersbeger et al., 2000).

## Neurofeedback

Green and Green (1989), at the Menninger Clinic, developed the first portable electroencephalography (EEG) biofeedback unit. This unit provided sound feedback varying with the percentage of alpha, theta, or beta EEG rhythms and was used to treat adults with seizures and children with attention-deficit/hyperactivity disorders (ADHD). Lubar (1991) reported the successful application of neurofeedback for children with ADHD. In our behavioral pediatrics clinics, we used the Menninger Clinic unit clinically for children with intractable seizures and also for children with ADHD. We found neurofeedback training to be helpful to some of these children. There are now many clinical studies reporting reduction in symptoms of ADHD during neurofeedback training. Most training protocols require 30–40 training sessions (Fox, Tharp, & Fox, 2005; Fuchs, Birbaumer, Lutzenberger, Gruzelier, & Kaiser, 2003). Baena and colleagues (2021) did a systematic review to analyze the effects of neurofeedback interventions in children with ADHD. They identified nine randomized controlled trials published within the preceding 5 years. They concluded the neurofeedback improved behavior, allowed greater control of impulsivity and increased sustained attention. They did not describe specific neurofeedback protocols and noted that the nine studies varied substantially in the number of training sessions for children with ADHD.

A review of neurofeedback for autism spectrum disorders concluded that neurofeedback is an intervention that is possibly efficacious for symptoms of autism (Coben, Linden, & Myers, 2010); however, there is a need for well-designed studies that address issues of randomization, blinding, placebo controls, and multiple variables.

## Movement Disorders

Electromyographic (EMG) feedback has been used clinically to treat some children with movement disorders; however, we are not aware of any controlled studies in this area. The primary dystonias of childhood (Moskowitz, 1991) improve with relaxation, hypnosis, and rest, but EMG feedback might also be helpful to children with dystonias. Children with cerebral palsy have benefited from visual feedback of muscle stretch reflex sensitivity and from auditory feedback for gait training (Flodmark, 1986; Nash, Neilson, & O'Dwyer, 1989).

## Hypertension

Biofeedback and hypnosis have been used to help adults and adolescents increase awareness of the contribution of feelings (e.g., worry, tension, excitement, distress, frustration) to blood pressure recordings. Benson (1990) described the ability of adults, through the relaxation response, to lower blood pressure; the methods used have been demonstrated to reduce sympathetic nervous system activity, thereby decreasing cardiac output and lowering blood pressure (Ewart et al., 1987). It has also been noted that operant heart rate speeding and slowing are associated with changes in cardiac vagal tone (Hatch, Borcherding, & Norris, 1990).

Self-regulation techniques are useful in the nonpharmacological treatment of adolescents and adults with borderline high blood pressure and those with hypertension (Achmon, Granek, Golomb, & Hart, 1989; Barr, Pennebaker, & Watson, 1988; Blanchard, 1990; Crowther, 1983; Ewart et al., 1987; Patel & Marmot, 1987; Southam, Agras, Taylor, & Kraemer, 1982). An assessment of the physiological concomitants of stress and anxiety was completed by observing the heart rate and blood pressure of preschool children who had been assigned stressful tasks. The tasks elicited measurable changes in heart rate and blood pressure across subjects (Boyce et al., 1990). Increases in blood pressure and cardiac output are viewed as resembling the classical defense reaction, and it has been suggested that this pattern prevails in the early stages of hypertension (Freyschuss, Hjemdahl, Juhlin-Dannfelt, & Linde, 1988). In a study examining the heart rate and blood pressure of 395 healthy children, it was postulated that anxiety reactions may operate as a mechanism in the development of elevated blood pressure (Murphy, Alpert, & Walker, 1991).

Pediatric hypertension management guidelines note that "stress reduction techniques involving meditation, relaxation, or biofeedback are part of non-pharmacologic management" and are "often effective in the young" (Jung & Ingelfinger, 1993). It is clear that the control of blood pressure and cardiovascular reactivity in children at risk for hypertension and its cardiovascular sequelae is of major importance.

In a study by Kohen and Ondich (2004), 100 normal children with no history of hypertension were divided into four groups. Twenty-five children in one group were previously familiar with relaxation and mental imagery (self-hypnosis) for some clinical problem and were instructed to use that skill to lower their blood pressure to a healthy level. Seventy-five additional children were randomly assigned to one of three groups: (1) children in the experimental group listened to an audiotape of a hypnotic induction with specific instructions to lower their blood pressure; (2) children in the waking suggestion control group listened to a tape that gave them similar suggestions to lower their blood pressure but without a hypnotic induction; and (3) those in the control group listened to a tape that asked them to rest quietly during the experiment/measurement time. All children had blood pressure measurements taken during three 10-minute trial periods at week 1 and again at week 2. None of the children had hypertension or were at risk for hypertension. Children did not see their blood pressure recordings. Each group had some children who were able to change their blood pressure, but no group demonstrated significantly more subjects with this skill. Distinguishing characteristics of those individuals from each group who were most able to alter their blood pressure voluntarily in this experiment have yet to be defined. The individual differences provide a focus for future investigation and understanding of voluntary blood pressure control.

We have clinical experience with many adolescents who came to a teen medical clinic to undergo physical examinations, mandated by a variety of circumstances. For many, the circumstances were stressful; that is, they were brought in from a crisis center after running away from home, or they came in for a first pelvic examination or a sports physical. In such situations, the initial blood pressure was often elevated, and a simple relaxation or imagery exercise resulted in decreased blood pressure. An example of the spontaneous intervention follows (italicized words emphasize pacing or represent positive expectancy-based hypnotic suggestions):

> You'll probably *be surprised* to discover how *easy* it is for this kind of *slight* increase in blood pressure to *get lower* by *just* using your imagination. So, just *let* your eyes close … that's right … take a deep breath. *When* you let it out, *notice* the relaxation that *automatically* begins at your shoulders *naturally* as they go down … and, *as* the relaxation moves down your arms and chest gradually or quickly – either is okay – *let* your mind's imagination *drift off* to somewhere where you are *very comfortable and happy, because when your mind is relaxed, imagining being somewhere that's just right, the body listens.* When you are very comfortable and can notice the sights and sounds and what you are doing in your imagined place, then let me know, and I'll check the blood pressure again while you remain very comfortably relaxed.

Often such an approach results in a reduction in the blood pressure that was elevated in association with anxiety in the clinic environment. In such situations, the patient is well aware of the blood pressure cuff and often watches the recording of the follow-up measurement (visual biofeedback) at the end of the hypnotherapeutic suggestions.

It is well known that the reaction to stressful circumstances can also raise heart rate and blood pressure to unhealthy levels (Chesney et al., 1987; Crowther, 1983; Ewart et al., 1987; Menkes, Matthews, Krantz et al., 1989). It is appropriate to consider preventive management by avoidance of the stressors, as well as by the development of skills to manage the physiological sequelae of stressors that are unavoidable. Although the best ways to accomplish this are not yet clear, it seems appropriate to learn intentional modulation of autonomic functions such as heart rate and blood pressure and to practice these skills, especially during distressing times. This may be of lifelong significance with respect to cardiovascular health (Jung & Ingelfinger, 1993). We believe that it may be prudent to train children from hypertension-prone families in the self-regulation of blood pressure.

## Biofeedback Research with Children

There is a great need for further research in these areas. Miniature telemetry devices may make it possible to provide biofeedback to children in school and on the playground. With respect to biofeedback of autonomic responses as a general adjunct to hypnosis, we believe that individual differences should dictate which type of feedback is chosen; however, research data do not yet allow us to do that. Personality types, learning styles, interests, likes, and dislikes of children must also be significant factors in determining whether or not biofeedback should be used and what type of equipment is most likely to interest a given child.

### *Nonpharmacologic Interventions Related to Biofeedback*

The process of teaching self-regulation with biofeedback nearly always involves instructions to direct one's thinking to a focus on breathing or on progressive relaxation or on imagery or mindful meditation. Our experience is that most of these instructions lead to a hypnotic state. An article on non-mindfulness-based interventions includes 43 different non-mindfulness-based interventions, including biofeedback (Xia, Hu, Seritan, & Eisendrath, 2019). Authors state that "the line between MBIs and non-MBIs is not well defined" and that "future studies will be needed to understand the mechanism that pervades all interventions on this mindfulness spectrum." Moss and Khazan (2019) were editors for a special issue on integrating mindfulness training with clinical biofeedback. The issue described this integration for a number of chronic clinical conditions. Clinicians should develop a tolerance for uncertainty with respect to definitions of non-pharmacologic self-regulation interventions. The current confusion in nomenclature is evident in clinical research protocols where it sometimes appears that hypnosis is being compared with hypnosis. A review study on combining biofeedback with stress management interventions (progressive relaxation, rhythmic breathing, and relaxation) noted similar interventions in most of the control groups (breathing protocols, muscle relaxation, and combination of muscle relaxation and mindfulness). The control groups also demonstrated improvement in psychological and physiological responses (De Witte, Buyck, & Van Daele, 2019). Daily practice was required in both the experimental and control groups. In those studies where the stress management interventions were similar in both groups, e.g., breathing protocols or relaxation, and study subjects also did daily practice, it is likely that they were learning self-hypnosis.

## Eye Movement Desensitization and Reprocessing for Children

Eye movement desensitization and reprocessing (EMDR) requires a narrowing and focusing of attention just as hypnosis does. Most reported studies of EMDR have been conducted with children with posttraumatic stress disorder (PTSD) as a result of motor vehicle accidents, natural disasters, or manmade disasters (Chemtob, Nakashima, & Carlson, 2002). A meta-analysis (Rodenburg, Benjamin, deRoos, Meijer, & Stams, 2009) demonstrated EMDR efficacy when effect sizes were based on comparisons between the EMDR and the non-established trauma treatment or no-treatment control groups; however, efficacy was reduced when the comparisons were between the EMDR and established cognitive behavioral trauma treatment.

A randomized clinical trial of EMDR, fluoxetine, and placebo in PTSD (Van der Kolk et al., 2007) included 88 PTSD subjects, of whom one third had child-onset trauma. Subjects were followed for 6 months. For most childhood-onset trauma patients, no treatment produced complete symptom remission. In Sweden, Ahmad and colleagues (Ahmad, Larsson, & Sundelin-Wahlsten, 2007) conducted a randomized controlled trial of EMDR treatment for 33 children with PTSD compared with untreated children in a wait-list control group. The reduction in re-experiencing symptoms was the most significant between-group difference.

Another study in Sweden (Oras, de Ezpeleta, & Ahmad, 2004) reported successful treatment with EMDR of 13 refugee children with PTSD. In Hawaii, Chemtob and colleagues (Chemtob et al., 2002) conducted a study of 32 children with disaster-related PTSD. The children were taught EMDR a year or more after the disaster. Treatment resulted in substantial reductions in the Children's Reaction Inventory and in modest reductions in the Children's Depression Inventory and Children's Manifest Anxiety Scale. Gains were maintained at 6 months. A study in Australia (Kemp, Drummond, & McDermott, 2010) reported substantial reduction in PTSD symptoms of 27 children who had been in a motor vehicle accident. These children had four EMDR sessions, and positive results were maintained at 3- and 12-month follow-ups. A study by De Jong, Andrea, and Muris (1997) compared 22 spider-phobic girls with 21 girls who were not spider phobic. The phobic girls were tested before and after treatment, which consisted of 1.5 hours of EMDR and 1.5 hours of exposure to spiders *in vivo*. A decline in the fear of spiders was observed after the treatment. The number of EMDR training sessions reported varied from three to eight. There are no reported studies in children comparing hypnosis or biofeedback with EMDR.

## References


Achmon, J., Granek, M., Golomb, M., & Hart, J. (1989). Behavioral treatment of essential hypertension: a comparison between cognitive therapy and biofeedback of heart rate. *Psychosomatic Medicine, 51*, 152–164.

Ahmad, A., Larsson, B., & Sundelin-Wahlsten, V. (2007). EMDR treatment for children with PTSD: results of a randomized controlled trial. *Nordic Journal of Psychiatry, 61*, 349–354.

Andrasik, F. & Holroyd, K.A. (1980). Test of specific and non-specific effects in the biofeedback treatment of tension headache. *Journal of Consulting and Clinical Psychology, 48*, 575–586.

Baena, L.S., Canadas-Dela Fuente, G.A., Martos-Cagrerea, M.B., Gomez-Urquiza, J.L., Albendin-Garcia, L., Romero-Bejar, J.L., & Suleiman-Martos, N. (2021). Effects of neurofeedback in children with attention-hyperactivity disorder: a systematic review. *Journal of Clinical Medicine, 10*, 3797. 10.3390/jcm10173797

Barr, M., Pennebaker, J.W., & Watson, D. (1988). Improving blood pressure estimation through internal and environmental feedback. *Psychosomatic Medicine, 50*, 37–45.

Basmajian, J.V. (1989). *Biofeedback: Principles and Practice for Clinicians*. Baltimore, MD: Williams & Wilkins.

Benson, H. (1990). *The Relaxation Response*, 2nd ed. New York: Avon Books.

Blanchard, E.B. (1990). Biofeedback treatments of essential hypertension. *Biofeedback and Self-Regulation, 15*, 209–228.

Boyce, W.T., Chesney, M.A., Kaiser, P., Alkon, A., Eisenhardt, M., Chesterman, E., & Tschann, J. (1990). Development of a protocol for measuring cardiovascular response to stress in pre-school children. *Journal of Developmental and Behavioral Pediatrics, 11*(4), 214.

Brown, B. (1974). *New Mind: New Body*. New York: Harper & Row.

Burke, E.J. & Andrasik, F. (1989). Home vs. clinic-based biofeedback treatment for pediatric migraine: results of treatment through one-year follow-up. *Headache, 29*, 434–440.

Chemtob, C.M., Nakashima, J., & Carlson, J.G. (2002). Brief treatment for elementary school children with disaster-related PTSD: a field study. *Journal of Clinical Psychology, 58*, 99–112.

Chesney, M.A., Agras, W.S., Benson, H., Blumenthal, J.A., Engel, B.T., Foreyt, J.P., Kaufmann, P.G., Levenson, R.M., Pickering, T.G., Randali, W.C., & Schwartz, P.J. (1987). Task Force 5: non-pharmacologic approaches to the treatment of hypertension. *Circulation, 76*(Suppl. 1), 104–109.

Christie, N. H. (2009). I ntegrating biofeedback into a pediatric neuroscience department. *Biofeedback, 378*, 126-128.

Coben, R., Linden, M., & Myers, T.E. (2010). Neurofeedback for autistic spectrum disorder: a review of the literature. *Applied Psychophysiology and Biofeedback, 35*, 83–105.

Crowther, J. (1983). Stress management training and relaxation imagery in the treatment of essential hypertension. *Journal of Behavioral Medicine, 6*, 169–186.

Culbert, T. (2017). Perspectives on technology-assisted relaxation approaches to support mind-body skills practice in children and teens: clinical experience and commentary. *Children, 4*(4), 20. 10.3390/children 4040020

De Jong, P.J., Andrea, H., & Muris, P. (1997). Spider phobia in children: disgust and fear before and after treatment. *Behaviour Research and Therapy, 35*, 559–562.

De Witte, N.A.J., Buyck, I., & Van Daele, T. (2019). Combining biofeedback with stress management interventions: a systematic review of physiological and psychological effects. *Applied Psychophysiology and Biofeedback, 44*, 71–82.

Dikel, W. & Olness, K. (1980). Self-hypnosis, biofeedback, and voluntary peripheral temperature control in children. *Pediatrics, 66*, 335–340.

Ewart, C.K., Harris, W.L., Iwata, M.M., Coates, T.J., Bullock, R., & Simon, B. (1987). Feasibility and effectiveness of school-based relaxation in lowering blood pressure. *Health Psychology, 6*, 399–416.

Flodmark, A. (1986). Augmented auditory feedback as an aid in gait training of the cerebral-palsied child. *Developmental Medicine and Child Neurology, 28*, 147–155.

Fox, D.J., Tharp, D., & Fox, L.C. (2005). Neurofeedback: an alternative and efficacious treatment for attention deficit hyperactivity disorder. *Applied Psychophysiology and Biofeedback, 30*, 365–373.

Freyschuss, U., Hjemdahl, P., Juhlin-Dannfelt, A., & Linde, B. (1988). Cardiovascular and sympathoadrenal responses to mental stress: influence of beta blockade. *American Journal of Physiology, 255*, 1443–1451.

Fuchs, T., Birbaumer, N., Lutzenberger, W., Gruzelier, J.H., & Kaiser, J. (2003). Neurofeedback treatment for attention deficit hyperactivity disorder in children: a comparison with methylphenidate. *Applied Psychophysiology and Biofeedback, 28*, 1–12.

Grayson, P. (2009). The biofeedback program at children's mercy hospitals. *Biofeedback, 37*, 137–140.

Green, E. & Green, A. (1989). *Beyond Biofeedback*. Fort Wayne, IN: Knoll Publishers.

Hatch, J. P., Borcherding, S., & Norris, L.K. (1990). Cardiopulmonary adjustments during operant heart rate control. *Psychophysiology*, 27, 641–648.

Hogan, M., MacDonald, J., & Olness, K. (1985). The effects of hypnosis on brainstem auditory responses in children. *American Journal of Clinical Hypnosis, 27*(3), 91–94.

Jung, F.F. & Ingelfinger, J.R. (1993). Hypertension in childhood and adolescence. *Pediatrics in Review, 14*, 169–179.

Kagan, J. (1994). *Galen's Prophecy*. New York: Basic Books.

Kemp, M., Drummond, P., & McDermott, B. (2010). A wait-list controlled pilot study of EMDR for children with PTSD symptoms from motor vehicle accidents. *Clinical Child Psychology and Psychiatry*, 15, 5–25.

Koechlin, H., Kossowsky, J., Lam, T.L., Barthel, J., Gaab, J., Berde, C.B., Schwarzer, G., Linde, K., Meissner, K., & Locher, L. (2021). Nonpharmacological interventions for pediatric migraine: a network meta-analysis. *Pediatrics, 147*(4), e201194107.

Kohen, D.P. & Ondich, S. (2004). Children's self-regulation of cardiovascular function with relaxation/ mental imagery (self-hypnosis): report of a controlled study. *Hypnos: The Journal of European Society of Hypnosis in Psychotherapy and Psychosomatic Medicine, 31*(2), 61–74.

Lee, L. & Olness, K. (1995). Impact of imagery changes on autonomic reactivity in children [abstract]. *Archives of Pediatrics and Adolescent Medicine, 149*, 47.

Lubar, J.F. (1991). Discourse on the development of EEC diagnostics and biofeedback for attention-deficit/ hyperactivity disorders. *Biofeedback and Self-Regulation, 16*, 201–226.

MacIntosh, A., Desailly, E., Vignais, N., Vigneron, V., & Biddiss, E. (2020, June 22). A biofeedback-enhanced therapeutic exercise video game intervention for young people with cerebral palsy: a randomized single-case experimental design feasibility study. *PLoS One. 15*(6), e0234767.

Mauersberger, K., Atz, K., Duncan, B., & Gurgevich, S. (2000). Can children with spastic cerebral palsy use self hypnosis to reduce muscle tone? *Integrative Medicine, 21*, 93–96.

Menkes, M.S., Matthews, K. A., Krantz, D. S., Lundburg, U. , Mead, L. A., Qagish, B., Liang, K. Y., Thomas, C. B., & Pearson, T. A. (1989). Cardiovascular reactivity to the cold pressor test as a predictor of hypertension. *Hypertension*, 14, 524–530.

Miller, N.E. (1969). Learning of visceral and glandular responses. *Science, 163*, 434–445.

Moskowitz, C.B. (1991). The primary dystonias of childhood. *Journal of Neuroscience Nursing, 23*, 175–178.

Moss, D., Cyr, L., & Culbert, T.P., Eds. (2005). Hypnosis and biofeedback in pediatrics (special issue). *Biofeedback, 33*, 2.

Moss, D. & Khazan, I. (2019). Special issue: integrating mindfulness training with clinical biofeedback: practical applications. *Biofeedback, 47*, 49.

Mullinix, J.M., Norton, B.J., Hack, S., & Fishman, M.A. (1978). Skin temperature biofeedback and migraine. *Headache, 17*, 242–244.

Murphy, J.K., Alpert, B.S., & Walker, S.S. (1991). Stability of ethnic differences in children's pressor responses during three annual examinations. *American Journal of Hypertension, 4*, 630–634.

Nash, J., Neilson, P.D., & O'Dwyer, N.J. (1989). Reducing spasticity to control muscle contracture of children with cerebral palsy. *Developmental Medicine and Child Neurology, 32*(4), 471–480.

Olness, K. (1990). Reflex sympathetic dystrophy syndrome: treatment of children with cyberphysiologic strategies. *Swedish Journal of Hypnosis in Psychotherapy and Psychosomatic Medicine, 17*, 15–18.

Olness, K. & Conroy, M. (1985). A pilot study of voluntary control of transcutaneous $PO_2$ by children. *International Journal of Clinical and Experimental Hypnosis, 33*, 1–5.

Olness, K., MacDonald, J., & Uden, D. (1987). A prospective study comparing self-hypnosis, propranolol, and placebo in management of juvenile migraine. *Pediatrics, 79*, 593–597.

Olness, K., McParland, F.A., & Piper, J. (1980). Biofeedback: a new modality in the management of children with fecal soiling. *Journal of Pediatrics, 96*, 505–509.

Olness, K. & Rusin, W. (1990). Cyberphysiology in children and its relationship to self-regulatory control. In L.P. Lipsitt & L.I. Mitnick, Eds., *Loss of Self-Regulatory Control: Its Causes and Consequences* (pp. 241–256). Norwood, NJ: Ablex Press.

Olton, D.S. & Noonberg, A.R. (1980). *Biofeedback: Clinical Applications in Behavioral Medicine.* Englewood Cliffs, NJ: Prentice-Hall.

Oras, R., de Ezpeleta, S.C., & Ahmad, A. (2004). Treatment of traumatized refugee children with eye movement desensitization and reprocessing in a psychodynamic context. *Nordic Journal of Psychiatry, 58*, 199–203.

Osterhaus, S.O.L., Passchier, J., van der Helm-Hylkema, H., de Jong, K.T., Orlebeke, J.F., de Grauw, A.J.C., & Dekker, P.H. (1993). Effects of behavioral psychophysiological treatment on schoolchildren with migraine in a nonclinical setting: predictors and process variables. *Journal of Pediatric Psychology, 18*(6), 697–715.

Patel, C. & Marmot, M.G. (1987). Stress management, blood pressure, and quality of life. *Journal of Hypertension, 5*(Suppl. 1), 21–28.

Rodenburg, R., Benjamin, A., deRoos, C., Meijer, A.M., & Stams, G.J. (2009). Efficacy of EMDR in children: a meta analysis. *Clinical Psychology Review, 29*, 599–606.

Schwartz, M.S. & Olson, R.P. (2003). A historical perspective on the field of biofeedback and applied psychophysiology. In M.S. Schwartz & F. Andrasik, Eds., *Biofeedback: A Practitioner's Guide* (pp. 3–19). New York: The Guilford Press.

Schwartz, N.M. & Schwartz, M.S. (2003). Definitions of biofeedback and applied psychophysiology. In M.S. Schwartz & F. Andrasik, Eds., *Biofeedback: A Practitioner's Guide* (pp. 27–40). New York: The Guilford Press.

Smith, M.S. (1991). Biofeedback. *Pediatric Annals, 20*, 128–134.

Smith, M.S., Womack, W.M., & Pertik, M. (1987). Temperature feedback and hypnotic ability in children and adolescents. *International Journal of Medicine and Health, 3*, 91–99.

Southam, M.A., Agras, W.S., Taylor, C.B., & Kraemer, H.C. (1982). Relaxation training: blood pressure lowering during the working day. *Archives of General Psychiatry, 39*, 715–717.

Thomson, L. (2022). Hypnotherapy for complex regional pain syndrome. *American Journal of Clinical Hypnosis, 64*, 195–205.

Van der Kolk, B.A., Spinazola, J., Blaustein, M.E., Hopper, J.W., Hopper, E.K., Korn, D.L., & Simpson, W.B. (2007). A randomized clinical trial of EMDR, fluoxetine, and pill placebo in the treatment of posttraumatic stress disorder: treatment effects and long-term maintenance. *Journal of Clinical Psychiatry, 68*, 37–46.

Wang, Y. & Morgan, W.P. (1992). The effect of imagery perspectives on the psychophysiological responses to imagined exercise. *Behavior and Brain Research, 52*, 167–174.

Xia, T., Hu, H., Seritan, A., & Eisendrath, S. (2019). The many roads to mindfulness: a review of nonmindfulness based interventions that increase mindfulness. *The Journal of Alternative and Complementary Medicine, 25*, 874–889.

# 17

# SELF-HYPNOSIS

## A Tool for Prevention and Prophylaxis

Prevention has long been intrinsic to pediatric research and practice. Immunization programs, anticipatory guidance in pediatric clinics, nutrition programs, and school programs, as well as laws related to newborn screening, are designed to prevent diseases (Christopherson, Finney, & Friman, 1986; Miller, 1985; Wasserman, 2021). Child health programs also focus on prevention of behavioral problems. A collaborative multidisciplinary approach is essential to a successful prevention program (Bass et al., 1993; Creer, Stein, Rappaport, & Lewis, 1992; Irwin, Cataldo, Matheny, & Peterson, 1992; Schor & Bergman, 2021). Where does self-hypnosis fit into such approaches? Developing skills in self-regulation and control is important to healthy development, and self-hypnosis is a tool that facilitates acquisition of these skills (Olness, 2009).

## Infants

The application of self-hypnosis for prevention of infant morbidity can begin in pregnancy and continue through the life of the child. Several authors have noted that the use of self-hypnotic techniques for relaxation during pregnancy, labor, and delivery has been found to be helpful to both mother and child (Beevi, Low, & Hassan, 2017; Catsaros & Wendland 2020; Cooper, Shafter, & Tyndall, 1986; Vadurro & Butts, 1982). Mothers who practice self-hypnotic strategies often require less medication during labor and delivery, thus reducing potential harmful effects on the infant. Self-hypnosis has also been helpful in facilitating breastfeeding, which has many benefits for the child. Prolonged infant crying due to presumed colic triggers much stress in families. Although the cause of colic is not clear, both parents and infants may benefit from hypnotic strategies to reduce the anxiety of parents.

## Toddlers

Anticipatory guidance might well include training of parents to use phrases that encourage a young child to use his or her natural gift of imagery in positive ways. By means of simple games, young children can become aware of sensory imagery (auditory, visual, gustatory, or olfactory), which they can learn to apply as distracters during procedures such as diaper changing and

DOI: 10.4324/9781003243687-19

dressing. By 3 or 4 years of age, a young child can learn that, by thinking in certain ways, he or she can change physiologic responses such as peripheral temperature or other physiologic responses by means of simple feedback or can even alter breathing patterns associated with illness such as asthma (Kohen & Wynne, 1997). Prospective studies are necessary to determine whether early development of these skills facilitates maintenance or enhancement of physiological self-regulation in adulthood. We have received feedback from many young adults to whom we taught self-hypnosis when they were preschoolers. They tell us that they continue to use self-hypnosis skills as adults and for various purposes (e.g., during dental visits). Kuttner (1989) produced an impressive documentary of eight young adults who had learned self-hypnosis skills during treatment of their cancers. All indicated that they continued to benefit from the self-regulation skills learned during their cancer treatment. They emphasized the sense of personal control they had acquired from being given the tool of self-hypnosis. Kohen (2010) reported the long-term follow-up of children who had originally learned self-hypnosis for successful management and relief of recurrent headaches. Participants were surveyed many years following treatment and contact. Eighty-five percent of respondents reported continued use of self-hypnosis for relief of headache; but perhaps more importantly, half of respondents described their spontaneous use of self-hypnosis for life stresses including other types of pain, difficulty with sleep due to stress (school/test anxiety), sports, and other performance anxiety (Kohen, 2010; see also Chapter 13). Pediatricians and other child health professionals might teach young children prophylactic pain control, which the child can apply in unexpected emergency room visits, during dental procedures, and in other stressful situations.

## Compliance with Medical Regimens

Existing studies of chronic illnesses, such as hemophilia, diabetes, recurrent abdominal pain, juvenile migraine, and malignancies, provide data to support the recommendation that children so diagnosed should learn self-regulation strategies as soon as possible to reduce morbidity, lessen their symptoms, and enhance mastery and comfort (Accardi & Milling, 2009; Agle, 1975; Dinges et al., 1997; Gelernter et al., 2015; Hoekman et al., 2021; Kaiser, Kohen, Brown, Kajander, & Barnes, 2018; Kohen, Colwell, Heimel, & Olness, 1984; Kohen & Kaiser, 2014; Kumari, Bahuguna, Garg, & Yeluri, 2021; Kuttner, 1989; Nunns et al., 2018; Olness, MacDonald, & Uden, 1987; Richardson, Smith, McCall, & Pilkington, 2006; Rutten et al., 2017). Self-hypnosis is helpful in facilitating compliance with injections (e.g., for diabetes or allergy), special diets, nebulizer or inhaler regimens, frequent oral medications or nutritional supplements, special exercises, and other procedures. Fear of injections can be prevented or mitigated by parent education, including assessment of parental anxiety and teaching parents comfort strategies including self-hypnosis. Also, at medical visits not involving injections young children can be taught to play breathing games or distraction methods that can be used when they have subsequent visits for injections. Thomas (2017) developed a video to help children understand pain and to prepare them for procedures such as injections or pokes.

## School-Age Stress

Bothe, Grignon, and Olness (2014) conducted a study of a stress management intervention in a third-grade classroom. In this controlled prospective longitudinal study, teachers led daily practice of 1 minute of diaphragmatic breathing, 4 minutes of simple stretching, another 1 minute of diaphragmatic breathing and 4 minutes of guided imagery (self-hypnosis). This practice continued for 4 months during which time the teacher of the control class read to the children for 10 minutes each day. A standardized anxiety scale and heart rate variability was measured in each child before the 4-month intervention, immediately after 4 months, and 1 year later. The children who participated in the experimental group showed significant reductions in total anxiety at 4 months and at the 1-year follow-up. The control group showed no improvements. Qualitatively, children reported that they continued to do the breathing and guided imagery during stressful times at home and at school after the study ended.

There are hundreds of books and apps marketed to parents to help children address stress. Some of them include terms such as "guided imagery," "mindfulness meditation," "progressive relaxation," "belly breathing exercises," or "virtual reality relaxation." It is important to recognize that these are all closely related to self-hypnosis. Storytelling is a very effective and favored form of hypnosis and engaging children in self-hypnosis. Several authors have contributed substantially to this, including Brett (1986, 1992) and Garth (1991, 1993, 1995, 1997). We believe that the use of such resources is maximized by parental consultation with child health professionals who can provide informed support, reinforcement, and guidance in the most appropriate utilization of such materials.

## Performance Anxiety

All children must perform during family, school, religious, creative, and sports events. Many overcome performance anxiety by means of self-hypnosis training. Prophylactic training in this skill is recommended for all children who perform in some way. School children may learn these techniques to maximize their athletic potential. With the increased social awareness, popularity, and success of sports psychologist consultants for Olympic and professional athletes and entire teams, universities and even some high school athletic teams similarly have engaged various health professionals to consult with and coach young athletes in self-hypnosis-like techniques. Minimally, the expectation with such training is to reduce, eliminate, or prevent performance-interfering stress. Optimally, such strategies might also promote improved performance through, for example, focused imagery of desired outcomes. In Sweden, Unestahl and colleagues (Unestahl, Bundzen, Gavrilova, & Isakov, 2004) have worked with sports teams to investigate what mental aspects or processes are necessary for the ideal performance state. Unestahl's work identified four essential factors: self-image, attitude, goal-image, and emotion (the right feeling). Earlier, in his doctoral thesis, Unestahl (1973) concluded that regular, systematic, and long-term self-hypnosis training was superior to heterohypnosis. His research has led to programs for grade-school children in Sweden who are taught self-regulation techniques in physical education classes. Unestahl (2018) described the positive responses of Olympic competitors who practiced sports hypnosis. He also described how self-hypnosis training is available in most areas of Swedish society, including schools, businesses, sports, and health settings and has been practiced by millions of Swedish people, from childhood to retirement.

## Reduction of Morbidity from Allergies

Clinical reports and prospective intervention studies indicate that self-regulation training in children can reduce morbidity with respect to asthma, hives, and eczema (Kohen, 1986; Kohen & Wynne, 1997). Current research may allow therapists to be more precise in setting up appropriate times and strategies for self-hypnosis practice for children who have allergies.

## Cost Reduction

Existing studies in clinical applications of therapeutic hypnosis in children suggest that one can anticipate a significant reduction in overall health-care costs for children who learn and use these techniques (Kohen et al., 1984). The average number of visits for treatment of habit problems is four, and long-term follow-up indicates that relapses are rare. Children with chronic problems such as asthma require fewer emergency room visits. Overall, children who use self-regulation strategies can be expected to require fewer medications, to miss fewer school days, and to make fewer demands on parental time for clinic and hospital visits.

## Coping and Happiness

People who practice self-hypnosis to regulate body processes learn that directing one's own thoughts not only brings about rapid physiological responses but also affects feelings, emotions, attitudes, expectations, and overall perceptions of comfort and satisfaction. Images produce feelings; feelings are preceded by specific thinking patterns. Humans can change their feelings by changing their thoughts. In the past, American children have been taught that a feeling simply *is*, that it is good to express feelings, whether they are angry or happy or sad. This concept can lead to frustration and feelings of helplessness. If children are taught early that feelings can respond to changes in thinking and that they can be controlled, or at least modulated, this provides them with a basic tool for coping and mastery. If children learn to control or change thoughts, life can become easier and happier.

## Some Guidelines for Teaching Self-Hypnosis

In each encounter with a child or adolescent that involves hypnosis we assume that the teacher or coach will emphasize that the child should practice by himself or herself. To emphasize that the child or adolescent is in control and owns the self-hypnosis skill is to give him or her a great gift. Guidelines for the child health professional who is teaching self-hypnosis include:

- Provide the child with choices about when and where he or she will practice.
- Ask parents not to remind the child about practice or to ask the child what he or she is doing.
- Encourage children to teach their parents their methods of self-hypnosis when they are ready to do so.
- Give the child a choice about what approach to use and the preferred mental imagery.
- Be sure the therapeutic suggestions are consistent with the child's wishes and previous explanations.
- Ask the child if he or she would like to have a recording of the practice conducted in your office. If so, suggest that the child use it only occasionally.
- Provide the child with options for recording progress in his or her practice and achievement of therapeutic goals.
- Tell the child to contact you if he or she has questions, forgets something, or is bored with the practice.

## Self-Hypnosis for Child Health Professionals

Child health professionals can personally gain from regular practice of self-hypnosis. They may enjoy self-hypnosis simply for relaxation or to be comfortable during a dental or medical procedure. They may choose to use self-hypnosis to help manage undesirable habits or chronic pain or overcome writer's block. In the process of becoming expert in personal self-hypnosis, child health professionals also become more expert in helping child and adolescent patients learn self-hypnosis.

## References


Accardi, M.C. & Milling, L.S. (2009). The effectiveness of hypnosis for reducing procedure-related pain in children and adolescents: a comprehensive methodological review. *Journal of Behavioral Medicine, 32,* 328–339.

Agle, D. (1975). Psychological factors in hemophilia: the concept of self-care. *Annals of the New York Academy of Sciences, 240,* 221–225.

Bass, J.L., Christoffel, K.K., Widome, M., Boyle, W., Scheidt, P., Stanwick, R., & Roberts, K. (1993). Childhood injury prevention counseling in primary care settings: a critical review of the literature. *Pediatrics, 92*(4), 544–550.

Beevi, Z., Low, W.Y., & Hassan, J. (2017). The effectiveness of hypnosis intervention for labor: an experimental study. *American Journal of Clinical Hypnosis, 60,* 172–191.

Bothe, D., Grignon, J., & Olness, K. (2014). The effects of a stress management intervention in elementary school children. *Journal of Developmental and Behavioral Pediatrics, 35,* 62–67.

Brett, D. (1986). *Annie Stories.* Victoria, Australia: McPhee Gribble Publishers Pty Ltd.

Brett, D. (1992). *More Annie Stories* – Therapeutic Storytelling Techniques. New York: Magination Press.

Catsaros, S. & Wendland, J. (2020). Hypnosis-based interventions during pregnancy and childbirth and their impact on women's childbirth experience: a systematic review. *Midwifery, 84,* 102666. 10.1016/jmidw.2020.102666

Christopherson, E.R., Finney, J.W., & Friman, P.C., Eds. (1986). Prevention in primary care [special issue]. *Pediatric Clinics of North America, 33,* 743–1009.

Cooper, W., Shafter, W.L., & Tyndall, C.S. (1986). Shortening labor with hypnosis as an adjunct to Lamaze [abstract]. *American Journal of Clinical Hypnosis, 28,* 193.

Creer, T.L., Stein, R.E.K., Rappaport, L., & Lewis, C. (1992). Behavioral consequences of illness: childhood asthma as a model. *Pediatrics, 80*(5, Pt. 2), 808–815.

Dinges, D.F., Whitehouse, W.G., Orne, E.C., Bloom, P.B., Carlin, M.M., Bauer, N.K., & Gillen, K.A. (1997). Self-hypnosis training as an adjunctive treatment in the management of pain associated with sickle cell disease. *International Journal of Clinical and Experimental Hypnosis, 45,* 417–432.

Garth, M. (1991). *Starbright: Meditations for Children.* New York: Harper One.

Garth, M. (1993). *Moonbeam: A Book of Meditations for Children.* New York: Harper One.

Garth, M. (1995). *Sunshine: More Meditations for Children.* New York: Harper Collins.

Garth, M. (1997). *Earthlight: New Meditations for Children.* New York: Harper Collins

Gelernter, R., Lavi, G., Yanai, L., Brooks, R., Bar, Y., Bistrizer, Z., & Rachmiel, M. (2015). Effect of auditory guided imagery on glucose levels and on glycemic control in children with type 1 diabetes mellitus. *Journal of Pediatric Endocrinology and Metabolism.* 10.1515/jpem-2015-0150

Hoekman, D.R., Vlieger, A.M., Stokkers, P.C., Mahhmod, N., Rietdijk, S., de Boer, N.K., de Meij, T.G., Frankenhuis, C., D'Haens, G.R., & Benninga, M.A. (2021). Hypnotherapy for irritable bowel syndrome-type symptoms in patients with quiescent inflammatory bowel disease: a randomized, controlled trial. *Journal of Crohn's & Colitis, 15*(7), 1106–1113.

Irwin, C.E., Cataldo, M.F., Matheny, A.P., & Peterson, L. (1992). Health consequences of behaviors: injury as a model. *Pediatrics, 90*(5, Pt. 2), 798–807.

Kaiser, P., Kohen, D.P., Brown, M.L., Kajander, R.L., & Barnes, A.J. (2018). Integrating pediatric hypnosis with complementary modalities: clinical perspectives on personalized treatment. *Children, 5*(108), 1–25. 10.3390/children5080108

Kohen, D.P. (1986). Applications of relaxation/mental imagery (self-hypnosis) to the management of asthma: report of behavioral outcomes of a two-year, prospective controlled study [abstract]. *American Journal of Clinical Hypnosis, 28,* 196.

Kohen, D.P. (2010). Long term follow-up of self-hypnosis training for recurrent headaches: what the children say. *International Journal of Clinical and Experimental Hypnosis*, *58*(4), 417–432.

Kohen, D.P., Colwell, S.O., Heimel, A., & Olness, K.N. (1984). The use of relaxation/mental imagery (self-hypnosis) in the management of 505 pediatric behavioral encounters. *Journal of Developmental and Behavioral Pediatrics*, *5*(1), 21–25.

Kohen, D.P. & Kaiser, P. (2014). Clinical hypnosis with children and adolescents – what? Why? How?: origins, applications, and efficacy. *Children*, *I*, 74–98. 10.3390children1020074

Kohen, D.P. & Wynne, E. (1997). Applying hypnosis in a preschool family asthma education program: uses of storytelling, imagery, and relaxation. *American Journal of Clinical Hypnosis*, *39*, 2–14.

Kumari, S., Bahuguna, R., Garg, N., & Yeluri, R. (2021). Immersive and non-immersive virtual reality distracxtion on pain perceptioi to intraoral injections. *Journal of Clinical Pediatric Dentistry*, *45*(6), 380–394.

Kuttner, L. (1989). Management of young children's acute pain and anxiety during invasive medical procedures. *Pediatrician*, *16*, 39–44.

Miller, N.E. (1985). Some professional and scientific problems and opportunities for biofeedback. *Biofeedback and Self Regulation*, *10*, 3–24.

Nunns, M., Mayhew, D., Ford, T., Rogers, M., Curle, C., Logan, S., & Moore, D. (2018). Effectiveness of non-pharmacological interventions to reduce procedural anxiety in children and adolescents undergoing treatment for cancer: a systematic review and meta-analysis. *Psychooncology*, *8*, 1889–1899.

Olness, K. (2009). Self-control and self-regulation: normal development to clinical conditions. In W.B. Carey, A.C. Crocker, W.L. Coleman, E.R. Elias, & H.M. Feldman, Eds., *Developmental-Behavioral Pediatrics* (chap. 46). Philadelphia, PA: Saunders.

Olness, K., MacDonald, J., & Uden, D. (1987). A prospective study comparing self-hypnosis, propranolol, and placebo in management of juvenile migraine. *Pediatrics*, *79*, 593–597.

Richardson, J., Smith, J.E., McCall, G., & Pilkington, K. (2006). Hypnosis for procedure-related pain and distress in pediatric cancer patients: a systematic review of effectiveness and methodology related to hypnosis interventions. *Journal of Pain and Symptom Management*, *31*, 70–84.

Rutten, J.M.T.M., Vlieger, A.M., Frankenhuis, C., George, E.K., Groeneweg, M., Norbruis, O.F., Tjon, A., Ten, W., van Wering, H.M., Dijkgraaf, M.G.W., Merkus, M.P., & Benninga, M.A. (2017). Home-based hypnotherapy self-exercises vs individual hypnotherapy with a therapist for treatment of pediatric irritable bowel syndrome, functional abdominal pain, or functioinal abdominal pain syndrome: a randomized clinical trial. *JAMA Pediatrics*, *171*(5), 470–477.

Schor, E.L. & Bergman, D. (2021). Pediatric preventive care: population health and individualized care. *Pediatrics*, *148*(3), e2020049877. 10.1542/peds.2020-649877

Thomas, J. (2017). Project director, primary consultant: "you are the boss of your brain: learning how to manage pain during medical procedures" (13 min.) produced by Stanford children's health and Lucile Packard children's hospital. https://www.youtube.com/watch?v=UbK9FFoAcvs; https://www.Meg Foundation's new Provider Kit is now ready; https://www.Pain Champions Guide for parents; https://www.SuperMeg Comfort Plan Builder for kids

Unestahl, L.E. (1973). Hypnosis and posthypnotic suggestion. PhD thesis, Uppsala University, Orebro, Sweden.

Unestahl, L.E., Bundzen, P., Gavrilova, E., & Isakov, V. (2004). The effects of integrated mental training on stress and psychosomatic health. *Hypnos*, *31*, 83–88.

Unestahl, L.-E. (2018). Alert, Eyes-Open Sport Hypnosis. *American Journal of Clinical Hypnosis*, 61, 159–172. 10.1080/00029157.2018.1491387.

Vadurro, J.F. & Butts, P.A. (1982). Reducing the anxiety and pain of childbirth through hypnosis. *American Journal of Nursing*, *82*, 620–623.

Wasserman, R.C. (2021). The future(s) of pediatric primary care. *Academic Pediatrics*, *21*(3), 414–424.

# 18

# PSYCHONEUROIMMUNOLOGY

## Introduction

In 1979, before the term *psychoneuroimmunology* had appeared in print, we conducted a pilot study of voluntary control of white cell function in five children and six adults. Three of these children, who had prior experience in self-hypnosis, demonstrated changes in neutrophil chemiluminescence in the requested direction. This pilot study stimulated us to continue the difficult research in this area. Because studies of voluntary regulation of other autonomic processes indicate that children achieve such control more quickly than adults, we believe that it is reasonable and important to study voluntary immunoregulation in children. The developing immune system of the child is complex (Stiehm & Johnston, 2005). It may be particularly responsive to behavioral effects. Early conditioning of the immune system, whether intentional or not, may have profound long-term effects on immune capacity (Schleifer, Scott, Stein, & Keller, 1986). Many studies in psychoneuroimmunology, involving both animals and humans, were reported in the 1980s and 1990s, but relatively few in humans since then.

In the first edition of his book *Psychoneuroimmunology*, Ader (1981) did not provide a definition for the title. The nearest he came to a definition was with this sentence: "There is a growing awareness of an intimate and relatively unexplored relationship between the immune system and the central nervous system, and an analysis of this relationship might reveal much about the operation of the immune system and the brain" (p. xxi). Other attempts to define the term implied the existence of intentional immunomodulation by humans, something that was not yet proved. The majority of Ader's *Psychoneuroimmunology* (Ader, 1981, 1991) is devoted to animal experiments; however, in the second edition, Ader became a little bolder and more assertive with respect to the relationship between the immune and central nervous systems:

> There [are] now abundant data documenting neuroanatomical, neuroendocrine, and neurochemical links to the immune system. … The existence of bidirectional pathways of communication between nervous and immune systems provides an experimental foundation for the observation of behavioral and stress-induced influences on immune function and, conversely, the effects of immune processes on behavior. (p. xxvi)

DOI: 10.4324/9781003243687-20

## Conditioning of Immunosuppression and Immunoenhancement

The essence of Ader's exciting discovery was that the linking of a taste stimulus to an immunosuppressive drug, cyclophosphamide, led, after relatively few pairings, to conditioning of the physiological effects of that drug, including immunosuppression. This was a serendipitous discovery in rats. Ader was actually studying a model for conditioned taste aversion that might be relevant for humans who developed taste aversions while undergoing treatment for cancer. Dozens of animal studies have confirmed Ader's observations.

Immunoenhancement has also been conditioned in animals. A most impressive study (MacQueen, Marshall, Perdue, Siegel, & Bienenstock, 1989) conditioned rats to effect an immune response – the secretion of rat cell protease II by mucosal mast cells. The original unconditioned stimulus was the injection of egg albumin, which is known to elicit a mast-cell response. The stimuli to be conditioned were flashing lights and the sounds of fans. After only two pairings, the mast-cell response to the flashing lights and sounds of fans was equivalent to that in animals injected with egg albumin on the test trial. Mast cells are recognized as increased and hyperactive in a number of human diseases. It is possible that some mast-cell functions in humans are inadvertently conditioned to environmental stimuli that happen to be concurrent with the presence of an antigen that would ordinarily trigger mast-cell responses. There are numerous reports of urticaria, a mast-cell-mediated phenomenon in humans, that seem conditioned to a sight or sound. Possibly, an inadvertent conditioning occurred in those individuals sometime in the past when that sight or sound happened to be paired with an allergen, which then triggered mast-cell responses. Shertzer and Lookingbill (1987) reported that hypnosis was successful in the treatment of urticaria.

One of the authors (KO) saw an 11-year-old girl, Cindy, who was unable to participate comfortably in ice skating competitions because she developed generalized hives whenever she got on the ice. She had a history of a number of allergies and had previously taken antihistamines but was afraid they might interfere with her ability to skate. Several members of her family had used self-hypnosis successfully for various problems, and she asked about this for herself. I began by teaching Cindy a progressive relaxation exercise while I monitored her peripheral temperature. She was pleased to note that her temperature increased as she became more comfortable. I explained to her the mechanism of hives and told her that mast cells were much less likely to release substances causing hives under conditions of relaxation. I also asked her to think about a control system in her brain that she could use to shut down the mast-cell response when necessary. She thought of a joystick that would move in "on" and "off" directions. I also asked her to imagine skating a favorite routine and enjoying knowledge that her brain sent directions for skating that her muscles and nerves followed perfectly. I asked her to imagine that she had finished a performance, and she was feeling very comfortable, very pleased with how well she did, and delighted that the problem of hives had disappeared. I asked her to practice this exercise at home twice daily and saw her once for review 2 weeks later. In a 1-year follow-up, Cindy had no further problems with hives in connection with ice skating. She said that, on one occasion, she felt a few hives appearing, but she quickly moved the joystick to the "off" position.

It has been demonstrated in several human studies that conditioned immune responses are developed quite easily in humans; for example, a study in Germany (Buske-Kirschbaum, Kirschbaum, Stierle, Lehnert, & Hellhammer, 1992) demonstrated this phenomenon in 24 university students. A neutral sherbet was paired four times with a subcutaneous injection of 0.2 mg epinephrine. Subsequently, conditioned subjects showed significantly increased natural killer (NK) cell activity after re-exposure to the sherbet alone. A control group in which the sherbet was paired with subcutaneous saline showed no similar increases in NK cell activity. A study of conditioning of anticipatory nausea in women receiving cyclic chemotherapy for ovarian cancer found that they demonstrated not only conditioned nausea but also conditioning of cellular immune responses. Inasmuch as hypnosis can facilitate the deconditioning of negative physiological responses (e.g., tachycardia associated with the sight of a dog), it seems reasonable that it can be applied to de-conditioning of undesirable immune responses, such as those of the ice skater, Cindy.

## Pharmacological Conditioning

Ader extended the principle of conditioned immunosuppression to pharmacological conditioning. His work in lupus-prone mice found that animals could be trained, via pairing of a taste such as chocolate milk or saccharin flavored water with cyclophosphamide, to elicit a life-lengthening immunosuppression (Ader, 1989); that is, the response to the conditioned stimulus was equivalent to that of the drug. There is one clinical report of application of this principle to treatment of an adolescent female suffering from life-threatening lupus erythematosus (Olness & Ader, 1992). The patient had 2 years of prior experience using self-hypnosis for relief of pain and anxiety related to her disease. Cyclophosphamide was paired with the taste of cod liver oil and a pungent rose perfume over a 3-month period. Subsequently, the cod liver oil and pungent rose perfume were used as the conditioned stimuli once monthly. The patient improved clinically but, after 15 months, refused further cod liver oil because it triggered unpleasant nausea, a side effect of cyclophosphamide. She said that she continued to imagine a rose and believed that this image had become a conditioned stimulus for the desirable immunosuppressive effects of cyclophosphamide. It is intriguing to consider that the imagined visual image or smell or taste could be the equivalent of a tangible conditioned stimulus in effecting certain physiological responses.

## Effects of Stress and Relaxation on Immune Responses

Most of the studies in this area have been done with adults. A meta-analytic study on the effects of stress and relaxation on the *in vitro* immune response in humans (Van Rood, Bogaards, Goulmy, & van Houwelingen, 1993) reviewed 24 stress studies and 10 relaxation studies. The weakness of the meta-analysis was that it assumed parity among interventions that were, in fact, very different; for example, some studies included in the relaxation group asked subjects to focus on changing specific immune parameters, and some asked subjects merely to relax. The two requests are very different. Other studies in this meta-analysis included imagery with relaxation. The authors concluded that there were immunological changes in association with either stressors or relaxation, but confusion about interventions makes the changes difficult to interpret.

The first study in the English language medical literature to ponder an association between stress and the clinical expression of an infectious agent in children was published in 1962 (Meyer & Haggerty, 1962). This article found that children in stressful environments were more likely to have clinical symptoms associated with group A streptococcal infection than were children in less stressful environments. Boyce and colleagues (1993) undertook a study in 1989 to assess immunological changes that might occur at kindergarten entry. Their study protocols focused on individual differences that might mediate responses to stress. Twenty children were enrolled, and blood for immune measures was drawn 1 week before they began kindergarten. Two weeks later, this was repeated. At enrollment, mothers completed a variety of psychometric instruments to evaluate problem behaviors, stressful life events, child temperament, and family environment. During the 12-week follow-up period, the incidence, severity, and duration of respiratory illnesses were assessed from parent interviews done every 2 weeks. At 6 weeks, the Loma Prieta earthquake struck the San Francisco area where the study was in process; therefore, data assessment was divided into two periods, before and after the earthquake. Six weeks following the earthquake, the Child Behavior Checklist (CBL) was readministered along with a Child Earthquake Experience Checklist and a Parent Earthquake Impact Scale.

Broad variability in change scores was observed for the three immune measures: helper/suppressor ratio, pokeweed mitogenesis, and antibody responses to Pneumovax®. This was also true for respiratory illness incidence. Upregulation of the helper/suppressor ratio and pokeweed mitogenesis were associated with increased respiratory illness incidence following the earthquake. Change in behavior problems was significantly related to scores from the Parent Earthquake Impact Scale and inversely associated with pokeweed mitogenesis; that is, high earthquake-related parental distress and low immune reactivity were predictive of an increase in parent-reported problem behaviors. With low parental distress, neither highly nor minimally reactive children experienced a marked change in respiratory illness incidence. By contrast, under conditions of high parental distress, highly reactive children showed a marked increase in illness while minimally reactive children showed a decrease.

Boyce wrote that the health effects of psychologically stressful events are best predicted by an interaction between the intensity of environmental stressors and the biological reactivity of the individual host. Only a subset of children within any given population are truly at risk under environmental stress and adversity. Past studies using hypnotic interventions for a variety of problems have not considered the variables of biological reactivity and intensity of environmental stressors. This failure may explain results that are variable or inconsistent as reflected in existing studies of intentional immunomodulation by humans.

## Is There Evidence for Intentional Immunomodulation by Humans?

The short answer to this question is *yes*, but it is a qualified yes because most reported studies are essentially laboratory studies in normal humans. Clinical implications are not yet clear. Of the more than 30 reported studies in the English language, most are studies of adults (Beahrs, Harris, & Hilgard, 1970; Black, Humphrey, & Niven, 1963; Gruzelier, 1999; Halley, 1991; Kiecolt-Glaser, Glaser, Stain, & Stout, 1985; Locke et al., 1994; Smith, McKenzie, Marmer, & Steele, 1985). Many of these studies relate to the impact of hypnosis on delayed cutaneous hypersensitivity responses. A study by Locke and colleagues (1994) is an example. They studied 24 college students, selected for their high hypnotizability and ability to change skin temperature with hypnotic suggestions. Students were assigned randomly to undergo a predetermined sequence of four different experimental conditions, with each condition including varicella (VZ) skin testing: (1) hypnosis with suggestions to enhance the delayed-type hypersensitivity (DTH) response to VZ antigen, (2) hypnosis with suggestions to suppress the DTH response, (3) hypnosis with suggestions for relaxation only, and (4) skin testing without hypnosis. They found no significant effects on the area of the DTH response. Limitations of the study included use of a standardized script and induction technique, hypnotic suggestions given after injection of the antigen, and the assumption that high hypnotizability and skin temperature changes were predictors for success. Some individuals did achieve changes in the suggested directions, and these should be studied carefully to guide experimental methods in future studies of intentional immunomodulation.

## Intentional Immunomodulation in Children

Ma, Serbin, and Stack (2018) compared self-reported anxiety and diurnal variations of salivary IgA across successive periods from ages 9–12 to ages 12–15, and from ages 15–18. Worries in the first group significantly predicted lower cumulative daily levels of salivary IgA 3 years later. These lower levels were then predictive of higher anxiety at ages 15–18. Inasmuch as salivary IgA is a first line of defense against illness, it would seem that interventions to reduce anxiety, such as training in self-hypnosis, would be associated with higher salivary IgA levels and more resistance to infectious illness. Two research studies demonstrate that children who practice self-hypnosis can increase salivary IgA levels.

In a prospective, controlled study with 57 children ages 6–12 years, children who were assigned randomly to a 30-minute self-hypnosis practice associated with specific instructions to increase salivary immunoglobulin A (SIgA) demonstrated significant increases in SIgA compared to attention controls and to children who practiced the relaxation only (Olness, Culbert, & Uden, 1989). The children were seen twice, once for a baseline collection of saliva and to watch a puppet video that explained the immune system and once for the experimental intervention. No significant increase in immunoglobulin G was observed within or across groups, nor was any correlation with outcome and performance on the Stanford Children's Hypnotic Susceptibility Scale evident.

Hewson-Bower (1995) replicated our work that demonstrated SIgA increases in children who practiced relaxation and imagery. She took this information into the clinical arena in an exceptionally complex and excellent thesis study of 45 children with recurrent upper respiratory infections and a wait-list control group (Hewson-Bower & Drummond, 1996). She taught one group relaxation and imagery techniques focused on increasing SIgA and a second group relaxation and imagery techniques, problem-solving, and coping skills. Both interventions were equally effective in reducing the number of days of upper respiratory illness in children with recurrent infection problems in comparison to the control group. Hewson-Bower and Drummond 2001 then did a follow-up study that combined the two treatments described above. Combination treatment resulted in reduced days of upper respiratory illness in children with a history of recurrent colds and flu (both within subjects compared to a pretreatment baseline and cross sectionally with a matched control group). Twelve-month follow-up indicated that treatment gains persisted for days of illness. Hewson-Bower included psychometric assessments of subjects and families as well.

We also conducted controlled prospective studies of intentional modulation of neutrophils in 45 adolescents who were assigned randomly to one of three groups. Group A (the control group) had blood samples taken before and after a rest condition for two sessions spaced 1 week apart. Peripheral temperature and pulse recordings were also taken before and after the rest intervention. Group B (the untrained experimental group) had blood, peripheral temperature, and pulse recordings taken before and after a self-regulation exercise, with imagery focused on increasing neutrophil adherence, a measure of white cell function. Group C was an experimental group that received four training sessions prior to their attempts to increase neutrophil adherence. The immunology results from this study revealed that neither control group A nor the untrained experimental group B demonstrated increased neutrophil adherence in either session. Only the experimental group that received prior self-hypnosis training demonstrated a statistically significant increase in neutrophil adherence for the second session. These studies were conducted in a clinical research center with controls for time of day, no prior experience with hypnosis, and no immunological disorders. There were no changes in total numbers of neutrophils or chemiluminescence but only in the specific parameter they had been asked to change (Hall, Minnes, Tosi, & Olness, 1992). Although the practice of a self-hypnosis exercise was associated with success, the most successful subjects did not demonstrate physiological evidence of relaxation, whereas the resting group did (Hall, Minnes, & Olness, 1993). This suggests that some cognitive effort is associated with intentional changes in neutrophil adherence. The control group, who simply rested, did demonstrate physiological evidence of relaxation. The amount and type of practice related to outcomes in these studies as is true of other clinical hypnosis studies, especially with adolescents and adults. Young children learn quickly and seem to require less practice to achieve success.

Nassau and colleagues (Nassau, Tien, & Fritz, 2008) published a review of the literature on pediatric psychoneuroimmunology in chronic illness. They included only four articles related to hypnosis or hypnosis-like interventions in children with chronic conditions. Two of the studies were the previously mentioned studies by Hewson-Bower. A third was a study of 35 Venezuelan children (Castes et al., 1999); 19 of them were taught relaxation, which focused on developing mental images to suppress mast-cell degranulation and open airways. They were followed for 6 months and showed decreased immunoglobulin E responses to allergens in comparison to the 16 control subjects. They also had fewer asthma episodes and improved pulmonary function compared to the control group. The fourth study (Kern-Buell, McGrady, Conran, & Nelson, 2000) involved teaching biofeedback-assisted relaxation to 16 subjects with asthma, of whom a few were adolescents. Training in eight sessions included autogenic relaxation, progressive muscle relaxation, and deep breathing training; four of the sessions included biofeedback. The group learning biofeedback-assisted relaxation had reduced asthma severity and improved pulmonary function.

## Mast-Cell Function and Hypnosis in Juvenile Migraine

We did a study of mast-cell activation in children with migraine because mast cells contain many neurotransmitters known to be associated with the symptoms of migraine (Olness, Theoharides, Hall, Schmidt, & Rozniecki, 1999), and mast-cell products are known to be increased in the urine of adult migraneurs (Theoharides, 2002). We randomized 30 children with migraine to learn self-hypnosis or to remain in a control group that would later learn self-hypnosis. Tryptase and histamine levels were measured. Results confirmed earlier studies that self-hypnosis practice led to a substantial reduction in migraine episodes. This was associated with decreased levels of urine tryptase, suggesting that the mechanism of reduced migraine episodes was due to stabilization of mast cells. It is possible that the regular practice of self-hypnosis can reduce the likelihood of mast-cell degranulation.

## Warts

Numerous clinical reports have been published regarding warts remitting in association with nonpharmacological treatments, including hypnotherapy (Ewin, 1992; Goldstein, 2005; Noll, 1994; Spanos, Stenstrom, & Johnston, 1988; Tasini & Hackett, 1977). We have had many clinical experiences similar to the one we describe here.

Andy, a 10-year-old boy, had a total of 27 warts on both hands, his right arm, and abdomen. They had been present for 2 years, and he had been seen by his pediatrician and dermatologists who had prescribed topical therapy followed by cryotherapy. Some of the warts would get smaller for a period and then grow to a larger size. Andy had no prior experience with hypnosis and was intrigued with the possibility that he could make his warts disappear. He and his mother completed a questionnaire about his likes, interests, skills, fears, and imagery. He was a good student, was taking piano lessons, and enjoyed basketball, his favorite sport. During the first hypnosis session, I monitored his peripheral temperature, electrodermal activity, and heart rate to document for him that changes in thinking could effect physiological changes. He noted that the lines on the computer screen that reflected his heart rate and electrodermal activity jumped immediately when he thought of something exciting. I suggested he begin his hypnosis training by imagining himself standing at the free-throw line and shooting a free throw with great ease. He could note the connections between his brain and muscles that are involved in throwing the basketball and enjoy imagining the basketball swishing through the net. I asked him to repeat this ten times and then to imagine himself in a comfortable place, enjoying the feeling of having done so well with the free throws. I asked him to lift a "yes" finger when he was in a comfortable place. Within 2 minutes, Andy lifted his right index finger. I then said:

> You're doing very well. I can tell by the monitor. Your temperature has gone up, and your heart rate has gone down. That means you're comfortable and relaxed. Now, when you are so comfortable, it's a good time to program your body to get rid of the warts. So, when you're ready, very easily, just once, tell yourself to stop feeding the warts on your hands, stop feeding the warts on your arm, and stop feeding the warts on your abdomen. And, when you have told yourself that, continue to enjoy your comfortable, pleasant place in your imagination a little while longer, and when you're ready, slowly, and easily, you can open your eyes and enjoy the rest of today.

After Andy opened his eyes, I asked if he had questions, and I asked him to practice this exercise twice a day at home. I reminded him that he could telephone me if he had additional questions and that one would review with him in 2 weeks. When he returned in 2 weeks, he had only 10 warts left, and they were much smaller. He called a month later to report they were gone. There was no recurrence in a 1-year follow-up.

Meineke and colleagues (Meineke, Reichrath, Reinhold, & Tilgen, 2002) in Germany reported that a suggestion-based therapy (simulated x-ray treatment of children with warts) was associated with elimination of the warts. We conducted a 4-year consortium study of non-pharmacological management of warts that involved collaboration among six institutions (Felt et al., 1998). Children between the ages of 6 and 12 years who had warts on their hands and arms were randomized to topical or self-hypnosis or attention-control treatment for the management of warts. Each child completed a questionnaire related to likes, dislikes, interests, preferred imagery, and activities. Each child saw a video that explained about warts. Children also chose a signal wart that would be photographed and measured over the course of the study. Each child was seen four times over a 3-month period and followed over an additional 6 months. Signal warts were photographed at each visit. Children in the hypnosis group were taught a standardized self-hypnosis exercise. Group data analysis found no significant differences among groups, although there was evidence of wart regression in each group, and some children in the hypnosis group had dramatic wart regression. Children in the hypnosis group had 50% less recurrence of warts than the topical therapy group, and 78% of children in the hypnosis group reported continuing their self-hypnosis practice a year later. Many said that they used their self-hypnosis skills to reduce stress or help them prepare for exams and other performance activities such as soccer games. This study was limited by the need to use a standardized method of self-hypnosis and the large amount of attention paid to warts (e.g., photographing warts) in all groups.

Thomas (1979) wrote, "We will understand more about tumors if we could understand what goes away and in what order when warts are hypnotized away." We are still a long way from that ideal.

## The Future in Pediatric Psychoneuroimmunology

This is an exciting and important area in which progress has been very slow. Substantial evidence suggests that stress impacts the human immune system over a lifetime (Graham, Christian, & Kiecolt-Glaser, 2006; Morag, Morag, Reichenberg, Lerer, & Yirmiya, 1999). Danese and Lewis (2017) stated, based on experimental animal models and observational human studies, that PNI of early life stress offers a framework to understand and treat psychopathology associated with childhood trauma. Early life stress predicts inflammation. They demonstrated that cumulative exposure to child maltreatment led to increased inflammatory responses 20 years later (Danese, Pariante, Caspi,

Taylor, & Poulton, 2007). Danese and Lewis (2017) have also written that nonpharmacologic strategies like psychotherapy and meditation can reduce inflammation and buffer early life stress effects.

Although it is too early to make definitive statements about the clinical applications of research described in this chapter, there is merit in encouraging the pure laboratory group, the pure clinical group, and the mixed group of researchers to move forward concurrently. This has happened in other areas of medical science in which medications were used long before their mechanisms of action were clear. Nassau, Tien, and Fritz (2008) described challenges for conducting research on the effects of psychological interventions on immunity in children. These include choosing reliable and relevant immune markers, recruiting adequate samples of blood from children, gaining parental consent and child assent to blood draws, and conducting blood draws without causing undue distress. O'Connor, Moynihan, and Caserta (2014) have advanced a developmental model of psychoneuroimmunology and described the potential advantages of integrating this model into clinical research.

From designing many protocols over the years, we recognize that conventional protocol design does not lend itself easily to self-regulation interventions. Protocol review committees prefer that interventions are "constant and equal" for each child, yet we know that intrinsic thinking processes, imagery preferences, and learning styles vary (Olness, 1990). As noted in the research of Boyce and colleagues (1993), intrinsic differences in immunological reactivity also exist. By using the same coaching for each subject in a study, we ensure some failures. Data analysis of the Children's Cancer Study Group (CCSG) assumes that children in the study received the same intervention – that is, medication dictated by the protocol. But clinicians who work with these children are aware that, depending on the personality of the child and the innate persuasion skills of physicians, nurses, or parents, some medications reach the alimentary tract of the child and some go under the mattress or into the toilet bowl. The same principle applies in training for self-hypnosis. Clinically, we observe that coaching that varies according to developmental stage, interests, and learning style of a given child results in more predictable receipt of the intervention. Research protocols should consider:

- Quality and quantity of behavioral interventions
- Amount and type of self-hypnosis practice, if required
- Quality and quantity of antigenic stimulation
- Temporal relationship between interventions and antigenic stimulation
- Nature of the immune response
- Host factors such as age, sex, genes, intrinsic immune reactivity, sleep requirements, diet, and life experiences
- Chronobiological factors

It is also important that the possibility of inadvertent conditioning of immune responses be kept in mind and that researchers should follow children over long time periods.

Solomon (1993) stated in his thesis that psychoneuroimmunology represents a conceptual breakthrough that offers the opportunity to approach the body, in health and sickness, from a new theoretical perspective. It is tempting to speculate about how voluntary immunomodulation might occur in children. Persinger (1987) noted that any condition that enhances temporal lobe lability will increase recruitment of immune processes. Children have enhanced temporal lobe lability, especially during the school-age years (Carey & Diamond, 1980). Of relevance to the voluntary control of immune processes is the interaction between the cerebral cortex and hippocampus. The hippocampus provides access to the imagery of memory presumably stored in the cortex. In children, the typical adult distinction between the imagery of memory and the imagery of experience is less clear (Kail, 1984). As a result, verbal instructions can induce imagery as strong as emotional memories. This is documented in the physiological changes noted when children are encouraged to think in different ways (Lee & Olness, 1995). The capacity of children to show enhanced voluntary control of immune regulation through programmed imagining (suggestion) would be facilitated by the interdependence of imagination and memory (Persinger & De Sano, 1986).

Some practical questions in clinical areas that derive from research done in the area of pediatric psychoneuroimmunology include:

- Can inflammation induced by early trauma be reversed by frequent practice of self-regulation targeted at immune responses?
- What stressors may predispose to streptococcal infections?
- What stressors trigger recurrent herpes? Can their efforts be reversed via training in self-hypnosis?
- Will anticipatory guidance for families include information about how parental distress impacts on the immune responses of their children?
- Will we be able to recommend self-hypnosis practice for both children and parents to prevent undesirable immune responses?
- How might immunosuppression or immunoenhancement be conditioned inadvertently in children? How could this be reversed?
- How does winning (or losing) impact immunity?
- Is nonpharmacological treatment of warts less expensive than pharmacological treatment?
- Are responses to immunizations less effective if children are stressed?

In all of this, we must resist the temptation to overstate the clinical applications of psychoneuroimmunology research by making claims that are not grounded in sound data (Solomon, 1993).

## References

Ader, R., Ed. (1981). *Psychoneuroimmunology*. New York: Academic Press.

Ader, R. (1989). Conditioned immune responses and pharmacotherapy. *Arthritis Care Research, 2*, S58–S64.

Ader, R., Ed. (1991). *Psychoneuroimmunology*, 2nd ed. New York: Academic Press.

Beahrs, J.O., Harris, D.R., & Hilgard, E.R. (1970). Failure to alter skin inflammation by hypnotic suggestion in five subjects with normal skin reactivity. *Psychosomatic Medicine, 32*, 627–631.

Black, S., Humphrey, J.H., & Niven, J.S. (1963). Inhibition of the Mantoux reaction by direct suggestion under hypnosis. *British Medical Journal, 6*, 1649–1652.

Boyce, W.T., Chesterman, E., Martin, N., Folkman, S., Cohen, F., & Wara, D. (1993). Immunologic changes occurring at kindergarten entry predict respiratory illnesses after the Loma Prieta earthquake. *Journal of Developmental and Behavioral Pediatrics, 14*, 196–203.

Buske-Kirschbaum, A., Kirschbaum, C., Stierle, H., Lehnert, H., & Hellhammer, D. (1992). Conditioned increase of natural killer cell activity in humans. *Psychosomatic Medicine, 54*, 123–132.

Carey, S. & Diamond, R. (1980). Maturational determination of the developmental course of face encoding. In D. Caplan, Ed., *Biological Studies of Mental Processes*. Cambridge, MA: MIT Press.

Castes, M., Hagel, I., Palenque, M., Canelones, P., Corao, A., & Lynch, N.R. (1999). Immunological changes associated with clinical improvement of asthmatic children subjected to psychosocial intervention. *Brain, Behavior and Immunity, 13*, 1–13.

Danese, A. & Lewis, S.J. (2017). Psychoneuroimmunology of early-life stress: the hidden wounds of childhood trauma? *Neuropsychopharmacology, 42*, 99–114.

Danese, A., Pariante, C.M., Caspi, A., Taylor, A., & Poulton, R. (2007). Childhood maltreatment predicts adult inflammation in a life-course study. *Proceedings of the National Academy of Sciences of the United States of America, 104*, 1319–1324.

Ewin, D. (1992). Hypnotherapy for warts (*Verruca vulgaris*): 41 consecutive cases with 33 cures. *American Journal of Clinical Hypnosis*, *35*(1), 1–10.
Felt, B.T., Berman, B., Broffman, G., Coury, D., Dattner, A., French, G., Hall, H., Kohen, D.P., Schmidt, W., Young, M.H., & Olness, K. (1998). Wart regression in children: comparison of relaxation-imagery to topical treatment and equal time interventions. *American Journal of Clinical Hypnosis*, *41*(2), 130–138.
Goldstein, R.H. (2005). Successful repeated hypnotic treatment of warts in the same individual: a case report. *American Journal of Clinical Hypnosis*, *47*(4), 259–264.
Graham, J.E., Christian, L.M., & Kiecolt-Glaser, J.K. (2006). Stress, age, and immune function: toward a lifespan approach. *Journal of Behavioral Medicine*, *29*, 389–400.
Gruzelier, J.H. (1999). Hypnosis from a neurobiological perspective: a review of evidence and applications to improve immune function. *Anales de Psicologia*, *15*, 111–132.
Hall, H.R., Minnes, L., & Olness, K. (1993). The psychophysiology of voluntary immunomodulation. *International Journal of Neuroscience*, *69*, 221–234.
Hall, H.R., Minnes, L., Tosi, M., & Olness, K. (1992). Voluntary modulation of neutrophil adhesiveness using a cyberphysiologic strategy. *International Journal of Neuroscience*, *63*, 287–297.
Halley, F.M. (1991). Self-regulation of the immune system through biobehavioral strategies. *Biofeedback and Self-Regulation*, *16*, 55–74.
Hewson-Bower, B. (1995). Psychological Treatment Decreases Colds and Flu in Children by Increasing Salivary Immunoglobulin A. PhD Thesis, Murdoch University, Perth, Western Australia.
Hewson-Bower, B., & Drummond, P.D. (1996). Secretory immunoglobulin A increases during relaxation in children with and without recurrent upper respiratory tract infections. *Journal of Developmental and Behavioral Pediatrics*, *17*, 311–316.
Hewson-Bower, B., & Drummond, P.D. (2001). Psychological treatment for recurrent symptoms of colds and flu in children. *Journal of Psychosomatic Research*, *51*, 369–377.
Kail, R. (1984). *The Development of Memory in Children*, 2nd ed. New York: W.H. Freeman.
Kern-Buell, C.L., McGrady, A.V., Conran, P.B., & Nelson, L.A. (2000). Asthma severity, psychophysiological indicators of arousal, and immune function in asthma patients undergoing biofeedback assisted relaxation. *Applied Psychophysiology and Biofeedback*, *25*, 79–91.
Kiecolt-Glaser, J.K., Glaser, R., Stain, E.C., & Stout, J.C. (1985). Modulation of cellular immunity in medical students. *Journal of Behavioral Medicine*, *9*, 5–21.
Lee, L. & Olness, K. (1995). Impact of imagery changes on autonomic reactivity in children [abstract]. *Archives of Pediatrics and Adolescent Medicine*, *149*, 47.
Locke, S.E., Ransil, B.J., Zachariae, R., Molay, F., Tollins, K., Covino, N.A., & Danforth, D. (1994). Effect of hypnotic suggestion on the delayed-type hypersensitivity response. *Journal of the American Medical Association*, *272*, 47–52.
Ma, D., Serbin, L.A., & Stack, D.M. (2018). Children's anxiety symptoms and salivary immunoglobulin A: a mutual regulatory system? *Developmental Psychobiology*, *60*, 202–215.
MacQueen, G.M., Marshall, J., Perdue, M., Siegel, S., & Bienenstock, J. (1989). Pavlovian conditioning of rat mucosal mast cells to secrete rat mast cell protease. II. *Science*, *243*, 83–85.
Meineke, V., Reichrath, J., Reinhold, U., & Tilgen, W. (2002). Verrucae vulgares in children: successful simulated x-ray treatment (a suggestion-based therapy). *Dermatology*, *204(4)*, 287–289.
Meyer, R. & Haggerty, R. (1962). Streptococcal infections in families: factors altering individual susceptibility. *Journal of Pediatrics*, *29*, 539–549.
Morag, M., Morag, A., Reichenberg, A., Lerer, B., & Yirmiya, R. (1999). Psychological variables as predictors of rubella antibody titers and fatigue: a prospective, double blind study. *Journal of Psychiatric Research*, *33*, 389–395.
Nassau, J.H., Tien, K., & Fritz, G.K. (2008). Review of the literature: integrating psychoneuroimmunology into pediatric chronic illness interventions. *Journal of Pediatric Psychology*, *33*, 195–207.
Noll, R.B. (1994). Hypnotherapy for warts in children and adolescents. *Journal of Developmental and Behavioral Pediatrics*, *15(3)*, 170–173.
O'Connor, T.G., Moynihan, J.A., & Caserta, M.T. (2014). Annual research review: the neuroinflammation hypothesis for stress and psychopathology in children: developmental psychoneuroimmunology. *Journal of Child Psychology and Psychiatry*, *55*, 615–631.

Olness, K. (1990). Pediatric psychoneuroimmunology: hypnosis as a possible mediator—potentials and problems. In R. Van Dyck et al., Eds., *Hypnosis: Current Theory, Research, and Practice* (pp. 71–81). Amsterdam: Free University Press.

Olness, K.&Ader, K. (1992). Conditioning as an adjunct in the pharmacotherapy of lupus erythematosus. *Journal of Developmental and Behavioral Pediatrics*, 13, 124–125.

Olness, K., Culbert, T.P., & Uden, D. (1989). Self-regulation of salivary immunoglobulin A by children. *Pediatrics, 83*, 66–71.

Olness, K., Theoharides, T.C., Hall, H., Schmidt, W., & Rozniecki, J. (1999). Mast cell activation in child migraine patients before and after training in self-regulation. *Headache, 41*, 130–138.

Persinger, M.A. & De Sano, C.F. (1986). Temporal lobe signs: positive correlations with imaginings and hypnosis induction profiles. *Psychological Reports, 58*, 347–350.

Persinger, M. A. (1987).The Neuropsychological Bases of the God Experience. New York: Praeger.

Schleifer, S.J., Scott, B., Stein, M., & Keller, S.E. (1986). Behavioral and developmental aspects of immunity. *Journal of the American Academy of Child Psychiatry, 26*, 751–763.

Shertzer, C.L. & Lookingbill, D.P. (1987). Effects of relaxation therapy and hypnotizability in chronic urticaria. *Archives of Dermatology, 123*, 913–916.

Smith, G.R., McKenzie, J.M., Marmer, D.J., & Steele, R.W. (1985). Psychologic modulation of the human immune response to varicella zoster. *Archives of Internal Medicine, 145*, 2110–2112.

Solomon, G.F. (1993). Whither psychoneuroimmunology? A new era of immunology, of psychosomatic medicine, and of neuroscience. *Brain, Behavior, and Immunity*, 7, 352–366.

Spanos, N.P., Stenstrom, R.J., & Johnston, J.C. (1988). Hypnosis, placebo, and suggestion in the treatment of warts. *Psychosomatic Medicine, 50*, 245–260.

Stiehm, E.R. & Johnston, R.B. (2005). A history of pediatric immunology. *Pediatric Research, 57*, 458–467.

Tasini, M.F. & Hackett, T.P. (1977). Hypnosis in the treatment of warts in immunodeficient children. *American Journal of Clinical Hypnosis, 19*, 152–154.

Theoharides, T.C. (2002). Mast cells and stress: a psychoneuroimmunological perspective. *Journal of Clinical Psychopharmacology, 22*, 103–108.

Thomas, L. (1979). *The Medusa and the Snail.* New York: Viking Press.

Van Rood, Y.R., Bogaards, M., Goulmy, E., & van Houwelingen, H.C. (1993). The effects of stress and relaxation on the in vitro immune response in man: a meta-analytic study. *Journal of Behavioral Medicine, 16*, 163–181.

# 19

# APPLICATIONS OF HYPNOSIS WITH CHILDREN GLOBALLY

## Introduction

The World Bank classified countries into several categories. It assigns economies to four income groups – low, lower-middle, upper-middle, and high-income countries – based on gross national income per capita in current USD. Lower-middle income as of July 1, 2021, is $1,046–4,195. High income is more than $12,695. Seventy percent of the world's population are in the lower-middle or upper-middle categories (World Bank, 2022). Over the past decade increasing numbers of children in middle- and high-income countries have had opportunities to learn hypnosis. However, there remains a great need to increase hypnosis training, especially in low- and lower-middle-income countries. This need is especially huge with respect to nonpharmacologic pain management in areas where there is a general lack of effective medications. In 2021, the world had 2.53 billion children under 18 years. Five hundred million live in the low-income countries (UNICEF, 2022). These are areas where both infant and under-five mortality is high and where children are at greater risk for diseases or accidents involving pain or painful procedures. These include conditions such as sickle cell disease (Africa), thalassemia (Southeast Asia), injuries, burns, male and female circumcision, toothaches, and many painful infectious diseases. Some children will experience childhood cancer and the pain associated with the disease, as well as diagnostic and treatment procedures. As a result of inadequate pain management, untold numbers of children and the adults they have become will experience posttraumatic stress symptoms related to their experience of severe pain. Many children in resource poor areas will suffer early and permanent brain injury from malnutrition, iron deficiency, infectious diseases, alcohol use during pregnancy, or exposure to toxins such as lead or organophosphates (Olness, 2003). This often leads to learning disabilities that may complicate training in hypnosis.

A study by Green and colleagues (Green, Page, Rasekhy, Johnson, & Bernhardt, 2006) studied attitudes and beliefs about hypnosis across four samples of college students at the University of New South Wales, Australia; Dortmund University, Germany; The Ohio State University, United States; and Shaheed Beheshti University of Medical Sciences, Iran. Two hundred eighty undergraduate students were surveyed. Responses to some items varied by country but views about hypnosis were generally similar. About half of all students believed that hypnosis involved "giving up free will to the hypnotist." Most students also believed that hypnosis could force people to tell the truth and also to remember things they could not otherwise remember. Iranian

DOI: 10.4324/9781003243687-21

students, compared to the US and German students, were more likely to associate hypnotic responding with mental instability and to be more afraid of hypnosis. Overall, it was clear that there were many misconceptions about hypnosis and therapeutic hypnosis in college students from these four countries. Such misconceptions undoubtedly contribute to the fact that hypnosis training is limited in many countries and does not exist at all in some countries.

In terms of sheer numbers of child health professionals (per 1,000 population) who have been trained in how to teach children hypnosis, Germany leads. For many years, Dr. Bernhard Trenkle, a psychologist, and current past-president of the International Society of Hypnosis has organized every 2 years child hypnosis congresses in Heidelberg, with more than 1,000 attending each conference. In contrast, child hypnosis workshops at the Annual Workshops in Clinical Hypnosis in the United States had a beginning attendance of about 50. The Sixth European Child Hypnosis Congress held in Heidelberg from October 29 to November 1, 2009, took place in the Stadthalle, a wonderful old building situated adjacent to the Neckar River in Heidelberg. Attendance at the Sixth Congress was 1,800, with more than 100 faculty. Dr. Daniel Kohen taught three intermediate/advanced-level workshops on disorders of elimination, hypnosis for asthma, and self-hypnosis training for habit problems in children and adolescents. Other English-language workshops included Joyce Mills' workshop on "Changing Woman: An Honoring Approach for Adolescent Girls and Women," Julie Linden's workshop on "Hypnosis and Parenting," Maggie Phillips' workshop on "Saving the Velveteen Rabbit: Ericksonian Approaches to Pain Management with Children and Adolescents," and Heather Hays and Wayne Raiter's workshop on "Using Paradoxical Intention to Intervene with Addicted Adolescents." The Congress included a large book display and store, an exhibition and sale of puppets, and a variety of other healing methodologies. All the faculty presentation materials were provided to participants on a CD to encourage active listening by participants. This state-of-the-art Congress in Germany is an example of what can be accomplished by increasing the number of child health professionals who know how to teach hypnosis to children. Drs. Siegfried Mrochen and Karl Ludwig Holtz, leading German child psychologists, have been major teachers at this annual Congress. Their writings have inspired many in Germany who work with young people (Holtz & Mrochen, 2005; Mrochen, Holtz, & Trenkle, 1993). Dr. Mrochen's enthusiasm and seminal work with puppets and therapeutic hypnosis have influenced many who offer ongoing training in child hypnosis throughout Germany. Also at the Congress were Drs. Hiltrud and Alfred Bierbaum-Luttermann, who operate a Kinderhypnose clinic, a "Kid-Hyp" training curriculum and psychology training institute in Berlin; we have had the privilege of teaching workshops with them and learning from them on many different occasions over the past 30 years. Dr. Kohen has also provided pediatric hypnosis workshop training in many other cities in Germany: as part of many Child Hypnosis Congresses (Heidelberg, Wurzburg), as part of an International Society of Hypnosis Triennial Congress (Bremen), as invited 2–3 days workshops in Ravensburg, Rottweil, Krefeld, and Luneburg.

Pediatricians, nurse clinicians, psychiatrists, and other child therapists in the Netherlands have contributed substantially to our understanding and practice of clinical hypnosis in general and specifically with children. In the past and in more recent years, Drs. Kuttner, Sugarman, and Kohen have each taught child hypnosis workshops in Amsterdam with our Dutch colleagues and with strong support from psychiatrist Dr. Eric Vermetten, recent past president of the Dutch Society of Hypnosis and of the International Society of Hypnosis. Based in Nieuwegein, Dr. Arine Vlieger and colleagues (Vlieger, Menko-Frankenhuis, Wolfkamp, Tromp, & Benninga, 2007) published the first randomized controlled study describing the efficacy of hypnosis for recurrent abdominal pain or functional abdominal pain in children (see also Chapter 13).

Pediatricians and subspecialists (gastroenterology, neurology) from Israel have also contributed important understanding of applications of hypnosis in a variety of childhood problems including inflammatory bowel disease (Shaoul, Sukhotnik, & Mogilner, 2009), pediatric dentistry (Peretz, 1996a, 1996b; Peretz & Gluck, 1999), and school refusal (Aviv, 2006; see also Chapters 8 and 13).

## Therapeutic Hypnosis with Children and Adolescents in Norway

When Karen Olness went to Norway in 1977 to visit relatives, she met Dr. Inger Helene Vandvik, a child psychiatrist who was a faculty member at the Rikshospitalet of the University of Oslo. Dr. Vandvik consulted with the Department of Pediatrics and was interested in determining how therapeutic hypnosis might be helpful to children with such problems as needle phobia and enuresis (Vandvik, 1994). Dr. Vandvik kindly provided the information here about hypnosis in Norway.

The Norwegian Association for Clinical and Experimental Hypnosis (NACEH) was founded in 1979, 14 years after the Swedish Hypnosis Association was formed (Nielsen & Vandvik, 1981). Since 1977, the Faculty of Psychology at the University of Bergen has twice-yearly offered an elective course in hypnosis for its graduate students. This has regularly attracted about 90% of the students in the clinical psychology training program. From 1983 to 1998, the Faculty of Medicine at the University of Bergen, in collaboration with the Norwegian Medical Association, offered an annual 3-day postgraduate seminar in clinical hypnosis to physicians; however, at the present time, hypnosis is not included in the curriculum at any of the Norwegian medical faculties.

Over the past 40 years, a number of workshops on hypnosis with children have been held, although hypnosis is still underutilized in pediatric settings and in child psychiatry in Norway. A review in Norway of the literature regarding hypnosis in child psychiatry revealed no randomized or controlled trials or prospective, planned research studies using hypnosis for child psychiatric disorders (Huynh, Vandvik, & Diseth, 2008). After a small study regarding hypnosis in the treatment of ten boys with enuresis was published in the *Journal of the Norwegian Medical Association* (Diseth & Vandvik, 2004), the authors received more than 400 requests from colleagues and parents requesting help for a child with enuresis. In 2008, the Regional Center for Child and Adolescent Mental Health under the direction of Vandvik and Diseth in Oslo undertook a 1-year educational program on hypnosis with children and adolescents for physicians and psychologists, the two professional groups who are permitted to practice hypnosis by Norwegian legislation (Lindheim & Helgeland, 2017). The program includes four 2-day seminars that feature lectures, demonstrations, and group practice. There are also four meetings with supervision in groups of six to eight participants. Between seminars, the students work with mentors. Each participant must present a written paper at the end of the year. This must include two medical case histories and describe the application of hypnosis in clinical practice. Most participants have been psychiatrists or psychologists. Evaluations have been generally excellent.

## Self-Hypnosis around the World

Dr. Lars-Eric Unestahl has been a leader in teaching hypnosis to athletes, including Olympic contenders (Dobbin, 2006). His doctoral thesis work documented that self-hypnosis, if practiced over the long term, is more effective than heterohypnosis (Unestahl, 1973). He developed methods for teaching Swedish children self-hypnosis as part of their physical education programs in grade school, and his integrated mental training program has been used throughout the world.

Hypnosis has been taught to children in France and England for the past two centuries, and many child health professionals in Canada teach hypnosis to children (Rogovik & Goldman,

2007). An expert in pain management in Canada is Dr. Leora Kuttner, a child psychologist who began working with children who had cancer in the 1980s. She produced two extraordinary documentaries, *No Fears, No Tears: Children with Cancer Coping with Pain* and *No Fears, No Tears: 13 Years Later* (Kuttner, 1986, 1998), which have been used as superb teaching tools in hypnosis workshops and in pediatric oncology units around the world (see also Chapter 13).

Many experts on hypnosis with children can be found in Australia (Hewson-Bower, 1995; Jaaniste, Hayes, & von Baeyer, 2007; Mackenzie & Frawley, 2007), Canada (Kuttner, 1986, 1988, 1989, 1991, 1998, 2003, 2007; Kuttner & Catchpole, 2007; Kuttner, Bowman, & Teasdale, 1988; Jaaniste et al., 2007; Rogovik & Goldman, 2007), England (Liossi & Hatira, 1999, 2003; Liossi & White, 2001; Liossi, White, & Hatira, 2006), Italy (Astuto, Favara-Scacco, Crimi, Rizzo, & Di Cataldo, 2002; Fasciana 2009, 2014), and Indonesia (Lesmana, Suryani, Jensen, & Tiliopoulos, 2009), all of whom have contributed substantial research and publications related to hypnosis with children. A few child health professionals in Saudi Arabia and Turkey teach self-hypnosis to children for problems such as enuresis, functional abdominal pain, and habit problems (Al Sughayir, 2007).

An ideal program to make self-hypnosis training available to children with pain was developed in Khon Kaen, the capital of Khon Kaen Province in northeast Thailand, the poorest province in the country. Children are referred from throughout the largely rural province to Srinagarind Hospital at Khon Kaen University for treatment of complex problems such as cancer or hemoglobinopathies. Prior to 2003, children with cancer were subjected to outpatient procedures such as bone marrow aspirations or chemotherapy without local anesthesia, sedation, or psychological preparation. The hospital had insufficient numbers of anesthesiologists to monitor sedating medications in the outpatient areas. Few families could afford to pay for an indwelling intravenous catheter; therefore, children had to endure the placement of a new intravenous cannula each time chemotherapy was required. In the local university hospital, liquid narcotics were occasionally available to children with chronic pain associated with cancer, but oral narcotic preparations were rarely available at rural health stations. Many children manifested symptoms of PTSD after experiencing painful procedures. Two pediatric faculty members in Khon Kaen had been trained in developmental behavioral pediatrics in the United States and had taken hypnosis and biofeedback workshops. A nurse who received her doctorate in the United States also took hypnosis workshops. In 2003 and 2004, they arranged three training sessions for a total of 68 child health professionals working in the hospital. These sessions provided guidelines for pain assessment in children that were introduced into every pediatric ward, including the intensive care units.

In 2005, the Department of Pediatrics of Khon Kaen University organized a national workshop on pediatric pain management; 80 child health professionals attended from throughout Thailand. Since then, a collaborative effort between Khon Kaen University and Dalhousie University in Canada has resulted in the completion of several studies assessing parental attitudes, beliefs, and experiences concerning child pain and pain management and the prevalence of pediatric pain in northeast Thailand hospitals. These studies found that 81% of pediatric patients suffered moderate to severe pain and received little or no pharmacological pain treatment. As a result of these findings, the Khon Kaen pediatric pain management team established guidelines for the management of pain in children throughout the province. These guidelines have now been implemented, including education for all health-care workers, commitment to respond quickly to patients when they report pain, accountability for pain management by child health professionals, and continuing evaluation to improve the quality of both pharmacological and nonpharmacological pain management.

A member of the pain management team meets with every child newly diagnosed with cancer to explain the plans and procedures to the child and his or her family; also, training in self-hypnosis and biofeedback is offered. The training is similar to well-known meditative techniques in Thailand and is generally well received. As one example, an 8-year-old girl with leukemia learned to use self-hypnosis prior to her diagnostic procedures and treatments. She imagined herself in her mother's kitchen, anticipating the good food that her mother was preparing for her. She remained relaxed and comfortable throughout the procedures.

In 2013, Ben Furman, a child, adolescent, and adult psychiatrist, arranged for a 2-day pediatric hypnosis workshop to be presented in his home, Helsinki, Finland. It was the first pediatric hypnosis workshop ever presented there. While the hope, expectation, and promotion of the workshop was to child health clinicians, and therefore hoped to attract pediatricians, in fact the 50–60 participants were primarily psychologists and other psychotherapists, with but a few pediatricians and a couple of child psychiatrists. The author of over 12 books (all focused upon "kids' skills" especially for schoolteachers), Dr. Furman agreed that much of what he has developed and taught is very closely aligned to solution-oriented psychotherapy, which we and others understand to be analogous to, or a form of, clinical hypnosis. Recently Dr. Furman invited Dr. Kohen to be a guest interviewee about Pediatric Hypnosis for his YouTube Educational Channel (2021).

In 2014, Vibha Krishnamurthy, developmental behavioral pediatrician, organized a 3-day pediatric hypnosis workshop for her staff at the Ummeed Child Development Center in Mumbai. Self-hypnosis training emphasizing self-regulation and self-control has been very helpful to the many children with developmental disabilities who are cared for at this remarkable center (Ummeed, 2022).

The Japanese Society of Biofeedback Research recently published an article on their programs. These include a description of a stuffed animal bear containing a paced breathing device to help children learn relaxation by adjusting their breathing according to the movement of the bear's abdomen. The purpose is to help children acquire stress tolerance. It would be interesting to compare this relaxation system with training in self-hypnosis.

## An Example of a Culturally Appropriate Hypnosis Intervention in Bali

Lesmana, Suryani, Jensen, and Tiliopoulos (2009) studied 226 children, ages 6–12 years, who experienced the terrorist bomb blasts in Bali in 2002 and were diagnosed later with posttraumatic stress disorder (PTSD). Forty-eight children received spiritual hypnosis assisted therapy (SHAT) and 178 received no therapy. Children were followed for 2 years. The 48 children were divided into two groups, and the therapy was conducted one time in the group setting. SHAT included a meditation–trance induction. Children were instructed to meditate with their eyes closed. After 5 minutes, they were asked to breathe deeply through their nose and slowly exhale through their mouth for 1 minute. The researcher monitored cues such as arm rigidity and immobilization, eye catalepsy, and inability to communicate, which were considered to be indicators of a hypnotic state. When in trance, children were guided to be sensitive to their own spirit and advised to identify and reframe the meaning of traumatic memories that may have obscured their spirit. They were asked not to imagine or visualize the traumatic moment of the bomb blast but to let the process happen in a natural way. They were told that they could express undesirable feelings by crying, shouting, or inhaling deeply and exhaling slowly. They were told that the trauma was in the past and that what happened would enable them to face new challenges in life without the burdens of the past trauma.

Of the children treated with SHAT, 77.1% improved, compared to 24% of the control group. Mean PTSD symptom scores were significantly lower in the SHAT group. Results did not correlate with age or sex. All children were offered the option of individual hypnosis or psychotherapy but none elected this option. Results were remarkable, considering that each child had only one therapeutic intervention. All of the children in this study were from families who were Hindus, who believe that all humans consist of mind, body, and spirit. The spirit is a source of energy, personal awareness, and knowledge. The authors of this study recommended further research, using a multisite randomized design with cross-cultural variables, to assess the generalizability of the SHAT intervention across sites, situations, and cultures.

## Therapeutic Hypnosis in the Netherlands

In the Netherlands several National Pediatric Hypnosis Training Institute (NPHTI) faculties (Drs. Kuttner, Kohen, Sugarman) have taught pediatric hypnosis workshops in Amsterdam since the late 1990s/early 2000s. One very exciting outcome of this has been the participation of several Dutch clinicians in NPHTI workshops, notably Dr. Arine Vlieger and Ms. Carla Frankenhuis, a pediatrician and nurse clinician, respectively. Ms. Frankenhuis later was one of the "Facilitating Facilitators' Facilitation" (FFF) trainees (see Chapter 22 on Teaching Child Hypnosis) and participated not only in training participants in NPHTI workshops, but also "back home" she and Dr. Vlieger developed training workshops in Amsterdam as described further. In recognition of her significant pediatric hypnosis research Dr. Vlieger (see Chapter 13) was an invited guest faculty for NPHTI workshops in 2017. Ms. Frankenhuis and Dr. Vlieger expanded training to many surrounding towns and pediatric hospitals. In 2019 Ms. Frankenhuis and Dr. Vlieger started a foundation: "Hypnosis for children" and have since offered a free membership for all their former students who have followed the basic and advanced courses they have provided for hypnosis with children. Soon thereafter 72 people had registered. This organization publishes a newsletter which includes "hypnosis news," notice of training opportunities, and reports of results of ongoing research. One result of these efforts is that many of their Dutch child health professional colleagues and learners have in turn come to the United States for more advanced training with NPHTI, in Minneapolis, both at our fundamentals workshop and at the utilization level workshop. Beyond their clinical expertise and expansion of training to many other child health clinicians, they have been leaders in developing many research protocols and publishing results of RCT's, notably in controlled studies demonstrating the efficacy of therapeutic hypnosis for children with FAP, RAP, and IBS (see Chapter 13). In a recent communication (Frankenhuis, 2022, personal communication) documented the outstanding scope of their training in pediatric hypnosis for child health professionals:

> We teach a 3-day beginners course called "Hypnosis for children in a medical setting" and a 3-day advanced course "Hypnosis for children in a medical setting." Because we are a small country the 3 days are spread out over 3 months.
>
> Participants get homework assignments like reading articles before and during the course. After the first day of the beginner's course, they have to record a self-hypnosis exercise. Every participant must hand in a recording of a hypnosis session with a patient/client by the end of the course. We listen to each one (some during the day) and they get feedback.
>
> Participants in the advanced course must hand in a video recording of a hypnosis session. It is mandatory to receive credits for the course.
>
> We started teaching in 2009 and have taught so far 1,203 health-care professionals: MDs, nurses, psychologists, psychiatrists, dentists, social workers, counselors, child life workers, physical therapists, physician assistants, medical students.
>
> Before 2019 you (DK), Leora (Kuttner) and Laurence (Sugarman) came to the Netherlands to teach.
>
> You were our mentors.

Participants asked for a 1-day training so their colleagues could learn the distraction techniques and hypnotic language.

So we started teaching a 1-day course named skills4comfort in 2019. This is described at the website www.skills4comfort.nl

This is a course we mainly teach in hospital. A few times a year we organize it ourselves so health-care workers from all over the country can join. The course is designed for health-care workers in paediatrics as well as the adult population. https://skills4comfort.nl/referenties/

Here you can see all the hospitals we have been teaching so far.

These are the main academic paediatric hospitals where we teach: AMC Emma Kinderziekenhuis, is the academic children's hospital in Amsterdam where we are currently training all of their nurses: 168.

UMC Beatrix Kinderziekenhuis Groningen is the academic children's hospital in the North of Holland where Elroly lives. She has trained about 600 people there so far.

LUMC Willem Alexander Kinderziekenhuis Leiden. Wilhelmina Kinderziekenhuis Utrecht

We are also teaching in 2 major hospitals for burn patients.

Even with 2 lockdowns we have taught an estimate of 1,730 and are fully booked till

Summer (2022). Except for one pediatric oncology hospital where the training was sponsored by a very generous benefactor, all of the hospitals have funded the training for their clinicians.

We have translated Dr. Jody Thomas' video "you are the boss of your pain" into Dutch and Dr. Vlieger recorded it.

We also put together a brochure for parents: "how you can help your child during a medical procedure?" It basically tells parents how to prepare their child, helpful language and unhelpful language. The brochure has been translated into English, Turkish, and Arabic.

## Therapeutic Hypnosis in Switzerland

A group of pediatricians in Zurich and surrounding communities in Switzerland have learned pediatric hypnosis from workshops provided by Dr. Kohen in 2000, 2005, and 2017 and on a regular, recurring consultative basis also by Dr. Leora Kuttner. In 2017, a child hypnosis workshop was presented in Zurich to a group of nearly 50, comprised mainly of psychologists along with other psychotherapists, some pediatricians, and psychiatrists.

Very recently (Ceppi, 2021, personal communication) a group of four Swiss pediatricians – previously trained in pediatric hypnosis with NPHTI – provided a highly regarded inaugural pediatric hypnosis training workshop. Dr. Ceppi wrote:

> Kinderärzte Schweiz, the Swiss Pediatric Society and the Pediatric Society for Intensive Care Medicine have recognised that it is worth knowing about hypnosis and implementing it in everyday medical practice. Wonderfully so. This means that I receive invitations for presentations from various interested parties and continue to promote paediatric hypnosis! In September (2022) I will be able to give a seminar on paediatric hypnosis at the annual congress. (Ceppi, 2021, personal communication)

Most recently we also had an email from NPHTI "graduate" friend, colleague and NPHTI Faculty, Dr. Camilla Ceppi in Zurich. Understating her own pride and joy at the significance of her announcement she sent a photo of the 20 participants in the first pediatric hypnosis workshop presented *by* Swiss pediatrician *for* Swiss pediatricians noting "… by Your scholars" (Drs. Ines Baruffol, Mercedes Ogal, Birgitta Thomann, & Camilla Ceppi). We note indeed with pride that each of these pediatricians participated in all three levels of workshop training with NPHTI, i.e., fundamentals, utilization, and individualized consultation; and now have successfully launched their own training program, continuing expansion to reach greater numbers of children and families.

## Therapeutic Hypnosis and Education in Germany

As noted, under the guidance of Bernhard Trenkle, president of the MEG in Rottweil Germany, and ex-president of the ISH, the Kindertagung Child Hypnosis Congress has been presented every 2 years since the 1990s, and typically attracts well over 1,000 participants, primarily from European countries but also from China, Japan, Mexico, South Africa, the United States with over 100 faculties also from many different countries. As a result, a very large number of child health professionals have learned hypnosis skills which they have appropriately passed on to their young patients/clients.

## Conclusion

Few countries have a sufficient number of child health professionals trained to teach hypnosis to children. Due to the laudable efforts of Dr. Bernhard Trenkle, Germany is a leader in teaching hypnosis skills to child health professionals. Through the enthusiastic leadership and commitment of Clinical Nurse Specialist Carla Frankenhuis and Dr. Arine Vlieger of Amsterdam, The Netherlands has developed ongoing training workshops in hospitals and communities throughout the country over the past 13 years, reaching thousands of nurses, physicians and other child health clinicians Norway is unique in having developed a course which, over 1 year, provides 80 hours of training on hypnosis with children and adolescents. As described, The Netherlands have developed quite a large network of pediatric hospitals for which senior clinicians (including NPHTI faculty) have provided training. Analogous growth of training of child health professionals in pediatric hypnosis is occurring now in Switzerland.

There remains a great need for increased training in child hypnosis, especially in resource poor countries where children who suffer pain often have little or no access to pharmacological or nonpharmacological treatment. A model for such training has been developed in northeast Thailand. We recommend that child health professionals who have expertise in hypnosis should consider volunteering their skills to teach their colleagues in resource poor countries.

## References

Al Sughayir, M.A. (2007). Hypnotherapy for irritable bowel syndrome in Saudi Arabian patients. *Eastern Mediterranean Health Journal*, *13*, 301–308.

Astuto, M., Favara-Scacco, C., Crimi, E., Rizzo, G., & Di Cataldo, A. (2002). Pain control during diagnostic and/or therapeutic procedures in children. *Minerva Anestesiologica*, *68*, 695–703.

Aviv, A. (2006). Tele-hypnosis in the treatment of adolescent school refusal. *American Journal of Clinical Hypnosis*, *49*(1), 31–40.

Ceppi, C. (2021). Personal communication.

Diseth, T.H. & Vandvik, I.H. (2004). Hypnoterapi ved behandlingsrefraktaer enuresis nocturna. *Tidsskrift for Den norske Lægeforening*, *124*, 488–491.

Dobbin, A. (2006). Lars-Eric unestahl and mental training: an appreciation. *Contemporary Hypnosis*, *23*(3), 111–114.

Fasciana, L.M. (a cura di). (2009). "L'ipnosis con I babini e gli adolescent – tecniche psicoterapeutiche in eta evolutive" FrancoAngeli s.r.l., Milano, Italy.

Fasciana, L.M. (a cura di). (2014). "Storytelling – Storie terapeutiche per aiutare bambini e genitori ad aiutarsi" FrancoAngeli s.r.l., Milano, Italy.

Frankenhuis, C. (2022). Personal communication. www.skills4comfort.nl

Furman, B. (2000–2020). *Solution stories*. www.KidsSkills.org

Furman, B. (2021). *Interview with Dr. Daniel Kohen – Pediatric Hypnosis*. Furman, Ben - You Tube Channel.

Green, J.P., Page, R.A., Rasekhy, R., Johnson, L.K., & Bernhardt, S.E. (2006). Cultural views and attitudes about hypnosis: a survey of college students across four countries. *International Journal of Clinical and Experimental Hypnosis*, *54*, 263–280.

Hewson-Bower, B. (1995). Psychological treatment decreases colds and Flu in children by increasing salivary immunoglobulin A. PhD thesis, Murdoch University, Perth, Western Australia.

Holtz, K.L. & Mrochen, S. (2005). *Einfuhrung in die Hypnotherapie mit Kindern und Jugendlichen*. Heidelberg: Carl-Auer-Systeme Verlag.

Huynh, M.E., Vandvik, I.H., & Diseth, T.H. (2008). Hypnotherapy in child psychiatry: the state of the art. *Clinical Child Psychology and Psychiatry*, *13*, 377–393.

Jaaniste, T., Hayes, B., & von Baeyer, C.L. (2007). Effects of preparatory information and distraction on children's cold-pressor pain outcomes: a randomized controlled trial. *Behavioral Research and Therapy*, *45*, 2789–2799.

Kuttner, L. Director/Producer. (1986). *No Fears, No Tears: Children with Cancer Coping with Pain*, DVD available from BC Children's Hospital (http://bookstore.cw.bc.ca; 1-800-331-1533, ext. 3).

Kuttner, L. (1988). Favorite stories: a hypnotic pain reduction technique for children in acute pain. *American Journal of Clinical Hypnosis*, *30*(4), 289–295.

Kuttner, L. (1989). Management of young children's acute pain and anxiety during invasive medical procedures. *Pediatrician*, 16, 39–44.

Kuttner, L. (1991). Helpful strategies in working with preschool children in pediatric practice. *Pediatric Annals*, *20*(3), 120–127.

Kuttner, L. Director/Producer. (1998). *No Fears, No Tears: 13 Years Later*. DVD available from BC Children's Hospital (http://bookstore.cw.bc.ca; 1-800-331-1533, ext. 3).

Kuttner, L. Director/Producer. (2003). *Making Every Moment Count*. 38-minute documentary available from The National Film Board of Canada (1-800-267-7710; 1-800-542-2164).

Kuttner, L. (2007). Hypnosis and palliative care. In W.C. Wester II and L.I. Sugarman, Eds., *Therapeutic Hypnosis with Children and Adolescents* (pp. 453–466). Bethel, CT: Crown House Publishing.

Kuttner, L., Bowman, M., & Teasdale, M. (1988). Psychological treatment of distress, pain, and anxiety for young children with cancer. *Journal of Developmental and Behavioral Pediatrics*, *9*, 374–381.

Kuttner, L. & Catchpole, R.E.H. (2007). Developmental considerations: hypnosis with children. In W.C. Wester II and L.I. Sugarman, Eds., *Therapeutic Hypnosis with Children and Adolescents* (pp. 25–44). Bethel, CT: Crown House Publishing.

Lesmana, C.B.J., Suryani, L.K., Jensen, G.D., & Tiliopoulos, N. (2009). A spiritual-hypnosis assisted treatment of children with PTSD after the 2002 Bali terrorist attack. *American Journal of Clinical Hypnosis*, *52*(1), 23–34.

Lindheim, M.O. & Helgeland, H. (2017). Hypnosis training and education: experiences with a Norwegian one-year education course in clinical hypnosis for children and adolescents. *American Journal of Clinical Hypnosis*, *59*, 282–291.

Liossi, C. & Hatira, P. (1999). Clinical hypnosis versus cognitive behavioral training for pain management with pediatric cancer patients undergoing bone marrow aspirations. *The International Journal of Clinical and Experimental Hypnosis*, *47*, 104–116.

Liossi, C. & Hatira, P. (2003). Clinical hypnosis in the alleviation of procedure-related pain in pediatric oncology patients. *The International Journal of Clinical and Experimental Hypnosis*, *51*, 4–28.

Liossi, C. & White, P. (2001). Efficacy of clinical hypnosis in the enhancement of quality of life of terminally ill cancer patients. *Contemporary Hypnosis*, *18*, 145–160.

Liossi, C., White, P., & Hatira, P. (2006). Randomized clinical trial of local anesthetic versus a combination of local anesthetic with self-hypnosis in the management of pediatric procedure-related pain. *Health Psychology*, *25*, 307–315.

Mackenzie, A. & Frawley, G.P. (2007). Preoperative hypnotherapy in the management of a child with anticipatory nausea and vomiting. *Anaesthesia and Intensive Care*, *35*, 784–787.

Mrochen, S., Holtz, K.L., & Trenkle, B. (1993). *Die Pupille Des Bettnassers: Hypnotherapeutisches Arbeit Mit Kindern und Jugendlichen.* Heidelberg: Carl-Auer-Systeme.

Nielsen, G. & Vandvik, I.H. (1981). Hypnose anno 1980. *Tidsskrift for Den Norske Lægeforening*, *4*, 101.

Oikawa, L.O., Hirota, A., Uratani, H., & Sakakibara, M. (2021). History and recent advances of the Japanese Society of Biofeedback. *Applied Psychophysiology and Biofeedback*, *46*, 309–318.

Olness, K. (2003). Effects on brain development leading to cognitive impairment: a worldwide epidemic. *Journal of Developmental & Behavioral Pediatrics*, *24*(2), 120–130.

Peretz, B. (1996a). Confusion as a technique to induce hypnosis in a severely anxious pediatric dental patient. *The Journal of Clinical Pediatric Dentistry*, *21*, 27–30.

Peretz, B. (1996b). Relaxation and hypnosis in pediatric dental patients. *The Journal of Clinical Pediatric Dentistry*, *20*, 205–207.

Peretz, B. & Gluck, G.M. (1999). Reframing: reappraising an old behavioral technique. *The Journal of Clinical Pediatric Dentistry*, *23*, 103–105.

Rogovik, A.L. & Goldman, R.D. (2007). Hypnosis for treatment of pain in children. *Canadian Family Physician*, *53*(5), 823–825.

Shaoul, R., Sukhotnik, I., & Mogilner, J. (2009). Hypnosis as an adjuvant treatment for children with inflammatory bowel disease. *Journal of Developmental & Behavioral Pediatrics*, *30*(3), 268.

Ummeed. (2022). www.ummeed.org (accessed February 7, 2022)

Unestahl, L.-E. (1973). Hypnosis and posthypnotic suggestions. PhD thesis, Uppsala University, Orebro, Sweden.

UNICEF. (2022). Research and Reports, www.unicef.org

Vandvik, I.H. (1994). Collaboration between child psychiatry and paediatrics: the state of the relationship in Norway. *Acta Paediatrica*, *83*, 884–887.

Vlieger, A.M., Menko-Frankenhuis, C., Wolfkamp, S.C., Tromp, E., & Benninga, M.A. (2007). Hypnotherapy for children with functional abdominal pain or irritable bowel syndrome: a randomized controlled trial. *Gastroenterology*, *133*(5), 1430–1436.

World Bank. (2022). New World Bank country classification by income level: 2021-2022. www.worldbank.org

# 20

# ETHICS: LEGAL CONSIDERATIONS, CHILDREN, AND HYPNOSIS

## Legal Considerations, Children, and Hypnosis

Ethics refers to the discipline dealing with what is good and bad, and with moral duty and obligation. It also refers to a set of moral principles or values. Ethical behavior in the context of a health profession refers to conforming to accepted professional standards of conduct. The American Society of Clinical Hypnosis (ASCH, 2000), the Society for Clinical and Experimental Hypnosis, and the International Society of Hypnosis each has written ethical guidelines for its members and has active ethics committees. It is understood that each member of these societies is expected to conform to the ethical guidelines of his or her professional society or association (e.g., national or state medical or dental society, psychological association). Also, all persons who use hypnosis should adhere to published guidelines related to probing memories with hypnotic methods and should not probe memories until one has substantial experience with clinical hypnosis at the intermediate or advanced level.

A basic principle to keep in mind with respect to any therapeutic intervention is non-maleficence: "First, do no harm." Another basic principle is beneficence. Does what I am doing benefit the child? Is what I am doing in the best interests of the child and the family? The ethics of how one utilizes hypnosis must be guided by the ethics of one's individual clinical profession. Child health professionals should only recommend hypnosis for a particular diagnosis or condition if they are qualified and experienced in treating that diagnosis or condition with other non-hypnosis methods. The child health professional who teaches hypnosis should be able to do a careful diagnostic evaluation and to explain to families if some other treatment is more likely to be efficacious.

Partial truths have no place in hypnosis. Their use perpetuates myths about hypnosis, such as the power of the clinician facilitating the hypnosis or that the patient will do whatever the clinician teaching the hypnosis suggests. Clinicians should identify themselves as teachers or coaches who will help the child or adolescent to develop his or her own skill. It is important that the child or adolescent and family understand that *imagery*, *visual imagery*, *relaxation*, and *relaxation mental imagery* are part of the hypnosis process and that patients are expected to use these techniques by themselves and to practice this skill. From the beginning of the training, the therapist/clinician should emphasize that the child is in control, can choose when to practice self-hypnosis, and can change his or her mental images at any time. It is essential that the therapist obtain feedback from the child or adolescent and be prepared to modify the hypnosis approach as necessary.

DOI: 10.4324/9781003243687-22

It is necessary to obtain informed consent if one is using hypnosis in forensic situations, when it is important to inform patients or clients that, once they have been in hypnosis, the likelihood of having testimony accepted by a court is very low. A relevant case history follows.

In 1979, one of the authors (KO) was asked by the county attorney and the state Bureau of Criminal Apprehension to meet with an 11-year-old boy who had witnessed the murder of his mother and three siblings. He could not remember specifics about the murderer, and I (KO) was asked to teach him self-hypnosis and to determine if this would help him remember. I met with the child and his therapist on three occasions over 3 weeks. The sessions were videotaped, and the tapes were given to the county attorney. A representative from the State Patrol office reminded the child just before the meeting with me that he would not be required to testify in court about any part of any information he might remember while doing self-hypnosis. I taught him progressive relaxation and asked him to focus on riding or driving to a favorite place. I also taught him ideomotor signaling. He seemed very comfortable throughout the first session and indicated, via ideomotor signals, that he did not know who had committed the murder.

He was asked to practice self-hypnosis daily, which he did. His therapist also did two practice sessions with him. During the second and third visits, he again preferred to communicate with ideomotor signals and was able to give no specific information about the murderer; he again indicated that he did not know the person. He continued to practice the self-hypnosis for some months after the third visit. The murder case went cold. The boy was raised by his aunts, and he later joined the military, married, and had two children. Twenty years later, I received a phone call from the County Attorney's office. They reported that they now had solid evidence that identified the murderer; however, because of a new Minnesota law that precluded any evidence obtained with hypnosis, they needed my testimony to assure the jury that I had obtained no information related to the man now accused of the murders. I appeared in court and testified that no information related to the murderer was obtained. The suspect was convicted of four counts of first-degree murder. He was already in jail and serving two life sentences for two previous murder convictions. The case was unique, and its story was told on the television program *48 Hours*. Given the current Minnesota state law related to forensic use of hypnosis, we would not recommend that therapists help solve crimes by teaching hypnosis to potential witnesses.

Hypnosis should never be used by clinicians for entertainment, and in general we do not approve of or recommend live demonstrations with child subjects or patients even in a workshop or comparable training environment. This is because we do not believe that it is ethically appropriate; that is, we do not think that the ordinary power differential that exists between children and adults in our modern society allows for true informed consent and autonomous decision-making by a child – which, of course, would be most appropriate and essential for a live demonstration of hypnosis.

The *Belmont Report*, written by the National Commission for the Protection of Human Subjects of Biomedical and Behavioral Research (1979), emphasized respect for the research subjects, careful consideration of beneficence, and justice; for example, a distributive justice question asks if there is a fair distribution of the benefits and burdens of research. The Declaration of Helsinki, an international statement on research, stated that medical research is justified only if there is a reasonable likelihood that populations in which research is carried out stand to benefit from results of the research (World Medical Association, 2004).

A review of ethical considerations was provided in a publication by Etzrodt (2013) in the *American Journal of Clinical Hypnosis*. Much as we emphasized throughout this volume, Etzrodt emphasized the importance of a developmental perspective and evaluation of all child and adolescent patients in consideration not only of the how, when, and why of a clinical hypnosis approach, but also of the ethical considerations related to the nature of children. Notably, she emphasized that children have limited decision-making capacities commensurate with their developmental maturation and accordingly special attention should be paid to their rights and welfare. She considers special ethical concerns regarding children and hypnosis, including competence (to understand and make decisions), supervision and informed consent (by proxy of parent/guardian), confidentiality, and respect for appropriate boundaries (Etzrodt, 2013). We have referred to and emphasized various aspects of all of these throughout this text as we have reviewed the variety of considerations integral to the thoughtful, fair, reasonable, and appropriate approach to therapeutic hypnosis across the age and developmental ability and lifespan of children and adolescents.

We re-emphasize here that particularly in the context and appreciation of the developmental differences between children and adolescents and adults, clinicians wishing to work with children and adolescents with hypnosis must have specific training not only within the scope of child and adolescent health in their clinical specialty (pediatrics, psychology, dental, etc.), but also most definitively must have specific training in child hypnosis. While excellent training in Clinical Hypnosis is available through the American Society of Clinical Hypnosis, Society for Clinical and Experimental Hypnosis, International Society of Hypnosis, and accredited national organizations in other countries, these workshop trainings do not provide child-specific and child-oriented education and experiential training in pediatric hypnosis such as that provided by the National Pediatric Hypnosis Training Institute (NPHTI, www.nphti.com) and its now 35 year history of providing annual pediatric hypnosis training workshops. We also note that viewing of a training video on ethical considerations in pediatric hypnosis is integral to the fundamentals (introductory) workshop of the NPHTI training curriculum.

We cannot over-emphasize these requirements; and as Ezrodt also notes "The ethical use of hypnosis means only providing services to populations, such as children in those areas that are within the boundaries of competence based on one's "education, training, supervised experience consultation study or professional experience" (APA, 2002; Etzrodt, 2013).

A recent Internet search (Google Scholar, PubMed) did not identify any more recent publications beyond Etzrodt's (2013) review. Readers are referred to this review for further discussion of the history of the development of laws regarding who can/should practice clinical hypnosis, and issues surrounding informed consent, confidentiality, and boundaries as regards ethical consideration and therapeutic hypnosis with children and youth.

## References

American Psychological Association (APA). (2002). American Psychological Association ethical principles of psychologists and code of conduct. Retrieved from http://www.apa.org/ethics/code2002.html [Google Scholar]

American Society of Clinical Hypnosis (ASCH). (2000). American Society of Clinical Hypnosis code of conduct. Retrieved from http://www.asch.net/ [Google Scholar]

Etzrodt, C.M. (2013). Ethical considerations of therapeutic hypnosis and children. *American Journal of Clinical Hypnosis*, *55*(4), 370–377.

National Commission for the Protection of Human Subjects of Biomedical and Behavioral Research. (1979). *The Belmont Report: Ethical Principles and Guidelines for the Protection of Human Subjects of Research*. Bethesda, MD: National Institutes of Health, Office of Human Subjects Research.

World Medical Association. (2004). *Declaration of Helsinki: Ethical Principles for Medical Research Involving Human Subjects*. Helsinki, Finland: WMA General Assembly.

# 21

# HELPING CHILDREN IN DISASTERS AND PANDEMICS WITH HYPNOSIS

## Introduction

Disasters include man-made disasters such as war, terrorism, or chemical events. They also include natural disasters such as earthquakes, hurricanes, floods, or pandemics. Any disaster can lead to serious acute and long-term effects for both adults and children. The stressors experienced by relief workers and parents are likely to increase the morbidity experienced by children in disasters (Olness, 2015; Harkensee, Olness, & Esmaili, 2021). In disasters hypnosis may provide primary or adjunct benefits for children with respect to psychological challenges, problems with pain, and chronic issues plus stress reduction for parents and relief workers.

Both man-made and natural disasters may lead to displacement of children, loss of parent figures, and loss of familiar routines. The reactions of children will vary according to the child's developmental stage, the duration of displacement from home or community or school, and the type of trauma experienced. The most vulnerable are those children who have experienced the death of parents or are separated from parents.

A useful assessment tool early in a disaster situation is PsySTART (Schreiber, 2022). Children are rated at more or less risk for psychological trauma depending on what they have experienced, e.g., loss of parent, loss of a home, seeing a dead person. This evidence-based, objective assessment can be completed by non-mental health workers. Children with high scores should be monitored closely and referred for more extensive mental health evaluation if they develop psychological symptoms of concern. This is the ideal. In fact, in most disaster situations it is difficult to access mental health expertise. For this reason, it is helpful if relief workers such as physicians and nurses are able to teach self-hypnosis to children and adolescents with or without the assistance of additional biofeedback apps. This teaching should always emphasize the child's ability to cope and to self-regulate. Relief workers should be aware of programs and activities available to facilitate resilience. Culbert (2017) designed Comfort Kits with items appealing to children. The items include stress squeeze balls, pinwheels, finger puppets, and small toys. These had specific therapeutic benefit, and the kits include guidelines for relief workers or parents to facilitate belly breathing, guided imagery, and blowing, all intended to provide self-soothing and comfort. These have been used many times, including after the tsunami in SE Asia in 2006, the Haiti earthquake of 2010 and severe floods in Laos in 2018. Instructions for printing the guidelines and assembling the kits can be downloaded from the website of the International

DOI: 10.4324/9781003243687-23

Pediatric Association. Other programs to help children who experience disasters include the Return to Happiness program originally developed by UNICEF (Herran, 2021) and the Child-to-Child program begun by Professor David Morley in 1978 (Srour, 2021).

Another useful resource for children who experience pain in disaster situations is found on the website of the Meg Foundation for Pain (Thomas, 2017; https://www.youtube.com/watch?v=UbK9FFoAcvs).

Suitable medications for pain are often lacking or in short supply in disaster settings. Relief workers can download these free programs to their phones or laptops and offer them to children who experience either acute or chronic pain.

Relief workers are often over worked and experience stress. They benefit from learning and practicing self-hypnosis to enhance confidence, reduce stress, and sleep problems. Ideally, they should become facile in self-hypnosis prior to working in disaster situations. Harkensee et al. (2021) have recommended that relief workers consider learning self-regulation strategies from the Center for Mind Body Medicine (2022); https://cmbm.org/self-care. This website provides guidelines on guided imagery (self-hypnosis) and soft belly breathing for self-care.

## The COVID-19 Pandemic

The COVID-19 pandemic is an example of a disaster that has affected families and children in every country of the world. Since this pandemic began there have also been numerous weather and man-made events that have been compounded by the additional risk of COVID-19. The training of relief workers emphasizes the importance of resuming in person school for children who are displaced after disasters. They are urged to arrange for makeshift schools, if necessary, because school is a stabilizing factor for the majority of children (Chinnapha, 2021; Pairojkul, Siripul, Prateepchaikul, Kusol, & Puytrakul, 2010). There is now much evidence about the destabilizing effects of school absence following disasters, including COVID-19. Other stressors induced by the COVID-19 pandemic include limitations on contacts with friends and family members outside of school, deaths among family members and loss of employment for some parents. Several very recent publications have documented the substantial negative impact of COVID-19 on the mental health of children and youth in various countries around the world. These have included a report in the *Journal of the Canadian Academy of Child and Adolescent Psychiatry* (Mactavish et al., 2021) describing the "broad psychological impact on youth of the COVID-19 pandemic" and the need to safeguard children's mental health and the US surgeon general's warning that young people are facing "devastating mental health effects as a result of the challenges experienced by their generation, including the coronavirus" (Murthy, 2021). Murthy's 53-page report was described as a "rare public health advisory" and cited how "the pandemic intensified mental health issues that were already widespread by the Spring of 2020," noting significant increases in self-reports of depression, anxiety, and emergency room visits for mental health challenges. In a systematic review and meta-analysis Chai et al examined 12 studies and reported on the prevalence of mental health problems for Chinese Children and Adolescents during COVID-19 in China (Chai et al., 2021). They found the pooled prevalence of mental health problems to be 28%, with 22% for depression and 25% for anxiety. Reporting in *JAMA Pediatrics* in August 2021, Racine and associates (Racine et al., 2021) examined 136 full text articles and 3,094 abstracts to identify prevalence rates of clinically elevated depression and anxiety symptoms in youth. Twenty-nine studies including 80,879 participants met inclusion criteria. Pooled prevalence estimates of clinically elevated depression symptoms were 252% and anxiety symptoms were 20.5%.

Depression symptoms were higher in older children; and clinically elevated depression and anxiety symptoms were higher in studies collected later in the pandemic, and in girls.

The investigators concluded that one in four youth globally is experiencing clinically elevated symptoms of depression, and one in five is experiencing clinically elevated anxiety symptoms; and that these represent *double* of pre-pandemic estimates.

For some children the COVID immunization is a stressor. In addition, children who contact COVID-19 themselves may have long-lasting symptoms.

In early 2022, one of our NPHTI colleagues, pulmonologist, Dr. Lewis Kass, posted to the NPHTI Listserve describing how a long-term patient of his, well-versed in self-hypnosis for other challenges, had spontaneously applied self-hypnosis to challenges he experienced with COVID-19. After communicating how he had helped himself with self-hypnosis to his therapist, Dr. Kass shared this compelling report on the NPHTI Listserve (Kass, 2022) and it is reproduced here with permission (Kass, January 19, 2022, personal communication) Dr. Kass wrote:

> Hi All, I'm not sure I would have suggested such "assurances" regarding this insidious, opportunistic, ever-changing, deadly, scary bug (COVID-19) but this 16-year-old patient of mine who has been using hypnosis successfully and independently for 8+ years now, came up with this and I just felt like sharing …
>
> His Mom says: The link (photo) is his version of a physical lock (See Figure 21.1 below).
>
> When he does it, he recites:
>
> "I don't want it (Covid) – I don't have it – I'm not gonna get it."
>
> I just learned of this, because the Mom texted me describing how last weekend, this fully vaccinated family of 2 parents and 3 kids all tested themselves multiple times last weekend and this week because they all felt sick. The parents and 2 kids tested positive for COVID. This young man remained healthy and negative.
>
> Interestingly enough, this young man is chronically ill, suffering from POTS, requiring nighttime mechanical ventilation because of his autonomic dysfunction, excessive sleepiness, asthma, Ehlers-Danlos syndrome, laryngo-malacia and chronic pain. In most situations (prior to learning hypnosis) he would've been the first to get sick, would've stayed sick the longest and knocked backward the furthest.
>
> Over the past 8 years, he has used self-hypnosis, mostly on his own, to manage pain, sleepiness, breathlessness and even voice-cracking during puberty when singing The Star-Spangled Banner at his little league games!
>
> And now … ? Do we dare to believe? Preventing COVID-19?
>
> My response to Mom's multiple texts: WHEN (not if) that continues to work he will need to teach the rest of the world!
>
> I was just so proud of my guy, that I wanted to share! As my mom would have said, I was k'velling! (Really [friggin'] proud!)
>
> Best Always,
> Lewis
> (Pediatric Pulmonology and Sleep Medicine)

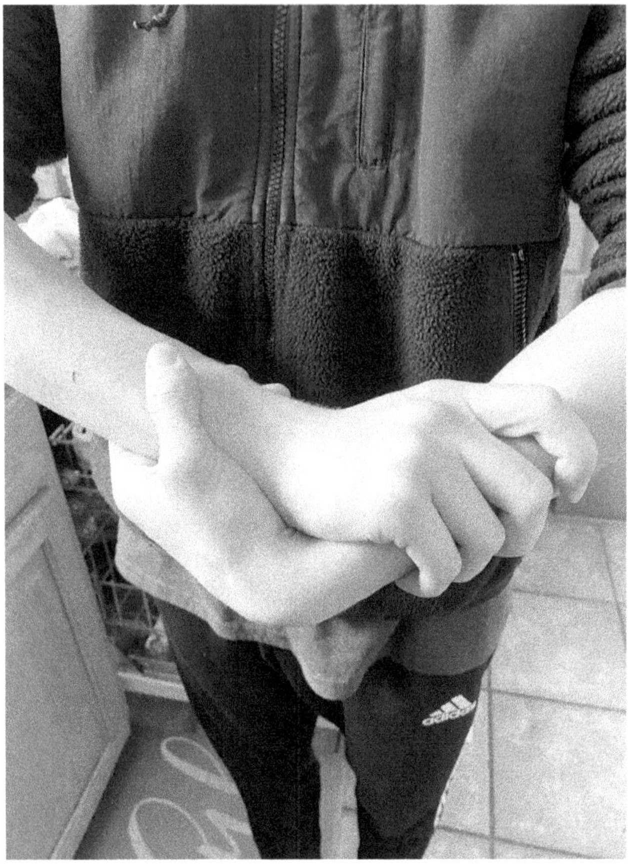

FIGURE 21.1 Photo of patient named "physical lock" to prevent COVID-19

The following case histories demonstrate how our colleague and very recent NPHTI workshop learner (Fundamentals and Utilization Workshops past 3.5 years), Dr. Alejandra Sencion, of Montevideo, URUGUAY has successfully taught patients effective and dramatic application of self-hypnosis for management of the long-term effects of COVID-19, i.e., parosmia/anosmia.

Dr. Sencion was prompted to post her experience in response to a question posted by long-term colleague, original developer and manager of the NPHTI Listserve, and emeritus NPHTI faculty, Dr. Bob Deutsch. Dr. Deutsch wrote on February 9, 2022:

> Hello all,
>
> I would greatly appreciate your suggestions/thoughts regarding a new patient I will be meeting this week. He presents with "*long COVID parosmia*" which I have no experience treating. I am hoping to benefit from the cumulative wisdom of this group.
>
> First, a bit of context:
>
> I will soon be working with a young adult, who was diagnosed with leukemia and then contracted Covid-19 two months later. For nearly two years, he has experienced what is known as: "long COVID", "COVID long haul syndrome", or "post-COVID syndrome" (PCS). He has been treated in a hospital setting.

> With much appreciation! (Published NPHTI Listserv February 9, 2022 with permission by Dr. Bob Deutsch)

While this side effect has been both unpredictable and often reported to have lasted for several months in many patients (Yan, Qiu, Liu, Guo, & Hu, 2021) to our knowledge this is the first reported case of the effective use of self-hypnosis training for the elimination of this very disturbing side effect. It is especially notable that the patient(s) described were novices with learning and utilizing self-hypnosis, unlike Dr. Kass's patient described above, who had many years of successful application of self-hypnosis.

After Dr. Sencion posted her case to the NPHTI Listserve, we contacted her and asked her permission to include this case description in this fifth edition of our text. She graciously agreed and is currently preparing a manuscript with a comprehensive description of her cases to submit for publication for a broad readership. From the NPHTI Listserv (NPHTI Listserv, Sencion, February 9, 2022, personal communication):

> Hi to everyone and specially this is a reply for Bob!
>
> I've seen 3 patients with parosmia lately and the 3 of them are getting better in their symptoms.
>
> As you said, anxiety does play a very important role in this matter. Approaching anticipatory anxiety as the first "move" will work really well. To have parosmia for 2 years implies that the patient is used to have this horrible experiences time after time … so to activate his parasympathetic system will help him to re-learn the tastes and smells as well.
>
> The technique that has worked for me in the 3 of my patients is to do a regression to the time when he/she enjoyed food, specially his/her favourite food (the one that the patient is so motivated to eat again but can't in the present). Make suggestions about colours, smells, textures, taste ( multisensory suggestions) and then invite the patient to go to the future, picture themselves enjoying that special meal.
>
> I had one patient that in only 1 session started eating almost everything, he was so grateful and surprised how quickly his brain was connected.
>
> One teenager said literally: "I think my brain is confused", and in fact that made so much sense to me … so I started a brief self-hypnosis exercise: to make the "memory game": Before having any food she had to spend at least 1 minute picturing the food, imagining the taste, the smell, the texture and then eat it. Like the memory game that kids play, you take a card and you have to find the "same card" in your mind. "Because your memory has all the knowledge, all the information you need, you just have to re connect again to that knowledge."
>
> This seemed to help a lot and she started eating food that she hasn't been eating in 3 months!
>
> Also I found it really interesting when I was making the first interview in which my 3 patients talked about "trying to eat" food. And I suggest instead of saying "trying" (as if tasting it for the first time) the message is: I'm going to eat this food, because I already know how it tastes, I've eaten this food many times before… .
>
> I hope this will help Bob and others in similar scenarios. Also if any of you would like to reach me you already have my mail!
>
> All the best and good luck!!!

> Alejandra
> Dr. Alejandra Sención.
> General Pediatrician.
> Private practice at the Centro de Hipnosis Uruguay
> http://hipnosisuruguay.com/

This is indeed an elegant and creative utilization of metaphor, careful listening to the patients' own description of their experience, re-framing, and the combination of time regression and progression to the future to develop alleviation and elimination of a complex and enduring problem.

A Swiss colleague and NPHTI faculty, Dr. Camilla Ceppi, offered the following thoughtful and instructive analysis of the therapeutic hypnosis elements which Dr. Sencion so ably applied and communicated to the over 800 members of our NPHTI Listserve:

> Your two case studies are excellent, rich and well thought out. Thank you so much for sharing them. You effectively link the different hypnotic techniques so that the two patients could access their old competencies and therefore experience self-efficacy in the present. The connecting to bodily abilities, to former bodily competencies, is purposeful. Brilliant!
>
> It is remarkable that you first addressed the aspect of negative expectations linked to fear. By addressing the fear issues, you open the ground for calm, relaxation, confidence and activation of the parasympathetic nervous system. And the next [therapeutic hypnosis] steps that lead to a sense of achievement and to change follow more easily.
>
> I think that the topic of parosmia is an important one because it affects a numerous cohort. Medical-therapeutic successful strategies do not yet really exist. This raises the question of whether your case reports should be made accessible to a broader, interested professional audience? How about a publication in a professional journal?
>
> So far I have only briefly read that there are specialists who offer aromatherapy.

Like Dr. Ceppi, and as noted above, we have recommended Dr. Sencion prepare her case presentations for potential publication and a much larger child health clinician readership. We understand that preparation of such a manuscript is underway and could potentially ante-date the publication of this text! For additional information regarding anosmia and taste dysfunction among children with COVID-19 infection, readers may consult the work of Yan and associates (2021).

We are grateful to Drs. Kass, Deutsch, and Sencion and their young patients for sharing their wonderful stories and allowing us to share them in this volume. We are also very grateful to Dr. Ceppi for her insightful commentary and recommendations.

## Summary

Man-made and natural, including pandemic, disasters impact millions of children throughout the world. Children who have experienced disasters benefit from learning self-hypnosis to enhance their sense of control, to reduce anxiety and enhance comfort.

Relief workers often sleep deprived and stressed, also benefit from practicing self-hypnosis. Although we have had little experience offering hypnosis to children who have had COVID-19, we have included the foregoing two case histories from colleagues who have worked with young people and families who have had COVID-19.

## References

Center for Mind Body Medicine. (2022). https://cmbm.org/self-care

Chai, J., Xu, H., An, N., Zhang, P., Liu, F., He, S., Hu, N., Xiao, X., Cui, Y., & Li, Y. (2021, October 6). The prevalence of mental problems for Chinese children and adolescents during COVID-19 in China: a systematic review and meta-analysis. *Frontiers in Pediatrics.* 10.3389/ped.2021.661796

Chinnapha, J.M. (2021). How can schools and teachers help displaced children? In C. Harkensee, K. Olness, & B.E. Esmaili, Eds., *Child Refugee and Migrant Health* (pp. 37–45). Switzerland AG: Springer.

Culbert, T. (2017). Perspectives on technology-assisted relaxation approaches to support mind-body skills practice in children and teens: clinical experience and commentary. *Children, 4*(4), 20. 10.3390/children 4040020

Deutsch, R. (2022). Personal communication. Published online NPHTI Listserve 2.9.22.

Harkensee, C., Olness, K., & Esmaili, B.E. (2021). *Child Refugee and Migrant Health.* Switzerland AG: Springer.

Herran, M.I. (2021). The return to happiness program. In C. Harkensee, K. Olness, & B.E. Esmaili, Eds., *Child Refugee and Migrant Health* (pp. 29–36). Switzerland AG: Springer.

Kass, L. (2022). Use of hypnosis to prevent COVID-19? – personal communication. Published online NPHTI Listserve, January 19, 2022.

Mactavish, A., Mastronardi, C., Menna, R., Babb, K., Battaglia, M., Amstadter, A.B., & Rappaport, L.M. (2021). Children's mental health in Southwestsern Ontario during Summer 2020 of the COVID-19 pandemic. *Journal of the Canadian Academy of Child and Adolescent Psychiatry/journal de l'Academie Canadienne de psychiatrie de l'enefant et de l'adolescent, 30*(3), 177–190.

Murthy, V.H. (2021). Surgeon general warns on "devastating" mental health effects young people are facing. *New York Times.* 12.7.2021 in AAP Daily Briefing, American Academy of Pediatrics AAPDailyBriefing@aap.bulletinhealthcare.com December 8, 2021.

Olness, K., Mandalakas, M., & Torjesen, K. (2015). *How to Help the Children in Disasters,*4th ed. Kenyon, MN: Health Frontiers.

Pairojkul, S., Siripul, P., Prateepchaikul, L., Kusol, K., & Puytrakul, T. (2010). Psychosocial first aid: support for the child survivors of the Asian Tsunami. *Journal of Developmental and Behavioral Pediatrics, 31,* 723–727.

Racine, N., McArthur, B.A., Cooke, J.E., Elrich, R., Zhu, J., & Madigan, S. (2021, August 9). Global prevalence of depressive and anxiety symptoms in children and adolescents during COVID-19: a meta-analysis. *JAMA Pediatrics.* 10.1001.jamapediatrics.2021.2482

Schreiber, C. (2022). Psychological simple treatment and rapid triage (PsySTART). www.PSYSTART.net and www.oregon.gov (accessed March 12, 2022)

Sencion, A. (2022). A case of post-COVID-19 anosmia treated successfully with self-hypnosis. Published online NPHTI Listserve, February 9, 2022.

Srour, M.L. (2021). Child health promotion for refugees and other vulnerable populations. In C. Harkensee, K. Olness, & B.E. Esmaili, Eds., *Child Refugee and Migrant Health* (pp. 171–186). Switzerland AG: Springer.

Thomas, J. (2017). Project director, primary consultant: "You are the boss of your brain: learning how to manage pain during medical procedures" (13 min.). Produced by Stanford Children's Health and Lucile Packard Children's Hospital. https://www.youtube.com/watch?v=UbK9FFoAcvs

Yan, Q., Qiu, D., Liu, X., Guo, X., & Hu, Y. (2021). Prevalence of smell or taste dysfunction among children with COVID-19 infection: a systematic review and meta-analysis. *Frontiers in Pediatrics, 9,* 686600. 10.3389/fped.2021.686600

# 22

# TEACHING PEDIATRIC CLINICAL HYPNOSIS TO CHILD HEALTH CLINICIANS

*The greatest of teachers, when his work is all done, the people (children) all say, "We have done it ourselves."*

– *Old Chinese proverb*

## Introduction

By the time of the expected 2022 publication of this volume, it will have been 46 years since the teaching of the initial pediatric hypnosis workshop. The first comprehensive, 3-day pediatric hypnosis workshop was presented in 1976 in Philadelphia. A few years later, another 3-day pediatric hypnosis workshop was sponsored by the International Society of Hypnosis (ISH) at its triennial meeting in Melbourne, Australia in 1979. In 1987, we were privileged to provide what we believe was one of the first introductory pediatric hypnosis workshops to become an annual offering, as part of the annual meeting of the Society for Behavioral Pediatrics, now the Society for Developmental and Behavioral Pediatrics (SDBP). The meeting was held at the Disneyland Hotel in Anaheim, California. Disneyland seemed an especially appropriate place to promote the value of imagination to the healthy lives of children, and the workshop received excellent evaluations. For the following 23 years, this training workshop became a regular feature of the annual meetings of the SDBP. In 1988, we were asked to provide intermediate-level workshop training for those who had participated in the previous year's introductory course and wanted to learn more. These companion workshops continued, and at the 1994 annual meeting in Minneapolis we added an advanced-level workshop for the first time. Over 60 child health professionals participated in the 1994 training, and over 1,100 attended these hypnosis workshops between 1987 and 2009. In 2010, the NPHTI was founded by members of our teaching faculty to formalize our philosophical and educational commitment to advancing the role of strategic and therapeutic child hypnosis in the care of children and adolescents in health and in illness. The commitment of NPHTI to offer at least annual skill development workshop training in clinical therapeutic pediatric hypnosis led to the inaugural NPHTI-sponsored introductory, intermediate, and advanced (individual consultation) workshops held in Minneapolis in 2010. These were co-sponsored by the Minnesota Society of Clinical Hypnosis; the University of Minnesota, Department of Pediatrics; and the University of Minnesota, Department of Continuing Medical

DOI: 10.4324/9781003243687-24

Education. Ongoing visits to the NPHTI website (www.nphti.com) will keep the reader apprised of NPHTI's efforts, significant research and publications in pediatric hypnosis, innovative regional and national learning opportunities, research endeavors, and ways of supporting the work of NPHTI to bring self-regulation skills to our youth.

## Why Teach Child Hypnotherapy?

As reflected in our review of the literature, in discussions of our and others' clinical experiences, and in our considerations and recommendations in this narrative, we have an abiding belief in the value of training children in cyberphysiologic (self-regulation) strategies. Perhaps our only greater faith is in children themselves, in their intrinsic worth, their unabashed curiosity, their often apparently limitless energy, and their potential. Childhood and adolescence are journeys toward mastery, and relaxation and mental imagery (RMI) and self-hypnosis facilitate mastery, so they are natural partners. We believe that all children ultimately should have the opportunity to learn these strategies and techniques with [self] hypnosis so that they may apply them to foster their healthy growth and development and the realization of their potential. To continue to reach toward this dream, we have come to believe that therapeutic and self-hypnosis, like other diagnostic and therapeutic skills, should be part of the armamentarium of all healthcare professionals who work with children. Toward this end, we began working with and teaching hypnosis skills to various child health professionals more than 46 years ago (Olness, 1977).

## Who Are the Learners?

Beyond our child patients and their parents, those to whom we have taught child hypnosis represent an ever-widening spectrum of those who provide health and illness care for children and their families. In Table 22.1, we note the spectrum of child physicians who have over the years sought our assistance with their patients or have availed themselves of training in clinical hypnosis, either to better understand and facilitate our consultative efforts or to employ clinical strategies themselves in integrating hypnosis into their practices. In Table 22.2, we highlight other child health-care providers who have referred patients or sought training in pediatric therapeutic clinical hypnosis for the children and families with whom they work.

**TABLE 22.1** Physicians Referring Patients for Child Hypnosis

| *Pediatricians* | ***Other Pediatric Specialists*** | ***Other Physicians*** |
|---|---|---|
| Developmental/Behavioral pediatricians | Pediatric nephrologists | Family physicians |
| Pediatric gastroenterologists | Pediatric neurologists | Child and adolescent psychiatrists |
| Pediatric pulmonologists | Pediatric subspecialists | Ophthalmologists |
| Pediatric intensivists | Pediatric rheumatologists | Allergists/immunologists ear, nose, and throat specialists |
| Pediatric emergency room physicians | Orthopedists | Emergency room/urgent care physicians |
| Pediatric hematologists/oncologists | Neurologists | |
| | Physical medicine and rehabilitation specialists (physiatrists) | |

**TABLE 22.2** Child Health Professionals Seeking Training in Hypnosis/Hypnotherapy

| ***Pediatric Nurses, Advanced Practice Pediatric Nurses (APRN), And Other Therapists*** | *Occupational Therapists And Others* |
|---|---|
| Pediatric nurse practitioners/associates | Physical therapists |
| Pediatric clinical nurse specialists | Respiratory therapists |
| School nurses | Child-life specialists |
| Child psychologists (including school psychologists) | Speech pathologists |
| Clinical social workers (including school social workers) | Marital and family therapists |
| Clergy (e.g., hospital chaplains, pastoral counselors) | Educators |

## Historical Perspectives

We began many years ago teaching RMI skills to nurses on the inpatient units of a children's hospital (then Minneapolis Children's Health Center/Minneapolis Children's Medical Center, now Children's Hospitals and Clinics – Minneapolis). As a natural extension of our work with individual children, nurses learned techniques to facilitate and reinforce what the children had been taught. Their greater and in some ways more natural accessibility to the children made this a perfect fit, and in the process most nurses discovered that they were not so much learning new techniques as they were defining a structure and a nomenclature into which to fit and expand their natural orientation to caring, positive expectancies, and flexibility to find the right words and strategy to meet the special or particular needs of a given child in a given predicament.

In the late 1970s and early 1980s, we extended our teaching and involvement of nursing personnel to the ambulatory setting and primarily to the emergency room, with specific workshop and seminar training for emergency room nursing staff. Challenged with the immediacy and urgency of saying and doing the things that will help the acutely ill or injured and highly stressed child (and family), nurses and other emergency department personnel focused on the special circumstances of hypnosis in emergencies (Kohen, 1986; see also Chapter 13).

Also, beginning in the late 1970s, for 10 years we hosted a weekly hypnosis seminar for practitioners of clinical hypnosis. The Tuesday afternoon, 4:30–5:30 p.m., slot provided a welcome ending to the day to which all participants looked forward. As an ongoing, interdisciplinary, mutual/peer supervision group, it provided a forum for discussion of difficult cases (not limited to child hypnosis), an opportunity for sharing information learned from a recent conference or seminar, a safe proving ground for new ideas, a review of interesting articles or books, and an opportunity for group self-hypnosis practice for comfort, relaxation, and positive reinforcement. Though not as enduring as the foregoing weekly seminars, analogous groups were also instituted at the University of Minnesota for a couple of years, at Case Western Reserve University, and in Rochester, New York; and we strongly recommend this process for the value noted.

During the 1970s and 1980s, while the interest and demand for education in clinical hypnosis grew nationally and while regional American Society of Clinical Hypnosis (ASCH) workshops and national ASCH and Society for Clinical and Experimental Hypnosis (SCEH) workshops experienced increasing popularity, attention to the uniqueness of pediatric clinical hypnosis was inconsistent. Activism on the part of national committees and organizational lobbying succeeded in including teaching in child hypnosis in intermediate and advanced hypnosis workshops during some ASCH and SCEH workshops, but there was less success in consistently integrating adequate amount of training in child hypnosis into introductory clinical hypnosis workshops. On a regional level, a brief (1–1.5 hours) presentation on pediatric clinical hypnosis had been a part of the University of Minnesota/Minnesota Society of Clinical Hypnosis Introductory course since the 1970s, though for reasons unclear in recent years this has been reduced to a 45-minute presentation. Inclusion of substantive education in pediatric clinical hypnosis has not been true in a consistent fashion for either regional or national ASCH or SCEH workshops. The ASCH's *Standards of Training in Clinical Hypnosis* (Hammond & Elkins, 1994) notes no requirement for training in child hypnosis other than to recommend that students in an introductory course be made aware of the above-average hypnotizability of children from 9 to 12 years of age and of the Stanford Hypnotic Clinical Scale for Children. While the recently updated ASCH *Standards of Training in Clinical Hypnosis* – Level 1 (American Society of Clinical Hypnosis Education and Research Foundation – ASCH-ERF, 2020 www.asch.net) makes a concerted effort to define appropriate content for training in pediatric hypnosis, from our perspective they are significantly unrealistic. That is, while stated expectations are to achieve a comprehensively developed and outlined set of legitimate learning objectives, the time period within which these are expected and required to be achieved is woefully inadequate and, therefore, highly unrealistic.

In contrast, however, ASCH, SCEH, and the ISH have for the past 25–30 years provided opportunities in their *advanced* workshops for the presentation of both intermediate level and advanced level pediatric hypnosis workshops. For more than 35 years, we have been privileged to teach in these workshops with an ever-growing number of pediatric, developmental–behavioral pediatric, nursing, and psychology colleagues. Although this forum has been unique and commonly has attracted clinicians interested specifically in children, it has also been an immense challenge, as often participants represent a wide spectrum of prior knowledge and experience in child hypnosis. More often than not, however, many to most participants have had introductory or additional general clinical hypnosis training and have clinical practices (medicine, psychology, dentistry) with a large percentage of children though they have had no prior specific training in child hypnosis. Often, therefore, these billed as "advanced" pediatric hypnosis workshops have often become, accordingly, very basic and quite introductory in focus and content.

These experiences led us to develop child-clinician-specific training in clinical hypnosis, initially building on our knowledge and experience with general hypnosis workshop training and our training with hospital personnel. In 1979, we taught an informational and descriptive 2-hour workshop on pediatric hypnosis at the Annual Meeting of the Ambulatory Pediatric Association (APA, now the Academic Pediatric Association). We believe that this was the first such workshop to be taught as part of a major national pediatric meeting. A reprise of the same workshop was taught the following year at the APA annual meeting, and similar workshops were taught by Dr. Olness at two annual meetings of the American Academy of Pediatrics. Since the turn of the century, analogous introductory pediatric hypnosis workshops (1.5–2 hours) have been taught by Dr. Kohen and colleague(s) at the American Academy of Pediatrics annual meetings.

In 1987, we were asked by the Child Life Staff and Hematology–Oncology nursing staff of St. Paul Children's Hospital (now Children's Health Care–St. Paul) to provide training in pediatric clinical hypnosis specific to their needs. We presented a 14-hour seminar over 5 days (4 hours on Monday and Friday, and 2 hours each on Tuesday through Thursday), built into which was a commitment to provide ongoing supervision and review for 1–2 hours monthly. The success of that workshop training has been beyond our wildest dreams; monthly supervision (one morning a month for 1.5 hours) continued uninterrupted for the next 10 years. At their request we have shared the curriculum of this training with several pediatrician colleagues across the United States who had been part of our Introductory Pediatric Hypnosis training workshops and wanted ideas on how to provide skill development training to the child life and nursing staffs of their hospitals.

Over the ensuing decades, a former student and now senior colleague of many years, Dr. Laurence Sugarman, developed and conducted "Preparing Bright Futures: Experiential Workshop in Basic Pediatric Hypnosis," initially in Rochester, New York, in 1998, followed by

Kansas City in 2005. In 2001, 2002, 2004, 2006, 2008, and 2010, the workshops were presented at the SUNY Upstate Medical University in Syracuse, New York, with the able collaboration of Dr. Ran Anbar. Providing both introductory and intermediate/advanced education and skill development training, these workshops have allowed introductory learners in a fall workshop (SDBP and now NPHTI) to receive intermediate/advanced level training available in the spring of the following year; and conversely, those completing introductory training with this group in the spring were able to avail themselves of next-level training at a NPHTI fall workshop.

In 2008, former students and now teaching colleagues of ours – pediatric nurse practitioners Linda Thomson and Becky Kajander and pediatric nurse practitioner and psychologist Pamela Kaiser – presented the first-ever introductory pediatric hypnosis workshop during the National Meeting of the National Association of Pediatric Nurse Associates and Practitioners (NAP–NAP). It was a resounding success, and many who studied in that workshop have already participated in next-level (intermediate) training. Although we are not surprised at this wonderful success of our former students, we are thrilled as only proud parents and grandparents can be, and our expectation is for continued growth and success of this significant endeavor that advances this arena in so many ways.

While completing the extensive research required to put together this volume, 11 years after publication of the fourth edition (Kohen & Olness, 2011), we have been especially cognizant of the continually growing and significant role that nursing colleagues have played in the research, practice, and teaching of child hypnosis. We reviewed well over 250 papers in preparation for this updated edition. Of the 170 new references added, over 6% are in nursing journals, and they represent publications in critical care, palliative care, hospice, intensive care, pain, and perioperative care.

## Creating an Interest in Learning

As we have utilized therapeutic hypnosis strategies with our patients and observed what children are capable of doing and achieving via these strategies, we have resolved to bring this to the awareness of other professionals. Professionals with whom we have had contact have become aware of hypnosis and its potential value for children in a variety of ways, leading some of them to pursue further formal training in pediatric clinical therapeutic hypnosis. Medical students, pediatric residents, and family practice residents have observed us working with hypnosis with individual children patients as part of general pediatric learning rotations in our respective hospital inpatient or outpatient settings. As such, they may have witnessed hypnosis with a patient in the emergency room who has an acute episode of asthma, an adolescent using hypnosis to help endure another bone marrow examination, an adolescent female using hypnosis to ease her discomfort during her first pelvic examination, a child practicing self-hypnosis for enuresis, or any of a myriad of other situations. Medical students at Case Western Reserve University have had the opportunity to choose an elective in clinical hypnosis, a course offering that was frequently full.

Since 1988, pediatric residents, during an obligatory month's rotation in Developmental–Behavioral Pediatrics at the University of Minnesota, have joined us in many sessions of pediatric hypnosis with a variety of patients and have also viewed videos of hypnotic interventions. Sugarman's video, *Hypnosis in Pediatric Practice: Imaginative Medicine in Action* (Sugarman, 1997/2007), and Kuttner's *No Fears, No Tears: Children with Cancer Coping with Pain* (1986) and *No Fears, No Tears: 13 Years Later* (1998) DVDs remain today as required viewing for this rotation experience.

Pediatric and family practice residents as well as practicing clinicians have had the opportunity to take an elective in pediatric hypnosis at our respective institutions since 1977. These are usually limited to those who have already had introductory workshop training in clinical hypnosis. Only a few residents per year avail themselves of these opportunities. Over time, many of our NPHTI faculty who are hospital based have had medical students, pediatric residents, and pediatric fellows (in various subspecialty disciplines) request "special rotations" with them to learn more about pediatric clinical hypnosis. Clinicians have had their interest piqued by presentations of case conferences featuring one or several children who have benefited from clinical hypnosis or by pediatric grand rounds describing clinical or research efforts in pediatric hypnosis. (Many of our NPHTI faculty are actively engaged in teaching about pediatric clinical hypnosis in these "Grand Rounds" type of venues and teaching workshops in pediatric clinical hypnosis around the United States and internationally. Rather than seeking to name or list all of such teachers we invite readers to view the NPHTI website at www.nphti.com and notably take a look at sections "About Us," "Training Opportunities," and "Other Resources," for video resources.)

Others have read reports of clinical cases or research, or review articles about applications of hypnosis in various mainstream pediatric journals. Some professionals have had their curiosity and interest aroused by inquiries or urgings for information from patients or their families who either have heard of hypnosis or related self-regulation strategies helping someone they knew or have seen something in the media, which intermittently re-arouses interest in alternative therapies (Coleman & Gupin, 1993; Furman, 2021; Kuttner, 2013; Moyers, 1993; Thomas, 2017).

## A Recommended Plan of Study for Therapeutic Pediatric Clinical Hypnosis

Just as we believe that there are many right ways – not merely one or two – to effectively do most things, we have also come to believe that certain approaches to learning pediatric clinical hypnosis seem to work, so we commend them to the reader and clinician for consideration.

### *Education Theory*

Unfortunately, most child health professionals have not had formal training in educational theory. Most tend to teach by emulating teachers and educational processes that they themselves have experienced. Prior to planning an educational program, the professional should consider several important points:

- The word "education" derives from the Latin *educere* ("bring forth"). And, after all, the word doctor (*doctor*) means teacher. Our task is to stimulate the learner, to encourage the learner, but not to cram in facts without attention to solid and tested principles of learning. This is especially true with respect to adult learners.
- Who is the learner? How does he or she [best] learn? There is considerable individual variability in learning styles. Some people learn best by watching, others by reading, some by listening, and still others by doing. When possible, the teacher should consider his or her *own* learning styles and ask about those of the students.
- What are the overall goals for the educational experience? An example of a goal would be "to increase the number of child health professionals who are knowledgeable regarding pediatric therapeutic clinical hypnosis." A lesser goal, but one that is often present, is for the teacher "to gain experience as an educator in pediatric clinical hypnosis."
- What are the specific objectives for components of the program? The teacher must indicate these. An example would be, "The participant will be able to learn to do their own self-hypnosis easily."
- What are the means of implementing the objectives? An example would be, "Each participant must have the opportunity to practice coaching eight colleagues into and through a hypnotic state." The teacher must consider what types of technical support will facilitate implementation of objectives (e.g., PowerPoint presentations, videos, live demonstrations, real-time practice/rehearsal with colleagues).

- How will you know if you have achieved your goals and objectives? There must be an evaluation plan. These can be simple or detailed, but they must be reviewed and heeded. We believe such evaluations are most useful when they are bilateral, i.e., reciprocal. Thus, learners should receive feedback evaluation from teachers (e.g., how well they conducted a hypnotic invitation and process, and what language worked well and what did not), and teachers should receive feedback from learners about all aspects of the teaching experience – whether objectives have been met and evaluations of the milieu, handout materials, technical support, and the style, demeanor, and attitude of the teacher. These are what lead to improved programs and improved teaching skills. Additionally, we invite and expect our faculty teachers to conduct and provide self-evaluation following training workshops. These should be submitted to training directors for review.

Ultimately, the children are our best teachers, and we are at our best as teachers when we let our students and colleagues know that, and we know how to learn from the children. As we work with them, our learning comes from their feedback – that is, asking them, "What works?" "What did you like the most?" "What helps?" "What did I say or do that you didn't like or didn't help you help yourself?" The best learning, therefore, comes from doing, from making notes of how the process unfolded and then reviewing and discussing them with our patients, our colleagues, our students, and our mentors. Given the ready access to smartphones and video capability often clinical sessions can be video-recorded and clinicians are encouraged to review them later for review of the encounter, to benefit future clinical sessions, and for self-review of all communication, verbal and non-verbal. Finally, the teacher must keep in mind an old Chinese saying: "But of the best leaders, when their task is accomplished, their work is done, the people will remark: 'We have done it ourselves.'" Indeed, that represents true success as a teacher.

## *Introductory and Foundational Learning in Pediatric Hypnosis*

Introductory learning in pediatric hypnosis should be in the context of a 3-day workshop to which we now refer as fundamental workshop in pediatric clinical hypnosis; either first learning general clinical hypnosis followed within 2–3 months by a 3-day workshop in pediatric hypnosis or preferably, first attending a 3-day fundamental workshop in pediatric clinical hypnosis. Although we have known colleagues over the years who have learned in other formats, we believe that this approach provides the most effective beginning. As distinguished from a 10-week university course or an apprenticeship learning opportunity, the 3-day intensive workshop training model offers the following advantages:

- Curricular-based training over a specified period (3 days) with focused concentration.
- Exposure to several different, experienced faculty educators (representing developmental–behavioral pediatrics, pediatric psychology, pediatric social work, and pediatric nursing)
- Opportunity for learning through a variety of proven educational experiences: didactic presentations, demonstrations (of first-time invitation [aka induction] of hypnosis, phenomenology, techniques, language), modeling (by faculty, video demonstrations, and small group practice sessions with colleague learners), and mentor supervision and consultation
- Freedom from distractions (other coursework, daily work, "on-call" etc.)
- Opportunity for informal learning and questions and answers during breaks

The content of such a fundamentals workshop is reflected in the schedule of our 3-day NPHTI workshop: fundamentals in pediatric clinical hypnosis, presented in Table 22.3.

**TABLE 22.3** Fundamental Workshop in Pediatric Clinical Hypnosis

| **Day 1** | **Teaching Activity** |
|---|---|
| All Times Are US Central Standard Time – C.S.T | |
| 7:00 a.m.–7:55 a.m. | Registration; breakfast buffet, socialization |
| 8:00 a.m.–8:25 a.m. | Introduction: course overview, faculty introductions |
| 8:30 a.m.–9:25 a.m. | Hypnosis: definitions, theories, myths |
| 9:25 a.m.–10:15 a.m. | Hypnosis structure and elements |
| 10:15 a.m.–10:35 a.m. | Refreshment break |
| 10:35 a.m.–11:15 a.m. | hypnosis: the many right ways |
| 11:15 a.m.–11:35 a.m. | Overview: format for small group practice |
| 11:35 a.m.–11:50 a.m. | #1 Demo: invitation: special place (dissociation): intensification: multisensory imagery |
| 11:50 a.m.–1:00 p.m. | Lunch with colleagues & faculty |
| 1:00 p.m.–2:40 p.m. | #1 SmGrp Practice: invitation: special place (dissociation) – intensificatioin: multisensory imagery – alert – debrief (4–6 learners per faculty) |
| 2:40 p.m.–3:00 p.m. | Refreshment break |
| 3:00 p.m.–3:15 p.m. | #2 Demo: invitation: the breath intensification: muscle relaxation |
| 3:15 p.m.–4:50 p. m. | #2 SmGrp Practice: invitation: the breath, intensification: muscle relaxation – re-orient – debrief |
| 4:55 p.m.–5:45 p. m. | Hypnosis: developmental considerations |
| 6:00 p.m.–7:30 p.m. | Welcome complimentary cocktail reception and keynote speaker |
| **Day 2** | |
| 7:00 a.m.–7:55 a.m. | Breakfast buffet |
| 8:00 a.m.–9:10 a.m. | Formulating suggestions: language, utilization/communication options |
| 9:10 a.m.–9:25 a.m. | #3 Demo: invitation: magnet fingers<br>Intensification: utilization give suggestions, reorient – debrief |
| 9:25 a.m.–9:45 a.m. | refreshment break |
| 9:45 a.m.–11:00 a.m. | #3 SmGrp practice: invitation: magnet fingers |
| 11:05 a.m.–11:30 a.m. | Intensification: utilization, incorporate language, and suggestions; reorient, debrief |
| 11:30 a.m.–12:40 p.m. | #4 Demo: explaining hypnosis to child and parents w/video |
| 12:40 p.m.–1:30 p.m. | Lunch on your own. |
| 1:35 p.m.–2:25 p.m. | #4 SmGrp practice: explain hypnosis to child and parent(s)<br>Choosing goals and suggestions for hypnosis session |
| 2:25 p.m.–2:40 p.m. | Refreshment break |
| 2:40 p.m.–3:40 p.m. | Choosing hypnosis goals and suggestions: self-regulation for worry, fears, anxiety, and pain |
| 3:40 p.m.–3:55 p.m. | #5 Demo: Invitation and intensification (learner's CHOICE), goal-driven suggestions |
| 4:00 p.m.–5:30 p.m | #5 SmGrp practice: invitation and intensification (learner's CHOICE) goal-driven suggestions, reorient and debriefing |
| 5:30 p.m. | Adjourn for the day |

(*Continued*)

**TABLE 22.3** (Continued)

| | |
|---|---|
| **Day 3** | |
| 7:00 a.m.–7:55 a.m. | Breakfast buffet |
| 8:00 a.m.–8:50 a.m. | Goals and suggestions: sleep disturbances |
| 8:50 a.m.–9:50 a.m. | Goals and suggestions: acute and chronic pain |
| 9:50 a.m.–10:10 a.m. | #6 Demo: magic glove technique + video |
| 10:10 a.m.–10:25 a.m. | Refreshment break |
| 10:25 a.m.–11:30 a.m. | #6 SmGrp practice – magic glove technique |
| 11:30 a.m.–12:45 p.m. | Lunch on own – KEYNOTE SPEAKER |
| 12:50 p.m.–1:05 p.m. | Self-hypnosis: learning, teaching, and questions |
| 1:05 p.m.–1:20 p.m. | Self-hypnosis: Large group experience/debrief |
| 1:25 p.m.–2:05 p.m. | #7 Demo: teach SH and do SH |
| 2:05 p.m.–2:20 p.m | #7 SmGrp practice: teach SH, do SH |
| 2:20 p. m.–3:30 p.m. | Refreshment break<br>#8 Breakout groups (participant's choice)<br>Planning a hypnosis session: goals and suggestions<br>1. Pain<br>2. Anxiety<br>3. Primary care<br>4. Chronic conditions |
| 3:35 p.m.–3:55 p.m. | Continued learning and resources beyond Monday: NPHTI next level training, other ongoing education and organizations |
| 3:55 p.m.–4:05 p.m. | Beyond today – what's left to learn? |
| 4:05 p.m.–4:15 p.m. | Special closure – all faculty group hypnosis with all levels' participants |
| 4:15 p.m. | Adjourn/submit evaluations |

*Source*: National Pediatric Hypnosis Training Institute, www.nphti.com.

### *Utilization (Level 2, Formerly "Intermediate"), Individualized Consultation (IC, Formerly "Advanced"), and Continuing Learning in Therapeutic Pediatric Clinical Hypnosis*

Some years ago, one of us (KO) developed a set of slides to present at the end of an introductory lecture or course in pediatric clinical hypnosis as a guide for further learning. These form the outline of what we present here as a menu of options for ongoing training or self-education in pediatric therapeutic hypnosis:

- After taking a fundamentals (introductory) workshop, professionals should seriously consider a follow-up course no longer than 3–6 months later. This could be a second introductory course in pediatric clinical hypnosis for the learner who desires additional opportunities for supervised small group practice or utilization or level II (intermediate) training such as is available through the NPHTI or workshops through ASCH. We also recommend that child health clinicians have solid grounding in adult hypnosis in order to be able to competently respond to questions about hypnosis from parents and other adults. Such training, available through ASCH, SCEH, or regional organizations such as the Minnesota Society of Clinical Hypnosis, the New England Society of Clinical Hypnosis, North Carolina Society of Clinical Hypnosis or other regional "component" sections of ASCH. These could also reasonably be taken either before or soon after a fundamental workshop in pediatric clinical hypnosis. As noted above, we wish to emphasize that since the NPHTI fundamental workshop is a uniquely child-focused workshop, we believe that either before or after the NPHTI fundamentals, a solid grounding in clinical hypnosis should include an adult-focused fundamentals workshop such as provided through ASCH or SCEH or related organizations indicated.

- Practice the personal use of self-hypnosis daily for 2–3 months for relaxation, stress reduction, or some other personal need. We believe that such a personal experience with hypnosis affords the clinician an intimate understanding of its phenomenology and that this leads to greater effectiveness in presenting hypnosis to his or her patients and families.
- Begin working with hypnosis in one or two specific areas, making sure that they are areas in which the clinician is already comfortable and confident, if not expert, with the usual applicable diagnostic and therapeutic approaches.
- Be certain – especially as psychotherapists or others who are neither nurses nor physicians – those patients have had the usual, necessary diagnostic studies for their problems, especially if a patient is being referred expressly for hypnosis. This is critical in order to reduce or to avoid missed or misdiagnoses (Olness & Libbey, 1987).
- Assess the patient's willingness to practice self-hypnosis. Most who do not or will not practice still believe that the change or ability for it somehow resides in their idealized or fantasized view of the all-powerful therapist. It is, in turn, usually an unproductive and unsatisfying trap to buy into their fantasy that they need only do [their self-] hypnosis when they come to the office and that you are there to do it to or for them.
- Consider making audio and video recordings of your work to analyze yourself.
- Consider using approaches, language, style, etc., that carefully take into account the patient's personality, interests, learning style, fears, knowledge, and experience.
- Consider the family's knowledge, interest, and support, and with the patient agree whether the family will or will not be involved (e.g., reminding the patient to practice self-hypnosis).
- Be flexible and creative; remember to ask the patient what was helpful and not helpful.
- Be permissive; do not seek to force ideas or imagery.
- If uncertain how to proceed, call or ask a colleague for help as you would in any diagnostic or therapeutic dilemma.
- Become involved in ongoing continuing education opportunities in hypnosis, both adult and pediatric.

The following sections focus on the evolution of our teaching program and the variety of learning/teaching experiences in which we have been involved and found to be meaningful for us as educators and learners and for those working with and learning from us. Each methodology or forum is described and discussed briefly.

## The Evolution of our Teaching Program

Following the 24 years of teaching pediatric hypnosis under the auspices of the Society for Developmental and Behavioral Pediatrics (1987–2009) and the creation of the NPHTI in 2010 (see section on "Historical Perspectives" above) our NPHTI faculty has continued to review, evaluate, evolve, innovate, and refine our workshop training to be the best it can be. To do so we have relied on careful creation of evaluation tools for our learners to utilize and consistently urge workshop participants to not only evaluate what they have experienced, but to also let us know please what they would like to learn more about, what was perhaps "missing" or insufficiently focused upon in their workshops. Beyond reminders to "Please make notes about evaluation and comments and suggestions *during* the workshop as well as at the end," we also assure participants that we read and utilize their evaluations and suggestions as we review our own presentations and success as educators. We have also encouraged our faculty to conduct a self-evaluation after each workshop and to share that with NPHTI's director(s) of education.

Over time our Workshops have evolved considerably from what they were before there was a NPHTI, and even following the first few years of NPHTI programming. In 2017, we published "State-of-the-Art Pediatric Hypnosis Training: Remodeling Curriculum and Refining Faculty Development" (Kohen, Kaiser, & Olness, 2017) to describe and document in detail the ways in which some of the content has changed significantly. We sought to also present the reasoning and decision-making processes that were involved in creating the changes which became part of the new curriculum. As we plan our annual workshops, we continue to carefully review evaluations from our most recent previous training programs, to understand what our colleague learners wish to have included in future educational workshops and webinars, to know both who and what was done well. With the challenges of COVID-19, we were obliged to cancel in-person workshops that had been in planning stages for over a year. These included international training workshops in Australia initially planned for 2020 but postponed to 2021, then postponed again to 2022, and now still "on hold." As of August, 2022 plans are now in place to provide NPHTI International Workshops in Australia during the latter part of 2023. We also postponed our usual tri-level annual workshops, last held in the Fall, 2019; and these have now recently been presented as the 11th NPHTI Workshops in October 2022. Other workshops were also re-scheduled, postponed, or canceled. As a whole our faculty met by ZOOM and agreed that we could and should develop a monthly webinar program to remain viable, visible, and valuable to those who have trusted and appreciated NPHTI pediatric hypnosis education since 2010.

Our Monthly Webinar Program in 2020–2021 and now "season 2" 2021–2022 has been very successful, attracting viewer-participants not only from around the United States but from Australia, Switzerland, Germany, Norway, Uruguay, Canada, and others.

Faculty development was also a focus of our recent manuscript (Kohen et al., 2017) and describes our special 1-day training workshop to develop faculty small group mentors to facilitate the small group practice sessions which are the backbone of fundamentals workshops. We are proud of having re-envisioned our curriculum to provide seven small group practice sessions during our 3-day fundamentals workshop. While "trading down" some didactic presentations in favor of more supervised/mentored "hands on" practice sessions, these have been universally appreciated and these sessions annually continue to receive the highest evaluation kudos. We are sure that this in part a function of the high quality of mentorship of the small group facilitators, many of whom have become facilitators by reason of completing the training workshop "Facilitating Facilitators' Facilitation" (FFF) taught initially by Drs. Wark and Kohen (Wark & Kohen, 1998) and later by Drs. Kohen and Kaiser. This "FFF" workshop has been taught twice for NPHTI, first in 2012 and again in 2014, each time providing training for eight additional small group facilitators. In the next year or two, it will be time for another such workshop to sustain the infusion of young and committed faculty to our existing core group of faculty.

In the wake of the COVID-19 pandemic which continues worldwide unabated into 2022, our Fall, 2021 NPHTI in-person workshops, like most, were suspended due to the risks of contagion and limitations/risks of both domestic and foreign air travel. To maintain our commitment to teaching pediatric hypnosis education, NPHTI convened a ZOOM faculty meeting to brainstorm both commitment to and options for a NPHTI TeleHealth Education program. While many questions arose, the faculty was unanimous in a resolve to both develop and contribute to our monthly webinar program.

Like the annual Society for Developmental and Behavioral Pediatrics (SDBP) and NPHTI workshops described earlier, the creation, development, and maturation of these webinars require a considerable amount of time and a formidable commitment of energy to produce, maintain, and sustain. We are immensely grateful to Dr. Candace Erickson as the program director for the SDBP pediatric hypnosis workshops (1987–2009) and to Drs. Pamela Kaiser and Daniel Kohen for their time and energy as co-directors of education for NPHTI (2010–2020). While we urge our colleagues nationally and internationally to consider the development of analogous training opportunities, we emphasize the importance of careful, precise, and mindful attention to the significant amount of time, detail and ongoing colleague communication required to expect, evolve, and maintain successful programs.

## The NPHTI Webinar Program

The NPHTI Webinar Program began by soliciting suggestions from faculty for potentially desirable topics for presentation. Like our annual workshops, we were able to rely successfully upon the extensive evaluations, recommendations, and requests provided by prior workshop attendees; and, of course, upon various faculty volunteering to provide presentations. Reviewing the experience of other [new] health care webinar programs, we decided on a monthly program to be offered regularly on the third Tuesday of each month, from 11:00 a.m. to 12:15 p.m. Central Standard (or Daylight) Time (United States). Considering current understanding of differences in sustainability of attention via ZOOM or analogous video platforms, we encouraged our faculty to develop presentations of 45–50 minutes in length, and encouraged content to provide participatory involvement by learners, such as by intermittent "polling questions" and/or questions about a case example, viewing of a brief video vignette, or doing a brief (2–3 minutes) self-hypnosis exercise. Feedback from participants has been uniformly positive and excellent, and, as with our workshops, participants provide ideas about what future presentations they would prefer. The timing of webinars allows for 15–20 minutes of time for questions which are typed into a Q & A box. Answers are provided "live" by the presenter and/or by another faculty person who functions to introduce the webinar, and as a moderator is present (off camera) throughout, monitoring the Q & A, explaining the Continuing Medical Education (CME)/ Continuing Education Unit(s) (CEU) process, and contributing to discussion as appropriate.

For the record, the NPHTI Webinar Series for 2020–2021 and 2021–2022 are presented below. The program for 2022–2023 (beginning August or September, 2022) is currently in development and readers will find it in the Summer, 2022, on the NPHTI website (www.nphti.com), see Tables 22.4 and 22.5.

Readers are also encouraged to read further about the pediatric hypnosis curriculum in the forthcoming new book edited by Gary Elkins, PhD to which we have contributed an invited chapter on Fundamental Workshop Training in Pediatric Clinical Hypnosis (Olness & Kohen, 2022).

### *Independent Learning*

Reading and reviewing videotapes, DVDs, audiotapes, or CDs of pediatric therapeutic hypnosis are mainstays in providing ongoing information and stimulating our creativity. We believe we should all do this to complement and supplement our lifelong learning from our patients and other sources. Many of the resources we have found useful are referenced within this text and can also be found in the NPHTI Bibliography and Resources sections in the NPHTI website: www.nphti.com

### *Independent Learning with a Mentor*

Borrowed from our psychology colleagues, the methodology of supervision or clinical supervision has proven to be very well suited to refining skills in pediatric therapeutic hypnosis. As have our colleagues, we have conducted such experiences with many kinds of learners, including nurse clinicians and practitioners, pediatric residents, fellows in developmental–behavioral pediatrics, practicing clinicians on mini-fellowships, and practicing clinical psychologists. Though they vary in specifics, common features of this very personal learning approach include:

**TABLE 22.4** 2020–2021 NPHTI Webinar Series

**NPHTI**
National Pediatric Hypnosis Training Institute

*a 501(c)(3) nonprofit educational corporation*

**NPHTI Continuing Education in Pediatric Clinical Hypnosis**
**WEBINAR SERIES - 2020–2021**
**EACH Webinar: 11:00 a.m.–12:15 p.m. CDT (> CST)**

| | |
|---|---|
| **#1: July 21:** | **NPHTI Guidelines ....**<br>Karen Olness, MD, FAAP; Pamela Kaiser, PhD, CPNP; Daniel Kohen, MD, FAAP<br>**No** CME credit offered |
| **#2: August 18:** | **Resilience to Stress: Learning to Tolerate Uncertainty**<br>Pamela Kaiser, PhD, CPNP |
| **#3: September 15:** | **Procedural Pain: Using Interactive Technology to Expand Our Reach and Impact**<br>Jody D. Thomas, PhD |
| **#4: October 20:** | **Integrating Conversational Hypnosis into Clinical Encounters**<br>Robert Pendergrast, Jr., MD, FAAP |
| **#5: November 17:** | **Utilization in the Diagnosis and Treatment of Headaches**<br>Daniel Kohen, MD, FAAP |
| **#6: December 15:** | **Resilience to Anxiety: Fostering a Growth Mindset**<br>Pamela Kaiser, PhD, CPNP |
| **2021** | |
| **#7: January 19, 2021** | **Hypnosis with Teenagers: Individualizing Their Hypnotic Experience**<br>Leora Kuttner, PhD & Melanie Gold, D.O. |
| **#8: February 23, 2021** | **Sleep Dysregulation: How Hypnosis Can Help**<br>Eileen Poulin, MD, FAAP |
| **#9: March 16, 2021** | **Hypnosis for Pediatric GI Conditions**<br>Jeff Lazarus, MD, FAAP |
| **#10: April 20, 2021** | **Back to Basics: Cultivating a Beginner's Mind in Hypnosis with Children**<br>Adam Keating, MD, FAAP |
| **#11: May 18, 2021** | **Hypnotic Strategies for Neurodiverse Youth**<br>Andy Barnes, MD, FAAP |
| **#12: June 15, 2021** | **Activating Hypnosis: When Hypnosis is not Relaxation**<br>Laurence Sugarman, MD, FAAP |

- *Long-term learning.* Commonly, such supervision takes place over several months' time, often on a half-day or one-day-per-week basis. The now nearly universal access to and necessity for TeleHealth during the COVID pandemic has enabled the utilization of ZOOM and other video platforms – or audio conference calling – for not only 1:1 mentoring but also for small group mentoring and case discussions
- *Individual patient care review, consultation, supervision.* Usually the learner is engaged in working with patients with hypnosis and participates in the step-by-step process of diagnostic evaluation, treatment-plan evolution, and ongoing implementation of therapeutic hypnosis with his or her mentor. This aspect of the learning process provides the opportunity for precise

**TABLE 22.5** NPHTI Continuing Education in Pediatric Clinical Hypnosis Webinar Series – 2022

| | |
|---|---|
| Third Tuesday/Month – 11:00 a.m.–12:15 p.m. CST | |
| 2022 | |
| January 18 | Hypnosis for Pain – How to Use Technology to Help<br>*Jody Thomas, PhD* |
| February 15 | Planning Hypnotic Interventions for Chronic Pain<br>*Candace Erickson, MD* |
| March 15 | Social Emotional Health, Technology and Hypnotic Principles<br>*Lisa Lombard, PhD* |
| April 19 | Psychoneuroimmunology and POTTS Syndrome<br>*Howard Hall, PhD, PsyD* |
| May 17 | Self-Hypnosis for Self-Care<br>*Andy Barnes, MD, MPH, FAAP* |
| June 21 | Not Everything That Counts Can Be Counted: Therapeutic Scaling with Clinical Hypnosis<br>*Laurence Sugarman, MD, FAAP* |

review of process, language utilized, pacing and timing, and the formulation of indirect, direct, formal, and informal hypnotic behavior and suggestions through the use and review of audio recordings or video recordings of patient encounters. This teaching is also beneficial to the mentor. We have always found that the more we teach, the more we learn.

### *Group Supervision with a Mentor*

Such arrangements allow for both personal and more diversified learning by bringing the perspective of several learners to a group, varying the types of problems encountered and discussed, and inevitably encouraging more discussion and debate. It also tends to be more economically feasible. Such groups often meet monthly, for 1–2 hours, or perhaps longer.

### *Group Mutual Supervision*

These ongoing study groups or seminars offer the advantage of bringing together professionals from different disciplines (e.g., pediatricians, nurse clinicians/practitioners, social workers, psychologists) who are also at different stages in their own professional development, learning, expertise, comfort, and knowledge about therapeutic clinical hypnosis with children. Thus, rather than one experienced teacher with many novices, the group becomes one of many teachers teaching one another, sharing responsibility from session to session for leadership and perhaps for content and style, as well.

## Teaching Techniques, Strategies, and Styles

In hypnosis, as in any discipline, the nature, style, and strategy for effective teaching vary appropriately from teacher to teacher and with the same teacher from milieu to milieu and perhaps even from student to student. Approaches and strategies that seem to have served us best in the ongoing teaching of child hypnosis methodology beyond the fundamentals level include the following:

- *Didactic presentations*. Such presentations should be brief (e.g., 20–30 minutes) and be utilized primarily to introduce new ideas or material, such as the application of hypnosis to an area not previously described; to present results of pediatric hypnosis research; or to offer case report examples or demonstrations as triggers for discussion and brainstorming. Interspersal of video examples (e.g., integrated into a PowerPoint presentation) is a very effective method of illustrating an idea in almost real time.

- *Small group practice and role playing of specific case management.* We have found it very useful during utilization (intermediate) and individualized consultation workshops to prepare a series of five to seven case vignettes of common behavioral or medical pediatric problems with trigger questions for group consideration. Typically, these might take the form of:
- "A 7-year-old boy is brought by his parents for help with primary nocturnal enuresis. He is dry at night only once or twice a month, and his parents are wondering what to do. Can hypnosis help him? How would you proceed? What would you say?"
- "A 12-year-old girl has had recurrent abdominal pain and occasional vomiting off and on for 4 years. She has had a negative evaluation by a pediatric gastroenterologist and now is missing more school. The problem seemed to get worse when she started junior high school. Is hypnosis appropriate? How would you introduce it? What techniques might be effective?"

With a mentor present to facilitate the discussion, the participants of a small group (four to six participants) would be encouraged to respond to these or other sample cases through either discussion or role playing; thus, this type of learning resembles an advanced version of small group practice. The clinician and subject (albeit in a role-playing situation) discuss the hypnotic experience after a 5- to 7-minute practice session. Additional members of the group are solicited for their impressions, and finally the mentor gets the proverbial "last word" before the group moves on to another case discussion. Commonly, this evolves into discussions of the participants' own patients and dilemmas. Learners almost always give such experiences and opportunities high marks in feedback evaluations and discussions.

- *Group review of videotape examples of hypnotic work.* This is a particularly effective approach, especially when the teacher has previewed or edited the videos to allow the group to focus on and discuss specific teaching points, including specific language used, pacing demonstrated, spontaneous hypnotic behavior before any official or formal induction, various hypnotic phenomena during trance, or the nature and structure of hypnotic suggestions. This model has been the central feature and focus of our advanced workshops over the past 25 years. Participants in this now called Individualized consultation (IC) workshop apply to participate in a workshop, which takes place over 3 days and allots 0.5 day (3.5 hours) to each of a maximum of six participants. Each half-day session is focused upon the review of that half-day participant's submitted video case and is mentored by a member of the faculty carefully matched to the participant and to their case. The other participants serve as peer mentors in the process, each having their own "half-day" of focused attention and mentoring. It has been a highly valued and appreciated process.

We believe that this particular component of training is most closely aligned with the changes in teaching and learning in hypnosis proposed and advocated in recent publications (Alter & Sugarman, 2017; Hope & Sugarman, 2015; Sugarman, Schafer, Alter, & Reid, 2018) and we encourage the reader to examine these publications carefully to understand how they challenge what Sugarman et al. (2018) refer to as the "legacy model" Standards of Training in Clinical Hypnosis (SOTCH) (Elkins & Hammond, 1998) and recently updated SOTCH (ASCH-ERF, 2020).

- *Review of videotape examples of an individual's hypnotic work.* This form of supervised advanced learning is often the most powerful and important for many professionals. Although it seems to require a modicum of courage and self-confidence from professionals new to hypnosis to be willing to record their work with their newfound skill, at the same time it carries with it the strong promise of the highly positive reward of direct, precise, honest critique and feedback from experienced clinicians and teachers. Review of an individual's videorecorded interview, preparation for hypnosis, and therapeutic hypnotic intervention is an important, time- and labor-intensive endeavor with valuable outcomes. Such interactions are scrutinized for all aspects of the professional/patient encounter, before, during, and after hypnosis. Rigorous attention is paid to detail and subtleties in the interactional process, with feedback provided to the learner both positively and negatively regarding the pre-hypnosis interview, invitation/initiation, intensification, formulation of hypnotic suggestions, structure and use of language, posthypnotic suggestions, termination of the trance, teaching self-hypnosis, and closure of the interview. Feedback may be verbal or written, and time must be provided for discussion. The most employed and most effective teaching strategies in this form of learning include positive and negative feedback (written and oral), modeling (by the mentor), discussion of certain behaviors and language, and, to a lesser degree, didactic instruction. This format can be conducted 1:1 with a mentor in person, in small groups in person or via video conferencing as described, or in the context of an advanced or individualized consultation workshop as described above. Most recently we were delighted at the success of an individualized consultation workshop conducted with two participants and two mentors completely by ZOOM, and across continents, with one learner in Brisbane, Australia and one in Philadelphia, PA in the United States and one mentor in Vancouver, BC, Canada and another in Minneapolis, MN in the United States. All participants knew one another from prior in-person workshops, and all agreed afterward that everything "worked just great!" despite the huge time zone differences and expanse of oceans separating participants.

## Hypnosis Education in Other Countries

While we are aware that the model(s) we have described have been gradually evolved and are regularly re-evaluated and have been successful, we are also aware that there may be other successful methods of providing training in this vitally important area of child health care.

Amongst the most vibrant of such programs are found in the Kindertagung in Germany as developed by Bernhard Trenkle, the training opportunities throughout the Netherlands spearheaded by Carla Frankenhuis, R.N. and Arine Vlieger, M.D., and the program in Norway, all of which are also described in detail in Chapter 19. We encourage readers to contact colleagues in these countries and others through their noted leaders, through indicated websites, and/or through contact via the ISH (https://www.ishhypnosis.org) to learn more about their individual approaches to education in child hypnosis.

## Conclusion

We would be remiss if we didn't include recent publications which have thoughtfully challenged what they refer to as "the more dominant, ritualistic, hierarchical, induction based Standards of Training in Clinical Hypnosis" (Alter & Sugarman, 2017; Hope & Sugarman, 2015; Sugarman, Linden, & Brooks, 2020; Sugarman et al., 2018). We hope you will be curious and intrigued as you review and consider the messages of these publications.

In concluding these observations about education in child hypnosis, we direct the reader also to Chapter 19 for a discussion and review of the many ongoing and growing efforts around the world to educate our colleagues in the utilization and practice of therapeutic child clinical hypnosis. We take special note of, and have respect for, the largest venue in the world for teaching child hypnosis: the "Kindertagung" European Child Hypnosis Congress, conceived, organized, and directed approximately every 2–3 year in Heidelberg, Germany, by Bernhard Trenkle, clinical psychologist and director of the Milton Erickson Institute of Rottweil, Germany, and most recent former president of the ISH.

## References

Alter, D.S. & Sugarman, L.I. (2017). Reorienting hypnosis education. *American Journal of Clinical Hypnosis, 59*(3), 253–259.

American Society of Clinical Hypnosis Education and Research Foundation (ASCH-ERF). (2020). Standards of training, approved – 2019, revised – October, 2020. Level I: fundamentals of clinical hypnosis workshop. *American Society of Clinical Hypnosis Education and Research Foundation.* info@asch.net (accessed March 14, 2022).

Coleman, D. & Gupin, J., Eds. (1993). *Mind Body Medicine.* Yonkers, NY: Consumer Reports Books.

Elkins, G.R., & Hammond, D.C. (1998). Standards of training in clinical hypnosis: preparing professionals for the 21st century. *American Journal of Clinical Hypnosis, 41*(1), 55–64.

Furman, B. (2021). Interview with Dr. Daniel Kohen – Pediatric Hypnosis - Furman, Ben - You Tube Channel.

Hammond, D.C. & Elkins, G.R. (1994). Standards of training in clinical hypnosis. American Society of Clinical Hypnosis. Des Plaines, IL, USA.

Hope, A.E., & Sugarman, L.I. (2015). Orienting hypnosis. *American Journal of Clinical Hypnosis, 57*(3), 212–229. 10.1080/00029157.2014.976787

International Society of Hypnosis (ISH). (2022). https://www.ishhypnosis.org

Kohen, D.P. (1986). Applications of relaxation/mental imagery (self-hypnosis) in pediatric emergencies. *International Journal of Clinical and Experimental Hypnosis, 34*(4), 283–294.

Kohen, D.P., Kaiser, P., & Olness, K. (2017). State-of-the-art pediatric hypnosis training: remodeling curriculum and refining faculty development. *American Journal of Clinical Hypnosis, 59*(3), 292–310. 10.1080/00029157.2016.1233859

Kohen, D.P. & Olness, K. (2022). Hypnosis with children. In G.R. Elkins, Ed., *Introduction to Clinical Hypnosis: The Basics and Beyond.* Waco, TX: Mountain Pine Publishing.

Kohen, D.P. & Olness, K. (2011). *Hypnosis and Hypnotherapy with Children-Fourth edition.* New York, London: Routledge. Taylor & Francis Group.

Kuttner, L., Director/Producer. (1986). No fears, no tears: children with cancer coping with pain, DVD available from BC children's hospital (http://bookstore.cw.bc.ca; 1-800-331-1533, ext. 3).

Kuttner, L., Director/Producer. (1998). No fears, no tears: 13 years later, DVD available from BC children's hospital (http://bookstore.cw.bc.ca; 1-800-331-1533, ext. 3).

Kuttner, L. (2013). Dancing with Pain. DVD. Youth with Chronic Pain. (20 min). www.bookstore@bc.cw.ca

Moyers, B. (1993). *Healing and the Mind.* New York: Doubleday.

Olness, K. (1977). In-service hypnosis education in a children's hospital. *American Journal of Clinical Hypnosis, 20*, 80–83.

Olness, K. & Libbey, P. (1987). Unrecognized biologic bases of behavioral symptoms in patients referred for hypnotherapy. *American Journal of Clinical Hypnosis, 30*, 1–8.

Sugarman, L.I. (1997/2007). *Hypnosis in Pediatric Practice: Imaginative Medicine in Action [video and instructional manual].* Bethel, CT: Crown House Publishing.

Sugarman, L.I., Linden, J.H., & Brooks, L.W. (2020). *Changing Minds with Clinical Hypnosis – Narratives and Discourse for a New Health Care Paradigm.* New York: Taylor and Francis, Routledge.

Sugarman, L.I., Schafer, P.M., Alter, D.S., & Reid, D.B. (2018). Learning clinical hypnosis wide awake: can we teach hypnosis hypnotically. *American Journal of Clinical Hypnosis, 61*, 140–158.

Thomas, J. (2017). Project Director, Primary Consultant: "You Are the Boss of Your Brain: Learning How to Manage Pain during Medical Procedures" (13 min.) Produced by Stanford Children's Health and Lucile Packard Children's Hospital. https://www.youtube.com/watch?v=UbK9FFoAcvs

Wark, D.M. & Kohen, D.P. (1998). Facilitating facilitators' facilitation: experience with a new training model for teaching leaders of hypnosis practice groups. *American Journal of Clinical Hypnosis, 41*(1), 75–83.

# 23

# HELPING PARENTS HELP THEIR CHILDREN HELP THEMSELVES WITH SELF-HYPNOSIS

## Introduction

As we have noted throughout, helping children with self-hypnosis requires a definitive and, some might say, a unique set of skills in order to accomplish this teaching and enable their learning. We have emphasized how, of course, clinicians working with therapeutic hypnosis with children must be intimately familiar and conversant with normal and abnormal child development since the application and utilization of therapeutic hypnosis varies with, and is dependent upon, awareness of the developmental maturation level of the individual child or adolescent patient/client. Clearly, just as 2-year-olds are different from 4-year-olds are different from 6-year-olds, so it is that the ages of 8, 10, 12, 14, 16, 18, and 20 differ from one another. It is well understood by child health experts that some 8-year-olds are more like 5, 6, or 7 in their maturation and behavior, and others are more "advanced" in some aspects of their development, and may seem like they are 9 or 10. Thus, learning about a given child's developmental status is critical to being able to understand not only their problem but also to developing and optimizing an approach to helping them ("hypnotically" or otherwise) resolve the problems/challenges for which they have come to the clinician. Beyond these critical aspects of historical and in-the-moment evaluation of each child, each clinician must – as we have also emphasized in other sections (see Chapter 5 "Hypnotic Invitations for Children: Techniques, Strategies, and Approaches" and Chapter 7 "Facilitating Effective Interpersonal Relationships with Hypnosis -Language for Clinicians and Parents") – develop a rapport with their child/adolescent patients which is concordant with understanding who they are developmentally, and who they are in the context of their family, school, community.

The fundamental importance of these elements of history and rapport cannot be overemphasized. Furthermore, they must also be understood contextually, i.e., answering the questions: Who is/are the family members with whom the child lives? What is the "culture" (e.g., ethnicity, religious/spiritual history) within which they live? What is the community in which they live and function (e.g., neighborhood, school, etc.)? Depending upon a clinician's personal style, this information can often be gathered from the child/teen personally, as well as from "intake forms" completed by the parent(s), and certainly confirmed and affirmed in conversations with parents at both an initial an ongoing clinical encounters.

In so doing, it is always appropriate to learn from the child and parents – preferably in that order – their understanding, thoughts, feelings, and attitudes about why they come for the visit with the

DOI: 10.4324/9781003243687-25

clinician. Were they referred by another clinician? Were they referred "for" hypnosis or was hypnosis not mentioned at all? Or was it their own idea? What have they heard about and what do they know about hypnosis? We believe it is essential to give voice to these questions (and answers!) early in the initial encounter. Often this is easy, as many (but not all) children know what their problem(s) is/are and usually have "heard" something about the appointment. What they heard, how they heard it, and what they thought, felt, and came to expect, however, are only going to be learned from asking. We think it is important to direct these questions directly to the child before asking the parent, as this is far more likely to elicit the child's honest belief and reply. If the parent "goes first" even when the clinician addresses the child, one has (1) learned a lot about family dynamics! and (2) the child may perhaps be reluctant to share their view or thoughts, hesitance, etc. particularly if they are different from the parents. We tend to do the best we can to enable the child speaking and answering first, including talking to the parent "through the child." This might be to say something to the child like "I know I'm asking you this stuff FIRST on purpose, but I promise I won't leave your Mom/Dad out, they just get to go next ... in my office kids always get to go first." It has been rare indeed for parents to quarrel with this. Some are more impatient than others in getting to their "turn" to speak, but most parents are delighted to discover – sometimes for the first time! – and see and hear that their child can carry on a reasonable conversation with the clinician when they are approached respectfully and "at their level."

Allowing of course for individual needs and variations between children and families, we think it is essential that parents be partners with us in helping children learn to help themselves with self-regulation through learning self-hypnosis techniques and strategies. Dependent upon the presence or absence of fears about hypnosis, or mistaken understandings based on myths and misconceptions (or, sometimes, various religious teachings), approaching establishment of the "partnership" requires assurance that everyone is "on the same page" in understanding what hypnosis is and is not. There is no substitute for asking parents directly (after the child has given their opinion about what they believe, thought, learned about, e.g., from cartoons, friends, books, movies). Sometimes – more often than not – the answers are favorable and positive, and sometimes the parents themselves have learned self-hypnosis for any of a variety of personal issues – including "anxiety," "my uncle is a dentist and taught us how to be calm in the dentist's chair," "I used it to quit smoking," "I learned how to stop a nervous tic," etc.

As noted earlier in Chapter 4, Traphagen (1959) found a preponderance of positive attitudes toward hypnosis among parents (65%), higher than she expected. Likewise, we have found many positive attitudes among parents of our prospective child therapeutic hypnosis patients. Some parents are interested to discover that they have unknowing been using hypnotic-like techniques/ language with their children: one mother told us that "I taught all 3 of our children how to fall asleep easily by concentrating on their breathing – it really worked. Is THAT hypnosis?"

As described in Chapter 4, Katie, 12 years old, *used to* have problems with swallowing oral medications, until her mom taught her to focus upon her favorite foods instead of gagging. Katie then easily used favorite food imagery on her own and resolved the problem of taking medication.

Gardner (1974) described techniques designed to help parents who are reluctant about hypnosis to move from being obstacles to becoming allies in their children's treatment. The approach includes three basic steps: educational, observational, and experiential. Details of each of these steps follow:

- Begin with a relatively didactic discussion with the parents, pausing to allow and encourage questions. Hypnosis can be defined as basically a state of mind, usually combining relaxation with concentration on a desired point of focus so that other undesired thoughts or feelings can then fade into the background. Parents can easily experience this personally by asking them to focus upon sounds in the environment which they had not previously noted

> consciously, like, for example, the soft hum of the air conditioner. The heightened attention which characterizes hypnosis can be described in the context of everyday events such as a mother's ability to waken to her infant's cry while sleeping through other louder but far less significant noises. [Answers to other questions concerning hypnosis generally, can be found from the websites of the National Pediatric Hypnosis Training Institute (www.nphti.com) and the American Society of Clinical Hypnosis (www.asch.net).]

Such a beginning easily allows discussion to flow to talking about the specific reasons why hypnosis may be appropriate for a particular child. Parents may be told that the goal is to help the child focus on comfort so that pain will ease on feelings of well-being so that anxiety will diminish, or on pleasant hunger in order to counteract nausea and vomiting. A few basic principles of invitation strategies, such as relaxation training and favorite place imagery, can then be explained. In so doing, we would emphasize the need to tailor the invitation approach to the individual and unique needs of each child, and provide some understanding of simple physiological and psychological principles that account for the success of the techniques. Throughout, the parents' specific questions are answered, and misconceptions are clarified including such things as the distinction between hypnosis and sleep and concerns about spontaneous hypnosis or greater susceptibility to charlatans. The goals are (1) to teach the parents that hypnosis can be described in simple, everyday terms without myths or concepts suggesting magic or witchcraft, and (2) to help the parents understand that hypnosis may be a specifically useful treatment modality for their child. Like Dr. Gardner who first described these ideas, we find that following this kind of opening, early discussion, almost all parents are willing to proceed with their child experiencing a trial of therapeutic hypnosis. For those who are not [yet?] willing or ready there is no pressure to proceed.

If the parents become enthusiastic about the possible value of therapeutic hypnosis for their child, they have already accomplished a major step toward becoming an ally in promoting therapeutic hypnosis and facilitating their child's development of mastery of a self-hypnosis practice. Usually, children look to their parents for guidance and assurance when facing new situations, and if the parents communicate a confident and positive attitude toward hypnosis the child is much more likely to be trusting and to be cooperative and enthusiastic learning, practicing, and utilizing self-hypnosis

For those parents who permit therapeutic hypnosis for their children, a second phase of parent education and guidance may consist of having them observe their children in hypnosis. On an individual basis, this may occur as early as a first visit (especially with a younger child under 7 or 8 years old) when as "let's do an experiment together" the parents and child are invited to learn to experience hypnosis. Without any mention of the problem of the child, the clinician may then invite parent(s) and child to simply

> Just close your eyes and pretend you're not here. I don't know where you will imagine or pretend that you are, because YOU are the boss of your imagination. Maybe it will be in a favorite room in your house, or on a family vacation, or riding bikes, or going for a walk or a picnic, or something else. But, wherever it is, really enjoy it, notice where you are, whether inside or outside, whether the weather is winter, summer, Fall or Spring, make it just right for you, and notice the smells there, and maybe pretend you're having a snack of your favorite food and you can enjoy it right now *just as though you were really having it BECAUSE you ARE really having it in your IMAGINATION. (Pause) You probably noticed that while you have been doing this EXACTLY RIGHT that your breathing got slower kind of all by itself BECAUSE when the MIND is RELAXING, the BODY LISTENS and breathing slows*

> *down ... and you probably also noticed that your muscles started relaxing, especially in your face and neck getting all loose and soft and comfy BECAUSE when the MIND relaxes and the BODY relaxes by BREATHING SLOWER, the BODY muscles also relax. AND you can let the muscle relax automatically even more every time you breathe OUT because it feels so good to relax all the way down to your toes.*
>
> *You are [each or all] doing this SO well, it's so nice to learn a QUICK and EASY way to get CALM and COMFORTABLE when you want and need to. So, now before we FINISH this nice experiment, I'll be quiet for a few moments and you can enjoy the quiet, and when you're ready, slowly open your eyes and bring the good, relaxed feelings back with you to this room.*

Such an exercise almost universally evokes smiles in all, and glances of wonderment to and from parent and child. Often, they are happy to share what they each were imagining about, and happy to discover that each had a DIFFERENT and unique response to the clinician's open-ended suggestions.

For older children it may be preferable to postpone parental observation until sometime following the initial invitation and therapeutic hypnotic experience, as this is often the point of maximum concern for both the child and the clinician regarding whether a state of hypnosis can be achieved and whether it will be effective for the presenting problem. Gardner (see Chapter 4 "Correlates of Childhood Hypnotic Responsiveness") noted that having any third-party present (e.g., parent, doctor, or nurse), could increase the likelihood of anxiety about successful performance. This anxiety could in turn interfere with success, as it may deflect attention away from the task and replace intended and desired relaxation with tension. Even with an older child, occasionally the parents may be invited to have the foregoing kind of group "experiment" if the child is particularly anxious and wants his parents to stay with him.

Once rapport has been established and it is clear that the child can use hypnosis to alleviate his problem, then with the child's permission the parent may sometimes be invited to observe a hypnotic session. In so doing, parents may witness with joy that the child can be in control both of beginning and ending the hypnosis session. Once it is clear to the patient and clinician that the child has practiced and is confident with his/her self-hypnosis, the session with the parents present may begin with the clinician offering a simple invitation like "Okay, just go ahead and begin your self-hypnosis and give yourself the messages you want your mind and body to have inside your mind ... and we'll be quiet and right here. Take your time and when you're done, you'll be finished."

If biofeedback is used concurrently, parents are commonly pleased to see that their child can change physiologic responses while practicing self-hypnosis.

A significant part of the parental observation session is the parents listening to and watching the clinician and their use of verbal and non-verbal communication. This allows the child to respond both verbally and nonverbally during hypnosis. In some cases, parents may be encouraged in advance to take such cues from the clinician and utilize their own hypnotic rapport to communicate with the child.

Gardner noted that such an

> ... exercise helps assure the parent that the child is in contact with his surroundings and in control of the hypnotic state as much as necessary. Parents who initially went along with the idea because of desperation or 'blind faith' now have keener understanding and are able to be even more supportive, both in sessions with the therapist and when the child is asked to practice self-hypnosis for use with a chronic condition or for repeated painful procedures or unpleasant experiences where the therapist may not always be available. (See Chapter 4)

Since publishing her paper on parental attitudes, Gardner (1974) continued the educational and observational steps of parent training but decreased the frequency of having parents actually experience formal hypnotic invitation. Moreover, when parents did request formal hypnosis for themselves, Gardner asked that the child not be present, at least initially. This change developed when it became clear that some parents – even in brief hypnosis – might use the opportunity to experience grief or other feelings whose full expression might be inappropriate in front of the child. An alternative, of course, is to refer the parent to a colleague who works primarily with adults learning hypnosis, particularly if the parent has been intrigued by their child's success and wishes to work on a problem of their own.

The process and value of parental involvement have been wonderfully enhanced in recent years by the availability of books written for parents and children with the specific intention of teaching parents how to tell and utilize storytelling to facilitate hypnotic experiences, responsivity, and reduction or resolution of symptoms/conditions of various kinds. Most notably, Linda Thomson's stories of *Harry, the Hypno-potamus* (Thomson, 2005, 2009) have intrigued and helped a multitude of families. Other writers (Hudson, 2009; Lyons, 2015; Reznick, 2009) have also recently published very user-friendly books accessible to therapists and parents alike to help children develop their innate imaginative skills to solve and resolve problems related to stress, illness, and discomfort.

And, the work of the Meg Foundation (www.megfoundation.com) and founder Dr. Jody Thomas (2017) has gone a long way to creatively educate and involve parents and children together in their wonderful and engaging YouTube options (www.megfoundation.com) (Thomas, 2021).

## References


Gardner, G.G. (1974). Parents: obstacles or allies in child hypnotherapy? *American Journal of Clinical Hypnosis, 17*, 44–49.

Hudson, L. (2009). *Scripts and Strategies in Hypnotherapy with Children: For Young People Aged 5 to 15*. Bethel, CT: Crown House Publishing.

Lyons, L. (2015). *Using Hypnosis with Children: Creating and Delivering Effective Interventions*. New York, NY: W.W. Norton and Company.

Reznick, C. (2009). *The Power of Your Child's Imagination: How to Transform Stress and Anxiety Into Joy and Success*. New York: Penguin Group.

Thomas, J. (2017). Project director, primary consultant: "You Are the Boss of Your Brain: Learning How to Manage Pain during Medical Procedures" (13 min.) Produced by Stanford Children's Health and Lucile Packard Children's Hospital. https://www.youtube.com/watch?v=UbK9FFoAcvs

Thomas, J. (2021). The Meg Foundation. www.megfoundation.com

Thomson, L. (2005). *Harry the Hypno-potamus: Metaphorical Tales for the Treatment of Children*. Bethel, CT: Crown House Publishing.

Thomson, L. (2009). *Harry the Hypno-potamus: More Metaphorical Tales for Pediatric Problems*. Bethel, CT: Crown House Publishing.

Traphagen, V. (1959). A survey of attitudes toward hypnotherapy with children. *American Journal of Clinical Hypnosis, 2*, 138–142.

# 24

# LOOKING TO THE FUTURE

## Introduction

We have brought together a variety of ideas concerning hypnotic responsiveness in childhood and the use of hypnosis in childhood disorders. In our attempt to integrate clinical observations with research studies, we have found that many have significant methodological shortcomings, including some of our own! The weight of evidence suggests that most children are responsive to hypnosis, and it can be useful in their treatment. At the same time, the data often raise more questions than they answer. A great deal of work remains to be done; however, many published articles do address evidence-based practice in clinical hypnosis, such as those in a special issue of the *International Journal of Clinical and Experimental Hypnosis*, devoted to evidence-based clinical hypnosis for psychosomatic disorders, chronic pain, sleep disorders, medical procedures, eating disorders, cancer symptoms, and labor and delivery (Alladin, 2007). Several Cochrane Reviews have addressed the benefits of clinical hypnosis, including one on needle-related procedural pain and distress in children and adolescents, which concluded that hypnosis was effective and the most promising of procedures reviewed (Uman, Chambers, McGrath, & Kisely, 2006). A literature review on the impact of hypnosis on psychophysiologic measures concluded that hypnosis leads to a physiological relaxation response in adults (Fernandez, Urwicz, Vuilleumier, & Berna, 2021). There has been progress in understanding the neurophysiology and neuropsychology of hypnosis, but the vast majority of studies relate to adults (Acunzo, Oakley, & Terhune, 2021; De Benedittis, 2021).

Since the first edition of this book was published, the terms *alternative medicine*, *alternative therapies*, *complementary alternative medicine*, and *integrative medicine* have entered the general vocabulary (Culbert & Olness, 2010). Studies have documented that Americans use many types of complementary and alternative and/or integrative therapies and spend billions of dollars yearly on them (Eisenberg et al., 1993; Murray & Rubel, 1992; Spigelblatt, Laine-Ammara, Pless, & Guyver, 1994). Under pressure from Congress, the National Institutes of Health created an Office of Alternative Medicine in 1992, followed by the National Council on Complementary and Alternative Medicine (NCCAM) in 1998, and now the National Center for Complementary and Integrative Health (NCCIH). The mission of NCCIH "is to determine, through rigorous scientific investigation, the fundamental science, usefulness, and safety of complementary and integrative health approaches and their roles in improving health and health care" (NCCIH, 2022). NCCIH has funded a wide variety of research studies, primarily focused on mind and body

DOI: 10.4324/9781003243687-26

practices, natural products, and pain. Relatively little of this has related to hypnosis with children. The NCCIH provides health information for the public on its website. A summary on "children and the use of complementary health approaches" states that studies have looked at many complementary health approaches for children with different conditions, but the evidence generally isn't strong enough to show what works and what doesn't. This statement is, of course, discouraging.

Gellert (1994), in analyzing the credibility problem of complementary and alternative medical therapies, stated that a critical factor is the tendency of alternative practitioners to globalize their therapies – that is, to advance them as cure-alls that can resolve all disease phenomena. He also observed that the experiential model engenders strong resistance from conventional medical practitioners, although an initial empirical observation regarding an alternative therapy may have value. Gellert pleaded for a sharpening of the focus of the experiential model through a narrowing of global explanations and expansion of conventional research interest. In this way, the alternative and conventional medical communities might gravitate toward the other's perspectives. It is essential that we avoid globalization and, if anything, design protocols with more care than we might in the conventional arena. We now present issues of research methodology, pointing out some technical considerations that should enhance the value of future research. Finally, we address specific problem areas in which we expect future research to provide clarification.

## Research Methodology

Although we cannot attempt a full discussion of methodological issues in child hypnosis research, we would like to mention several problems that come up repeatedly in the studies previously cited. For a thorough review of the technical aspects of hypnosis research, we refer the reader to the excellent book *Contemporary Hypnosis Research* (Fromm & Nash, 1992); almost every chapter contains ideas that are relevant to child hypnosis research. Two other excellent books, *Behavioral Pediatrics: Research and Practice* (Russo & Varni, 1982) and *Hypnotherapy of Pain in Children with Cancer* (LeBaron & Hilgard, 1984), both describe specific protocols involving hypnosis with children. The monograph by Dienstfrey (1992) addresses whether or not psychosocial influences on health can be demonstrated and discusses significant methodological problems that relate to all research in the mind–body area. Nassau, Tien, and Fritz (2008) reviewed studies of pediatric psychoneuroimmunology and identified problems in research design and implementation. The *International Journal of Clinical and Experimental Hypnosis* published a special issue on contemporary research in hypnosis in October 2019. Although this issue related to adult research, it contains articles relevant to common issues in both clinical and laboratory research. Lynn and colleagues (2019) include a 40-year perspective on clinical and research foundations of hypnosis, hypnotic phenomena and hypnotic responsiveness. These authors emphasize the importance of defining terms such as a "trance" or "altered state" in research protocols.

In August 2015, the International Society of Hypnosis and Confederation Francophone d'hypnose et Therapies Breves so-sponsored a meeting among 13 hypnosis researchers. Subsequently they published a paper (Jensen et al., 2017) in which they summarized key advances in hypnosis research during the previous two decades and made recommendations for future research agendas. They noted the importance of laboratory hypnosis researchers taking care about how they assessed hypnotic suggestibility in studies and the importance of research protocols clearly delineating the roles of inductions and specific suggestion. They recommended data sharing and a focus on the efficacy of hypnotic treatments for clinical conditions as well as the neurophysiological underpinnings of hypnotic phenomena. Although their recommendations and references related to adults, their summary points also related to pediatric hypnosis research.

Some of the recurrent design issues in protocols involving child hypnosis include controlling for individual variables, inability to develop double-blind crossover trials, contamination of subjects by other people during the course of a study, and the problems with standardization of a hypnotic intervention. With respect to individual variables, it is probable that we do not yet know all that are significant. We have noted that there are intrinsic differences in preferred mental imagery, in biobehavioral reactivity, in personality, and in learning styles; for example, there are augmenters and reducers with respect to pain perceptions, and vast differences in children's past experiences may make them more or less responsive to hypnotic interventions. Churchill, Persinger, and Thomas (1994) described recent research indicating that some individuals are more responsive to geomagnetic field changes and that these changes impact on mental processing. Many of the studies we have cited have lumped school-age children and adolescents. We believe that age is an important variable and one that can be easily controlled in studies.

Individuals, including children, vary in preferred mental imagery, and rarely does one encounter a child who denies imagination altogether. If a standardized protocol mandates progressive relaxation cued to breathing or autogenic relaxation and the subject is most comfortable with detailed visual imagery, he or she may find the instructions boring and dull and will lose interest in the whole experiment. A child with superb auditory imagery and poor visual imagery is not likely to respond well to a prescribed focus on specific visual images. We have found repeatedly, to our dismay, that research review committees recommend that the intervention be constant for each child, and they request written descriptions of detailed instructions. The best way to handle this and respond to individual preferences is to offer a protocol such as:

> The best way to enjoy hypnosis is to pretend you're in a favorite place doing what you like to do there, in a special, comfortable place. If you like, you can imagine seeing things you enjoy seeing there or hearing things that you enjoy hearing or just feeling good, just the way you would feel if you were actually there.

We believe that protocols should control for differences in imagery preferences, personality type, and autonomic fingerprints. This requirement often leads to a requirement for large numbers of subjects, thus increasing the cost and duration of studies.

Another research problem intrinsic to protocols involving hypnosis is that one cannot randomize interventions because the child who is in the hypnotic intervention group and the child who is in the resting or attention group will each know what group he or she is in. If one were to begin with a hypnotic intervention and then cross over to a medication, it would be impossible to prevent the subject from continuing the hypnotic intervention during the medication trial. It is true that sham biofeedback can be given but no one has developed a viable sham protocol for hypnotic inductions with children.

Perhaps a major problem encountered by many experts who have done research with hypnosis is contamination of the control groups. Children in control groups may either learn something about hypnosis by chance from other children or their parents or even from meeting someone in the waiting room who is in the experimental group. In the case of Santer's (1990) study of hypnosis in emergency settings, parents were inadvertently giving subjects hypnotic invitations. Spontaneous hypnosis occurs frequently in children. Kohen (1986) and Hall, Minnes, Tosi, and Olness (1992) encountered this problem in prospective, "controlled" studies. In one study (Plotnick, Payne, & O'Grady, 1991), it was necessary that parents see the hypnosis invitation protocol prior to providing consent. Although they were asked not to share this information with their children prior to the experiments, it is likely that some children learned in advance of the experiments.

## Hypnotic Responsiveness

We described hypnotic rating scales for children in Chapter 3. Although some subsequent research has included a fantasy scale (LeBaron, Zeltzer, & Fanurik, 1988; Plotnick et al., 1991), the existing scales do not allow predictions about which children might be most successful in the therapeutic application of hypnosis. It may be that there are other surrogate markers for hypnotic responsivity that we are missing. It is possible that the existing scales are unsuitable for children with certain personality traits or learning styles or with certain types of autonomic reactivity. We look for more sophisticated research on other correlates of hypnotic responsiveness and strongly urge our colleagues to continue research on the role of imagination in childhood hypnotic responsiveness. Substantial research, using such techniques as 3T (3 Tesla) functional magnetic resonance imaging, has demonstrated that it is possible to identify which areas of the brain respond to which imagery tasks (Ganis, Thompson, & Kosslyn, 2004; Thompson, Slotnick, Burrage, & Kosslyn, 2009). The potential for use of portable functional near-infrared spectroscopy (fNIRS) to assess brain activity changes during hypnosis is described by Halsband and Wolf (2021).

## Clinical Research

We have been happy to note increasing numbers of clinical studies of hypnosis with children in print and to see them published in a variety of professional journals, including those for pediatrics, psychology, nursing, dentistry, and social work. Much good laboratory research with humans has evolved from clinical observations. The careful reporting of clinical observations is much needed in this area, and we encourage readers who are clinicians to do this. To the best of our knowledge, there is still a great lack of literature on applications of hypnosis with children in many areas, including various types of procedures, dermatological problems, learning problems, ophthalmologic problems, otolaryngological applications, child abuse, and in orthopedics. We hear clinical anecdotes from colleagues at workshops and meetings about creative, successful applications of hypnosis in some of these areas, but these need to be published. In all research studies, both negative and positive results should be reported, and special attention should be given to communicating effectively in oral presentations and in published reports.

## Consortium Research

In 1986, we began organizing a group of colleagues who were interested in designing consortium studies involving nonpharmacological therapy, such as hypnosis and biofeedback. The initial hope was that such consortium studies could do what the Children's Cancer Study Group has done for many years – that is, assemble groups of comparable patients and study interventions more rapidly than would be possible at any one institution and by any one individual. We also hoped to overcome the criticism that successful application of hypnosis or biofeedback was a phenomenon of individuals or settings. Initially, interested colleagues found times to meet and brainstorm research protocols at national scientific meetings. Later, the W.T. Grant Foundation provided a few thousand dollars to allow a planning meeting to be held in Cleveland in 1988. At this meeting, numerous possible protocols were discussed. Eventually, the group decided to focus on a protocol on nonpharmacological treatment of warts and a protocol on Tourette's syndrome.

As is true with most protocols, it is far easier to write them than to obtain funding. Eventually, the wart protocol, involving seven institutions, was funded by the Fetzer Foundation for a total of $50,000. It was evident that this could not cover investigator salaries, so all professional time was donated. In implementing the protocol, investigators found many unexpected complications.

They learned that dermatologists had not established absolute classifications for describing warts and that there was no agreement on the immunological aspects of wart growth and regression. One of the investigators negotiated with the Edison Sensor Technology Center in Cleveland to design a wart sensor. The hope was that this sensor would allow some monitoring of physiological changes at the base of the wart that might be associated with or predict regression. This plan delayed the whole project. A sophisticated sensor was developed, but there were never enough sensors for each site. It turned out to be very complicated to get seven investigators at different sites to photograph warts in comparable ways. Thus, the initial study took 4 years instead of the projected 2 years (see Chapter 16).

Despite these difficulties, the consortium has learned a great deal and provides a basis for designing additional studies involving multiple institutions. The protocol for a comparison of hypnosis and Haldol® in Tourette's syndrome was completed but turned down for funding several times. We continue to be supportive of such consortium research and encourage colleagues to get involved. One of the benefits is that younger, inexperienced researchers can learn about research from such collaborations.

## Topics for Future Research

### *Consciousness and Imagination*

We have taken the position that hypnosis is a different state of consciousness and that it provides a treatment modality distinct from other forms of medical and psychological therapy and that it has unique benefits for many child patients. It is possible that we are wrong on both these points. It is possible that a generic common denominator in a number of mind body (such as mindfulness, progressive relaxation) strategies exists and remains to be defined. If we are correct about hypnosis as a worthy treatment modality, we would hope to be able to increase the level of confidence of ourselves and our colleagues through research in several areas: the nature of consciousness in general; the nature of altered states of consciousness, how these are best achieved, and how they vary in terms of potential value; the nature of imagination and how imagery skills can be fostered and preserved; and the process that connects changes in mental imaging to physiological responses.

Future research concerning child applications of hypnosis and related strategies must take into account why childhood imagery skills peak and subsequently fade as the child moves into adulthood. Imagery is intrinsic to child hypnosis; it is also an important part of child development, play patterns, creativity, and adult achievements. Plato, in *The Republic*, was keenly aware of the tremendous influence of imaginative involvement on child development. He argued, for example, that children should be exposed to certain kinds of literature, drama, and music, whereas other kinds should be suppressed; otherwise, children would learn inappropriate values and behave as adults in ways that would be harmful to themselves and to society. Plato may have been right; we certainly hear similar arguments today, especially with respect to children's television programming and computer games. Indeed, an important area for research relates to what types of images are triggered in young minds by television and the lag period from absorbing the image until acting on it.

Although most parents and teachers would agree that imagination in children should not be stifled, our society seems to be producing a reverse situation. Children are allowed access, with few restrictions, to a plethora of visual and auditory stimuli through constant access to television, computer games, and cellphones. Many children are allowed little time and receive no direction or encouragement to enjoy their own internal creative images. Bronowski (1974) wrote: "All great civilizations have failed in one regard. They have limited the freedom of imagination of their young."

This idea is old. William Blake, writing in 1788, lamented the loss of childhood imagination to the repressive forces of reason and expressed hope that "the real man, the Imagination" would be found again (Kazin, 1974, p. 83). Holton, in *The Creative Imagination* (1978), noted that antecedents of scientific discoveries made in adulthood were to be found in the childhood experiences of scientists. He provided many examples of this; for example, Einstein, as a child, imagined himself riding on a beam of light and tried to envision what the world would look like as he rode on that beam. He believed that this inspired his idea of the theory of relativity later in life.

We all think we know what imagination is, yet scientists are still trying to define it. There are many questions. Is imagination essentially a single process, or is it a set of discrete skills? Why does it persist in some people and drop out in others? Why do some people use it adaptively and others maladaptively? Because it appears to be of great value in dealing with certain potentially devastating situations, such as when one is a hostage or a prisoner of war, why don't we make a greater effort to teach people to preserve it, to use it for relatively minor problems as well as for major ones? Who should be the teachers, and how should they teach? How is imagination related to eidetic imagery, a skill present in about 6% of children but only rarely in adults (Haber, 1980). If imaginative skills facilitate hypnotic responsiveness, might it also be true that experience with hypnosis fosters the development and preservation of imaginative skills? Should all children be taught self-hypnosis? Are children who are familiar with self-hypnosis better able to adapt to life's challenges and to develop their own assets? Is creative use of imagination facilitated by reading or telling stories to children? Is it facilitated or thwarted by television? This last point is an important issue, because the average preschooler in the United States watches television for more than 30 hours a week.

### *Links between Mental and Physiological Processes*

Substantial evidence suggests that voluntary changes in mental processing or imaging are associated with significant physiological changes even when the individual is not following a prescribed mind body strategy. For example, adults and children can deliberately increase and decrease peripheral temperature. How does this happen? Every adult human body contains 100 trillion cells. These fundamental components of living things were first discovered in the 17th century. Since then, we have learned much about what happens inside cells but very little about how it happens. Researchers ponder why genes in individual cells appear to switch themselves on and off and perform differently in varying circumstances. Why, for example, does messenger ribonucleic acid (mRNA) not always transmit the complete messages that it carries from deoxyribonucleic acid (DNA)? The whole issue of regulation of the function of the 100 trillion cells has thousands of scientists working on it. There is no clear explanation for how microtubules transmit instructions between cell nuclei and surfaces. Does some of the regulation of cell behavior evolve from messages of thoughts or mental images? We now know that cytokines, mediators of inflammation, are synthesized not only by immunocompetent cells that permeate the blood–brain barrier and enter the brain but also by microglia and by neurons. The numerous cytokines have many effects, including the alteration of behavior and cognitive function. We know that both the amygdala and hippocampus have direct neural connections to hypothalamic nuclei and that they mediate affective and cognitive processes. How do the affective processes impact on the amygdala and hippocampus? What type of energy is associated with a thought? Are there specific cell receptors for this energy, and do they set off a conformational change that is passed along to an ion channel, setting off a cascade of movement from cell to cell and eventually to hypothalamic nuclei? Tracing transmission of thoughts to the cell and through cells and using that knowledge to alleviate the human condition must be a central task for the remainder of this century.

## Role of the Therapist in Hypnosis

It seems logical that mental processes – affect, imagery, and expectations – of therapists are related to treatment outcomes. Some studies (e.g., Rutter, 1980) have found a relationship between teacher expectations and student performance, independent of IQ levels. Many people have had the experience of feeling worse if a friend or neighbor says, "You don't look well. Are you sick?" What happens when the therapist anticipates a poor treatment outcome? What are the cues by which such an expectation gets communicated to a patient? The "hanging crepe" phenomenon, first described as a problem in the medical profession by Siegler (1975), should be studied with regard to hypnosis.

What about chronobiology issues, fatigue, family concerns, and other variables in therapists? It is possible that we will develop objective measures of these variables that will enable us to decide that we should not work with children at certain times. Do some clinicians work more successfully with their patients than others? Which people are most suited to be therapists and which least? How do we assess relationship factors between clinicians and children? Linden (2019) has described healthy therapist responses that are timed to match the absorbed receptivity of the child. Do therapists always have healthy responses to children? Should we discourage some clinicians from working with children at certain times? Should we be more selective about whom we accept for training? How and to what extent should clinicians communicate their own imagery to patients? How should we foster and direct our own imaginative processes so as to be of maximal help to our patients? Answers to any of these questions are relevant to all therapeutic interactions with children and adolescents.

## Role of the Child in Hypnosis

We hope that in future years a more prescriptive approach to hypnosis will be seen. By this we do not mean a "cookbook" approach but one basing diagnosis and treatment on data about important individual variables. The design of a hypnotic approach for a particular child must take into account such factors as age, developmental level, verbal and imaginal fluency, activity level and other temperamental variables, personality factors such as motivation, internal–external locus of control, mechanisms of coping and defense, needs and conflicts, biobehavioral reactivity, anxiety level and the manner of its expression, learning styles and disabilities, and physical strengths. We must consider the child's roles in the family, the school, and other social settings that may have direct or indirect influences on treatment. We might find it important to measure autonomic responses or neurotransmitter levels before teaching hypnosis or making practice recommendations. We already have some data suggesting that children respond differently to different kinds of hypnotic invitations/initiations. It is also likely that children respond differently to different kinds and amounts of hypnotic suggestions.

Which children benefit most from direct suggestion? Which do better with more indirect, symbolic approaches? Which children need a special emphasis on self-hypnosis? Which require more therapist contact? Which children do best with which therapists? Which children benefit most from treatment in groups and which from individual sessions? When a child wants to master a problem, at what specific points is hypnosis likely to be helpful? If learning is state dependent (Tart, 1986), how can we ensure that a review of learning will occur in a state comparable to that when it was first learned? What about the child who has experienced a significant trauma early in life that may not be mentioned to the clinician? Will that impact a child's response to learning hypnosis? In a child with maladaptive anxiety regarding learning and performance, should we teach hypnosis before learning begins, during initial learning, during review of learned material, before performance, during performance, or at several of these points? How can we predict these variations in response so that treatment programs can be designed more effectively and carried out with minimal cost of time and money?

## The Future and Professional Hypnosis Organizations

The Society for Clinical and Experimental Hypnosis (SCEH), American Society of Clinical Hypnosis (ASCH), International Society of Hypnosis (ISH), and European Hypnosis Society (ESH) have, for many years, provided forums for health-care professionals who were interested in hypnosis. Increasingly, hypnosis and other related strategies have been taught in other societies for health-care professionals. The role of the ASCH and SCEH is changing somewhat from providing only professional education to also providing public education and leadership with respect to ethical and public policy issues. An unfortunate fact of life for many clinicians, including those in child health who use hypnosis, is that reimbursement for teaching hypnosis is inadequate. Third-party and government payers, for example, are usually willing to pay for expensive procedures, such as MRI scans for children with migraine, or for untested medications, but may balk at reimbursement for training a child in self-hypnosis, a therapeutic intervention documented to be more effective than many medications. This is an area in which the SCEH, ASCH, and other professional societies supporting nonpharmacological interventions can provide leadership and assistance to clinicians. Research is needed on the cost effectiveness of teaching hypnosis.

## Art and Science

As we learn answers to questions raised in this chapter and to other questions not yet raised, we will become better able to employ both research and therapeutic child hypnosis in the scientific context of prescriptive treatment. The application of approaches found to have particular value will be expanded, and useless approaches will be eliminated. Cultural changes may require changes in approaches. We will learn how best to combine hypnosis with other treatment modalities. We will question basic assumptions and define new problems. We believe that hypnosis will continue to involve art as well as science. Intuition and hunches may continue to be important, but we hope that scientific developments will lead to more creative and effective use of intuition. We also hope that tolerance for uncertainty will prevail. Most of all, we hope that our synthesis of available observations and information will provide inspiration, clues, and nuggets for those who wish to expand the frontier of child hypnosis. The future involves a lot of hard work. It also contains the potential for excitement and satisfaction as we use our own skills to find better ways of allowing children to develop their potential to the fullest, to be all that they really are.

## References

Acunzo, D.J., Oakley, D.A., & Terhune, D.B. (2021). The neurochemistry of hypnotic suggestion: review. *American Journal of Hypnosis*, *63*, 355–371.

Alladin, A., Guest Ed. (2007). Special issue: evidence-based practice in clinical hypnosis, Part II. *International Journal of Clinical & Experimental Hypnosis*, *55*, 251–371.

Bronowski, J. (1974). *The Ascent of Man*. Boston, MA: Little, Brown.

Churchill, D.R., Persinger, M.A., & Thomas, A.W. (1994). Geophysical variables and behavior: increased geomagnetic activity and decreased pleasantness of spontaneous narratives for percipients but not agents. *Perceptual and Motor Skills*, *79*, 387–392.

Culbert, T.P., & Olness, K., Eds. (2010). *Integrative Pediatrics*. New York: Oxford University Press.

De Benedittis, G. (2021). Neurophysiology and neuropsychology of hypnosis. *American Journal of Hypnosis*, *63*, 291–293.

Dienstfrey, H., Ed. (1992). Can we demonstrate important psychosocial influences on health? *Advances: The Journal of Mind–Body Health, 8*, 5–45.
Eisenberg, D.M., Kessler, R.C., Foster, C., Norlock, F.E., Calkins, D.R., & Delbanco, T.L. (1993). Unconventional medicine in the United States. *New England Journal of Medicine, 328*, 246–252.
Fernandez, A., Urwicz, L., Vuilleumier, P., & Berna, C. (2021). Impact of hypnosis on psychophysiological measures: a scoping literature review. *American Journal of Clinical Hypnosis, 64*, 36–52.
Fromm, E. & Nash, M.R., Eds. (1992). *Contemporary Hypnosis Research.* New York: Guilford Press.
Ganis, G., Thompson, W.L., & Kosslyn, S.M. (2004). Brain areas underlying visual mental imagery and visual perception: an fMRI study. *Cognitive Brain Research, 20*, 226–241.
Haber, R.N. (1980). Eidetic images are not just imaginary. *Psychology Today, 14*, 72–82.
Hall, H.R., Minnes, L., Tosi, M., & Olness, K. (1992). Voluntary modulation of neutrophil adhesiveness using a cyberphysiologic strategy. *International Journal of Neuroscience, 63*, 287–297.
Halsband, U., & Wolf, T.G. (2021). Current neuroscientific research database findings of brain activity changes after hypnosis. *American Journal of Clinical Hypnosis, 63*, 372–388.
Holton, G. (1978). *The Creative Imagination.* New York: Cambridge University Press.
Jensen, M.P., Jamieson, G.A., Luz, A., Mazzoni, G., McGeown, W.J., Santarcangelo, E.L., Demertzi, A., De Pascalis, V., Banyai, E.I., Romiger, C., Vuilleumier, P., Faymonville, M., & Terhune, D.B. (2017). New directions in hypnosis research: strategies for advancing the cognitive and clinical neuroscience of hypnosis. *Neuroscience of Consciousness, 3*, 1. 10.1093/nc/nix004
Kazin, A., Ed. (1974). *The Portable Blake.* New York: Viking Press.
Kohen, D.P. (1986). Applications of relaxation/mental imagery (self-hypnosis) to the management of asthma: report of behavioral outcomes of a two-year, prospective controlled study [abstract]. *American Journal of Clinical Hypnosis, 28*, 196.
LeBaron, S., & Hilgard, J.R. (1984). *Hypnotherapy of Pain in Children with Cancer.* Los Altos, CA: William Kaufmann.
LeBaron, S., Zeltzer, L., & Fanurik, D. (1988). Imaginative involvement and hypnotic susceptibility in childhood. *International Journal of Clinical and Experimental Hypnosis, 36*, 284–295.
Linden, J. (2019). Relationship factors in the theater of imagination: hypnosis with children and adolescents. *American Journal of Clinical Hypnosis, 62*, 60–73.
Lynn, S.J., Green, J.P., Pouzzi, C.P., Ellenberg, S., Gautam, A., & Aksen, D. (2019). Hypnosis, hypnotic phenomena, and hypnotic responsiveness. *The International Journal of Clinical and Experimental Hypnosis, 67*, 475–511.
Murray, R.H. & Rubel, A.J. (1992). Physicians and healers: unwitting partners in health care. *New England Journal of Medicine, 326*, 61–64.
Nassau, J.H., Tien, K., & Fritz, G.K. (2008). Review of the literature: integrating psychoneuroimmunology into pediatric chronic illness interventions. *Journal of Pediatric Psychology, 33*, 195–207.
NCCIH. (2022). www.NCCIH.gov
Plotnick, A.B., Payne, P.A., & O'Grady, D.J. (1991). Correlates of hypnotizability in children: absorption, vividness of imagery, and social desirability. *American Journal of Clinical Hypnosis, 34*, 51–58.
Russo, D. & Varni, J.W., Eds. (1982). *Behavioral Pediatrics: Research and Practice.* New York: Plenum Press.
Rutter, M. (1980). School influences on children's behavior and development. *Pediatrics, 65*, 208–220.
Santer, L. (1990). Imagery use during laceration repair in children. Paper presented at the 41st Annual Scientific Meeting of the Society for Clinical and Experimental Hypnosis, Tucson, AZ.
Siegler, M. (1975). Pascal's wager and the hanging of crepe. *New England Journal of Medicine, 293*, 853–857.
Spigelblatt, L., Laine-Ammara, G., Pless, B., & Guyver, A. (1994). The use of alternative medicine by children. *Pediatrics, 94*, 811–814.
Tart, C. (1986). *Waking Up: Overcoming the Obstacles to Human Potential.* Boston, MA: New Science Library.
Thompson, W.L., Slotnick, S.D., Burrage, M.S., & Kosslyn, S.M. (2009). Two forms of spatial imagery: neuroimaging evidence. *Psychological Science, 20*, 1245–1253.
Uman, L.S., Chambers, C.T., McGrath, P.J., & Kisely, S. (2006). Psychological interventions for needle-related procedural pain and distress in children and adolescents [review]. *The Cochrane Database of Systematic Reviews*, Issue 4. Article No. CD005179.

# AUTHOR INDEX

Note: **Bold** page numbers refer to tables and *italic* page numbers refer to figures.

# SUBJECT INDEX

Note: **Bold** page numbers refer to tables and *italic* page numbers refer to figures.

For Product Safety Concerns and Information please contact our EU
representative GPSR@taylorandfrancis.com
Taylor & Francis Verlag GmbH, Kaufingerstraße 24, 80331 München, Germany

www.ingramcontent.com/pod-product-compliance
Ingram Content Group UK Ltd.
Pitfield, Milton Keynes, MK11 3LW, UK
UKHW052054230926
475702UK00026B/1212
* 9 7 8 1 0 3 2 1 5 0 6 8 0 *